Pediatric Occupational Therapy

Facilitating Effective Service Provision

Edited by

Winnie Dunn, PhD, OTR, FAOTA
Occupational Therapy Program
University of Kansas
Kansas City, KS

SLACK Incorporated, 6900 Grove Road, Thorofare, NJ 08086

Printed in the United States of America

Library of Congress Catalog Card Number: 89-043515

ISBN: 1-55642-014-5

Published by: SLACK Incorporated
               6900 Grove Rd.
               Thorofare, NJ 08086

Last digit is print number: 10 9 8 7 6 5 4 3 2

to Robert
my co-editor in spirit
for exemplifying the meaning of partnership

Contents

APPENDICES

Contributing Authors

As you read about the authors, the rich and substantive basis for the materials contained in this textbook will be very clear. Be sure to meet these colleagues when you have the opportunity to do so; they have enriched my life, and will enrich yours as you read; they are also delightful individuals to know.

Elizabeth A. Cada, MS, OTR/L is a general partner in Pediatric Rehabilitation Service, a private practice pediatric program in Lisle, Illinois. She obtained her BS in Occupational Therapy from Colorado State University and her masters degree in Administration and Organizational Behavior from George Williams College in Illinois. Beth has sixteen years of pediatric experience, emphasizing community-based intervention. She has emphasized a collaborative approach with other professionals, family members, and general health and education agencies that serve children and families. Both her service provision skills and continuing education experiences reflect these priorities. She has been certified to administer and interpret the Southern California Sensory Integration Tests Battery, and continues to incorporate her knowledge of sensory integration into her intervention strategies. Beth has had extensive involvement with state and national association activities, and presently serves as the Speaker of the Representative Assembly of the AOTA.

Philippa H. Campbell, Ph.D., OTR is the Director of the Family Child Learning Center of the Children's Hospital Medical Center of Akron, Ohio, and is Associate Professor for the Special Education and Speech Pathology Departments at Kent State University, in Kent, Ohio. She received her BS in Psychology from Susquehanna University, her masters degree in Special Education from the University of Pittsburgh, and her doctorate in Special Education and Psychology from Kent State University. She has twenty-five years of pediatric experience creating and implementing state-of-the-art services for individuals and their families. She is a strong advocate for integrated programing for individuals with all types of disabilities, and has written and taught extensively about programing for persons with severe and multiple disabilities. She also teaches intervention to therapists and teachers from a neurodevelopmental treatment perspective.

Jane Case-Smith, Ed.D., OTR is Chief of Occupational Therapy at Nisonger Center, and Assistant Professor at Ohio State University, Columbus, Ohio. She received her BS in Psychology from Kalamazoo College, her MS in Occupational Therapy from Western Michigan University, and her doctorate in Education from the University of Georgia, at Athens, Geor-

gia. She has ten years of pediatric experience in preschool and early intervention programs, and has had extensive involvement with families in her service provision. She is certified in both neurodevelopmental treatment and sensory integration, and incorporates this knowledge into her practice activities. She is presently the chair of the Developmental Disabilities Special Interest Section of AOTA, and serves on the AOTA Advisory Committed for Advanced Recognition for Pediatrics. Her speaking and writing both address the needs of early intervention, specifically regarding the NICU and feeding problems.

Terri Collier, MS, OTR is a Program Specialist at the Jackson County Respite Care Program in Kansas City, Missouri, and an instructor of Pediatrics at the University of Missouri and Kansas University. She obtained her BS in Occupational Therapy and her MS in Special Education from the University of Kansas. She has fourteen years of pediatric experience, providing consultative and direct services for individuals with developmental delays, behavior disorders, and learning disabilities. She has been certified to administer and interpret the Southern California Sensory Integration Tests battery, and has applied this information to other populations in her practice. Terri is well known for her expertise in oral motor development, feeding and eating interventions, positioning and handling, orientation, and behavior management. She provides continuing education in these areas for both caregivers and professionals.

Debra Galvin Cook, MS, OTR is Assistant Professor in Occupational Therapy for the University of Kansas Medical Center in Kansas City, Kansas. She has thirteen years of pediatrics experience, and has provided intervention for a wide range of children in early intervention, clinical, preschool, and public school programs. She received her Occupational Therapy degree (BS) and her Special Education degree (MS) from the University of Kansas. She is presently a member of the Developmental Disabilities Special Interest Section Steering Committee for the American Occupational Therapy Association. She has been certified to administer and interpret the Southern California Sensory Integration Tests, and the Brazelton Infant Assessment. She provides continuing education in the areas of service provision strategies, assessment, and autism, and has written about vestibular input as an effective intervention strategy, and about autism.

Martha Coutinho, Ph.D. is an Educational Research Analyst for the Office of Special Education Programs, Department of Education in Washington D.C., where she is involved with policy and directed research activities. She has a Bachelor of Arts degree in History Education from the University of Colorado, a master's degree in Special Education, and a doctorate in Educational Psychology from the University of Connecticut. She has fourteen years of experience in federal, state, and local agencies providing administrative, intervention, and research services. She formerly served as a teacher and a director of Special Education, and has more recently worked with the National Association of State Directors of Special Education. She has been involved in providing special education and related services within integrated settings, serving students with severe emotional disturbance. She wrote her chapter in her private capacity; no official endorsement by the Department of Education should be inferred.

Winnie Dunn, Ph.D., OTR, FAOTA is Professor and Chair of the Occupational Therapy Curriculum at the University of Kansas. She obtained her bachelors degree in Occupational Therapy and her masters degree in Special Education from the University of Missouri, and her doctorate in Neurosciences from the University of Kansas. She has sixteen years of experience in pediatrics, serving young children, school-aged children, and adolescents with a variety of handicapping conditions during that time. She has worked primarily in community-based agencies, such as preschool programs and public schools, emphasizing the integrative approaches to programing. She has written in the areas of service provision, development, functional assessment and intervention, and neuroscience foundations for performance. She also emphasizes these topics in continuing education. She continues to provide consultation within agencies and state programs to enable system level changes that advocate on behalf of children's needs.

Barbara E. Hanft, MA, OTR/L, FAOTA is Program Manager of the Early Intervention Project at AOTA and a consultant/trainer in a private practice in Maryland. She received her BS in Occupational Therapy from the State University of New York at Buffalo, and her masters degree in Counseling Psychology from the University of California at Santa Barbara. She has eighteen years of experience working with children, primarily in school systems and early intervention programs. She is faculty emeritus of Sensory Integration International, and has provided continuing education in this area, and in child development, family dynamics, and school system practice. Between 1984 and 1988, Barbara served as a lobbyist, advocating for the enactment of PL99–457 and the reauthorization of the Developmental Disabilities Act. She has also written in early intervention, legislation, and advocacy and practice.

Elizabeth J. Maruyama, MPH, OTR/L is a general partner in Pediatric Rehabilitation Services, a private practice in Lisle, Illinois. She earned her BS in Occupational Therapy from the University of Illinois, and her masters degree in Public Health from Illinois Benedictine College. She is certified in both the Southern California Sensory Integration Tests Battery and the Sensory Integration and Praxis Tests. She has fifteen years of experience in pediatrics, primarily within community-based agencies. She serves as a consultant to the American Lung Association of Illinois, and has established asthma ed-

ucation and summer camping programs for them. She provides continuing education for parents and other professionals on service provision and management.

Linda Haney McClain, Ph.D., OTR, FAOTA is Assistant Professor and Assistant Chair of Occupational Therapy Education at Kansas University Medical Center, Kansas City, Kansas. She received her BS in Occupational Therapy, her masters degree in Education, and her doctorate in Special Education from Kansas University. She has been very active in the Kansas Occupational Therapy Association, and the American Occupational Therapy Association, serving in both elected and appointed positions, including the nominations chair for the AOTA. She provides continuing education on documentation and clinical fieldwork supervision, and has written in these areas and in motoric and kinesiological applications to function and intervention. Most recently, she served as the guest editor for the *Occupational Therapy Practice Journal* for a special issue on motion and movement issues in practice.

Susan Merryfield, OTR is Director of Rehabilitation Services and an instructor at the University of Kansas Medical Center in Kansas City, Kansas. She has twelve years of experience in pediatric services to children in school settings, through outreach contracts with suburban and rural schools. She received her Occupational Therapy degree from Kansas University, and is presently completing her masters degree in Health Service Administration from Kansas University. She has been very active in state and national occupational therapy endeavors, and has served as an officer for the Council of State Association Presidents for the American Occupational Therapy Association. She served as one of the normative data gatherers for the Sensory Integration and Praxis Tests. She provides continuing education in pediatrics and management.

Mary Muhlenhaupt, OTR is Coordinator of therapy services for BOCES 2-Suffolk, in Patchogue, New York. She received her bachelor's degree in Occupational Therapy from Sargent College of Boston University. She has fourteen years of experience with children, primarily in school-based therapy services, and has been certified in administration and interpretation of the Sensory Integration Tests batteries. She is presently president of the New York State Occupational Therapy Association, and has been active in AOTA projects as well. She has written about school-based therapy; most notably she created a reference guide for occupational therapy in New York state. She is also involved in continuing education experiences for therapists who work in schools. Her views about interdisciplinary service provision are well respected within the field.

Patti Oetter, MA, OTR/L, FAOTA works with several programs in Alberquerque, New Mexico. She provides service to young children and their families in a private practice there, and serves as a team member at the University Affiliated Program, providing assessment and followup for children and families who are referred to the UAP through various state systems. She also participates in outreach programs to serve those who are unable to reach the center-based program.

She is faculty emeritus of Sensory Integration International, and has provided extensive continuing education in this area, particularly related to intervention. Patti has more than twenty years of pediatric experience, and has served children from birth through school ages throughout her career. Recently, she has had a particular interest in studying dysfunction in the sensory systems that leads to defensive reactions.

Lillian Gonzolez-Pardo, M.D., is Associate Professor in Pediatrics and Neurology at the University of Kansas Medical Center in Kansas City, Kansas. She has worked as a physician for twenty-seven years, and has worked in pediatrics for twenty years. She provides neurology expertise within the University Affiliated Program for those children and families who require this expertise to have a comprehensive evaluation and program plan. She provides many services within the midwest community, including serving as a pediatric neurology consultant to the Kansas Special Outreach Health Services of the Kansas Crippled Children's Program, and providing frequent continuing education experiences for her colleagues in areas particular to neurology and pediatrics. She has particular interests in the issues of epilepsy, and has worked closely with the Epilepsy League to provide accurate community information about seizures and seizure disorders. She has also been active as an advocate for children with learning disorders, and specific motor disorders of childhood. She is a strong advocate for the needs of children and families, and supports the involvement of occupational therapists to assist families and school personnel to meet their goals.

Charlotte Brasic Royeen, Ph.D., OTR, FAOTA is Editor of the Self-Study Series published by AOTA, and consultant for Research and Specialty Practice in a private practice in Virginia. She obtained her BS in Occupational Therapy summa cum laude from Tufts University, her masters degree in Occupational Therapy from Washington University, and her doctorate in Educational Evaluation and Research from Virginia Polytechnic Institute and State University. She has fourteen years of pediatric experience with school-aged children, and those with sensory integrative problems. She is faculty emeritus of Sensory Integration International, with a particular interest in the function and dysfunction of the somatosensory system. She provides continuing education for therapists on school-based practice and consultation, and has written several definitive works in research for the field.

Special Notes:

The following two special educators provided material for the early drafts of this text. Their views about special education services and the relationship between special education and occupational therapy services are embedded in the first section of this book. Their wisdom and insight have also contributed to the editor's professional growth throughout the years, and so their influence is pervasively represented as well.

Mary Ellen O'Hare, M.Ed.	Master Teacher Special School District St. Louis County, Missouri.
Susan Parks, M.Ed.	Education Specialist Platte Valley Educational Cooperative Smithville, Missouri.

The following occupational therapists are master clinicians who are well respected members of our professional community. They graciously shared their knowledge, insights, and pediatric expertise by contributing core material for the case studies contained in Chapters 4 and 7. They demonstrate the value of diversity within our profession, and point out to the reader that there are many ways to provide effective occupational therapy services to children and their families.

Rosemary Edell, OTR	Independent School District #535 Rochester, Minnesota
Patty Knutson, OTR	St. Joseph's Hospital Milwaukee, Wisconsin
Ellen Mellard, M.S., OTR	Northeast Kansas Education Service Center Lecompton, Kansas
Madonna Nash, OTR	Dupage Easter Seals Chicago, Illinois
Patti Oetter, MA, OTR/L, FAOTA	
Eileen Richter, MPH, OTR, FAOTA	
Karen Spencer, MA, OTR	Colorado State University Fort Collins, Colorado

Foreword

A quiet revolution has been occurring in occupational therapy during the last fifteen years. The ways in which occupational therapy services are provided for infants, toddlers, children, and youth has changed. Broadening out from its traditional models of hospital-based service provision, occupational therapy has shifted its services to community and school-based programs. Concomitant with this change is the need to reexamine methods of service provision, and develop new ways that best match the needs of the child within appropriate environments.

Currently, one-third of occupational therapists work in pediatrics, with half of these employed in school systems. Pediatric priorities have been modified dramatically to reflect the increasing concern for children at educational risk. Public and professional interests are evidenced by the Education for All Handicapped Children Act of 1975 (PL 99–142), and the more recent amendment PL 99–457, which provide incentives for states that provide intervention for handicapped infants and toddlers. These regulations affect both intervention models and standards for documentation.

Dr. Dunn, a recognized leader in pediatric occupational therapy, provides an integrated approach to examining the role of the occupational therapist in pediatric practice. She describes the particular expertise of the occupational therapist, and discusses how this can best be amalgamated into a holistic educational and intervention plan for the child. Dunn discusses different models of integration (peer, functional, and practice), and provides new meaning to the term "integration." The pros and cons of direct service, monitoring, and consultation models of service provision are highlighted, along with guidelines for selecting the appropriate service provision model.

As an academician, I have often thought about what it is that makes a great teacher. One aspect is the ability to produce the "aha" phenomenon. Suddenly the pieces fit together and the learner thinks to himself "Of course, that makes perfect sense. Why didn't I think of it?" Dr. Dunn's book is filled with "aha's." She provides a comprehensive guide for systematic observation and decision-making. She and her contributing authors provide an overall framework for action by clarifying the logical relationships among assessment, program planning, service provision, evaluation, and documentation. Through valuable charts, diagrams, and practical examples to illustrate ideas, Dr. Dunn helps the therapist structure services and provides models for decision making.

In my professional capacity, I have known few people who not only have the skills to teach both process and content, but also have the ability to shape an individual's way of thinking about intervention. Dr. Dunn is one of these individuals; through this textbook, she enhances clinical reasoning abilities and inspires others to share her vision of pediatric occupational therapy practice.

Sharon A. Cermak, Ed.D., OTR, FAOTA

Preface

Many pediatric textbooks address the frames of reference, assessment, and intervention strategies used by occupational therapists; but there has been little written material that addresses the underlying components of, and related factors to, the service provision process itself. In order to be effective in the next decade, therapists must know how to design and orchestrate services within interdisciplinary contexts and in a variety of environments, regardless of their frame of reference. Until now, therapists have had to rely on continuing education courses, or the opportunity to work with a colleague who is successful at operating within pediatric systems, if they wanted to learn these skills. When important information is only passed along through demonstration and discussion, the information takes on a "folklore" quality. The "folklore" process allows us to experiment with new ideas, but has limited usefulness for building the body of knowledge of occupational therapy. I created *Pediatric Occupational Therapy* to provide practicing occupational therapists and preservice students with a written record of important information about the service provision process.

I believe that occupational therapists have a lot to contribute to the quality of children's and families' lives. We value individual independence in life tasks, and have many skills to promote this independence. However, to be effective in reaching this goal, we must possess an expansive view of the contributions we can make in community-based services and natural life environments, rather than limiting ourselves to isolated service provision structures. The children we serve do not generalize skills to new tasks or settings easily, so we must be responsible for making sure that these skills develop in functional contexts in the first place. Our knowledge of sensorimotor, cognitive, and psychosocial performance components, and ability to analyze task and environmental variables, enables us to embed our expertise into every activity the child engages in throughout each day. When occupational therapists take this approach to service provision, the natural course of the child's day provides cues and reinforcement for functional performance, reducing the need for special services, and increasing the possibility for life independence. I hope this textbook is a contribution that enables us to move in this direction.

Acknowledgments

My ability to create and orchestrate the development of useful material is dependent on the dedication and labor of many individuals, a list that extends well beyond the contributing authors. My accomplishments are shared with all of these individuals. Their legacies live on in the pages of this book.

My deepest gratitude . . .

Bonnie Danley organized and managed this project, overseeing the production of materials for every draft.

Kevin Birchard created and adapted much of the visual material in the text.

Rebecca Conrad, Carolyn James, Jacquie Foster, and Dorie Shelton produced and edited many of the manuscripts.

Marion Marshall located primary sources when we needed them and offered cogent advice during a critical period of development.

The OT faculty at the University of Kansas worked with flexible schedules and continue to create a healthy, dynamic department; this environment provides the "soil" for growth and creativity.

James P. Cooney, Dean of the School of Allied Health at the University of Kansas, established both high expectations and consistent support to enable task completion.

Sarah Hertfelder, Randy Strickland, and Jim Hinojosa got me involved in critical association projects during a formative stage in my development.

Pip Campbell challenged me to broaden my views, and simultaneously validated the basic principles that guide my teaching, service provision, and research. She provided a multifaceted reflection of the application of knowledge to life's challenges.

Manley Vance recognized my "unusual ways of working" as talents to be nurtured.

Gloria Scammahorn reminded me repeatedly that each of us has a unique contribution to make to the development and growth of occupational therapy.

Many colleagues, families, and children taught me the core principles of service provision by their example.

Mary L. Wiese and Ignatius J. Wiese, my parents, created an environment that enabled my siblings and I to value equally the contribution of women (girls) and men (boys) to work and our culture, in an era when this was not the accepted practice. Without this unconditional expectation of acceptance and performance, I may not have chosen the paths I have since been willing and exhilarated to explore.

Erna Marxer, my grandmother, has loved me in every one of my roles.

My siblings and their families accept and rejoice in my idiosyncrasies, whether they produce something tangible or not:

Mary Ellen, Steve, Nicholas, Jamie, and Michael O'Hare;
Johnny, Kathy, Danielle and Jacob Wiese;
Gary and Susann Wiese; and
Michael Wiese and Susan McLaughlin

Robert Gregory Dunn, my husband, had recognized my skills and abilities long before they were discernable to those outside my family of origin. He values the concept of different, but necessary contributions to the same task, and therefore, rightly shares credit for my accomplishments. He provides a stable base from which I can create, produce, struggle, and complete tasks. He runs errands, cooks, cleans, does caretaking and laundry, so that I have more time to write, think, meet, etc.

Jessica, my youngest daughter, has always been flexible in her time, accommodating my sometimes difficult schedule so that we can still do things together. Her relentless expectation that we will be an integral part of each other's lives has provided necessary grounding for me about what is most important in life.

Jim, my son, has always celebrated my nontraditional nature as a mother, and found joy in my style of nurturing. His acceptance has provided strength during difficult times.

Introduction

Pediatric Occupational Therapy is designed to provide a comprehensive reference about the service provision process. It is organized so that it can be used to learn about the entire service provision process one part at a time, or as a guide for therapists who wish to improve a particular aspect of their service program. The chapters contain descriptions of the content area, examples illustrating the application of the content to pediatric situations, and sample forms and figures to assist therapists who wish to create specific plans for their settings. The text is divided into two major sections; Section I addresses the components of the service provision process, and Section II contains discussions of topics that support effective service provision.

Section I contains three general categories, which are part of the service provision process. The *identification process* is addressed in the first four chapters. The *Referral Process* (Chapter 1) explains the primary factors that must be considered when therapists establish referral procedures, and provides sample referral forms and checklists. The *Screening Process* (Chapter 2) outlines the steps involved in both system-wide and individual screening programs. It will be important for therapists to understand and participate in screening, as community agencies become more involved in early identification programs. Chapter 3 provides a comprehensive discussion of The *Assessment Process*. The author describes performance compnent (sensorimotor, cognitive, and psychosocial) and performance area (ADL, work, and play/leisure) assessment strategies, following the AOTA Uniform Terminology—second edition format. Finally, in Chapter 4, twelve case studies are presented to illustrate the application of identification processes to children from ages four months to 19 years, who have a variety of handicapping conditions.

The *intervention process* is described and illustrated in the next three chapters. Chapter 5 (The *Program Planning Process*) discusses the primary issues that must be considered to create program plans as part of a team, and within the child's natural environment. The *Service Provision Process* (Chapter 6) addresses methods for creating systematic service provision strategies, and points out the wide range of service provision options that are available to occupational therapists. Chapter 7 revisits the same twelve children who are introduced in Chapter 4, provides the reader with a description of their team's processes for making decisions, and illustrates sample portions of programing documents for each child.

The *recording process* is reported in the final two chapters of Section I. Chapter 8, *The Documentation Process*, provides the reader with a comprehensive description of documentation methods, including many examples to demonstrate the ways that therapists can keep track of information about children. Another critical aspect of recording involves *Program Evaluation* (Chapter 9). This chapter outlines the components of program evaluation and explains why this is a necessary aspect of all effective pediatric service provision programs.

Section II also contains three general categories that provide information to support and enhance effective service provision. A historical perspective is provided in Chapter 10 (*Impact of Federal Policy on Pediatric Health and Education Programs*). The author reviews federal policies that have affected pediatric services, and discusses the relationship between cultural patterns (as reflected in public policy) and the options available to occupational therapists. A business perspective is provided in Chapters 11 and 12. It is becoming more common for occupational therapy services to be contained in free-standing programs, which necessitates that therapists understand *Marketing the Pediatric Program* and *Financing the Pediatric Program*. A critical issue in the provision of effective pediatric services is the therapist's ability to work within interdisciplinary teams. The final four chapters of Section II address the perspectives of four primary groups with whom occupational therapists collaborate. *The Special Education Administrator's Perspective* reviews the impact of PL94–142 and PL99–457 on children's services, and discusses the roles of the occupational therapist as a service provider within these contexts. *The Family Perspective* provides a comprehensive review of the literature on families, and offers suggestions for successful interactions with families, acknowledging their priorities and needs. *The Medical Perspective* addresses the behavioral, cognitive, and motoric correlates of commonly prescribed drugs, furnishes a framework for dealing with children who have special health care needs, and proposes appropriate expectations for referrals to pediatric specialists. The final chapter, *Tests Used by Other Professionals*, reviews the interpretation methods for the most commonly used psychoeducational tests, and suggests a way for occupational therapists to use these data to verify or refute their own assessment results.

This comprehensive coverage of the service provision process furnishes the pediatric occupational therapist with many strategies for implementing effective services. The profession is best served when programs are designed, orchestrated, and evaluated in a systematic and ongoing manner. I hope that this contribution will serve to improve the systematic nature of pediatric services as we approach the next century.

The Service Provision Process

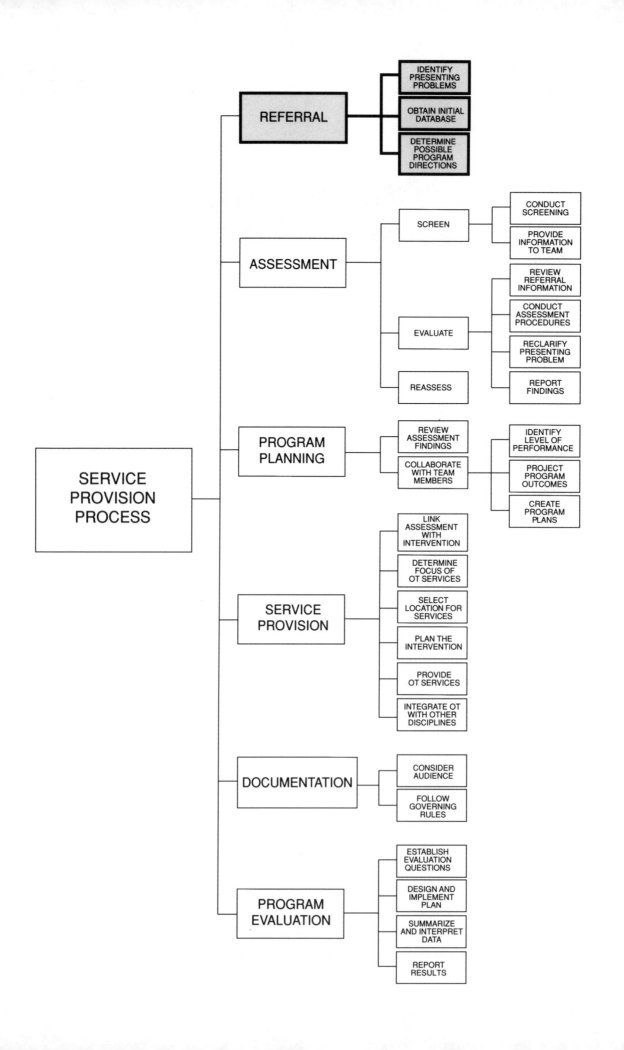

CHAPTER 1

The Referral Process

Susan Merryfield, OTR

"The first step in making a good referral is putting the problem in behavioral terms." Wodrich, 1984

When occupational therapists begin working in a pediatric setting, the referral process is often the least of their worries. Therapists tend to focus attention on determining what materials are needed, identifying which evaluations are to be given, and learning documentation procedures. However, the referral process is very important because it is the starting point for the process of providing pediatric services. Frequently, the policies and procedures for school districts, hospitals, or other community agencies will not include a written procedure for referrals, although professionals in the agency are knowledgeable about the referral process from their experience. Teachers, fellow therapists, or the administration can provide guidance, but may provide somewhat different information, each from their own perspectives. It is essential then for the occupational therapist to establish a specific standard operating procedure for referral to occupational therapy services, so individuals within the agency and the community will take a critical look at the children they serve and be sensitive to situations which would warrant a referral to occupational therapy. When the referral procedure is established, the therapist can then educate those who have the potential to refer and establish a mechanism to encourage appropriate referrals to occupational therapy.

DETERMINING THE REFERRAL PARAMETERS

When working in a pediatric setting, it is important to understand that decisions made regarding a child's education are often related to local traditions, professional relationships, and previous cases (White & Calhoun, 1987). When exploring the referral process for an agency, one must be aware of what the agency desires. The agency must be consistent with its own mission, comply with government regulations, and respond to the fiscal constraints of the agency to determine particular strategies for implementing its occupational therapy services (Dutton, 1986). This information allows the therapist to know which children and families can be served within the agency's structure. Therapists themselves must work within parameters as they comply with state regulations and professional standards. Clear knowledge and understanding of the various parameters that affect a specific pediatric practice enables therapists to construct effective referral strategies.

A number of regulatory agencies affect the parameters of referral to pediatric occupational therapy within various settings. These are discussed in more detail in Chapters 8 and 10.

Education of the Handicapped Act (Public Law 94-142) is the federal law which mandates education for all handicapped children. This law defines occupational therapy as a related service. For this reason, occupational therapy referrals occur after the child's special education needs have been identified. The implementation of PL94-142 occurs through state and local education agency plans. Therapists who work in public schools must be familiar with these documents to ensure that referral procedures are consistent with these policies and guidelines (Langdon & Langdon, 1983). Public Law 99-457 extends mandated services to infants, toddlers, preschoolers and their families, and specifies a family-focused referral process.

The Joint Commission of Accreditation for Hospitals Organization (JCAHO) accredits hospital facilities. To be in compliance with their regulations, the referral for service must come from a physician. Pediatric therapists who work for JCAHO accredited facilities follow this procedure within the hospital, but may also have to follow this procedure within community agencies. Clarification of expectations prior to accepting referrals is very important.

The *Committee on Accreditation of Rehabilitation Facilities* (CARF), certifies centers providing vocational and rehabilitation services, with many specialty rehabilitation certifications being provided. If one is employed or contracts with a CARF accredited center, a referral may go through a screening team. The therapists may or may not serve on this team.

Many states regulate occupational therapists through licensing and registration laws. Some state regulations determine who may make referrals to occupational therapy. For instance, in the State of Kansas, if one is employed in a hospital or any other type of community agency, a physician's referral is necessary for occupational therapy services; an exception is made for the therapists who are employed in school systems, and physician's referrals are not required. Occupational therapists need to know the requirements of their state regulations.

DESIGNING THE REFERRAL PLAN

The therapist's supervisor can be extremely helpful in providing useful information when designing the referral plan. When working within the public schools, the supervisor is usually the Director of Special Education; while in an agency, the supervisor may be the Director of Occupational Therapy or Director of Rehabilitation Services. First, the therapist and supervisor discuss the agency's interpretation of pertinent regulations. For example, PL94-192 classifies occupational therapy as a related service in schools, limiting services to those children with special education needs. A school system may want to use local money to provide services for children who have motor problems, but do not qualify for special education services. A hospital that fulfills community contracts might restrict referrals to only those received from a physician, even though the community-based contract would not require this.

Second, the therapist and supervisor identify financial issues that would limit or expand referral parameters. All agencies have financial parameters within which to work. The administration is concerned with the number of children who might require occupational therapy services, both from revenue generation and resource usage standpoints (Langdon & Langdon, 1983). The occupational therapist and the administrator must work together to provide services to the largest number of appropriate children. The manner by which referrals are handled will affect how services are provided.

The therapist and supervisor must also determine priorities for occupational therapy services, especially if the agency is designed to serve specific populations. The therapist will not want to cultivate new referral sources in areas that are incompatible with agency priorities. Other agency staff members also provide information about priorities and may also be able to generate occupational therapy referrals. The intake coordinator employed by the children's hospital may be able to screen occupational therapy referrals according to preset criteria. Arrangements such as these enable therapists to make the most efficient use of their time on behalf of the agency and its priorities.

Established agency policies and procedures provide information about the agency's focus and goals. Procedures for referral into the agency may already be established, but referral procedures for specific services such as occupational therapy may or may not be available. Although the basic guidelines are determined by federal and state regulations, each agency will design variations to accommodate their particular needs. In a small school district, the school counselor might coordinate all the referrals to specific services. In a large school system, there may be a referral team which evaluates all the referrals for the entire school system. It is important for the referral coordinator or the referral team members to be well acquainted with occupational therapy services so that they recognize appropriate times to include occupational therapy on the evaluation team.

DEVELOPING A STANDARD OPERATING PROCEDURE

With all the available information, the occupational therapist develops procedures for referral to occupational therapy services. Often the referral stage of providing services has been criticized for lacking sufficient safeguards to prevent inappropriate referrals (White & Calhoun, 1987). Inappropriate or too many referrals can be a resource-draining proposition. To be most effective, a referral process requires both a highly disciplined procedure for acquiring information and an equally disciplined process for analyzing the information (Mahan & Mahan, 1981).

First, there must be a delineation of who gets referred to occupational therapy; not all children who are referred need to be evaluated by the occupational therapist. The therapist lists the types of children and the characteristic behavior patterns that would make them likely candidates for occupational therapy services. Figure 1-1 provides an example of a very simple referral guide sheet. Agencies may then develop more specific referral criteria. In these cases, the therapist outlines the steps which the referring person should follow. There are two common strategies for a referral process: those that go to a team or centralized location and those that come directly to the therapist. When the child is referred to a centralized body, the evaluation coordinator usually determines whether to refer the child to specific services such as occupational therapy. The evaluation team coordinator must have a clear picture of occupational therapy services in order to decide whether a child should be seen by this service. If persons in this position do not know the many signs indicating occupational therapy needs, services may not be utilized efficiently. A referral form which specifies the amount and type of behaviors which warrant occupational therapy evaluation is helpful. Figure 1-2 displays an example of an Occupational Therapy Referral Checklist.

The child may also be referred to the occupational therapist directly. These referrals frequently come from community agencies, physicians, parents, or other professionals. In these cases, the occupational therapist has the responsibility to ensure that proper referral safeguards are followed (e.g., obtaining a physician's referral if required by the agency or state regulations).

It is important to remember that the standard operating procedure for the referral process works for the agency and other professionals, as well as the occupational therapist.

OCCUPATIONAL THERAPY REFERRAL GUIDE SHEET

1. Children who have *sensori*motor motor problems. They may have trouble with writing, or they cannot perform motor skills as peers do.
2. Children who have difficulties with caring for themselves, (e.g., Dressing, feeding, grooming, toileting), performing work (e.g., learning) or play/leisure tasks.
3. Children who have trouble moving their limbs for functional use.
4. Children who may be able to function more efficiently if adaptations were made.
5. Children who have difficulty with cognitive or behavioral skills.

Figure 1-1.   Children who demonstrate the above problems, can benefit from Occupational Therapy.

OCCUPATIONAL THERAPY REFERRAL FORM

_____ has been referred for an occupational therapy evaluation. To help with the evaluation, your input is very important. Please complete this questionnaire and return to the occupational therapist. The evaluation will be completed on _____
_____ . Thank you very much for your help!!!

Date of Referral: _____   Teacher: _____

Why do you feel this child should be evaluated by the occupational therapist? _____
_____
_____
_____

Formal Evaluations:
1.   I.Q./Name of Test: _____
      Data Given: _____
      Full Score: _____
         Verbal: _____
         Performance: _____
2.   Academic Levels:
      Reading: _____   Date of Assessment: _____
      Spelling: _____   Date of Assessment: _____
      Math: _____   Date of Assessment: _____
3.   Other Pertinent Evaluations:
      Speech Evaluation Results: _____
      _____
      Special Evaluations (Given by Counselor or Special Teacher of LD resource teacher):
      _____
      _____
      VMI: _____
      Peabody Picture Vocabulary Test: _____
4.   Health Evaluation:
      Medical Problems: _____
      _____
      Health Screening Results: _____
      _____
      _____
      Medications: _____
      _____

CHECKLIST FOR OCCUPATIONAL THERAPY

Please check (√) the statements which are pertinent to this child.

Gross Motor
_____ Seems weaker than other children his/her age
_____ Does not have the endurance other children his/her age have for an activity
_____ Difficulty with hopping, jumping, skipping, or running as compared with others his/her age.
_____ Appears stiff and awkward in his/her movements
_____ Clumsy, does not appear to know how body works, bumps into others or objects, never quite sits in chair correctly
_____ Does not seem to understand concepts such as right, left, front, or back as it relates to his/her body
_____ Shies away from playground equipment. May only play on one particular item
_____ Poor posture (always seems to be leaning against something, shoulders slump forward)

Fine Motor
_____ Difficulty with drawing, coloring, tracing
_____ Performs these activities quickly and result is usually sloppy
_____ Avoids fine motor activities
_____ Problem holding pencil, grasp may be very loose or very tight

Figure 1-2.   Occupational Therapy Referral Form and Behavior Checklist.

_____ Printing is too dark, too light, too large, too small
_____ Does not seem to have a dominant hand

Academic
_____ Distractible
_____ Restless
_____ Slow worker
_____ Disorganized, messy desk
_____ Short attention span
_____ Hyperactive
_____ Can't follow directions
_____ Never completes assignments

Tactile Sensation
_____ Withdraws from touch
_____ Tends to wear only certain types of clothing
_____ Touches everything
_____ Avoids being close to others (doesn't like to be hugged)

Vestibular Sensation
_____ Fearful of being off the ground
_____ Doesn't like playground equipment at the merry-go-round, slide
_____ Can't seem to stop moving, craves swinging, rocking

Auditory
_____ Has difficulty pronouncing words
_____ Does not appear to understand other people
_____ Tends to repeat things to himself/herself

Visual Perception
_____ Trouble discriminating shapes, letters, or numbers
_____ Can not complete puzzles appropriate for age
_____ Difficulty copying designs, letters or numbers
_____ Difficulty tracking (i.e., as in reading in a book or following teacher's arm movements)

Emotional
_____ Does not care to have routine changed
_____ Is easily frustrated
_____ Can not get along with others
_____ Accident prone
_____ Deals better with a small group situation or one-to-one
_____ Frequently involves self in other people's activities.

Additional Information:

Please attach a sample of the child's seatwork. An example of this would be a drawing or a printing exercise.

_____ Date: _____
(Signature of person completing form)

Figure 1-2. _Continued._

Professionals feel the referral process works when the administration is concerned, cooperative and encouraging with regard to the referral process (Harrington & Gibson, 1986). It is also important that the procedure be followed or adapted if there are problems, so the staff can work efficiently for the benefit of the children. An example of a Standard Operating Procedure for referrals is found in Figure 1-3.

DEVELOPING THE REFERRAL FORM

In either the team or the direct referral process, it is advantageous for the therapist to develop a referral form for occupational therapy. An occupational therapy form provides the necessary guidance for the referral source in defining a child's problem and whether occupational therapy can help. The information gathered on this referral form acknowledges that the informant is a valuable source of information for identifying those children whose performance deviates from that of other children (Clark & Allen, 1985). The referral form can also provide the occupational therapist with more detailed information which normally would take several visits to obtain.

Several components are included on the referral form to maximize its usefulness. First, basic demographic information is requested. Include items such as: the child's name, date

Title: Referral Procedure for Occupational Therapy
Date of Implementation:
Date of Review:
Procedure:

1. Children who demonstrate problems on the referral guidesheet are good candidates for referral to occupational therapy.
2. When a child meets the criteria noted above, the referral process is initiated.
3. The Occupational Therapy Referral Form must be completed by the referral source. A copy of the Form may be requested from the Director of Special Education, the school counselor, or the occupational therapist.
4. All parts of the Referral Form are completed and given to the occupational therapist.
5. The occupational therapist will review the referral and gather more information if necessary.
6. Based on the information, the occupational therapist will recommend one of the following alternatives:
   a. The child will be screened; the child will receive a complete evaluation if indicated by screening.
   b. The child does not meet screening criteria. The referral source is given feedback as to why the child will not be evaluated and examples of activities to enhance performance in the future are provided.
7. All referral statistics will be reported to the Director.

Figure 1-3. Standard operating procedure for referral process.

of birth, grade placement, the teacher's name, the source of referral, the date referral is made, and the date referral is received by the therapist. These data enable therapists to track the sequence of events (See Figure 1-2 for an example).

Next, the referral form includes a statement by the referral party regarding concerns about this child. With this statement, the therapist identifies the reasons why the informant is concerned and can begin to formulate a plan for addressing this need. Keep the space for this section short (e.g., two or three lines) so that the informant will summarize the major concerns and does not feel a long narrative is necessary.

The referral form may also include a section for reporting prior test results. Oftentimes children are evaluated by various professionals prior to the occupational therapy referral. In agencies that utilize a predictable set of tests, it is beneficial to list them on the form, to save time completing the referral. The therapist may also choose to list only those tests with results relevant to possible occupational therapy concerns. Tests which are often useful are: intelligence, language, perceptual, and developmental test data (see Chapter 16).

The referral form might also include behavioral information about how the child is presently functioning. A checklist format enables the informant to complete this section quickly. This section provides a mechanism to let the referral party know the focus of the occupational therapist's attention. The concerns listed in the checklist are related to the child's life tasks and must relate to the structure, limits, and expectations of relevant environments. For example, therapists who work in schools would focus on what one would see in the classroom. It is also helpful if one categorizes the questions or statements. By doing this, the teacher is alerted to characteristics which are related to each other (Turnbull, Strickland, & Brantley, 1982). The questions or statements are written clearly (refer to Chapter 8: Documentation).

Finally, it is useful to ask the referral party to provide any other information which may be pertinent to the current situation. The therapist may ask the teacher to provide examples of the child's handwriting, or samples of drawing projects. The parent may describe an anecdote which illustrates the concern. This section may also be passed on to other people who work with the child, so they may give their input. Speech/

language pathologists, reading specialists, adaptive physical education teachers, or social workers could contribute additional information in this section (See Figure 1-2).

DEVELOPING A REFERRAL NETWORK

Occupational therapists know their own capabilities, and should know the capabilities of the members of the interdisciplinary team in order to collaborate effectively (Florian & Sacks, 1985). The referral procedure will only work if the professionals develop a plan to integrate the referral process into the everyday activities of the agency. The occupational therapist within an agency must develop a networking system which will facilitate appropriate referrals within an efficient timeline. In private practice, development and nurturance of a referral network is an ongoing process (see Chapter 11, Marketing).

To facilitate occupational therapy referrals in an agency and its community, a therapist learns as much as possible about both of them. This background information helps the therapist frame occupational therapy priorities within the proper context to increase an understanding of occupational therapy and make it easier for others to make appropriate referrals.

The therapist must also know both the official and the functional line of authority, so that information reaches the proper places at the right times. For example, in a small community agency, the occupational therapist may report directly to the special services director, but the pediatric nurse practitioner may be the evaluation coordinator. Together, the therapist and the nurse may determine evaluation criteria which are then passed on to the director for administrative approval. These mechanisms are established to facilitate efficient work plans that are compatible with professional judgement and the agency's mission.

As a therapist coming into a new situation, the referral base may be small or may be only for children who traditionally receive therapy. In order to increase the referral base for therapy, the occupational therapist spends time with those sources that may be most instrumental in referring children. One may want to spend time with persons in the appropriate community agencies, assess their immediate needs, and then

---

INSERVICES FOR PARENTS AND PROFESSIONALS

1. Helping the child who has writing problems.
2. Good body mechanics in the classroom.
3. How to survive the holiday crazies.
4. The helping relationship (How Occupational Therapy can assist in inpatient unit or classroom activities).
5. What can you do for the clumsy child?

Figure 1-4. Topics which a therapist may use in designing inservices to meet the needs of both parents and teachers.

determine what help, if any, can be provided. For example, in a school system, the learning disabilities resource teacher may be viewed as a referral source for children with sensory integration problems. The therapist requests time to talk with this teacher, and find out more about the school population. When talking with the teacher, the therapist can discuss the problems she is having with the child in the classroom. From the discussion, the therapist may find that a large number of children are having visual perception problems. Suggestions may then be offered to the teacher to increase her activity base, and provide the therapist with more information regarding which children may have a sensory integration deficit. If this information leads the therapist to believe there are potential referrals, the therapist can then make these arrangements. This will foster the therapist's role as a resource to the teacher, in addition to creating and fostering a referral source.

When a potentially fruitful referral source provides an inappropriate referral, the therapist meets with the person involved and listens carefully to the concerns that are expressed, both in words and the tone of voice. The therapist can then guide the discussion to determine a clearer focus, and therefore a more successful solution. It is important to focus on the solution, and not the problem. Even if an occupational therapy referral is not needed, it is important to suggest options for the present situation. This interaction will foster a feeling that the therapist is supportive and can serve as a resource.

Not only does the therapist want to develop relationships with individual professionals, but also with groups within the agency. Offering inservice training to others is an excellent way to begin. The occupational therapist may suggest a list of topics that could be discussed (See Figure 1-4). Keep in mind when developing this list, that the topics should be of interest to the referral source. For example, an inservice to elementary teachers on ways to help improve handwriting skills would pique the teachers' interest. The inservice would be designed to help the teachers with individual problems they may be having, and provide better information about referrals for this particular problem.

Other effective strategies include attending staff and parent meetings, participating in special agency projects, or eating lunch with other staff members. These situations broaden others' view of the occupational therapist and offer opportunities for informal discussions.

Written communication can also increase a referral base. Timely responses to referrals encourage further interactions. Brochures or flyers (Chapter 12) can be distributed to potential referral sources. When referrals are not appropriate, alternate solutions can be offered. Documentation is important and can make a lasting impression. The occupational therapist may also develop information sheets and simple suggestions which can be given out to referral sources as they identify needs. These may include handouts on activities to increase dexterity or improve visual perception skills. Always note somewhere on the handout sheets who designed the

---

ACTIVITIES TO ENHANCE FINE MOTOR COORDINATION

Below you will find activities that you can incorporate into your classroom which will help with fine motor coordination. Please have _____ work on one activity each day. Thank you for your time, and if there are any questions, please let me know.

1. Get a paper plate or other flat surface, and modelling clay. Flatten out the modeling clay on the flat surface, until it resembles a slate or chalkboard. Now have the child use his/her pencil and draw in the clay. You can start out with shapes and work up to printed letters. To "clean" the board, have the child use their fingers to erase the lines drawn.
2. Take a pair of tweezers, lima beans, and a jar. Place the lima beans next to the jar. The child should use the tweezers to pick up the lima beans and place them in the jar. Once the child has mastered the task, he/she can have races against himself/herself, or against other kids in the classroom.
3. Give the child a deck of playing cards. Have him/her hold them in one hand and flip each card over and place in a pile as fast as he/she can. You may also like to lay out a red and black-faced card. The child can then sort the cards as fast as he/she can into the color groups.

Sue Merryfield, OTR
Occupational Therapist

Figure 1-5. An activity sheet designed for the classroom. The activities are designed to fit into the classroom routine. They do not require a lot of materials or instruction, but address a particular concern identified by the teacher.

activities, so the referral party has an immediate source of help. An example of a handout may be found in Figure 1-5.

SUMMARY

Although the referral process is not the first component an occupational therapist thinks about when starting a program, it is a vital part of the entire process. The referral process is designed so the agency takes a crucial look at young children with whom they interact, and is sensitive to situations in which a referral is appropriate (Peterson, 1987). The process also allows the occupational therapist to develop a procedure so the children who need therapy may be referred in a timely and efficient manner. It must be kept in mind however, that the therapist must work to initiate the referral process and develop a referral network which will meet the needs of everyone involved.

EXPAND YOUR NEWLY ACQUIRED KNOWLEDGE

1. Create a referral form which provides you with a complete picture of the concerns of the referring party. Be sure to include demographic information and pertinent questions about the child's history. Remember, the referral information you receive will direct the next steps in the assessment, program planning and service provision processes.
2. Tommy is a second grader who is not completing his seatwork in a timely manner. His teacher is concerned about this, and makes a referral to the special education team. Write questions you would want to ask the teacher to clarify the exact problem. List pieces of data you might look for in Tommy's records and files to clarify the referral issues.

References

Clark, P., & Allen, A. (1985). *Occupational therapy for children.* St. Louis, MO: C. V. Mosby Company.

Dutton, R. (1986). Procedures for designing an occupational therapy consultation contract. *American Journal of Occupational Therapy, 40*(3), 160–166.

Florian, V. & Sacks, D. (1985). Reasons for patient referral to occupational therapy units by health care professionals. *Journal of Allied Health, 14*(3), 317–326.

Harrington, R. G. & Gibson, E. (1986). Preassessment procedures for learning disabled children: Are they effective? *Journal of Learning Disabilities, 19*(9), 538.

Langdon, H. J. & Langdon, L. L. (1983). *Initiating occupational therapy programs within the public school: A guide for OT's and public school administrators.* Thorofare, NJ: SLACK, Inc.

Mahan, T. & Mahan, A. (1981). *Assessing children with special needs.* New York: Holt, Rinehart & Winston.

Peterson, N. (1987). *Early intervention for handicapped and at-risk children.* Denver: Love Publishing Co.

Turnbull, A., Strickland, B., & Brantley, J. (1982). *Developing and implementing individualized education programs.* Columbus: Charles Merrill Publishing Company.

White, R., & Calhoun, M. L. (1987). From referral to placement: Teachers' perceptions of their responsibilities. *Exceptional Children, 53*(5), 460–468.

Wodrich, D. L. (1984). *Children's psychological testing: A guide for non psychologists,* (p. 19–20). Baltimore: Paul H. Brookes Publishing Co.

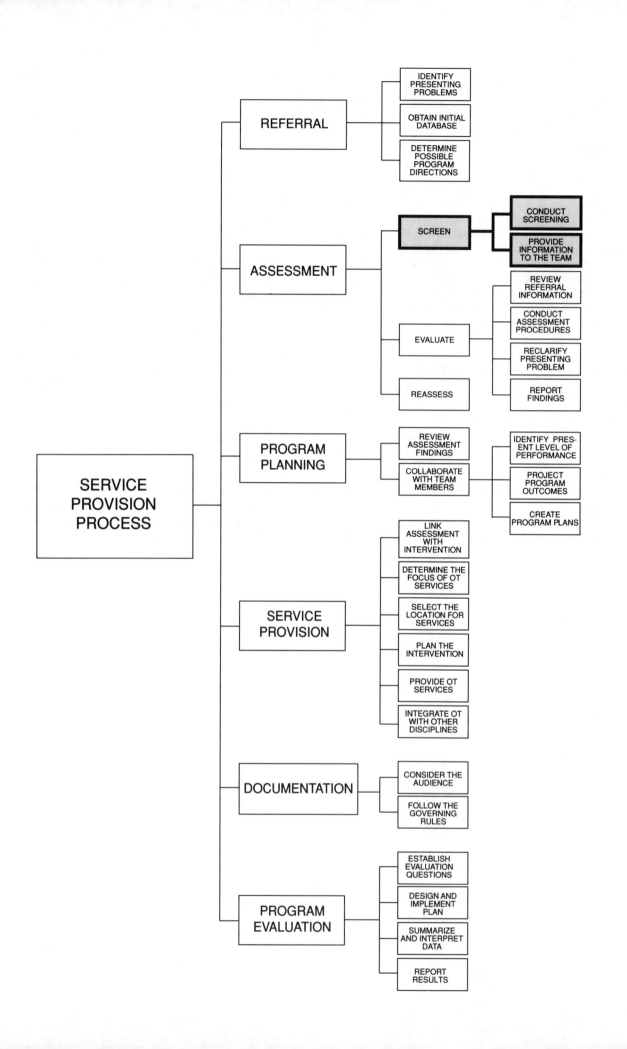

CHAPTER 2

The Screening Process

Terri Collier, MS, OTR

"Screening is a source of valuable information about the development of children, but it has its limitations in that it can only indicate the possible presence of an impairment." Cross, 1977

In the last decade there has been an increasing emphasis on early recognition and subsequent referral to intervention programs for children with developmental disabilities. School systems are mandated by law to set up mass community "child find" screening programs for the early identification of children with any signs of developmental lags or deviations. With the passage of the Education of the Handicapped Act (EHA) amendments (P.L. 99–457), school mandates have been extended to preschoolers and services to infants and toddlers and their families have been mandated, causing states to further define what constitutes a significant problem. Occupational therapists can play a part in this screening process, but first must understand what screening is, and what is involved in the screening process. There are several components of the screening process that must be understood in order to identify occupational therapy's potential roles in screening.

Screening is one aspect of the assessment process; sometimes screening results demonstrate that there is no cause for concern, and sometimes the results indicate the need for specialized assessment. Screening is a means of verifying if a child needs further diagnostic evaluation. Through the screening process, children who do not fall within normal ranges of development, as suggested by a broad estimate of their behavior, are identified as potential candidates for assessment and possibly intervention. Screening involves looking at a child's skills in a general, more broad sense to determine if they are within normal developmental expectations for children of the same age. Screening of developmental skills is typically a quick, easy look at a child within a limited amount of time. Generally, screening results place children into three groups: a) those whose developmental skills are within age expectation and therefore need no further special services; b) those children who demonstrate skills that cause concern and therefore require a more in-depth thorough look (evaluation); and c) those children who require periodic follow-up due to possible borderline developmental problems.

Many use screening to identify children during their preschool and early school years who may be asymptomatic, but who are highly likely to have problems that interfere with the expected sequence of normal growth and development. Positive (abnormal) screening results lead to diagnostic evaluation; if a disorder is confirmed, intervention is begun earlier than if the diagnosis were dependent on the later appearance of obvious symptoms. Even when screening test results are negative (normal), the quality of future life can be enhanced by a provision of anticipatory guidance. In this second situation, the professional provides caregivers with information about the next set of expectations, and sometimes offers suggestions about activities that would be useful to stimulate further development (Stangler, Huber, & Routh, 1980).

The major goals and objectives in setting up a good screening program were identified by Lessler (1972): a) to provide relevant information about life tasks of children for those who work with them; b) to utilize the screening information gained for the benefit of the child; c) to conduct ongoing evaluation which will ensure that all aspects of the screening program are contributing to the goal of screening; d) to promote primary preventative measures including health, education, family participation, and commitment to individual growth.

As a result of screening activities, the professional should have enough information about each child to decide: a) if the child is a candidate for more thorough diagnostic evaluation; b) if the child does not need additional services to maximize potential (indicating that the prognosis for success without intervention is very good); or c) if periodic followup would be useful to ensure that a potential problem is not manifesting itself.

SCREENING PROGRAM GUIDELINES

In the field of medicine, screening for serious conditions and/or diseases has been occurring for many years. Recently, medical screening has become more extensive and sometimes includes screening for various developmental disabilities. Frankenburg (1975) has listed ten criteria that should be considered in planning a screening program. In adapting these criteria for educational and developmental screenings, six major principles emerge as appropriate guidelines:

1. *Screening assumes a problem being screened (e.g., developmental delay, emotional maladjustment, or visual impairment) can be ameliorated or modified as a result of subsequent intervention programs.*

When establishing a screening program, the professional must consider the purpose of the program. Some early intervention studies (e.g., Weiner & Koppelman, 1987; Bricker & Bricker, 1976; Lillie, 1977) offer evidence which indicate that intervention provided in the early years produces better results. One must question the use of community resources for screening if there are no mechanisms for referral, follow-up evaluation, or intervention available to those families whose child is unable to perform adequately.

> 2. *One must assume intervention provided as a result of finding problems through early screening is likely to improve the condition more than intervention at a later date when the problem becomes more obvious.*

The best age for early intervention has not been clearly established. What we do have are some general indications, such as those offered by Bloom (1964), that the earlier the intervention the more there is potential for improvement. Bloom (1964) continues by stating that data can support the position that children must have certain behaviors or skills before higher level skills or behaviors can emerge. Thus the unidentified child who has difficulty learning the earlier or more basic skills or behaviors falls further behind in his development as growth occurs and more complex behaviors are expected.

> 3. *The problem or condition being screened for can be specifically diagnosed through further application of measurement procedures.*

In medical screenings, professionals are looking for conditions or variables that may form a pattern of a specific diagnosis through additional diagnostic work. In education, screening is frequently the first step in making decisions concerning needed interventions. The behaviors displayed, and their severity, are the critical variables in educational or developmental screening; generally, the physiological cause of the behavior is not addressed at this level.

> 4. *The necessary follow-up procedures must be presently or potentially available.*

The need for meeting this criterion has been debated. Should professionals screen, and thereby label certain children, if there are no services available to them? The identification procedure alone can set up altered expectations on the part of the parents, teachers, or any other individual that is aware of screening results. Consequently, the options given to the child can be shaped to correspond to those expectations, thus affecting other performance areas. Presently, the states that oversee state-wide screening programs argue that un-

less a population of children needing assistance is identified through screening, the necessary funds for providing services will not be allocated. Thus a delicate balance between identification and follow-up must be created and maintained.

Screening teams take responsibility for ensuring that there are options for appropriate further evaluations when situations warrant it. The effort and time given to screening should be questioned if there are no follow-up services or plans available to families. Screening programs are set up to provide information and options to families. Follow-up can be simple, such as the provision of a list of expectations and activities for a typical child's next stage of development, or complex, such as referrals for evaluation and intervention programs.

> 5. *The condition being screened for must either be prevalent in the population or the consequence of not discovering it must be very severe.*

This criterion is primarily a consideration of the cost/benefit ratio. Are the potential benefits derived from screening and placement of children worth the cost? If, in other words, you are screening for a relatively rare condition, is the benefit to the few children placed into programs worth the cost? Is the cost worth the results? If the potential number of children that will require treatment or education is small, but the benefits of the program alleviate the problem all together, it still may be worthwhile to conduct screening. For example, very few children actually have phenylketonuria (PKU), but the benefit of a known intervention which prevents the onset of severe retardation makes the cost of screening every infant justifiable.

> 6. *Measurement procedures to screen for the problem should be readily available and should be valid and reliable measures.*

When professionals use screening methods that have not been shown to be valid and reliable, there is a danger that errors will occur in the identification process. Some children may be labeled with a problem, when they really don't have one, while others may have a problem and yet not be identified by the measure (Dunn, 1989). This situation can be

| | | SCREENING OUTCOME | |
		OK	Problem
CHILD OUTCOME	**OK**	Valid & reliable tests will find a large number of children here. **True Negative** **A**	The screening test says the child has a problem, but the child is actually OK. **False Positive** **B***
	Problem	The screening test says the child is OK, but the child actually has a problem. **False Negative** **C***	Valid & reliable tests usually find a small number here, but those found will truly have problems. **True Positive** **D**

* These conditions do not match; the test would say one thing while the actual outcome for the child is different. Perfectly accurate tests find no children in either of these categories. In reality, a few children may be identified incorrectly.

Figure 2-1. Summary of possible findings from screening tools.

characterized by a four box grid, pictured in Figure 2-1. An unstable test would place children in Boxes B and C inappropriately.

Box B (false positive) findings can lead to needless parental anxiety, while Box C (false negative) findings may delay a child getting help for an unrecognized problem.

Whether to use standardized or non-standardized screening tools is a very controversial subject. Many school districts mandate the use of standardized instruments for screening; others use criterion-referenced or developmental checklists. It is important for the occupational therapist who participates in the screening process to collaborate with the director of the screening program, to determine the most appropriate options for the population and problems addressed in the screening program. A summary of a number of screening instruments used by occupational therapists is provided in Table 2-1.

CRITERIA FOR SCREENING TOOLS

Stangler, Huber, and Routh (1980) have outlined six criteria to assess the attributes of a screening procedure.

1. *Acceptability:* Screening tools must be acceptable to all who will be affected by them, including the children and family being screened, the professionals who receive results and referrals, and the community as a whole.
2. *Simplicity:* Screening tools should be relatively easy to teach, learn, and administer.
3. *Costs:* The cost of the screening tool includes cost of equipment, preparing and paying personnel, the cost of inaccurate results, personal costs to the individuals being screened, and the total cost of the test in relation to the benefits of early detection.

TABLE 2-1. Summary of Primary Characteristics of Screening Instruments Frequently Used by Occupational Therapists

	Ayres Clinical Observation of Sensory Integration	Miller Assessment for Preschoolers (MAP)	Developmental Profile II (Interview)	Denver Developmental Screening Test Revised (DDST-R)	Quick Neurological Screening Test	Therapist Generated Developmental Screening Checklists
AGE RANGE	5–8 years	2 years 4 months 5 years 8 months	0–9$^{1/2}$ years	0–6 years	5–18 years	typically 0–9 years
TESTING TIME (minutes)	20 minutes	20–30 minutes	20–40 minutes	5–7 minutes	20 minutes	15–20 minutes
SCORING TIME (minutes)			10–20 minutes	5 minutes	5–10 minutes	
MAJOR AREAS TESTED: personal/social			X	X		X
communication			X	X		X
cognition		X	X			
self help			X	X		X
gross motor		X	X	X	X	X
praxis	X	X			X	X
reflexes	X					X
fine motor		X		X	X	X
visual-motor integration		X			X	X
visual perception		X			X	X
tactile	X	X			X	X
vestibular	X	X			X	X
TYPE OF TEST: norm referenced		X				
criteria referenced				X		
informal/ structured		X			X	X
observation	X		interview		X	X
SCORES OBTAINED: age level			X	X		X
percentile		X		X		
standard						
quantified observations	X					

4. *Appropriateness:* Appropriateness of screening tools is based on the prevalence of the problem in the population to be screened, and/or its applicability to the population under consideration.
5. *Reliability (precision):* Screening tools must be capable of yielding consistent results in repeated trials or when administered by different screeners.
6. *Validity (accuracy):* Screening tests must be capable of giving a true measurement of the behavior, skill, or characteristic being tested.

THE SCREENING PROCESS

An article titled *Developmental Assessment and Early Intervention Programs for the Young Children: Lessons Learned from Longitudinal Research*, by Robert W. Chamberlin (1987), describes a two-stage screening approach that has been used very successfully to reduce the number of false positive findings produced in mass screenings. In his model, children with delays found in two consecutive screenings, three to six months apart, or children found in unstimulating and/or stressful living situations, are referred without further delay to a comprehensive assessment center for a more detailed look at child and family function. Chamberlin (1987) advocates that parents and professionals make a joint decision about whether to pursue comprehensive assessments immediately, or continue to repeat the screening in three to six months.

The American Occupational Therapy Association's *Guidelines for Occupational Therapy Services in School Systems* (1987, 1989a), advocates two types of screening. The first, called Type 1 screening, occurs prior to a formal referral procedure, and the second, Type 2 screening, occurs after the formal referral of a child for special education evaluation. They each serve different purposes and facilitate efficient use of professional resources.

Type I Screening

Type 1 screening is an initial and systematic approach to the identification of children who are at risk because of a specific developmental or educational problem. It allows the agency to collect baseline data, disseminate information about developmental expectations, and refer to evaluation or early intervention if indicated. Many Type 1 screening programs look at every aspect of the child's growth and development, including motor, language, cognition, social/adaptive behavior, and physical development, including vision, hearing, and physical status (e.g., the integrity of the spine for scoliosis screening). It is not necessary for the individuals who carry out components of Type 1 screening to be "professionals"; they can be well-trained volunteers who follow the prescribed screening procedure. Occupational therapists may or may not be directly involved in this type of screening. However, the occupational therapist is frequently used as a resource to design the screening program, train volunteers in proper procedural techniques, and as a follow-up referral source if specific problems are identified in the screening process.

Each state utilizes a statewide plan for early identification of children who may have special needs; in Kansas they call this program *Count Your Kid In* and it can be considered

Type 1 screening. Each school district is responsible for implementing a program in their geographic region; the screening program is carried out each spring in preparation for the next school year. They utilize the resources of their professional experts and enlist the help of community volunteers to conduct Type 1 screening of infants, toddlers, or preschoolers in their districts. Parents who are concerned about their child's development, or who wish to know more about their child from a developmental perspective, may call and make an appointment. Districts advertise the availability of this service through press releases such as the one pictured in Figure 2-2.

When parents call in for appointments, they are told about the screening program, and how long the screening will take. The person who takes the call schedules a time, and takes down the family's address and telephone number. Following this initial contact, the parent receives a student history form and a consent to screen form which are to be filled out and brought to the screening appointment. Figure 2-3 contains a sample scheduling grid, and Figure 2-4 contains a sample student history form.

Figure 2-5 contains an example of how screening team members in one school district have organized their Type 1 screening program. It is important to note that this district utilizes many professionals to carry out the screening program; this is not necessary in order to have a quality Type 1 screening program. Many school districts utilize one to two professionals to oversee the program, and supervise community volunteers for screening procedures; in this case, the occupational therapist may well be one of the supervising professionals, since the sensorimotor areas are so important in the early years of development.

It is also important for Type 1 screening programs to be efficient at moving children and families through the components in a timely manner; when there are a lot of delays, children become fatigued and inattentive to the tasks, and the parents can then become anxious. Figure 2-6 provides an example of one district's organizational structure for the screening day. Most screening teams use a selection of tests, skilled observation and interviews to gather their data. Figure 2-7 contains a sample list of screening procedures that might be chosen by a school district screening team. Several of the screening program tools are illustrated in Figures 2-7a, b, and c.

As each team member completes their screening component, they must briefly summarize their impressions. Many screening teams use a composite form such as the one pictured in Figure 2-8. It is important to identify both strengths and concerns, and to decide whether an in depth evaluation may be necessary in particular areas. Some states determine the level of delay that is necessary to identify an area as at-risk; local agencies may use state guidelines, or may set up their own, as long as they meet the minimum standard set by their state. For example, a district may determine that a six month delay is significant enough to warrant a further look at that area of development, while the state may only require intervention with delays of one or more years. It is important for professionals to know the standards for their particular agency, so that recommendations are consistent with the agency's position.

One person meets with the family at the end of a Type 1

Count Your Kid In

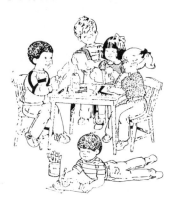

Many children are born with problems or develop them later. They may have trouble talking, seeing, hearing, thinking, or they may have problems doing things. Many of these conditions can be helped or completely corrected if parents recognize the problem early and seek help. *Count Your Kid In* is available to assist parents with questions about their child's development.

Free developmental screenings for infants and preschool children are offered by the Blue Valley Schools Department of Special Services. The screening includes vision and hearing examinations, a check on the developmental areas of language, speech, motor development and of general physical condition. The screening is to help parents identify potential problems and find help. *Count Your Kid In* because your child counts on you.

BLUE VALLEY PRESCHOOL SCREENING

On March 14 and 15, 1990, Blue Valley Schools will offer preschool screening for children in the Blue Valley district. Children eligible for the screening are those who will be under 5 years of age as of September 1, 1990, and who are demonstrating delays in one or more areas of development.

Parents who have a concern about their preschooler's development should call to arrange an appointment after March 1, 1990.

Please call:
MORSE ELEMENTARY SCHOOL
15201 Monrovia
681-4300

Figure 2-2.   Sample press release for availability of service. *Reprinted with permission.*

A.M.	Speech	O.T.	Vision/ Hearing	Conference
8:00 Group 1 (8:00–9:30)				
	8:00	8:30	9:00	
	9:00	8:00	8:30	
	8:30	9:00	8:00	
9:30 Group 2 (9:30–11:00)				
	9:30	10:00	10:30	
	10:30	9:30	10:00	
	10:00	10:30	9:30	
11:00 Group 3 (11:00–12:30)				
	11:00	11:30	12:00	
	12:00	11:00	11:30	
	11:30	12:00	11:00	

Figure 2-3.   Sample schedule sheet for district screening program.

STUDENT HISTORY FORM
CONFIDENTIAL

General

NAME _____ SEX _____ AGE _____
        (LAST)   (FIRST)   (MIDDLE)
ADDRESS _____ CITY/STATE _____ ZIP _____
PHONE _____ DATE OF BIRTH _____
AGE AT TIME OF HISTORY _____ PLACE OF BIRTH _____
FATHER OR GUARDIAN'S NAME _____ AGE _____
OCCUPATION _____ HEALTH _____
MOTHER'S NAME _____ AGE _____
OCCUPATION _____ HEALTH _____
CHILD'S PHYSICIAN _____ PHONE _____
RELATIONSHIP OF INFORMANT TO CHILD _____
HOME SCHOOL _____ SUBDIVISION _____

Family

A. Are parents separated? _____ Divorced? _____
B. Has either parent remarried? _____
                        Which one?
C. With whom does the child live? _____
D. Check one: (   ) Natural Child   (   ) Adopted Child   (   ) Foster Child
E. Name of children in family (eldest to youngest—giving age): _____
F. Others living in the home: _____

Developmental and Medical Background

1. Prenatal: Was there any illness, infection, or unusual condition of mother during pregnancy? _____
2. Birth: Length of pregnancy? _____ Weight at birth? _____
   Difficult or forced labor? _____
   Instrument delivery? _____
   Was there a delay in starting the baby to breathe? _____
   Other comments: _____
   Child's Health History:
3.
   A. Has the child ever had: Convulsions? _____ Seizures? _____
      Give details: (Identify illness being discussed with exact dates or ages when it occurred, etc.) _____
   B. Unexplained high fever: How high? _____ Duration? _____
      When? _____ Circumstances? _____
   C. Is your child on medication or has he/she been on any in the past? _____
      Type? _____ Reason? _____
      _____ Date? _____
   D. Present physical condition: Good _____ Fair _____ Poor _____
   E. Please list any preschools and/or special programs your child has attended including therapy for speech, motor, etc.:
      _____

Physical Factors

A. At what age was he/she potty trained? _____
B. Does your child now have or has he/she ever had any of the following conditions?
   Difficulty: Talking? _____ Seeing? _____ Hearing? _____
   Falls or accidental injuries? _____
   Does your child have trouble running or walking? _____
   How well does your child use:
              Scissors?   Good _____ Fair _____ Poor _____
              Pencils?   Good _____ Fair _____ Poor _____
              Crayons?   Good _____ Fair _____ Poor _____
              Right handed?   _____
              Left handed?   _____

Figure 2-4.   Legal guardian's report of student's history form. *Adapted from and used with permission of Blue Valley School District, Johnson County, Kansas.*

C. Has your child had any of the following?
   Serious accidents? _____ Date? _____
   Operations? _____ Date? _____
   Unusual illnesses? _____ Date? _____
   Unusual diseases? _____ Date? _____
D. To what things is the child allergic? _____
E. Has the child had any special problems in visual function? (Prolonged wandering of the eyes in infancy, crossed eyes,
   eyes turned out, drooped lids, failure to follow light or motions, reverses numbers or letters, i.e., sees "b" for "d" or "p"
   for "g", sees a "6" as a "9") _____
   Has vision been tested? _____ Date or age tested? _____
   Results: _____
F. Has the child even had his ears examined by a physician? _____
   At what age? _____ Results: _____
   Has hearing been tested? _____ Was an audiometer used? _____
   At what age? _____
   Has your child even had earaches/otitis media? _____
   How often? _____ Have these been reoccuring? _____
G. Medical treatment being given out; for what conditions and by whom? _____

Family and Home Situation
A. What types of discipline do you use most often in guiding your child? Give examples:_____
B. Are there any adults besides the parents who play an active part in guiding your child? If so, whom? _____
C. Is he/she afraid of certain things, persons, animals, or situations? _____
   Explain: _____
D. Has he ever had temper tantrums? _____ At what age? _____
   Explain: _____
E. What particular talents does your child have? _____
F. Are your child's sleeping habits regular? _____
G. Are your child's eating habits regular? _____
   Does your child have strong likes or dislikes toward food textures?
   Likes? _____ Dislikes? _____
H. How does your child respond to other siblings? _____
I. How do other siblings respond to this child? _____
J. Did he seem to understand what was said to him before he learned to talk? _____
K. Were the child's wants anticipated before he attempted to speak? _____
L. Did your child use much gesture or sign language? _____
M. Did anyone "baby talk" to your child? _____
N. Is your child easily distracted or does he/she have trouble functioning if there is a lot of noise around?

Figure 2-4. *Continued.*

screening to review findings and make recommendations, if appropriate. Many agencies formulate handouts which describe age-appropriate activities on the various areas of development, and give these to families as needed to address areas of concern; this procedure also streamlines the process for the families. Figure 2-9 contains examples of handouts that might be used. If recommendations include the need for comprehensive evaluation in one or more areas of development, one of the professionals meets with the parents to discuss this recommendation and obtain consent for further testing. Figure 2-10 contains a face sheet for a comprehensive evaluation permission form; these forms must also contain information about the parents' rights. This is mandated by state and federal legislation (e.g. Public Law 94.142).

Type II Screening

Type II screening occurs after the initial referral to a special service is developed. The purpose of Type II screening is to determine whether further assessments are indicated and if so, which diagnostic procedures would be appropriate for the particular child. This type of screening facilitates an efficient diagnostic process by enabling the therapist to choose only those procedures that are necessary to clarify the problem.

In order to conduct a Type II screening to determine whether a comprehensive occupational therapy assessment is indicated, the occupational therapist may review the child's medical, developmental, and familial history, observe the child, and/or discuss developmental concerns with caregivers and

COUNT YOUR KID IN
PREPARATION PROCEDURES CHECKLIST

<u>Initial Preparation of Team</u>

Meeting of the specialists to determine the date of C.Y.K.I.

A press release (Figure 2-2) is then distributed to:
—Elementary buildings for their newsletters
—Newspapers in the area
—Private preschools
—Grocery Stores
—Multipurpose Center

Developmental Council

Meeting of the principal and the preschool specialists to determine:
—rooms to be used
—date for staffings for those who qualify for the Special Needs Preschool Program after the C.Y.K.I. evaluation is completed.

<u>Individual Preparation</u>

Preschool Specialist

1. Review call-in procedures with secretary and give them the "office folder" with the basic information form, cover letter for appointment time, press release, social history form and time schedule.
   —Parents call in and C.Y.K.I. basic information form is filled out over the telephone.
   —A time is then assigned.
   —The secretary then sends the cover letter for appointment time and the social history form to be filled out and returned when they arrive.
2. Meet with other specialists assigned to evaluation during C.Y.K.I. to review procedures and give them a specialist's folder with:
   —date of evaluation
   —individual duties
   —place assigned for testing
   —list of children and times of each evaluation
   —copy of the press release form
3. Prepare each child's folder with information on Basic Information Form stapled inside the folder on the left side. Inside the folder are Consent for Evaluation form, Parent's Rights form, two Results forms (with carbon) and a Cover Letter for Results form.
4. Be sure enough extra Cover Letter for Results forms, Results forms, Social History forms, and Special Needs Preschool Information forms are available.
5. Have name tags for evaluators and children typed.
6. Have small prizes available for the children as they leave.
7. Be sure signs are made and put up directing parents to waiting area as they arrive.
8. Get camera and film.

Nurse (Vision)

1. Get eye chart and response forms and any other equipment ready.
2. Set up room for testing—measure for eye examination, etc.
3. Get handouts, if applicable.
4. Be sure table, chairs, etc., are set up inside and outside the room.

Audiologist (Hearing)

1. Get audiometer set up along with other equipment.
2. Get response forms.
3. Set up room for testing.
4. Get handouts, if applicable.
5. Be sure table, chairs, etc., are set up inside and outside the room.

Figure 2-5. Count Your Kid In (C.Y.K.I.). Preparation Procedures. *Used with permission of the Blue Valley School District, Johnson County, Kansas.*

Speech Pathologist

1. Get tests, other materials, and test forms.
2. Get speech/language evaluation forms.
3. Get handouts, if applicable.
4. Be sure table, chairs, etc., are set up inside and outside the room.

Psychologist, Guidance Counselor, or Designated Person

1. Get extra forms, name tags, and pens from Preschool Specialist.
2. Have handouts on behavior, discipline, thumb sucking, toilet training, etc., if applicable.

Occupational Therapist

1. Select screening tools and gather screening materials needed to perform the test.
2. Get screening tools ordered or copied and ready for screening.
3. Get handouts ready for a variety of problem areas a child might have (e.g., fine motor difficulty, gross motor, self-help, visual perceptual, etc.).
4. On the day of the screening, set up testing room for screening—table, chairs, testing instrument and materials.

Community Volunteers

1. Get waiting area for family and children set up (i.e., chairs—both for adults and children, table—so that children who are waiting can color, refreshment table, etc.).
2. Escort parent and child to each screening section.
3. Take folder with each screening result to each screening station.
4. Escort children to restroom, if needed.
5. Record screening information on forms, if asked by professional performing screening.
6. Set up games, toys, and fine motor activities in waiting room to help the time pass for children who are waiting for screening.

Figure 2-5. *Continued.*

COUNT YOUR KID IN DAY

Parents and children arrive and follow signs to waiting area.

Give out name tags and take picture of each child.

Psychologist, Guidance Counselor, or designated person checks for social history form, has consent signed, and gives out Parent's Rights form. Then that person is available to parents for questions or concerns about the child's social and cognitive development, kindergarten expectations, behavior discipline, thumb sucking, toilet training, etc.

Speech Pathologist, Occupational Therapist, and Nurse take the first child assigned to each of them for the first session.

Each professional finishes evaluating and writes results on the appropriate form and signs his or her name. If there is an area of concern and services may be warranted, a star is placed in the left margin.

Each professional briefly reviews their own results with the parent after the evaluation.

The child and his folder are then taken to the next evaluator with handout information, if applicable.

The last specialist reviews with parents. If an area of concern is noted, the parents are told that a call will be made to them after the specialists meet and determine what services or further recommendations would most benefit the child. Cover letter for results is attached to one copy of the results form for the parents to take with them.

The child chooses a small prize to take home.

The team meets at the end of the day to determine which children warrant services—either the Preschool Program or individual speech and/or occupational therapy. A representative from the school speech therapists attends to make any followup recommendations on children only needing speech services.

Parents are called with recommendations for areas of concern. If the Preschool Program is recommended, a time is set up for them to visit the classroom and arrange a staffing time.

Figure 2-6.   Count Your Kid in Day Procedure. *Used with permission from Blue Valley School District, Johnson County, Kansas.*

Summary of District Screening Battery			
Developmental Area Screened	Name of Screening Tool(s)	Length of time to administer	Who can perform this screening
Vision	*Vision Screening	5 minutes	Nurse
Hearing (Pure Tone Screening) (Tympanometry)	Report of Hearing Test	10 minutes	Nurse
Speech and Language	Goldman Fristoe (Articulation Screening)	10 minutes	Speech Pathologist
	The Communication Screen (language & articulation)	10 minutes	
	Bankson Language Screening Test (language)	10 minutes	
	Peabody Picture Vocabulary Test (PPVT)	10–15 minutes	
	Preschool Language Scale	10–15 minutes	
Motor (Fine and Gross Self-help)	Denver Developmental Screening Test (0–6 years)	5–10 minutes	Occupational Therapist Physical Therapist Physical Education Trained Volunteer
	Miller Assessment for Preschoolers (ages 2.9 years to 5.8 years)	20–30 minutes	Administered by professional or non professional, interpreted by professionals who have attended MAP seminar.
	*St. Lukes Gross, Fine, Self-help Screening, Checklist (2–5 years)	20 minutes	Occupational Therapist Physical Therapist
	Developmental Profile II (requires parent report) 0–9 1/2 years	20–40 minutes (all sections given) Areas that are screened are physical, self-help, social, academic & communication. (*Can do only sections of this screening)	Professionals or paraprofessionals
	*Blue Valley School District Gross Motor Screening	5–10 minutes	Occupational Therapist Physical Therapist
Behavior	*Informal observation of child during screening, observation of parent/ child interaction		Psychologist School Counselor

*Illustrated in Figures 2-7a–c.

Figure 2-7.   District Screening Battery. *Used with permission of the Blue Valley School District, Johnson County, Kansas.*

other professionals. The occupational therapist may also administer standardized or non-standardized screening tools. Specific screening areas may include sensorimotor development, psychosocial development, neuromuscular reflex maturation, neurophysiological status, adaptive behavior, work, leisure, and self-care skills (AOTA, 1989b). Table 2-1 summarizes primary characteristics of screening tools frequently used by occupational therapy. Screening must not replace assessment, which is individualized and in more depth. It is not cost effective to conduct a full assessment of all performance components; Type II screening allows the therapist to determine only those areas which may need further attention and analysis. Either informal observation or selecting a screening instrument can be considered a Type II screening. Let us consider an example.

John is a seven year old boy who is in the second grade.

His teacher, Mrs. White, has observed that John has poor pencil grasp, messy papers, letter reversals, and is always slow at his table work. Mrs. White has completed an Intervention Checklist (Figure 2-11) and submitted it to the Preassessment Team along with her referral concerns. This team consists of other classroom teachers, the principal and selected special service personnel; the team's purpose is to support teachers as they attempt to adapt the classroom to meet student needs. If successful, comprehensive special education assessment is not necessary. She hopes that with some extra help John can become more successful in his seat work, since several of the strategies she has tried have not resolved the problem. Mrs. White feels that John is becoming self-conscious, and more introverted in his interaction with his peers, as a direct result of his comparison of his paper and pencil work with his peers' work.

VISION SCREENING

Functional Assessment   Date _____

		OK	?

1. **Pupillary Response**   (right)   **constrict** _____ | _____
   (shine penlight into eye from 12″)   **dilate**   _____ | _____
                                           (left)   **constrict** _____ | _____
                                                        dilate

2. **Corneal Light Reflex**   **similar position**
   (penlight to bridge of nose from 14−16″) **of reflection**
                                            in each eye

3. **Blink Reflex**   **blink**   _____ | _____
   (hand moves toward face)

4. **Alternate Cover Test**   **right eye**   _____ | _____
                                           left eye   _____ | _____

5. **Tracking (14−16″)**   **right/left**   _____ | _____
                                           above/below   _____ | _____

6. **Visual Acuity-Lighthouse**   **lighthouse score** _____ | _____
   (if appropriate)

7. **Near point convergence**   **near point**   _____ | _____
   Comments:

Additional Observations

    Eyes crossed—turning in or out—at any time, or eyes that do not appear straight, especially when child is tired.

2. **Has reddened eyes or eyelids.**
3. **Turns the head to use one eye only.   L   R   (eye used)**
4. **Tilts the head to one side: L   R**
5. **Places an object close to the eyes to look at it.**
6. **Squints while looking at objects.**
7. **Blinks excessively.**
8. **Covers or closes one eye: L   R**
9. **Rubs eyes: L   R**
10. **Sits close to the TV.**

Figure 2-7a.   Vision Screening Form. *Used with permission of the Blue Valley School District, Johnson County, Kansas.*

Mary Lake, the occupational therapist, is part of the Preassessment Team. This group meets each week to go over any Intervention Checklists or other materials that have been submitted. In this meeting it is decided that the occupational therapist is the most appropriate specialist to observe John and suggest strategies for a six week preassessment period. Mary observes John in the classroom utilizing a classroom observation recording sheet (Figure 2-12). Mary then has the option to proceed with designing preassessment strategies which will help John and Mrs. White in the classroom, or may decide to screen John's fine motor skills a bit further, utilizing any of several informal screening checklists or screening instruments, documenting results using a simple screening write up form, such as the one illustrated in Figure 2-13. She then meets with Mrs. White to make suggestions about how to improve John's fine motor skills in the classroom. Mary provides Mrs. White with a triangle grip for his pencil, because she noticed that John had difficulty maintaining a stable pincer grasp when writing. His unstable grasping pattern caused him to drop his pencil frequently, make extra marks on his paper, and create poorly formed letters and numbers. Mary and Mrs. White also discuss allowing John to use either wider lined paper or unlined paper for writing tasks, to decrease errors and erasures which occur when he cannot control the writing utensil to stay within very small lines. Mrs. White pre-

ferred to try unlined paper, since larger lined paper was likely to elicit comments from other classmates about John using "baby paper" from earlier grades. (Other classroom adaptations that can be used in the preassessment process are listed in Figure 2-14; they correspond to common occupational therapy referral complaints.) Mary and Mrs. White then met after the third week to review progress. The occupational therapist documented this visit. At the end of six weeks, Mary and Mrs. White reviewed the referral concerns to measure the outcome of preassessment strategies. Mrs. White was very pleased with John's performance using these adaptations and felt no further evaluation was necessary.

Mary then reports the outcome of the preassessment strategies to the Team. If John's seat work had still been noticeably different compared to his peers', the team would then recommend that John would benefit from a comprehensive assessment. It is likely that the occupational therapist would conduct the fine motor skills component of this comprehensive assessment. John's parents are contacted to obtain consent to perform a comprehensive assessment. This permission to evaluate must be signed before the comprehensive testing occurs.

The process of providing support for children and teachers in regular classrooms is a proactive strategy. It facilitates success in the least restrictive environment, which is in chil-

Developmental Skills Screening

Name: _____   Examiner: _____

Birthdate: _____   Date: _____

B = requires assistance of examiner   A = accomplishes activity within normal time

Age	Gross Motor			
3 years	1. Gets up from floor with partial trunk rotation			
	2. No longer walks with arms outstretched and shows uniformity of heel-toe gait			
	3. Balances on one foot for 1 second			
	4. Crawls through objects			
	5. Walks backwards			
	6. Catches large ball with arms fully extended			
	7. Throws small ball with torso participation			
	8. Alternates feet going upstairs holding rail			
	9. Jumps from bottom step with feet together			
	Fine Motor			
	1. Inserts circle, square and triangle into formboard with rotations			
	2. Picks up cube without touching table			
	3. Builds 9-block tower			
	4. Imitates train of 3 or more blocks			
	5. Screws lid on jar			
	6. Demonstrates preferred hand using 3 fingers and thumb to grasp crayon			
	7. Copies circle			
	8. Copies horizontal line			
	9. Imitates cross			
	10. Uses scissors to snip at paper			
	Visual and/or Tactile			
	1. Hesitates at top of stairs when descending (depth perception)			
	2. Recognizes halves and fits together			
	3. Identifies familiar objects by touching and handling			
	Self-Help Skills			
	1. Undresses but needs help with fastenings			
	2. Puts on shoes and socks; may be incorrect			
	3. Unlaces shoes			
	4. Washes hands in appropriate sequence			
	5. Drinks from glass with one hand			
	6. Drinks through straw			
	7. No turning of spoon with minimum spilling			
	8. Pours from small container into glass with assistance			
	9. Uses fork to pierce food			
	10. Has BM and urinates in potty when reminders and assistance in wiping -- boys may stand			

Figure 2-7b.   Type I screening program tool. *Used with permission of St. Luke's Hospital of Kansas City.*

Developmental Skills Screening

Name: _____   Examiner: _____

Birthdate: _____   Date: _____

B = requires assistance of examiner   A = accomplishes activity within normal time

Age	Gross Motor			
4 years	1. Walks with long swinging steps			
	2. Gets up from floor with no trunk rotation			
	3. Hops on toes with both feet			
	4. Balances on one foot for 2-5 seconds			
	5. Can touch end of nose with finger			
	6. Gallops			
	7. Walks on 3½" walking board stepping off 3 times			
	8. Catches large ball with hands moving in accordance with ball			
	9. Throws ball with elbow movement and no torso involvement			
	10. Holds rail to walk downstairs alternating feet			
	11. No evidence of ATNR			
	Fine Motor			
	1. Adult grasp of pencil			
	2. Copies cross			
	3. Imitates square			
	4. Traces diamond			
	5. Cuts straight line			
	6. Draws man with 3 parts			
	7. Copies train of blocks			
	8. Copies bridge			
	9. Imitates gate			
	Visual and/or Tactile			
	1. Can identify closer of 2 objects			
	2. Matches identically shaped objects by size			
	3. Tactilly matches objects by size with vision occluded			
	Self-Help Skills			
	1. Undresses and unbuttons buttons			
	2. Puts coat on			
	3. Laces shoes			
	4. Identifies front and back			
	5. Uses fork appropriately			
	6. Pours from container without spilling			
	7. Blows nose			
	8. Goes to toilet on own — may need reminder to wipe			
	9. May call for mother at night for toileting			

Figure 2-7b. *Continued.*

Developmental Skills Screening

Name: _____   Examiner: _____

Birthdate: _____   Date: _____

B = Requires assistance of examiner   A = accomplishes activity within normal time

	Age		Gross Motor			
	5 years	1.	Arms held near body with narrow stance in gait			
		2.	Stands up without using hands for support			
		3.	Can change from sitting, standing and squatting in serial manner			
		4.	Makes 90 degrees pivot in standing			
		5.	Distinguishes between own right and left			
		6.	Walks full length of 3½" walking board			
		7.	Sits up straight in chair			
		8.	Skips on alternating feet			
		9.	Bounces ball			
		10.	May catch and kick ball simultaneously			
		11.	Walks up and down stairs on alternating feet without rail			
			Fine Motor			
		1.	Copies square			
		2.	Copies triangle			
		3.	Draws man with 6 parts			
		4.	Reach and placement of blocks show good accuracy			
		5.	Copies gate of blocks			
		6.	Cuts gate			
		7.	Cuts curved line			
		8.	Alternates supination and pronation irradically			
		9.	Serial opposition with overflow and poor rhythm			
			Visual and/or Tactile			
		1.	Differentiates square from rectangle			
		2.	Localizes tactile stimuli to specific body part (arm, leg, etc.)			
		3.	Mean of nystagmus to left – 8.9 seconds to right – 8.7 seconds			
			Self-Help Skills			
		1.	Fastens buttons that are within sight			
		2.	Washes and dries hands			
		3.	May dress without prodding, but needs help with back fasteners			
		4.	Brushes hair			
		5.	Brushes teeth			
		6.	SLow but independent feeding			
		7.	Uses knife to spread			
		8.	Needs reminders to wipe			
		9.	No longer needs night toileting			

Figure 2-7b. *Continued.*

```
                        Developmental Skills Screening

    Name: _____     Examiner: _____

    Birthdate: _____     Date: _____

    B = requires assistance of examiner    A = accomplishes activity within normal time
```

Age	Gross Motor			
6 years	1. Bows with feet together, legs and knees straight			
	2. Balances on one foot with eyes open			
	3. Walks on 1½" walking board with 2-3 falls			
	4. Jumps over one foot obstacles			
	5. Reaches for objects beyond arm's length with ease			
	6. Kicks ball from running start			
	7. Catches small ball and throws using optimal use of upper extremity			
	8. Jumps from bottom step on toes			
	9. Balances well on toes			
	10. TLR prone and supine held for 20-30 seconds			
	11. Body righting diminished			
	12. Heel-toe walks forwards			
	Fine Motor			
	1. Shows good thumb and index finger flexion in writing.			
	2. Draws square with sharp corners			
	3. Copies diamond			
	Visual and/or Tactile			
	1. Nystagmus mean to left – 10.5 seconds to right – 9.2 seconds			
	Self-Help Skills			
	1. Dresses self; may need minimal assistance			
	2. Ties shoe laces loosely			
	3. Bathes self except for head and neck			
	4. Uses fork to cut food to bite size			
	5. Toilets self completely			

Figure 2-7b. *Continued.*

dren's best interest. Occupational therapists have many skills to make preassessment more effective and must contribute these skills to decrease unnecessary referrals for comprehensive assessment.

SUMMARY

Early identification of deviations from the normal developmental process is an important purpose for the screening process. It is important that the occupational therapist involved in the process be very knowledgeable of the normal sequence of growth and development, enabling the occupational therapist to make appropriate decisions on whether a developmental problem does or does not exist for a child. The brief observation which occurs during screening enables the therapist to filter out areas that are of no concern, and to focus on those areas that may be a concern. Areas of concern can then be evaluated specifically utilizing a more in-depth diagnostic assessment process, which is described in detail in Chapter 3.

EXPAND YOUR NEWLY ACQUIRED KNOWLEDGE

1. Consider a district-wide Type 1 screening program. List three unique roles of the occupational therapist in a screening program such as this one; list three unique roles of other professionals in this endeavor.

2. Sandra is a three year, two month old who just completed Type 1 district screening activities. She performed within age expectations in language, cognition, fine motor and socialization, but was nine months delayed in gross motor and self care areas. Describe three activities that the parents could incorporate into home

---

PUPIL OBSERVATION AND PARENT INTERVIEW

Pupil's Name: _____

Age: _____

Date: _____

Interviewer: _____
  (Psychologist or school counselor)

Brief I counselor)

Brief summary of developmental and medical history:

Discussion with parent pertaining to their concern for bringing their child to Count Your Kid In:

Interviewer's observation of child during screening: (The interviewer at this time looked at how the child interacted with the examiner either in speech or motor screening. The interviewer looked at the child's attending skills, compliance, ability to follow directions, or any other appropriate or inappropriate behaviors observed during the screening.)

Interviewer's observation of the child's interaction with parent:

Summary of Interviewer's Observation of Parent-child Interaction and Child Interaction During the Screening:

Recommendations by Interviewer:

Review of Psychological Testing: (This section will be completed by the psychologist either by review of reports the parents have brought to screening or by interviewing the parent concerning any intellectual functioning questions the parent might have about the child during the screening.)

Figure 2-7c. Pupil observation and parent interview form. *Used with permission of the Blue Valley School District, Johnson County, Kansas.*

routines which would stimulate development in her areas of concern.

3. Jim is an eight year old who has been referred to the educational team because of his poor written work. The team agreed that occupational therapy services might be needed, and so ask you to become involved in Jim's case. Summarize three things that you could do as Type 2 screening PRIOR to conducting a comprehensive evaluation to determine whether further assessment would be necessary.

COUNT YOUR KID IN RESULTS FOR: _____
                                        (Child's Name)

                                  Date: _____

SPEECH/LANGUAGE _____ Speech/Language Pathologist
   Articulation:
   Language: receptive:
               expressive:

MOTOR _____ Occupational Therapist
   Gross motor:
   Fine motor
   Self help:

BEHAVIORAL _____ Psychologist
   Parent observations:
   Interactions:
   Interview data:

VISION _____ Nurse
   Functional assessment:
   Additional observations:

HEARING _____ Audiologist
   Audiometric:
   Tympanometric:

RECOMMENDATIONS:
   1.
   2.
   3.
   4.

REFERRAL DATES:

  *Denotes area(s) of concern. Person screening a child will use (*) to denote a concern or delay in developmental area being screened.

Figure 2-8. **"Count Your Kid In" results form.** *Used with permission of the Blue Valley School District, Johnson County, Kansas.*

Fine motor activities involve the use of the small muscles of the hands. Many school tasks such as writing, drawing, and cutting require good fine motor skills, so it is helpful if these skills can be stressed at home.

1. Paper provides a medium that has a lot of fine motor possibilities. Tearing, cutting, folding, coloring, and pasting are all good activities. Making paper chains requires cutting, folding, and pasting; making paper airplanes can include folding and coloring.
2. Clay or play play dough is fun to play with and requires strength and coordination. Have your child make shapes or structures; roll it out and cut shapes with cookie cutters.
3. Clothing fasteners such as buttons, shoe strings, snaps and zippers require hand control. Help your child practice fastening.
4. The use of simple tools may be motivating for some children, while developing fine motor control. Screw drivers, saws, manual egg beaters, or rolling pins can be used in play or to "help" mom and dad during activities.
5. Finger games like Teensie Weensie Spider, The Wheels on the Bus, Little Bunny Fu-fu, or any game that requires finger movements can be incorporated into travel time in the car.
6. Let your child sort small objects for you. Nails, screws, and bolts can be sorted at the tool bench; paper clips, safety pins, and rubber bands can be sorted from the desk.
7. Sewing cards require coordination of both hands and rely on the child being able to watch the hands as they move. Tube macaroni, cranberries, or popcorn can be strung as an alternative to purchasing sewing cards.
8. A number of commercially available toys require fine motor coordination; these make good gifts (e.g., Lite Brite, pot holder loom, pop beads, chalkboard, craft kits, simple model kits, blocks, puzzles).
9. Coloring books, dot-to-dot books, cut and paste books, and sticker books are useful; parents may need to guide these activities to ensure success.
10. Blow soap bubbles and pop them with different fingers or hand patterns.
11. Blow up a balloon or wad up a piece of paper and play games with it as if it were a ball; hit it into the air with a paddle, racquet, paper plate, or hands. These activities encourage development of eye and hand coordination.
12. Playing with marbles or jacks facilitates controlled hand movements.
13. Purchase a piece of Masonite with the holes in it and get some golf tees. Have your child put one golf tee into each hole to make patterns.
14. Purchase spring-type clothes pins. Let your child use them to clip things together or to secure notes around the house.

Figure 2-9a.   Activities which can aid in the development of fine motor skills.

Gross motor skills involve the coordinated and efficient use of the body in movement. Balance, control and patterns of movement are all part of gross motor development.

Controlled movements such as walking, jumping, hopping, and skipping are all good gross motor activities. Vary the activities so that your child remains challenged to master harder skills. For example, have your child:

- Jump over various sizes of objects, such as a book or a box.
- Jump off a step or box.
- Jump/hop with feet together around a box, table, the yard.
- Hop on one foot and then the other; change the speed; demonstrate a pattern and have your child repeat it.
- Hop into and out of objects such as hoops or a box.
- Walk on a 2" x 4" board, 8–10 feet long, positioned on the floor. Vary the method, such as walking sideways, backwards, or heel to toe.
- Gallop or skip around objects.
- Play hopscotch. Begin with simple hopscotch patterns; vary the pattern of boxes on the cement.

Construction toys with large pieces encourage the use of both hands, motor planning and imagination. Encourage your child to make anything; be creative; later guide him to make what is on the picture directions, by showing him the piece, then helping him find it, if necessary, and putting it together.

Ball or bean bag activities require gross motor coordination:

- Throw and catch a large ball. Adjust the distance, speed, and type of ball.
- Throw a ball or bean bag into a box or wastebasket.
- Bounce/dribble large ball with one hand and then the other hand; create patterns the child can copy.
- Kick balls of various sizes and weights; sometimes use stationary positions, other times roll or throw the ball.
- Set targets up, have your child throw bean bags toward the parts of the target.

Figure 2-9b.   Activities which can aid in the development of gross motor skills.

LAWFUL CUSTODIAN'S CONSENT FOR COMPREHENSIVE EVALUATION FORM

Date _____

Lawful Custodian Of: _____

| | Child's Name | School | Grade |

A referral for evaluation has been received from: _____

regarding: _____

_____

This referral is based on the following information: _____

_____

_____

EVALUATION PROCEDURE

Your consent is required in order for this comprehensive evaluation to be provided. The proposed evaluation may include the following:

Tests/Methods to be used:	Area Evaluated	Time Required	Approx. Date	Staff Name	Position
_____	_____	_____	_____	_____	_____
_____	_____	_____	_____	_____	_____
_____	_____	_____	_____	_____	_____
_____	_____	_____	_____	_____	_____
_____	_____	_____	_____	_____	_____
_____	_____	_____	_____	_____	_____
_____	_____	_____	_____	_____	_____

CONSENT FOR EVALUATION

You have the opportunity to request a personal conference concerning the reason for referral and an explanation of this proposed evaluation.

(1) I understand my rights to due process as described herein

(2) I understand the proposed evaluation procedure; and

PLEASE CHECK ONE

☐ I agree with the proposed evaluation and give my consent.

☐ I object to the proposed evaluation and request a conference to present my objections.

_____
Signature

_____
Date

Figure 2-10. Consent for evaluation. *Used with permission of the Blue Valley School District.*

STUDENT: _____   TEACHER: _____
SCHOOL: _____   CLASS/SUBJECT: _____
D.O.B.: _____   DATE COMPLETED: _____

INTERVENTION CHECKLIST
Classroom Teacher

What strategies have you tried to correct the problem? Please indicate those strategies you have applied to the problem and give an estimate of how long the strategy has been in effect in terms of days or weeks. Also comment on the success of these strategies in terms of "Yes" or "No":

Environmental Strategies	Specify:	Duration (Days/Weeks)	Success (Y-N)
1. Seating Change		_____	_____
2. Isolation (How often?)		_____	_____
3. Change to a different hour/same teacher		_____	_____
4. Change to a different teacher		_____	_____
5. Other		_____	_____

Organization Strategies

	Duration	Success
1. Setting time limits for assignments/completion during class	_____	_____
2. Questioning at end of each sentence/paragraph to help focus on important information	_____	_____
3. Allowing additional time to complete task/take test	_____	_____
4. Highlighting main facts in the book	_____	_____
5. Organizing a notebook or providing folder to help organize work	_____	_____
6. Asking student to repeat directions given	_____	_____
7. Other	_____	_____

Motivational Strategies

	Duration	Success
1. Checking papers by showing "C's" for correct	_____	_____
2. Sending home daily progress report	_____	_____
3. Immediate reinforcement of correct response	_____	_____
4. Keeping graphs and charts of student's progress	_____	_____
5. Conferencing with student's parents	_____	_____
6. Conferencing with student's other teachers	_____	_____
7. Student reading lesson to aide, peer tutor or teacher	_____	_____
8. Home/school communication system for assignments	_____	_____
9. Using tapes of materials the rest of class is reading	_____	_____
10. Student using tapes of materials at home or school	_____	_____
11. Classmate to take notes with carbon	_____	_____
12. Other	_____	_____

Presentation Strategies

	Duration	Success
1. Giving assignments both orally and visually	_____	_____
2. Taping lessons so student can listen again	_____	_____
3. Allowing student to have sample or practice test	_____	_____
4. Providing legible material	_____	_____
5. Immediate correction of errors	_____	_____
6. Providing advance organizers	_____	_____
7. Providing tests in smaller blocks of questions/wider spaced	_____	_____
8. Providing tests in small segments/student hands in at end of each segment and gets next	_____	_____
9. Providing modified tests, fewer questions, simpler material	_____	_____
10. Giving tests orally	_____	_____
11. Other	_____	_____

Figure 2-11.   Intervention checklist for the classroom teacher.

Curriculum Strategies

1. Providing opportunities for extra drill   _____   _____
2. Providing study guide (outline, etc., to follow)   _____   _____
3. Reducing quantity of material   _____   _____
4. Providing instructional materials geared to lower level of basic skills   _____   _____
5. Vocabulary flash cards   _____   _____
6. Vocabulary words in context   _____   _____
7. Special materials   _____   _____
8. Other   _____   _____

Are there any other strategies you have used that are not listed above? If "yes", please describe: (Duration and success):

_____
_____
_____
_____
_____
_____
_____

Figure 2-11. *Continued.*

STUDENT'S NAME _____   SCHOOL _____
DATE _____   TEACHER _____
ACTIVITY _____   GRADE _____

1. Height of chair and desk:
2. Placement of chair:
3. Organization of materials on desk:
4. Placement in room:
5. Writing tool:
6. Attention to task:
7. Grasp:
8. Manuscript:
    1. Handedness:
    2. Type of paper:
    3. Placement of paper on desk:
    4. Quality:
        1. letter formation:
        2. spacing:
        3. placement on lines:
        4. letter size consistency:
        5. letter or number reversals:
        6. print name correctly and legibly:
        7. ability to adapt letter size to space on paper:

Recommendations and Suggestions:

Figure 2-12. Classroom observation form.

NAME: _____   TEST DATE: _____

DATE OF BIRTH: _____   EXAMINER: _____

CHRONOLOGICAL AGE: _____

Behaviors Noted During Screening:

Gross Motor:
Screening Strategies Used:
Functional Level:
Comments:

Fine Motor:
Screening Strategies Used:
Functional Level:
Comments:

Self Care:
Screening Strategies Used:
Functional Level:
Comments:

Summary:

Recommendations:

Figure 2-13. Motor screening report form.

Classroom Adaptations to be Considered for Common Related Service Referral Complaints Prior to Comprehensive Assessment	
Referral Complaint*	Possible Adaptations**
Poor lunch skills/behaviors	Provide a wheeled cart to carry lunch tray Provide large handled utensils Clamp lunch tray to table to avoid slipping Serve milk in sealed cup with straw
Poor toiletting skills	Provide a smaller toilet Provide looser clothing Provide a step stool for toilet/sink
Can't stay in seat; fidgety	Allow student to lie on floor to work Allow student to stand to work Provide lateral support to hips or trunk (e.g., rolled towels) Adapt seat to correct height for work Be sure feet are flat on floor when seated Provide more variety in seatwork
Clumsy in classroom/halls; gets lost in building	Move classroom furniture to edges of room Send student to new locations when halls are less crowded Provide visual cues in hall to mark locations Match student with partner for transitions
Can't get on or off bus independently	Allow student to back down stairs Provide additional smaller steps
Can't get jacket/coat on/off	Place in front of student, in same orientation each time Provide larger size for easier handling
Drops materials; can't manipulate books, etc.	Place tabs on book pages for turning Provide small containers for items Place all items for one task on a lunch tray
Poor attention, hyperactive, distractible	Decrease availability of distracting stimuli (e.g., visual or auditory) Provide touch cues only when student is prepared for it Touch student with firm pressure Provide frequent breaks in seatwork

Figure 2-14. Classroom adaptations that can be used in the preassessment process.

Poor pencil/crayon use	Use triangle grip on pencil/crayon Use fatter writing utensil Provide larger sheets of paper Provide paper without lines Provide paper with wider-spaced lines
Poor cutting skills	Provide adapted scissors Provide stabilized paper: e.g., tape it down, use large clips, C-clamps
Unable to complete seatwork successfully	Provide larger spaces for answers Give smaller amounts of work Put less items per page Give more time to complete task Change level of difficulty
Loses personal belongings; unorganized	Make a map showing where items belong Collect all belongings and hand them out at the beginning of each activity
Doesn't follow directions	Provide written or picture directions for reference Provide cassette tape of directions Allow student to watch a partner for cues

* More serious problems usually require immediate involvement of the occupational and/or physical therapist.
** If these strategies are unsuccessful, involvement of the occupational or physical therapist is appropriate.
Dunn, W. (1989). Integrated related services for preschoolers with neurological impairments: Issues and strategies. *Remedial and Special Education*, *10*(3), 31–39. Reprinted with permission.

Figure 2-14. *Continued.*

References

American Occupational Therapy Association (1987). *Guidelines for occupational therapy services in school systems.* Rockville, MD: author.

American Occupational Therapy Association (1989a). *Guidelines for occupational therapy services in school systems* (2nd Ed.). Rockville, MD: author.

American Occupational Therapy Association (1989b). Uniform terminology for occupational therapy—Second Edition. *American Journal of Occupational Therapy*, *43*(12): 808–815.

Bloom, B. (1964). *Stability and change in human characteristics.* New York: John Wiley.

Bricker, W. A., & Bricker, D. D. (1976). The infant, toddler, and preschool research and intervention project. In T. D. Tjossem (Ed.), *Intervention strategies for high risk infants and young children.* Baltimore: University Park Press.

Chamberlen, R. W. (1987). Developmental assessment and early intervention programs for young children: Lesson learned from longitudinal research. *Pediatrics in Review*, *8*(8), 237–247.

Cross, L. (1977). An introduction. In L. Cross & K. Goin (Ed.), *Iden-tifying handicapped children: A guide to casefinding, screening, diagnosis, assessment, and evaluation* (6th ed.). New York: Walker & Co.

Dunn, W. (1989). Validity. *Physical and Occupational Therapy in Pediatrics*, *9*(1), 140–168

Frankenburg, W. K. (1975). Criteria in screening test selection. In W. K. Frankenburg and B. W. Camp (Eds.), *Pediatric screening tests.* Springfield, IL: Thomas.

Lessler, K. (1972). Health and education screening of school-age children-definition-and objectives. *American Journal of Public Health*, *62*, 191–198.

Lillie, David L. (1977). Screening. In L. Cross & K. W. Goin (Eds.), *Identifying handicapped children: A guide to case finding, screening, diagnosis, assessment and evaluation.* New York: Walker and Company.

Stangler, S. R., Huber, C. J., & Routh, D. K. (1980). *Screening growth and development of preschool children: A guide for test selection.* NY, McGraw-Hill.

Weiner, R., & Koppelman, J. (1987). *From birth to 5: Serving the youngest handicapped children.* Alexandria, VA: Capitol Publications, Inc.

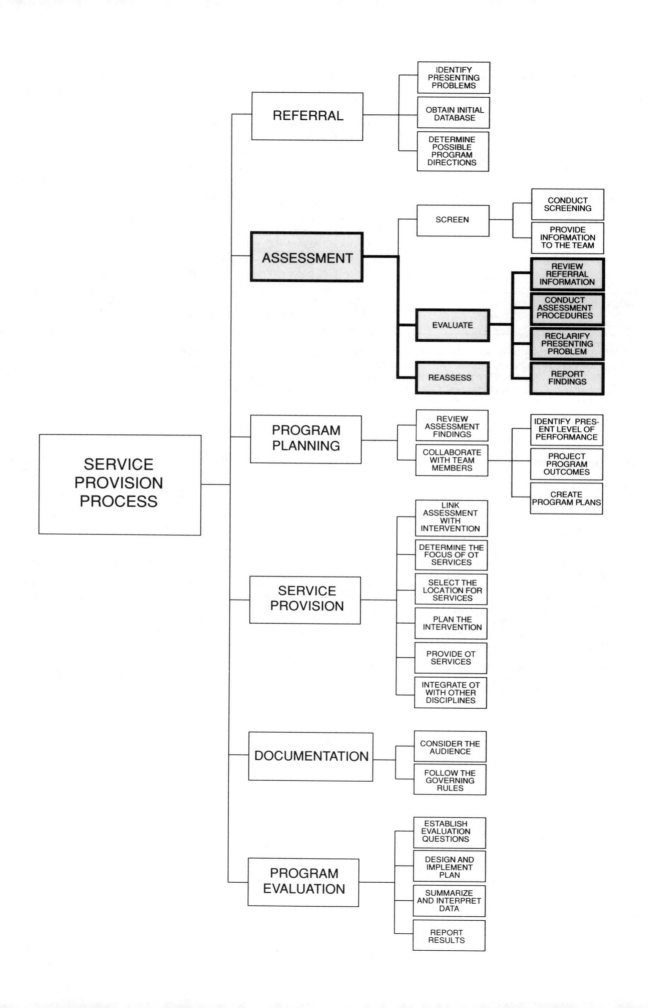

CHAPTER 3

The Assessment Process

Debra Galvin Cook, MS, OTR

"Assessing the intelligence and special abilities of children is a complex, demanding, and yet rewarding activity. It requires a variety of skills and talents. But these skills, however well established and integrated, pale before the one quality that perhaps is the most important and that provides the foundation for all of the others, namely, a liking of children." Sattler, 1982

Occupational therapists bring a wide and diverse background to the assessment process. We are uniquely trained to look at the continuum of development, and how that process fits into a particular environmental setting. Through didactic and clinical training in the social sciences, neurosciences, biomechanics, and study of occupational behavior, occupational therapists are well suited to assess the many variables that affect a child's performance and interaction with the environment.

Before engaging in the process of assessment, some basic ethical considerations must be addressed. In undertaking responsibility for the process and outcome of an evaluation, it is innately implied that the therapist is qualified and trained to address those areas being evaluated. Tests are powerful tools and must be thoroughly understood before they are used as assessment instruments (Sattler, 1982). Certain evaluations require specific training, while others require broad based knowledge of human development. Assessment is only useful as it assists professionals in planning for intervention to either resolve the problems identified, or create alternate strategies which minimize the effects of the problem. Standards of practice have been established by the American Occupational Therapy Association which outline the appropriate use of standardized tests and other evaluation techniques (Maurer, Barris, Bonder & Gillette, 1984).

Another ethical consideration is the impact that this newly gathered information will have on the client and family. Diagnosis and placement decisions will be shaped; family emotions, attitudes and expectations will emerge and will affect interactions and self perception (King-Thomas & Hacker, 1987). Confidentiality of the information is always maintained, along with an unquestionable respect for the human rights of clients and their families.

BASIC CONSIDERATIONS

For purposes of discussion, assessment is differentiated from evaluation. Assessment is the comprehensive process of obtaining information about an individual and family. Specific evaluation methods and ongoing evaluation during intervention are all considered part of comprehensive assessment. An assessment is comprised of measurable, data-based information gathered from several sources, and reported in an objective manner, so that it is an accurate description of the behavior exhibited. The intent is to assess concerns or weaknesses while also identifying strengths. Oftentimes identification of concerns and strengths can contribute to a diagnostic label. Figure 3-1 illustrates descriptors that do and do not comprise the end product of an assessment.

A screening helps determine whether any areas will need further attention, while an evaluation is a more thorough investigation of a client. An evaluation creates more specific information in many different areas. In the *Reference Manual of the Official Documents of the Occupational Therapy Association* (AOTA, 1986), evaluation is defined as:

"the process of obtaining and interpreting data necessary for treatment. This includes planning for and documenting the evaluation process and results. These data may be gathered through record review, specific observation, interview, and the administration of data collection procedures. Such procedures include, but are not limited to, the use of standardized tests, performance checklists, and activities and tasks designed to evaluate specific performance abilities (p. V-3)."

Therapists, clients, and families all participate in the assessment process; the end product may be a medical or educational diagnosis, a referral to another service, or the initiation of an intervention plan.

Figure 3-2 contains some specific examples of possible data gathering sources; they help define the parameters of an assessment. The more obvious choices of standardized or norm-referenced tests are clearly recognized as evaluation tools. Performance checklists, skilled observations, interviews and structured activities or tasks that are designed to evaluate specific performance abilities, are not clearly recognizable as objective data collection tools, but can be critical sources of data collection that will yield necessary assessment information. Therapists must maintain objectivity in using these non-standardized means of gathering data, so that accurate information can be applied to future planning.

The goal of compiling comprehensive information about a child's strengths and needs is best met through a team approach. A child's complex nature can be more successfully understood, and thus their needs more adequately addressed, when a group of professionals brings together their areas of expertise to identify an accurate diagnosis, and design an effective intervention strategy. While not a new concept, this team approach can bring together the diverse skills

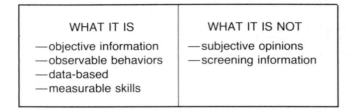

WHAT IT IS	WHAT IT IS NOT
—objective information	—subjective opinions
—observable behaviors	—screening information
—data-based	
—measurable skills	

Figure 3-1.   Descriptors of the assessment process.

and expertise of many professionals to provide more effective, better coordinated, and higher quality services for children (Golin and Ducanis, 1981).

The members of an assessment team can include such professionals as: a special educator, psychologist, speech pathologist, classroom teacher, physician, audiologist, occupational therapist, and/or a physical therapist. The setting most often influences the makeup of the assessment team. In a medical model, representatives are more inclined to represent medical orientations; while in an educational setting, team members are those focused on learning processes and products of those processes. Guidelines for assessment in a school setting are detailed in AOTA's *Guidelines for occupational therapy services in school systems* (1987, 1989).

The team approach and the concept of serving the "whole" child has been vigorously supported by legislative mandates such as Public Law 94-142 (Golin and Ducanis, 1981), and more recently, Public Law 99-457. These laws outline team membership and function, and the requirements for the development and monitoring of individualized plans.

There are several issues that occupational therapists face when functioning as members of an assessment team. Initially, the role of the occupational therapist, and the services that occupational therapy can provide for children, their families, and other professionals, need to be defined. This can be an ongoing educational process, because as team goals change, occupational therapists must redefine their role within the team. Occupational therapists address functional performance, and therefore evaluate those performance components which interfere with functional outcomes. How this occurs will be different in various settings, but the goal of addressing functional performance remains the same for all occupational therapists.

EXAMINER CHARACTERISTICS

Perhaps the most influential factor in the success of an evaluation are the personal characteristics of the examiner.

—standardized tests
—criterion referenced tests
—performance checklists
—skilled observations
—interviews
—structured activities/tasks

Figure 3-2.   Potential data gathering sources for an evaluation.

It is not enough to complete a formal or informal assessment according to the directions. It is essential that examiners identify their personal characteristics and then determine how these characteristics need to be shaped to produce a successful evaluation outcome. A key factor is the examiner's ability to establish rapport with the child and family members. The relationship the therapist develops with the family is of the utmost importance to the overall success of the evaluation. Sattler (1988) notes that certain examiner characteristics lead to good rapport, including empathy, genuineness, warmth, respect for children, and a sense of humor. Phares (1984) suggests that there are many ways to achieve good rapport with children, perhaps as many as there are clinicians. However, there is not a particular bag of tricks that substitutes for an attitude of acceptance, understanding, and respect for the integrity of the child and family. Regardless of the child's age and the setting in which the evaluation takes place, the child has an idea that something different is happening. Their "normal" environment is altered just by virtue of the examiner's presence. Often children will react negatively to being tested. I am reminded of a family who recalled the developmental evaluation session of their toddler. The parents reported that three therapists from various disciplines entered the evaluation room in white laboratory coats, with clip-boards, pencils and their kits. The child became apprehensive and withdrew, increasing the parents anxiety, and reducing the opportunity to establish rapport with the child or the family. It is not likely that accurate developmental data were obtained that day.

An examiner takes inventory of personal characteristics which might be used to establish rapport. It is quite useful to obtain feedback from other colleagues, or to watch oneself on a videotape, to gain a more objective view of one's interactional skills. Consider how you initially greet the child and family and engage in introductory talk. This initial introduction is important; however, as Sattler (1988) notes, the building and maintaining of rapport is a process that must continue and be interwoven with the assessment. The evaluator must gauge the amount of interaction-type talking, so that the child is not distracted from the test demands. While the child is working at the given task, it is important to observe inconspicuously, so as not to distract, irritate or even make the child feel self-conscious. Similarly, recording responses is also accomplished discreetly. When reinforcing a child for attempts at a particular task, it is very important that the child be encouraged for efforts, rather than for the results of efforts. Phrases such as: "I like the way you're working," or "You're really working hard," are more effective than those that denote a value judgment of the finished project, such as: "You did that correctly."

Because every child and examiner are different, it is the examiner's responsibility to adapt to the personality of the child. Often, inexperienced examiners will comment that a child was untestable or would not cooperate. Perhaps a more accurate statement is that the examiner was not able to adapt personal characteristics to fit the personality of the child. Just as each therapist spends time practicing and learning the particular instructions for administering an evaluation, it is also necessary to spend time examining one's own personality characteristics, and developing ways to adapt to fit the personality characteristics of the child and family.

VEHICLE FOR THE ASSESSMENT PROCESS THE REFERRAL

The vehicle which puts the assessment process into motion is the referral. The assessment process consists of reviewing the referral questions, observing behavior, and selecting, administering, scoring, and interpreting the test (Sattler, 1982). Referrals in pediatric practice most commonly occur through two models of providing service: a medical model and an educational model. In a medical model, a referral is usually received from a physician or other health care professional, such as a speech pathologist or physical therapist. Most medical model agencies require physician referrals. In school settings, the referral is more likely to be from a member of the educational team, which might include the school psychologist, the classroom teacher, or other related service personnel such as the physical education teacher or the speech-language pathologist. Some states require a physician referral in their licensure bill, regardless of the model of practice. In educational settings, a student is referred to the occupational therapist for assessment when there appears to be dysfunction in the performance areas and components (McGourty, Foto, Marvin, Smith, Smith, & Kronsnoble, 1989), which affect the learning process. Appendix 1 contains the revised Uniform Terminology for Occupational Therapy from the American Occupational Therapy Association (McGourty et al., 1989).

The appropriateness of a referral depends upon the setting in which it is made. Appropriate referrals in a medical model might include assessing a child with concerns regarding motor development and adaptive skills. In educational settings, appropriate referrals may include assessing pre-academic skills that deal with organizational behavior, perceptual skills, social skills, self help skills, and fine and gross motor skills. In an educational setting the referral concerns must be related to educationally relevant needs.

Regardless of who made the referral, or in what setting the referral was made, it is always essential to address assessment priorities in relationship to the referral complaint or concern. By focusing on the referral questions, the therapist can select appropriate evaluation tools and ensure that the original concern or question is indeed addressed. Evaluations may expand beyond the referral concern in cases where the therapist identifies a new area of concern, but this must be in addition to the initial target concerns.

Each setting establishes eligibility criteria for determining whether an assessment is warranted, and what type of evaluation may be necessary. Screening procedures help to define those variables which may bring a child and family to an assessment situation (See Chapter Two). It is not appropriate to evaluate every child that might be referred in a clinical or school setting. The therapist must decide if, in fact, occupational therapy assessment is warranted. The occupational therapist frequently contributes to the establishment of oc-

---

TEACHER QUESTIONNAIRE
REFERRAL FORM FOR OCCUPATIONAL THERAPY

Child's Name _____   Grade: _____

Date _____   Teacher: _____

School _____

Teacher making referral: _____

Teachers: Please check the following behaviors that correspond to the concerns you have regarding your student.

_____ 1. Demonstrates mixed hand dominance in classroom activities
_____ 2. Grasps pencil/crayon improperly
_____ 3. Does not perform desk work from left to right
_____ 4. Does not know left from right on self
_____ 5. Has difficulty staying on line & spaces when writing and printing
_____ 6. Has difficulty copying from board or text
_____ 7. Reverses letters/shapes in writing/drawing
_____ 8. Has difficulty completing activities on time
_____ 9. Has difficulty following verbal directions
_____ 10. Has difficulty following written directions
_____ 11. Has difficulty maintaining self in seat for reasonable length of time
_____ 12. Is clumsy at recess, gym, or in classroom
_____ 13. Avoids physical activities with peers
_____ 14. Has extreme reaction to being touched
_____ 15. Has excessively high overall activity level
_____ 16. Has excessively low overall activity level
_____ 17. Projects poor self image

Figure 3-3a.   Sample teacher referral questionnaire. *Adapted from: Gilfoyle, E.M. (Ed) (1981). Training: Occupational Therapy Educational Management in Schools. Rockville, MD: American Occupational Therapy Association. Used with permission.*

cupational therapy referral criteria. These criteria serve to educate other service providers and community members about the expertise of occupational therapy, and create a more efficient assessment process. Two examples of referral criteria checklists, which might be used to determine whether an assessment is warranted, are provided in Figures 3-3a and 3-3b.

TYPES OF ASSESSMENT

Initial Considerations

Before creating a particular assessment plan for a given child, several factors must be considered in order to make thoughtful and appropriate choices. The most important initial factor is the content of the referral concern. It provides a guide for the creation of the initial assessment plan. At the completion of the assessment, the therapist refers back to the initial concern as a frame of reference for interpretation

of the findings. The time and setting available to conduct the assessment are also important preliminary factors. For example, in a specialty or followup clinic, there may be only twenty to thirty minutes available to see the individual. In a school, several periods may be necessary to complete a comprehensive assessment. In contrast, a referral to a diagnostic team for data regarding placement may require up to two hours per team member to create a complete picture. Special skills of team members may also alter the assessment strategy. For example, if the special educator or psychologist thoroughly addresses visual perception, the occupational therapist can use these data and focus on other components of performance.

Other important factors to weigh when choosing specific evaluation tools include the validity of the tool (if it truly measures what it is intended to measure), it's reliability (the ability to be consistent), and the age range and population characteristics of the normative group. For example, a test may have high validity for detecting visual motor deficits, but low

---

REFERRAL FOR ASSESSMENT
BY OCCUPATIONAL THERAPIST

Name _____ School _____ Grade _____

D.O.B. _____ Teacher _____ Date _____

GROSS MOTOR

_____ Seems weaker than others his age
_____ Difficulty with hop, jump, skip or run
_____ Appears stiff and awkward in his movements
_____ Clumsy, seems not to know how to move body, bumps into things, falls   out of chair
_____ Tendency to confuse right and left

FINE MOTOR

_____ Poor desk posture (slumps, leans on arm, head too close to work, other   hand does not assist)
_____ Difficulty drawing, coloring, copying, cutting; avoidance of these activities
_____ Poor pencil grasp, drops pencil frequently
_____ Hand dominance
_____ Quality of written work—too faint, too hard; breaks pencil often

TACTILE SENSATION

_____ Seems to withdraw from touch
_____ Has trouble keeping hands to self
_____ Apt to touch everything he sees
_____ Dislikes being hugged

VESTIBULAR SENSATION

_____ Fearful of activities moving through space (swing, teeter totter)
_____ Avoids activities that challenge balance
_____ Excessive craving for swinging, bouncing, slides, etc.

VISUAL PERCEPTION

_____ Difficulty discriminating colors, shapes, doing puzzles
_____ Letter reversals after first grade
_____ Difficulty tracking—following objects with eyes holding head still
_____ Difficulty copying designs, numbers, or letters

ADDITIONAL CONCERNS OR COMMENTS:

Figure 3-3b. Sample referral checklist.

validity for detecting readiness for reading and writing skills. In addition, tests that were developed for use with specific age and population characteristics in mind are not used with children who fall outside those intended parameters. Deitz (1989), states that the issue of reliability centers around consistency of test scores and test administration procedures. Therapists must also be aware of a particular test's "interrater reliability," or the ability of two or more independent examiners to score a test the same way. As Deitz (1989), points out, "reliability is a prerequisite to validity, but it does not insure validity." Dunn (1989), notes that often therapists find themselves in clinical situations where the test is inadequate, thus requiring that the assessment tool be adapted in some way to yield pertinent data. Because the assessment process is largely based on the therapist's professional experience, valid and effective test use is left up to the examiner's expertise. The development of this expertise, otherwise known as "good clinical judgment," is a process acquired by skilled observers. "Over years, a therapist's diagnostic skills are likely to evolve considerably as a result of ongoing refinements in both assessment procedures and professional judgment. Through this process, both evaluation and treatment skills are strengthened. This ongoing process results in the validation of therapeutic practice" (Dunn, 1989).

It is the therapist's responsibility to have a clear understanding of the intended use of a particular evaluation tool, in addition to its appropriateness for the intended population. Typically, each assessment tool provides technical data on the validity, reliability, and the intended purposes. The therapist must be "consumer-wise" in judging if a particular tool is appropriate for a given situation. The occupational therapist must be aware, informed, and trained in the appropriate use of measurement tools. Therapists must also avoid improper use of tools due to a limited knowledge of the variety of assessment tools available for particular needs (Lewko, 1976; Campbell, 1985).

The ultimate consideration in test selection is the relevance of the test scores, or the data gathered for the original purpose of the assessment. Knowing that a child scored a year below his chronological age in fine motor skill development may not adequately address a referral concern of poor handwriting skills. In this case, the qualitative components which enable handwriting skills may be an important focus of the assessment. These components could include bilateral coordination, the ability to cross the midline, hand dominance, residual influence of non-integrated reflexes, and prehension patterns. Merely reporting scores, without qualifying their meaning, serves only to cause the consumer to wonder about the meaning behind the score. It is also essential that the results of the assessment are described in relation to the referral concern.

Test Instruments

Test instruments can be categorized into three groups: norm-referenced, criterion-referenced and informal tests. In two separate recent surveys, therapists from Iowa (Arends & Clark, 1989), and therapists employed in rural and urban settings (Dunn & Gray, 1988), reported the most frequently used assessment tools. Table 3-1 contains a summary of the characteristics of common test instruments used by occupational therapists.

Norm-referenced Assessments

Norm-referenced measurements are also called standardized or formal measurements. These assessment tools contain data on the expected performance of a specified population, called norms (Sattler, 1982). Since performance is compared to a "normal standard," the tester must ensure that each person has the same opportunity to perform, and therefore must adhere to a strict pattern of test administration. Alteration of items renders comparison to norms impossible.

The boundaries for use of norm-referenced or standardized assessment are usually specific. They traditionally are intended for certain populations, and are not appropriate for use with populations to which they were not intended. For example, the *Sensory Integration and Praxis Tests* (*SIPT*) were intended to be used on children with normal intelligence, and were not intended to be used on children with severe multiple handicaps. The content and administration procedures are predetermined, and may not be altered. Too often, violation of testing procedures occurs, but is not reported in the scoring or interpretation. This is an unacceptable practice, because one cannot compare an individual's performance to a standard if that individual was given a different opportunity to perform. If it becomes necessary to deviate from the standardized procedure, this is reported in the interpretation of the evaluation results, and standard scores are not calculated.

Norm-referenced assessments yield specific results directed at particular domain areas. These results are expressed in various types of derived scores. Those derived scores that fall into a bell shaped curve, as a statistical point of reference, are summarized in Figure 3-4. Percentiles, standard deviations and standard scores are frequently used in occupational therapy evaluation tools.

Percentile scores rank the number of subjects at or below a particular score. A score reported at the 60th percentile reflects that an individual scored as well as or better than 60 percent of those who made up the normative sample population. It also means that 40 percent of the norm sample scored better than the person who scored at the 60th percentile. While the simplicity of this score is appealing, because it can be easily understood, a major drawback to interpreting percentile ranks stems from the inequality to percentile units. This is because differences are smaller near the mean than the extremes (Sattler, 1982). Figure 3-4, which summarizes all standard scores, illustrates this inequality.

Standard scores are raw scores that have been statistically prepared to yield a mean and a standard deviation. They are interpreted in relation to their closeness to, or distance from, the center of the bell curve. Standard scores are the preferred scores, as they are designed to have a constant mean and standard deviation at all ages of the normative sample (Sattler, 1982).

Age-equivalent and grade-equivalent scores are also frequently used in developmental and educational tests. They are determined by locating the average score obtained by children of the specified age or grade placement. Age-equivalent scores are typically expressed in years and months,

TABLE 3-1 Assessment Tools Commonly Used by Occupational Therapists in Pediatric Practice

	Ayres Clinical Observation of Sensory Integration	Bayley Scales of Infant Development Mental and Motor Scales	Beery Developmental Test of Visual-Motor Integration (VMI)	Brazelton Neonatal Behavioral Assessment Scale	Brigance Diagnostic Inventory of Early Development	Bruininks-Oseretsky Test of Motor Proficiency	DeGangi-Berk Test of Sensory Integration	Developmental Programming for Infants and Young Children	Test of Visual Perceptual Skills (Non Motor) (TVPS)	Erhardt Developmental Prehension Assessment (EDPA)
AGE RANGE	5–8 years	2 mos–2½ yrs	2–15 years	0–1 month	0–7 years	4½ to 14 years	3–5 years	0–6 years	4–12 yrs	0–6 yrs
TESTING TIME (minutes)	20	45–50	10–15	20–30	30–60	45–60	30	20–30	10–20	30–60
SCORING TIME (minutes)	5–10	15–25	10	10	10–15	10	5–10	10	10	10
MAJOR AREAS TESTED:										
personal social		X		X				X		
communication		X			X			X		
cognition		X			X			X		
self help					X			X		
gross motor		X		X	X	X		X		
praxis	X					X	X			X
reflexes	X	X		X			X			X
fine motor		X		X	X	X	X	X		X
visual-motor integration			X			X		X		X
visual perception									X	
tactile	X			X						
vestibular	X			X			X			
TYPE OF TEST:										
norm referenced		X	X			X			X	
criteria referenced					X		X	X		X
informal/structured observation	X			X						
SCORES OBTAINED:										
age level			X			X		X		X
percentile			X			X			X	
standard		X	X			X			X	
quantified observations	X			X			X			X

TABLE 3-1. Continued.

	Gesell Preschool Test	Hawaii Early Learning Profile (HELP)	Learning Accomplishment Profile-Diagnostic Ed.	Learning Accomplishment Profile-Revised Ed (LAP-R)	Motor-Free Visual Perceptual Test (MVPT)	Movement Assessment of Infants	Peabody Developmental Motor Scales	Sensory Integration and Praxis Test (SCSIT) (SIPT)	Test of Visual Motor Skills (TVMS)
AGE RANGE	2½–6 yr	0–36 mos	12–72 mos	36–72 mos	4–8 yrs	0–12 mos	7 years	4 yr 0 mo to 8 yr 11 mo	2–12 yr
TESTING TIME (minutes)	40	30–36	1½–2 hours	2–2½ (hours)	10–20	15	40–60	75–100	10–15
SCORING TIME (minutes)	15–30	10–15	15	15	10	10	15	45–60	5–10
MAJOR AREAS TESTED:									
personal social	X	X		X					
communication	X	X	X	X					
cognition		X	X	X					
self help		X	X	X					
gross motor	X	X	X	X		X	X	X	
praxis							X	X	
reflexes						X			
fine motor	X	X	X	X			X	X	
visual-motor integration		X					X	X	X
visual perception					X			X	
tactile								X	
vestibular								X	
TYPE OF TEST:									
norm referenced	X				X		X	X	X
criteria referenced		X	X	X			X		
informal/structured observation						X			
SCORES OBTAINED:									
age level	X	X	X	X	X		X	X	X
percentile							X	X	X
standard							X	X	X
quantified observations				X		X			

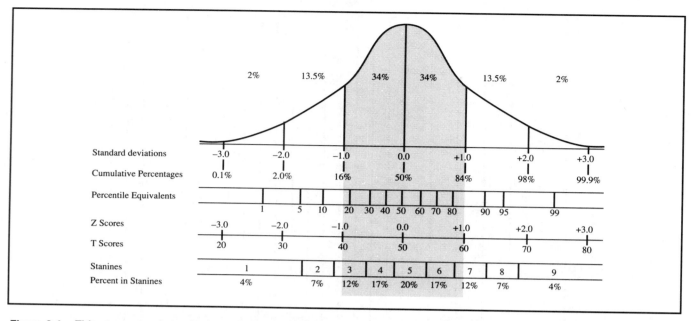

Figure 3-4.   This summary of standard scores in norm-referenced assessments illustrates the inequality to percentile units. *Sattler, J. (1988). Assessment of children, 3rd Edition. San Diego: Jerome M. Sattler Publisher. Used with permission.*

while grade-equivalent scores are expressed in tenths of a grade. For example, a 3.5 grade equivalent refers to performance expected midway through the third grade (Sattler, 1982). Age- and grade-equivalent scores are carefully interpreted. The scores may not reflect equal units of measurement and may not be topic sensitive, thus allowing for over interpretation of scores (Thorndike & Hagen, 1977; Sattler, 1982). For example, four-year-olds make much greater strides in fine motor skill development than thirteen-year-olds do, but both developmental periods are 12 months long.

In summary, interpreting the scores produced by norm-referenced assessments is an artful process. The task is more straightforward when all derived scores are compared to the bell curve for consistency.

Criterion-referenced Tests

Criterion-referenced tests compare a subject's performance to a previously established standard of performance. Individuals are compared to an established criterion, rather than to other individuals from a normative sampling (Sattler, 1982). These types of tests provide data on the mastery in particular domain areas, improvement in skill acquisition, and the child's readiness to proceed to the next level of development or instruction, and infer what materials or approaches might help towards mastery of skill development (Carver, 1972).

Criterion-referenced tests usually identify the intended population for which the tool might be used. *Developmental Programming for Infants and Young Children* (Schafer & Moresch, 1981) is appropriate for use with infants and children up through six years of age who may have developmental delays, while the *Callier-Azuza* assessment is especially useful for infants and preschoolers through age three who have severe, multiple handicaps. Typically, the administration procedures are suggested to the tester, rather than strictly outlined as in norm-referenced tests. Particular materials needed for test administration may or may not be supplied with the test kit, but frequently include common play or work items. The focus of a particular test item is centered on the degree of mastery the child exhibits. For example, the test item may call for the child to stack a tower of 8 one-inch cubes, but the way in which the examiner can ask, or present, the blocks may not be specifically stated.

Criterion-referenced tests yield data regarding the level of mastery for a particular task or skill; the criterion is used to describe the child's test performance (Montgomery & Connolly, 1987). For example, "Lois can match three of five geometric shapes," refers to Lois's level of shape-matching mastery, without reference to the performance level of other norm groups members (Sattler, 1982; King-Thomas & Hacker, 1987). Some criterion-referenced tests do yield derived standard scores; typically, age and/or grade equivalent scores are reported. Table 3-1 contains a summary of common criterion-referenced tests used by occupational therapists.

Table 3-2 summarizes the similarities and differences between norm-referenced and criterion-referenced tests. Criterion-referenced testing is most sensitive to individual gains, while norm-referenced testing is most sensitive to individual differences and comparison to the standard. Criterion-referenced testing usually complements norm-referenced testing (Sattler, 1982). Criterion-referenced scales usually are weighted towards the end of a continuum, or the point of mastery, while norm-referenced scales are weighted towards the mean or average of the normative group.

Informal Assessments

There probably is not a practicing occupational therapist who has not constructed or adapted a form to measure particular skills for assessment purposes. This type of data gathering

TABLE 3-2. Comparison of Norm-Referenced and Criterion-Referenced Tests

Norm-Referenced Tests	Criterion-Referenced Tests
1. Purposes: to examine individual performance in relation to a representative group; can be used to establish age levels; used for diagnosis and placement.	1. Purposes: to examine individual performance in relation to a criterion or external standard; used for program planning and evaluation because items are sensitive to effects of instruction (intervention).
2. Test construction: items developed from activities hypothesized to top specified skill or performance; test items usually not related to the objective of instruction (intervention).	2. Test construction: items developed from task analysis; test items are related to the objective of instruction (intervention).
3. Administration: must be administered in a standard manner as specified in test manual.	3. Administration: may or may not be administered in a standard manner.
4. Scoring: based on standards relative to a group; normal distribution, variability of scores (bell curve with means and standard deviations) is desired.	4. Scoring: based on absolute standards; variability of scores is not obtained because mastery of skills is desired.
5. Psychometric properties: test should demonstrate reliability and validity.	5. Psychometric properties: test should demonstrate reliability and validity.
6. Standards, or reference points are the average, relative points derived from the performance of a group.	6. Reference points are fixed at specific cut-offs which are predetermined by consensus of experts.
7. Evaluates individual performance in comparison to a group of persons; student competing against others.	7. Evaluates individual performance in relation to a fixed standard; student competing against self.
8. May or may not have a relationship to the specific instructional content.	8. Is content specific.
9. Tests may have a low degree of overlap with actual objectives of instruction.	9. Tests are directly referenced to the objectives of instruction.
10. Does not indicate when individuals have mastered a segment of the spectrum of instructional objective.	10. Identifies those segments of the spectrum of objectives the individual has mastered.
11. Designed to maximize variability and produce scores that are normally distributed.	11. Variability of scores is not desired; mastery is expected.
12. Designed to maximize differences among individuals	12. Designed to discriminate between successive performances of one individual.
13. Requires very good diagnostic and interpretive skill, otherwise a poor aid in planning instruction.	13. Geared to provide direct information for use in planning instruction.
14. Tests not sensitive to the effects of instruction.	14. Tests are very sensitive to the effects of instruction.
15. Is generally not concerned with task analysis.	15. Depends on task analysis.
16. Is more formative (used at various points during instruction) than summative though it can be used both ways.	16. Is more summative (used at the end of instruction) than formative or is strictly diagnostic.
17. Interpret test scores in relation to established norms.	17. Report which, or how many, of a set of specific achievement goals the individual has reached.
18. Broadly sample the domain of a particular achievement area.	18. Sample a limited number of specifically defined goals.
19. Provide a concise summary of overall outcomes of components of achievement and ability.	19. Report specific and detailed information on pupil achievement.
20. Encourage and reward individual excellence in achievement. Emphasize performance in relation to the reference group (e.g., age, group, males).	20. Emphasize mastery of specific subject matter by all pupils.
21. Treat learning as consisting of building a structure of numerous relations among concepts.	21. Treat learning as if it were acquired by adding separate, discrete units to the collection of things learned.

Adapted from: Gilfoyle, E.M. (Ed.) (1981). *Training: Occupational therapy education management in schools.* Rockville, Maryland: American Occupational Therapy Association.

can be classified as an informal assessment, and is a very important tool to help the therapists gain as much information as possible about the child. An informal assessment may take the form of structured clinical observations of neuromuscular development which are observed, elicited, and rated in a predictable manner, interviews of a parent, or observation of a child's behavior in a semi-structured or unstructured environment. The therapist can rate the occurrence or non-occurrence of particular domains of behavior in a checklist format, or record detailed descriptions of the behaviors observed for later interpretation with other data. The Uniform Terminology list (see Appendix 1) can be used as a template for focusing the therapist's attention on the various performance areas.

Just as there are guidelines for administering formal assessments, there are guidelines for administering informal assessments as well. These guidelines are comprised of those skills and areas of expertise most commonly referred to as "sound clinical judgment." Sound clinical judgment takes time, experience, and practice to acquire; and sometimes seems elusive to undergraduate students, beginning therapists, and even some seasoned practitioners.

Skilled Observation. A critical aspect of informal assessment is skilled observation. The professional must observe and record discrete, objective, specific behaviors as they are exhibited. The examiner must not become overly engaged in the environment, or the behavior of the child to an extent that it interferes with the ability to document what is observed in an objective manner. Over-engagement is a common problem among those developing observational skills; "cute" or "ornery" behaviors can be entertaining and the necessary information to be gathered is lost.

Second, it is important to be sensitive to environmental variables while conducting skilled observations. The examiner must be able to identify the impact of environmental events on the assessment session; if environmental variables are interfering, the examiner attempts to modify the situation. For example, the examiner may wish to decrease visual or auditory distractions to obtain the child's best performance. The setting must be described objectively; this description will provide additional, relevant data for interpretation. For example, the setting can be described as structured, semi-structured or unstructured. A structured setting may be a therapy clinic, school or day care center; an unstructured setting could be found in a shopping mall or a child's home. All relevant parameters of the setting must be described so that behaviors and expectations can be judged in the proper context.

Third, the professional must define the behaviors that occurred, and did not occur. Occupational therapists are well versed in the process of task analysis. This background enables the therapist to break down the components of a behavior or task, so that each facet of the skill can be analyzed and observed with regard to functional outcome. It is not considered "sound clinical judgment" to merely report that the child could not stack four blocks; the occupational therapist also describes the child's successful and failed attempts, analyzing the components of performance. These data lead to correct conclusions and eventually useful recommendations. Figure 3-5 summarizes the components which

COMPONENTS OF SKILLED OBSERVATION	
Components	Example
Setting	—structured setting—classroom
	—unstructured setting—home
	—range of environments on a given day—home, day care center, school, shopping mall
Behavior	—domain specifically identified
	—fine motor prehension skill
Quality	—performance delayed
	—performance in dysfunctional pattern
Frequency	—how many times the behavior occurs
Duration	—how long the behavior lasts

Figure 3-5. Summary of components which make up skilled observation.

make up skilled observation. Figure 3-6 is an example of an informal assessment tool which focuses on the sensorimotor components of specific functional life tasks. This particular tool, designed by two occupational therapists, allows for objective rating of various domain areas in terms of their quality, frequency and duration. The tool can be used across several settings (i.e., school, home, or clinic).

Interviewing. The process of interviewing a parent, caregiver, teacher, or child is an essential component of the assessment process. Not only does the interview process assist in gathering data, but it also serves to establish rapport between the therapist and the interviewee. Because rapport building is so essential to the amount, quality, and accuracy of the data that is gathered, the therapist must consider how best to establish rapport. An approach that works with one interviewee will not necessarily be the best for the next interviewee.

Careful selection of a specific type of interview, setting up and modifying the interview environment, all increase the likelihood of a productive and rapport-building process. Most agencies use a form which outlines the parameters for data collection. When the therapist uses such a form to ask the parent, caregiver, or teacher questions, there is an opportunity to build rapport while gathering important data. This benefit is lost when the therapist hands the form to the informant, and then never discusses the answers with the individual. Figure 3-7 provides one example of a questionnaire that a parent can fill out before the assessment, and then discuss later with the therapist.

Interviews can follow a general or more focused format (Bernstein & Bernstein, 1985). The information gathered may follow a funnel sequence where the questions start out broad and lead to more specific responses. For example, the therapist may begin by asking the parent to describe the family unit, which may lead to sibling interactions and parental feelings about the child with special needs. This, in turn, can lead to a more focused discussion of the parent's concerns, and a description of specific problems, such as eating difficulties. A reverse funnel sequence may sometimes be appropriate, where specific referral-oriented questions lead to more broad, expanded responses. For example, the therapist may begin by restating the referral complaint, request elab-

FUNCTIONAL BEHAVIOR ASSESSMENT FOR
CHILDREN WITH SENSORY INTEGRATIVE
DYSFUNCTION

SCORE SHEET

1 = lowest, most
dependent/dysfunction;
4 = highest, most
independent/functional

	Levels of Functioning			
	1	2	3	4

SELF CARE:
  MEALTIME ACTIVITIES
    Motor
    Posture
    Social
  DRESSING
    Fasteners
    Put On/Take Off
    Independence/Orientation
  BATHING
    Postural Balance
    Defensive Responses

BEHAVIOR:
  CONTROL AND MOTIVATION
  SOCIAL INTERACTION

APPROACH TO NEW ACTIVITIES:

TOUCH:
  RESPONSE TO HOLDING AND
  HUGGING
  SEEKING TOUCH INFORMATION

MEMORY:
  FOLLOWING COMMANDS
  (RECEPTIVE LANGUAGE)
  SEQUENCING EVENTS
  EXPRESSIVE LANGUAGE

SCHOOL ACTIVITIES:
  ACTIVITY LEVEL
  ATTENTION TO TASK/PERSON
  POSTURAL MUSCLE CONTROL
  ACADEMIC WORK
    Grade Level
    Rate of Progress
  PLAYGROUND ACTIVITIES
    Motor Coordination
    Response to Playground Equipment

GROSS MOTOR:
  BILATERAL MOTOR COORDINATION
  MOTOR PLANNING
  STATIC BALANCE
  DYNAMIC BALANCE

PERCEPTUAL/FINE MOTOR:
  GRASP
  CUTTING
  PRINTING
  ORGANIZATION
  HAND DOMINANCE

SENSORY MOTOR INTEGRATION:
  REFLEX INTEGRATION
    Flexion in Supine
    Prone Extension
    Protective/equilibrium Reactions
  MUSCLE TONE
  COCONTRACTION
  EYE MOVEMENTS
  RESPONSE TO TOUCH
  RESPONSE TO MOVEMENT

FAMILY
PARTICIPATION/UNDERSTANDING:

Figure 3-6. Example of a functional behavior tool.

oration, and then expand by asking if the person sees the problem in other situations.

Care is also taken in selection of open-ended and closed-ended questions. Words like "describe" and "explain" offer opportunities to elaborate on the topic, while fact-based, "yes or no" questions do not encourage this elaboration. The attitude the therapist projects is thoughtfully regarded and altered as needed. For example, responses that reflect a reassuring and understanding attitude may be appropriate during one part of the interview, while a probing and evaluative manner may be appropriate for another part of the same interview. Knowing when a particular technique is appropriate is an essential skill to an occupational therapist. Recognizing and understanding the choices is the first step in the therapist's acquisition of skill in this area.

Non-verbal communication is also critical to the interview form of evaluation. The way rapport is established and the manner through which the interview unfolds typically depends on the non-verbal responses the therapist employs. "Closed body language," such as crossed arms and legs, little eye contact, and posture turned away from the individual, can send a judgmental, non-involved message which diminishes the informant's motivation to share personal information. "Open body language," such as leaning forward, maintaining eye contact, and using facial expressions to respond to the information provided, encourages the individual to continue because there is a receptive listener.

AREAS TO CONSIDER IN A COMPREHENSIVE OCCUPATIONAL THERAPY ASSESSMENT

For the occupational therapist, the assessment process contains three major components: assessment of performance areas, assessment of the components of performance, and assessment of contextual variables that may affect performance. The goal of this data gathering is to create a profile of strengths and concerns that can be used to: a) identify a diagnosis, and b) formulate an effective intervention strategy; assessment is not a goal in itself (See Figure 3-8).

Selecting the areas that you will consider during a comprehensive assessment will be largely influenced by the referral questions and the service model (i.e., medical vs. educational). Regardless of the setting or the referral question, specific standards of practice are set forth (AOTA, 1986). The occupational therapist is concerned about the performance areas of work, self-care and play/leisure; therefore, assessment addresses functional abilities and deficits in these areas. See Appendix 1 for uniform terminology definitions (AOTA, 1989). The assessment also determines which performance components (sensorimotor, cognitive, psychosocial) are facilitating, and which are blocking the performance area(s) in question. For example, if a child is unable to complete school work (the performance area of work), the occupational therapist might evaluate the performance components of postural control, perceptual processing, visual motor control and memory to determine why the child is having difficulty. The occupational therapist also considers those environmental variables that might affect performance areas. In this example, the therapists would want to know whether the environment is distracting or quiet, and the methods used to

FUNCTIONAL BEHAVIOR ASSESSMENT FOR CHILDREN WITH SENSORY INTEGRATIVE DYSFUNCTION

Rating Guide

INSTRUCTIONS: This rating guide provides the descriptors needed to score the various functional behaviors on the accompanying score sheet. This assessment was intended for use by occupational therapists and physical therapists who utilize the sensory integrative frame of reference for assessment and treatment. The four point rating scale assists in initial identification of functional skills and can serve to document progress by measuring movement between the levels. Some sections (school activities, self care) may be completed through interview with parent and/or teacher.

	Level 1	Level 2	Level 3	Level 4
SELF-CARE **MEALTIME ACTIVITIES**				
Motor	Child has trouble holding or using fork or spoon and generally chooses to finger feed.	Child can manage fork and spoon. Occasionally uses fingers in conjunction with utensils.	Child consistently uses fork and spoon to feed self (can use knife to cut food but is messy).	Child manages all utensils well.
Posture	Child rarely remains in chair during meal and when he does, he wiggles, squirms, or slouches.	Child generally remains in his chair but does not sit still. May sit sideways, wrap leg around chair, etc.	Child remains in his chair but may need reminders to sit up. (Behavior in chair is not distracting.)	Child demonstrates good posture in chair.
Social	Does not interact in conversation or calls attention to self with inappropriate behavior (screaming, hitting, tugging, etc.)	Interacts in conversation when it is directed to him. May interrupt conversation by talking.	Initiates appropriate conversation but may occasionally interrupt.	Initiates interaction with family in appropriate conversation. Exercises control in waiting for turn to speak.
DRESSING				
Fasteners	Child needs assistance with most or all fasteners. May be able to zip, unzip and unlace but needs assistance or has much difficulty in tasks such as buttoning, snapping, buckling, and tying shoes.	Child can do basic fastenings except tying or untying shoes but takes an excessively long time and needs verbal cues. May also need help with separating zipper such as on jacket.	Child can independently and easily do all front fasteners including buckling and lacing. Can functionally tie shoes but they often come undone.	Child can do all fasteners, tie shoes, lock and close separating zipper with good coordination. Can also complete fasteners on back of clothes (bow, buttons, etc.), thread belt through loops when pants are on, etc.
Independence/ Orientation	Child needs physical assistance to dress and undress (pullovers, etc.).	Child is independent in undressing but may require minimal assistance in dressing. May require more assistance with difficult clothing such as tight turtlenecks. Needs to be told and shown right from left, front from back. Clothes must be turned right side out for him.	Child needs only supervision and occasional verbal cues. May occasionally have clothes reversed (wrong side out, front/back, right/left), and must be told that they are.	Child is completely independent in dressing and consistently gets clothes on correctly.
BATHING Postural Balance	Child requires physical assistance, seems fearful of getting into and out of tub.	Child needs to firmly hold on to someone for balance while getting into and out of tub.	Child needs to firmly hold on to something for balance while getting into and out of tub.	Child has no difficulty or hesitancy getting into or out of tub.
Defensive Responses	Cannot tolerate shower spray, does not dry off or allow someone else to dry him; doesn't use washcloth to scrub body or parts of body.	Dislikes shower spray and prefers bath because of that reason. Will dry or wash but does not allow anyone to do it for him because of aversion to touch.	Will dry or scrub self but reacts to shower spray, drying or scrubbing by another with grimacing, giggling, squirming, pulling away, verbal complaints, etc.	Shows no dislike of shower or drying or scrubbing done by self or other.
BEHAVIOR **CONTROL AND MOTIVATION**	Child does not control own behavior and does not respond to behavior control by others, including concrete rewards, punishment, or social praise.	Child may need to be disciplined before following through with an order. Demonstrates no self control and responds only to concrete outside controls (reward or punishment) as: getting to stay up past bedtime or having TV privileges taken away.	Child needs reminders to follow through with orders but generally behavior is controlled through social praise such as: "You did such a nice job cleaning your room." May occasionally require concrete control as in level 2.	Child is able to control own behavior, requiring only occasional social praise and concrete reinforcement. Child doesn't require immediate reinforcement and may delay rewards. For example: allowance at end of week, extra recess at end of week.
SOCIAL INTERACTION	Child does not participate in conversation or play with others. OR, Constantly dominates others inappropriately, breaks rules, exhibits excessive physical contact, yelling, etc. Involves others in inappropriate behavior.	In small groups (3–4), child participates in some conversation or play if someone else initiates. Will seek out children to play with in one-to-one situation. OR May occasionally be aggressive toward other children (pushing in line, hitting, etc.).	Child initiates some conversation and play in small groups. Generally follows rules, is good participant but not primary leader.	Child leads conversation and play appropriately in large and/or small groups. Peers may look to him for leadership, but it is not necessary that he is always the leader.
APPROACH TO NEW ACTIVITIES	Child refuses to try new activities. OR Child is reckless in approach which may result in danger to him or others.	Child is reluctant to perform new activities. May seem fearful, but with encouragement can be convinced to try. OR Child needs physical reminders to control himself. Example: put hands on his shoulders to slow him down.	Child is hesitant about performing new activities. May approach activity several times but will then attempt on own initiative—doesn't require encouragement from another person. OR Child needs verbal reminders for control. Example: "Slow down."	Child willingly approaches new activities.

Figure 3-6. *Continued*.

TOUCH

RESPONSE TO HOLDING AND HUGGING

Child will not tolerate being held or hugged, even by parent or familiar person.	Child will tolerate being held or hugged, sitting in lap, etc, if he is the one to initiate it. Child must be in control. Example: If you try to make him stay in lap, pull tightly, he'll resist and try to get away.	Child will tolerate and may enjoy being held or hugged, sitting in lap, etc. even if he is not the one to initiate it. After a short period of time or after you try to make him stay in lap, pull closer, hug tightly, child will give some indication of discomfort. Example: grimacing, squirming, etc.	Child does not resist attempt to hold or hug him. Seeks out affection—may crawl into parent's lap or spontaneously hug parent/familiar person.

SEEKING TOUCH INFORMATION

Child is constantly touching objects in his environment (even, objects which are unsafe) people, etc., to a much greater degree than most children. OR Refuses to touch objects/people in environment.	Child frequently touches objects/people inappropriately. OR Child frequently refuses to touch objects/people, but will if specifically verbally or physically prompted.	Child occasionally or infrequently touches objects/people inappropriately (example, only at home, but no where else). OR Child occasionally or infrequently refuses to touch object/people in acceptable environments, but will with verbal coaching.	Child seeks a normal amount of touch input.

MEMORY

FOLLOWING COMMANDS (RECEPTIVE LANGUAGE)

Can follow only simple and direct verbal instructions. Example: "Please shut the door."	Can follow basic two-step commands but may need to have instructions repeated. Example: "Please shut the door and take off your coat."	Can follow most verbal instructions but needs to have complex directions repeated.	Can follow complex verbal instructions and will ask for clarification when needed.

SEQUENCING EVENTS

Cannot sequence events of day.	With prompting can sequence routine events of the day but needs assistance to recognize errors.	With occasional prompting can sequence the routine events of the day and can recognize errors.	Can correctly sequence events of the day without prompting.

EXPRESSIVE LANGUAGE

Cannot repeat songs, rhymes, instructions, needs.	Watches other children and/or lags behind in songs, rhymes, expressing instructions and needs.	Looks to other children occasionally for clues in repeating songs, rhymes, instructions, expressing needs.	Can repeat songs, rhymes, instructions for others and express needs for self.

SCHOOL ACTIVITIES

GENERAL ACTIVITY LEVEL

Child lacks energy, is lethargic, and falls asleep in class. OR Is constantly moving around, cannot wait turn, etc.. Child distracts others.	Child frequently appears tired or sleepy and may be reluctant to engage in physical activity. OR Child appears anxious, tense. May shuffle feet, drum hands, etc.. Behavior may distract others.	Level of activity is generally appropriate to task but child may require period of time to adjust to changes in pace (playground back to class, when teacher leaves room, etc.)	Child is alert, appropriately energetic and controls activity level according to task (can lie still at nap time, quiets down after recess, etc.).

ATTENTION TO TASK/PERSON

Doesn't pay attention. Must be isolated and have one-to-one attention to stay with work.	Requires frequent verbal prodding to pay attention. Daydreams, is easily distracted by other children, does not stay with work, etc.	Requires only occasional reminders to pay attention or attend to work.	Directs attention to appropriate person. Can attend to assignment/task without being distracted by normal environmental occurrences

POSTURAL MUSCLE CONTROL

Child is unable to remain in chair and may prefer to work on the floor. Child may fall out of his chair and may miss seat when sitting.	Child is constantly moving, turning, shifting his weight in the chair, to the point of distracting others. He may slouch or lean back in chair and generally props himself up on elbows.	Child has trouble sitting still and may shift weight and fidget but is not distracting to others. Generally sits erect.	Child demonstrates good sitting posture and can sit still for expected period of time.

ACADEMIC WORK

These rating scales should be used for Reading, Writing, Spelling and Mathematics.

Grade Level	Child's performance is two or more semesters below expectations.	Child's performance is more than one semester below expectations.	Child's performance is up to one semester below expectations.	Child is performing work at or above grade level.
Rate of Progress	In the past three months, child's performance demonstrates either regression or no progress.	In the past three months, child's performance demonstrates less than 50% of expected progress. Example: less than 1.5 months period.	In the past three months, child's performance demonstrates 50% or more of expected progress. Example: 1.5 months to 2.9 months progress in a 3 month period.	In the past three months, child's progress is at least equal to time interval. Example: 3 months progress in 3 months period.

PLAYGROUND ACTIVITIES

Motor Coordination	Demonstrates poor eye-hand, eye-foot coordination in comparison to peers. May be able to kick stationary ball but cannot balance on one foot, cannot hit or catch or throw on target. Falls frequently during gross motor activities.	Child can perform motor skills from static position but accuracy is poor. Can kick moving ball not on target, can catch ball 50% of the time, can balance for at least two seconds on one foot. May jump and hop but performance is awkward and uncoordinated. Falls occasionally during gross motor activities.	Demonstrates good eye-hand, eye-foot coordination but must be fairly stationary. For example: Can kick ball with accuracy while standing or walking, can throw ball to target while standing still, can hit ball with bat. Can balance on one foot and hop on one foot with good control (stopping and starting). Can skip and jump rope but performance may be awkward and uncoordinated.	Demonstrates good skill during dynamic movement. For example: Can coordinate running with kicking ball. Demonstrates good eye-hand coordination for baseball. Can balance on one foot and pick up object such as in hopscotch. Demonstrates poor coordination in skipping, jumping rope.

Figure 3-6. *Continued*.

Response to Play-ground Equipment	Child is fearful of playground equipment and refuses to use it. Child avoids using almost all playground equipment, and does not seem to know what to do with it.	Child requires encouragement to use playground equipment and often assistance of an adult such as to hold hand down slide. help with climbing. or to stand nearby.	Child demonstrates some hesitation but will use equipment independently.	Child uses all playground equipment either without apprehension or with some hesitation regarding moving equipment (jumping into turning. jump rope. moving merry go-round).

GROSS MOTOR
MOTOR PLANNING

	In performing an unfamiliar motor planning activity (one he has not done before). child bumps into static obstacles and shows little indication of planning movement. In playing motor planning games such as dodge ball. obstacle courses. footprint sequences etc.. child may try to participate but action demonstrates little or poor planning. Child cannot succeed even with physical assistance and breakdown of activity into component parts.	In performing an unfamiliar motor planning activity (one he has not done before). child may bump into static obstacles because of under-estimation, or performance may be exaggerated due to overestimation of movement needed. In motor planning games (see #1). child attempts to plan action but cannot respond correctly according to stimulus. Child can perform activity when broken down into physical guidance or visual cues (with simpler activity).	In performing an unfamiliar motor planning activity (one he has not done before). child can make necessary adjustments in position of body to correctly move over, under, around and through. Performance may be slow and requires concentration. In motor planning games (see #1), child does make errors but can successfully perform some irregular movement patterns or parts of patterns slowly and with concentration. Child may require visual breakdown with more complex activities but does not require physical assistance for success.	In performing an unfamiliar motor planning activity (one he has not done before). child is able to maneuver easily and quickly in relationship to static obstacles. In motor planning games (see #1) child is able to quickly and successfully perform irregular motor patterns.

BILATERAL MOTOR COORDINATION

	Child cannot coordinate arms or coordinate legs when performing simple bilateral motor activity. For example: Child can barely clear floor when jumping in place (2 jumps in a row) and feet do not land together. Cannot jump from 6'' height with feet together.	Child can functionally perform simple bilateral activities but performance may not be smooth. For example: Child can perform consecutive jumps forward but feet do not land together. Can jump from 6'' height landing with feet together. Can separately move both arms or both legs for jumping jacks but motion is uneven and uncoordinated. Child is beginning to skip but trunk is rigid and there is little or no arm swing.	Child can perform simple bilateral activities well but may exhibit difficulty with higher level activities (bilateral and reciprocal) involving total body movement. For example: Child's feet land together when jumping forward but one foot leads when jumping sideways or backwards. Can put arm and leg movements together for jumping jacks but performance is not rhythmical and child may make error after a few repetitions. Child is beginning to skip with arm swing but performance lacks smoothness and requires concentration.	Child can coordinate two body parts for bilateral and reciprocal activities. For example: Child jumps in all directions with both feet even, can rhythmically coordinate arms and legs during jumping jacks and in skipping.

STATIC BALANCE

	Left foot _____ Right foot _____	Left foot _____ Right foot _____	Left foot _____ Right foot _____	Left foot _____ Right foot _____

All Levels: Record number of seconds child is able to stand on the left and right foot and rank performance to appropriate level.

DYNAMIC BALANCE

	Child can only walk on balance beam with one foot on and one foot off. Cannot maintain balance during movement activities.	Child can walk sideways on balance beam. Can walk forwards but may step off occasionally to regain balance for short periods during activities involving slow. predictable movement.	Child can walk forwards on balance beam but may have difficulty and/or step off going backwards. Can do the heel toe walk forwards with concentration. Child can maintain balance during activities involving moderate (including somewhat irregular) movements. Can become comfortable with balance abilities so as to be able to perform upper extremity activities involving reaching and trunk movements.	Child displays good control on balance beam and can heel toe walk backwards. Does not require observable cortical control. Can readily maintain balance during movement activities which vary in speed and regularity and call for upper extremity reaching. trunk movements. etc.

PERCEPTUAL/FINE MOTOR
GRASP

	Child displays gross grasp of pencil/crayon (generally holds it in fist). Cannot color or draw within the lines and lacks hand control for writing.	Child must position and re-position pencil in fingers with other hand. Has much difficulty manipulating and does not necessarily support arm on table. Written work is almost unintelligible.	Can pick up and position pencil in writing hand but still has some difficulty in manipulating (grasp may be tight and strained). Writing is inadequate for age level in respect to neatness. smoothness of lines.	Child demonstrates tripod (3 fingers) or well coordinated grasp. Can use wrist and finger movement to write. Writing is done neatly and smoothly.

CUTTING

	Is not able to manipulate scissors to cut with one hand and stabilize paper with the other.	Child attempts to cut with scissors but has no control over scissors and stabilizing paper with opposite hand.	Child cuts with scissors and stabilizes paper. but performance is somewhat jagged and inaccurate.	Cutting is done neatly and accurately.

PRINTING

	Child is unable to copy printing.	Child frequently reverses letters and/or is unable to form some letters properly. Is able to copy most letters directly next to one under sample.	Child occasionally reverses letters. Is able to copy printing from paper onto another. including single letters and words. Cannot copy from blackboard.	Child does not reverse letters. Can copy well from paper and blackboard.

ORGANIZATION

	There is no organization in fine motor tasks.	Child demonstrates through actions or verbalizations that he is attempting to organize materials in regard to space and planning but is not able to do so. Example: starting over. saying it's not right. etc.	Child organizes fine motor tasks correctly but spacing is uneven and inconsistent.	Child organizes fine motor tasks and work is spaced correctly.

Figure 3-6. *Continued*.

	Level 1	Level 2	Level 3	Level 4
HAND DOMINANCE	Child switches hands indiscriminately.	Child generally uses certain hand for one activity but may switch occasionally.	May use one hand to write, another for cutting, but does this consistently.	Hand dominance is well established and child clearly prefers either right or left.

SENSORY MOTOR INTEGRATION

REFLEX INTEGRATION

	Level 1	Level 2	Level 3	Level 4
Flexion in spine assessment	Child is unable to assume position or can hold from 0–9 seconds.	Child assumes and maintains position for 10–20 seconds with great exertion.	Child assumes and maintains position for 20 or more seconds with moderate exertion.	Child assumes position as in level 3 and can hold it against slight resistance.
	Child is unable to hold head up from floor even when placed.	Once head is placed in flexion, child can actively hold it in that position for 1–12 seconds.	Child can assume and maintain position of head flexion for 1–12 seconds.	Child can assume and maintain position of head flexion for 13–20 seconds.
Prone Extension	Child is unable to assume position or can hold from 0–9 seconds.	Child assumes and maintains position for 10–20 seconds with great exertion.	Child assumes and maintains position for 20–30 seconds with great exertion.	Child assumes and maintains position for 20–30 seconds with good quality and moderate exertion.
	Child is unable to life head, arms, and chest up off of floor.	Child is able to lift head, arms, and chest for 1–6 seconds.	Child is able to lift head, arms, and chest for 7–14 seconds.	Child is able to lift head, arms, and chest for 15–20 seconds.
Protective/Equilibrium Reactions	Child cannot maintain prone/supine position without holding on. Does not demonstrate protective reactions other than maintaining hold on board.	Child can maintain prone/supine position. Maintains sitting when using arms for support and is unsteady in all fours position.	Child can unsteadily maintain all positions utilizing trunk/limb reactions rather than using extremities for support. May demonstrate delayed or incomplete protective reactions.	Child is steady in all positions. Demonstrates good protective reactions.

MUSCLE TONE

	Level 1	Level 2	Level 3	Level 4
	Muscle tone is definitely hypotonic, hypertonic or unequal.	Muscle tone is moderately hypotonic, hypertonic, or unequal.	Muscle tone is slightly hypotonic, hypertonic, or unequal.	Child has normal muscle tone.

COCONTRACTION

	Level 1	Level 2	Level 3	Level 4
	Child is unable to cocontract muscles of upper extremities and neck.	Moderate deficiency is noted in ability to cocontract muscles of upper extremities and neck.	Slight deficiency is noted in ability to cocontract muscles of upper extremities and neck.	Child is able to cocontract muscles of upper extremities and neck.

EYE MOVEMENTS: Not to be scored on children under 5 years of age.

	Level 1	Level 2	Level 3	Level 4
	Child moves head when eye tracking and/or is unable to follow moving object.	Child can hold head still when directed and follow moving objects with eye but pursuits are smooth. May be obvious irregularity at midline.	Child does not need to be told to hold head still and eye pursuits are generally smooth. Slight irregularity may be seen at midline.	No irregularities observed in eye pursuits in general or across midline.

RESPONSE TO TOUCH

	Level 1	Level 2	Level 3	Level 4
	Child avoids all tactile contact whether imposed by self or others. Refuses to remove clothing during treatment (due to tactile defensiveness) and tolerates only tactile input which is inherent in the equipment (carpeted barrel, scooterboard, etc.). OR Child seeks intense stimulation.	Child will tolerate self-imposed tactile stimulation but shows defensive reactions through facial expressions, scratching, rubbing. Will tolerate direct tactile contact to body parts during disguised tactile activities but child still needs to be in control. Example: rolling in soft blanket with shirt off, pretending to dry body parts on softly carpeted floor.	Child shows no overt signs of defensiveness with self-imposed tactile stimulation or with non-aversive tactile stimulation from another (such as moderate pressure as opposed to light touch.) May demonstrate some laughing and giggling behavior. Will allow direct input imposed by another during games such as ghosts, pillow fights, drawing on back, rubbing with mitts, etc. Child reacts more strongly (through expressions, withdrawing, etc.) to unexpected touch from an unfamiliar person.	Child tolerates a normal amount and variety of obvious and direct tactile stimuli from light touch to deep pressure. Tactile responses remain the same if stimulation comes from unfamiliar person. Child will voluntarily choose tactile activities which incorporate tactile stimulation.

RESPONSE TO MOVEMENT

	Level 1	Level 2	Level 3	Level 4
	Child will tolerate only movement which is controlled by self. OR Child seeks and engages in excessive stimulation particularly involving much rocking and rotation such as in spinning.	Child will tolerate only slow back and forth movement which is controlled by self. OR Child will seek more than normal stimulation but will occasionally set limits, reach level of tolerance, etc.	Child tolerates a variety of input but demonstrates insecurity with much spinning, speed and/or changes in direction.	Child tolerates normal amount of vestibular stimulation in a variety of ways (scooter, barrel, hammock, etc.).

FAMILY PARTICIPATION/UNDERSTANDING

	Level 1	Level 2	Level 3	Level 4
	Child's family demonstrates no understanding of evaluation results and treatment program. Does not show evidence of willingness to participate in child's program.	Child's family attempts to understand child's problem but demonstrates little real knowledge of problem. Shows evidence of willingness to participate but follow-through is inconsistent or participation and support is inappropriate.	Child's family demonstrates basic understanding of child's problem and shows definite evidence of willingness to participate. May need continued education and suggestions for home treatment. Family's support is positive and appropriate.	Child's family demonstrates working knowledge of child's problem. Needs only general guidance to put knowledge into practice by adapting the environment or providing appropriate stimulation. Participation is consistent and appropriate.

Developed by: Carol McEnalty Lupton, OTR
Brendan Smith, OTR
Rehabilitation Institute
3011 Baltimore
Kansas City, MO 64108.

Adapted with permission by: Debra Cook, M.S., OTR, March, 1990.

Figure 3-6. *Continued.*

PARENT QUESTIONNAIRE

Name of Child _____

Address _____
Street   City   State   Zip Code

Home Phone Number _____ Parents' Work Phone _____
Date of Birth _____ Present Age _____
Referred by _____
Address _____
Father's Name _____ Birth Date
Occupation _____ Yearly Income
Mother's Maiden Name _____ Birth Date
Occupation _____ Yearly Income

Legal Relationship of Parents to Patient (please check):
   Natural Parent: Mother _____   Father _____
   Adoptive Parent: Mother _____   Father _____
   Step-Parent: Mother _____   Father _____
   Foster Parent: Mother _____   Father _____
   Relative: _____

All persons living in the home:

Name	Age	Relation to patient	Present School Grade or Highest Grade Completed

Parental Concerns

Please describe the major concerns you have in seeking help for your child. List your concerns in order of their importance to you.

1. (most important) _____
2. _____
3. _____
4. _____
5. _____

How can this facility help you most with these concerns?

MEDICAL HISTORY

Child's Pediatrician or Family Doctor _____
Address _____
Street   City   State   Zip Code

Please list any other doctors or clinics that have examined this child:

Name	Address	Purpose of Examination

Figure 3-7.   Sample demographic & history form. *Adapted from Children Rehabilitation Unit, University Affiliated Facility, University of Kansas Medical Center.*

PREGNANCY

While pregnant did child's mother have any of the following:

	Yes	No		Yes	No
German measles	_____	_____	Any severe emotional problems	_____	_____
Anemia (low iron)	_____	_____	Vaginal infection or bleeding	_____	_____
Diabetes	_____	_____	Have a high fever	_____	_____
Kidney Problems	_____	_____	Smoke cigarettes	_____	_____
High Blood Pressure	_____	_____	Drink alcohol	_____	_____

What medication did child's mother take during pregnancy? (include vitamins and iron):

_____

_____

Has child's mother ever experienced a miscarriage? _____

If yes, did miscarriage precede or follow pregnancy with this child? _____

BIRTH

Was the child born early _____ late _____ or on time?

Was child born by C-section? _____ Yes _____ No. If Yes, please give reason for C-section:

_____

About how long was mother in labor? _____

What was baby's birth weight? _____ length? _____

What was baby's condition at birth? _____

Has child ever had the following:

	Yes	No		Yes	No
Eye or vision problems	_____	_____	Anemia	_____	_____
Ear or hearing problems	_____	_____	Vomiting spells	_____	_____
Allergies	_____	_____	Frequent diarrhea	_____	_____
Asthma	_____	_____	Frequent colds	_____	_____
Convulsions or "Spells"	_____	_____	Strain on urination	_____	_____
Head injury	_____	_____	Meningitis	_____	_____

Has child had any other health problems not listed above? (Describe)

_____

_____

Does child take medication on a regular basis? _____ Yes _____ No

Please list medication taken and amount:

_____

_____

Please list below the name of the hospital where your child was born. Has child ever been hospitalized? Please list below:

Hospital	Address	Year	Reason
1. _____			
2. _____			
3. _____			

Figure 3-7. *Continued.*

DEVELOPMENT & SCHOOL HISTORY

DEVELOPMENT

At what age did child first:

Sit alone _____   Feed self finger foods   _____
Crawl (hands & feet) _____   Speak first real words   _____
Stand alone _____   Speak first real sentences   _____
Walk well _____   Become completely toilet trained _____

SCHOOL HISTORY

Is child currently enrolled in a school program? _____ Yes _____ No
If yes, please answer the following:

School Name: _____
Address: _____
Grade (if applicable): _____

Has child been evaluated by school diagnostic team? _____ Yes _____ No
If yes, when was evaluation completed? _____

Please describe child's performance at school. What subjects does he do well in; what subjects does he have difficulty with? _____
_____

Does child receive any special services to help him at school? _____
If YES, please describe _____
_____

SOCIAL-EMOTIONAL DEVELOPMENT

Does child exhibit behaviors at home or school that concern you? _____ Yes _____ No. If Yes, please describe the behaviors that concern you: _____
_____
_____

What methods are used to discipline child? _____
_____
_____

Are these methods effective? _____ Yes _____ No
What does child like to do to occupy his time? _____
_____

Does child have regular playmates or friends? _____ Yes _____ No

Person completing application _____

Relation to child _____

Date _____

Parent/Guardian
Signature _____

Figure 3-7. *Continued.*

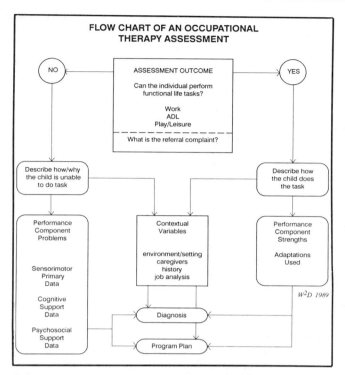

FLOW CHART OF AN OCCUPATIONAL THERAPY ASSESSMENT

W²D 1989

Figure 3-8. Flow chart of an occupational therapy assessment.

instruct the child. Further recommendations would be designed from these data.

Assessment of Performance Areas: Work, Activities of Daily Living, Play/Leisure

The referral complaint provides a frame of reference for assessment of performance outcomes. Teachers may be concerned that a student with severe disabilities can not eat or carry out personal hygiene tasks; vocational counselors are concerned that the adolescent will not be able to carry out a work assignment at the job site. Each of these concerns represents a functional life task that is important for independence, and therefore is an appropriate referral area for the occupational therapist.

It may also be appropriate for the occupational therapist to go beyond the specific referral complaint to determine the individual's ability to perform other functional life tasks. This decision to expand depends on the agency's mission (e.g., would this expansion still be within this agency's scope of work?), the time allotted for assessment, and the need for that information in diagnosis and intervention planning. Appendix 1 contains uniform terminology definitions for work, activities of daily living (ADL) and play/leisure, as defined by the American Occupational Therapy Association (McGourty et al., 1989). Figure 3-9 provides a grid for summarizing performance in appropriate ADL, work, and play/leisure tasks.

Occupational therapists primarily use skilled observation and interviews to identify the individual's ability to perform work, ADL and play/leisure tasks. Adaptive behavior scales are also available to evaluate performance outcomes; several scales have recently been created, or revised to be easier to use in a variety of settings (e.g., Vineland Scales of In-

dependent Behavior and AAMD Adaptive Behavior Scales). Please refer to Figure 3-10 for examples of areas covered in adaptive behavior assessments. Adaptive behavior is the individual's ability to engage in purposeful interaction with persons, objects, and situations in the environment. The focus of these adaptive behavior assessments is dictated by chronological age expectations, setting, and referral concerns. Adaptive behavior includes play and work skill development, communication skills, personal living or self help skills, and community living skills. Adaptive behaviors are the anticipated performance outcomes which form the goals of occupational therapy intervention. The occupational therapist investigates the reasons why the individual fails to demonstrate adaptive behaviors during the other parts of the assessment by evaluating the performance components.

The occupational therapist's assessment is not complete if it only includes data regarding mastery of work, ADL, and play/leisure. The occupational therapist's unique contribution to the diagnostic team is the ability to analyze how the individual was able to perform, what conditions were necessary to enable performance, and why the individual was unable to perform the functional life tasks. These decisions are made through an assessment of the components of performance (See next section).

In Figure 3-11 Jake demonstrates some difficulty combing Jessica's hair. In this example, it is not sufficient to comment only on his performance at this life task; the occupational therapist also describes the components of performance that are assisting him, and those that are inhibiting his performance. He demonstrates postural control, visual and tactile processing, and activity tolerance in this picture. His difficulties may be related to a number of performance components; without further observational opportunities, it is impossible to know the actual reasons. For example, poor tactile and proprioceptive processing, or fine motor dexterity, may be interfering with proper grasp of the brush; poor perceptual skills may make it difficult for Jake to discriminate the bristles from Jessica's hair. Lack of development of gross motor skills, such as pronated grasp, may be a primary factor. Occupational therapists contribute this type of valuable knowledge to team problem solving regarding life task performance.

Assessment of the Components of Performance

The second part of the occupational therapist's assessment process involves determining the integrity of the performance components, and their contribution to the success or failure in performing functional life tasks. The performance components fall into three major categories: sensorimotor, cognitive, and psychosocial. For clarity purposes, this text follows the sequences of Performance Components outlined in *Uniform Terminology Revised* (McGourty et al., 1989) (See Appendix 1). Figure 3-12 provides a grid to summarize findings regarding the integrity of performance components.

The occupational therapist provides primary expertise in the assessment of these abilities. In the areas of cognitive and psychosocial components, the role of the occupational therapist is typically to provide ancillary data to other professionals, such as the psychologist and special educator, in viewing the whole child. The occupational therapist does not

PERFORMANCE AREAS	Not applicable/not age appropriate	Performs task independently	Performs task independently with adaptations	Partially performs task, or requires assistance to complete	Performs isolated components of task incomplete even with assistance	Unable to perform task
ACTIVITIES OF DAILY LIVING						
1. Grooming						
2. Oral Hygiene						
3. Bathing						
4. Toilet Hygiene						
5. Dressing						
6. Feeding and Eating						
7. Medication Routine						
8. Socialization						
9. Functional Communication						
10. Functional Mobility						
11. Sexual Expression						
WORK						
1. Home Management						
2. Care of Others						
3. Educational Activities						
4. Vocational Activities						
PLAY/LEISURE						
1. Play or Leisure Exploration						
2. Play or Leisure Performance						

Figure 3-9. Grid to summarize performance in appropriate life tasks. *Reprinted with permission. Dunn 1988.*

usually provide primary expertise in the areas of cognitive and psychosocial components.

Sensorimotor Components

The therapist uses standardized and criterion-referenced tests, skilled observation, informal assessment, interviewing, and history-taking strategies to create a complete picture of the sensorimotor systems. Refer to Table 3.1 for a summary of standardized and criterion-referenced tests commonly used to assess sensorimotor performance components. Sometimes therapists use a specific frame of reference, such as sensory integration, or neurodevelopment, to guide this process, but a comprehensive evaluation may necessitate the use of several frames of reference to obtain adequate data. The therapist then begins to create a hypothesis about how the sensorimotor components of performance are enabling or interfering with functional life tasks, especially those addressed in the referral complaint.

Sensory Integration: Sensory Awareness/Sensory Processing. Our senses give us the foundation from which we gain information about our environments. Awareness precedes processing. This developmental sequence is important to consider during an evaluation. For example, an infant may neglect visual information such as faces and contrasting patterns. Upon further evaluation, this infant may have deficits in awareness of the stimuli due to congenital or acquired blindness. This deficit is in the awareness of the stimuli, not in the processing of them. In contrast, deficits in sensory processing deal with how incoming information is interpreted (i.e., hyper-responsiveness, or adequate processing). For example, an infant is able to receive visual information, but is overwhelmed by extraneous stimuli which cannot be inhibited in order to focus on what is important. Thus, the infant acts distracted, and is unable to be calmed unless placed in a darkened room. Basic responses to sensory input are observed in premies who have low tolerance for input (e.g., altered breathing pattern when picked up/moved).

EXAMPLES OF AREAS ADDRESSED IN ADAPTIVE BEHAVIOR ASSESSMENTS

American Association on Mental Deficiency Adaptive Behavior Scale, Revised Edition (1974).

Part One:
- Independent Functioning
- Physical Development
- Economic Activity
- Language Development
- Numbers and Time
- Vocational Activity
- Self Direction
- Responsibility
- Socialization

Part Two:
- Violent and Destructive Behavior
- Antisocial Behavior
- Rebellious Behavior
- Untrustworthy Behavior
- Withdrawal
- Stereotyped Behavior and Odd Mannerisms
- Inappropriate Interpersonal Manners
- Unacceptable Vocal Habits
- Unacceptable or Eccentric Habits
- Self-Abusive Behavior
- Hyperactive Tendencies
- Sexually Aberrant Behavior
- Psychological Disturbances
- Use of Medications

Vineland Adaptive Behavior Scales (1984)

Communication: receptive, expressive, written
Daily Living Skills: Personal, Domestic, Community
Socialization: Interpersonal Relationships, Play/Leisure Time, Coping Skills
Motor Skills: Gross and Fine

Woodcock Johnson Psycho-Educational Battery Scales of Independent Behavior (1984)

Motor Skills: Fine and Gross
Social and Communication Skills: Social Interaction, Language Comprehension, Language Expression
Personal Living Skills: Eating, Toileting, Dressing, Self Care, Domestic Skills
Community Living Skills: Time and Punctuality, Money and Value, Work Skills, Home and Community

Figure 3-10. Examples of areas addressed in adaptive behavior assessments.

When evaluating a child's sensory processing abilities, all sensory areas are considered. Figure 3-13 provides an example of a sensory history form that can be used to gather data.

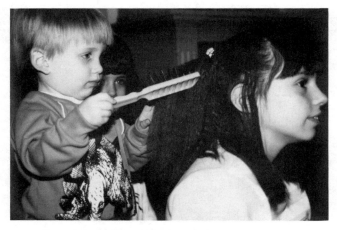

Figure 3-11. Jake understands how to perform the daily life task of combing, but demonstrates difficulty with certain performance components.

Tactile processing focuses on both discriminative and protective responses. In addition to specific test data which may yield information, the functional outcome must be considered. For example, a child with an impaired ability to process discriminative tactile information, may present safety concerns such as burning or cutting one's self. In contrast, a child which interprets tactile information as threatening, often has difficulty interacting with others due to frequent onset of fight-or-flight responses.

We relay *proprioceptive* information from the muscles and joints in our bodies to our brains. We use this information to direct our posture and movements. The effects of resistance (i.e., gravity and body weight) are considered in evaluating proprioceptive processing. Joint and muscle integrity provide clues to proprioceptive processing. When a joint is hypermobile, a muscle has low muscle tone, or the child seems to tire easily from tasks, poor proprioceptive processing might be suspected. Increased tone is sometimes indicative of overreactive proprioceptive mechanisms, resulting from a poor balance of power between higher and lower centers (Barnes, Crutchfield, & Heriza, 1977).

Nicholas demonstrates good use of proprioceptors of the hand, wrist, and forearm in Figure 3-14 as he holds the cards. The muscle tone that is required to maintain this position

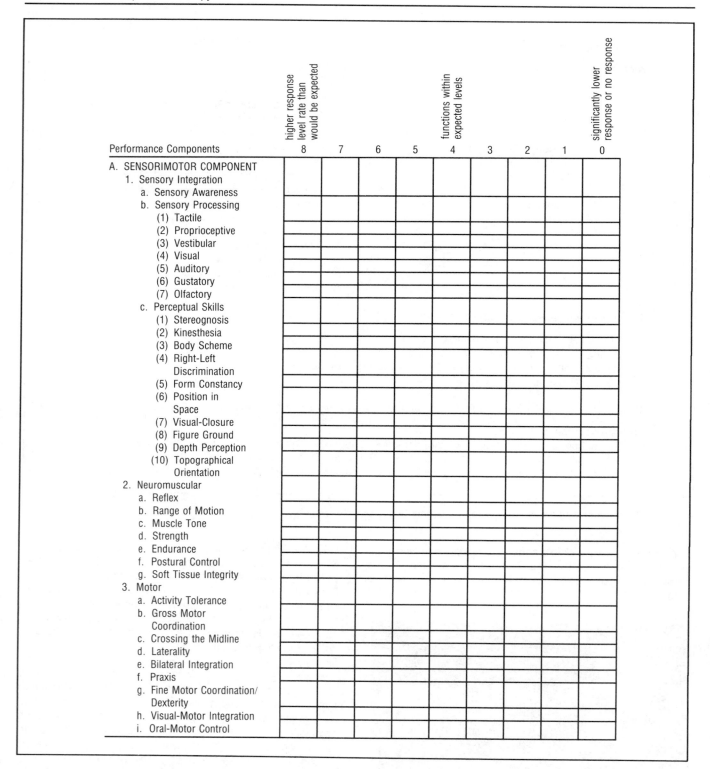

Figure 3-12. Grid to summarize performance component integrity. *Reprinted with permission. Dunn 1988.*

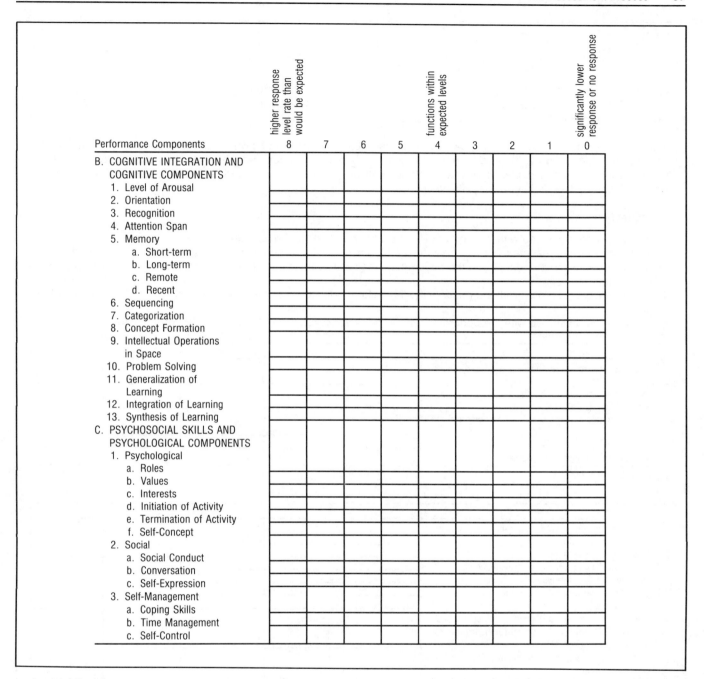

Performance Components	higher response level rate than would be expected				functions within expected levels				significantly lower response or no response
	8	7	6	5	4	3	2	1	0
B. COGNITIVE INTEGRATION AND COGNITIVE COMPONENTS									
1. Level of Arousal									
2. Orientation									
3. Recognition									
4. Attention Span									
5. Memory									
a. Short-term									
b. Long-term									
c. Remote									
d. Recent									
6. Sequencing									
7. Categorization									
8. Concept Formation									
9. Intellectual Operations in Space									
10. Problem Solving									
11. Generalization of Learning									
12. Integration of Learning									
13. Synthesis of Learning									
C. PSYCHOSOCIAL SKILLS AND PSYCHOLOGICAL COMPONENTS									
1. Psychological									
a. Roles									
b. Values									
c. Interests									
d. Initiation of Activity									
e. Termination of Activity									
f. Self-Concept									
2. Social									
a. Social Conduct									
b. Conversation									
c. Self-Expression									
3. Self-Management									
a. Coping Skills									
b. Time Management									
c. Self-Control									

Figure 3-12. *Continued.*

must be supported by proprioceptive feedback from the intrinsic muscles of the hand, the finger and hand joints, the wrist, and the forearm. Children with poor proprioceptive processing would be likely to: a) drop the card, b) have fingers spread loosely apart, c) prop forearms on the table, or d) display movement at the wrist.

Vestibular information can be processed as either accurate (normal), hyper-responsive, or hypo-responsive. In addition to specific tests which focus on how a child interprets vestibular or movement information, careful attention is also given to functional implications. For example, a child might avoid playground equipment, or crave car riding and swinging. Perhaps the most accurate data one can glean about a child's vestibular system, is through observation of interactions with the environment, particularly in the types of activities chosen for play.

Visual assessment typically is completed by an ophthalmologist. Occupational therapists can contribute data which leads to an appropriate referral to an ophthalmologist. The use of the eyes together to track and converge provide pre-

SENSORY HISTORY

Checklist

Child's Name _____   Person Competing Form _____
Date of Birth _____   Referral Source _____
Date Form Completed _____   Therapist _____

Instructions: Please check the response that best describes your child's behavior. Add any additional comments in the space after each category. If you are unable to comment because you have not observed the behavior, or feel that it's not applicable to your child, please draw a line through all the responses (————). Please do not leave any spaces blank. Use the following key in determining your response.

Key to responses:

1. *always*: when presented with the opportunity, the child responds in the manner every time, 100%.
2. *frequently*: when presented with the opportunity, the child usually responds in this manner, at least 75% of the time.
3. *occasionally*: when presented with the opportunity, the child sometimes responds in this manner, approximately 50% of the time.
4. *seldom*: when presented with the opportunity, the child usually does *not* respond in this manner, less than 25% of the time.
5. *never*: when presented with the opportunity, the child never responds in this fashion; 0% of the time.

Auditory	Always	Frequently	Occasionally	Seldom	Never
1. Responds negatively to unexpected or loud noises (i.e., vacuum cleaner, dog barking)					
2. Is distracted or has trouble functioning if there is a lot of noise around					
3. Enjoys strange noises/seeks to make noise for noise sake					
4. Enjoys music					
5. Appears to not hear what you say					

COMMENTS:

Visual	Always	Frequently	Occasionally	Seldom	Never
1. Expresses discomfort at bright lights (i.e. sunlight through window in car)					
2. Happy to be in the dark					
3. Looks carefully or intently at objects/people					
4. Puts puzzles together easily					
5. Hesitates going up or down curbs or steps					
6. Gets lost easily					
7. Has a hard time finding objects in competing backgrounds (i.e., shoes in a messy room, favorite toy in the "junk drawer")					
8. Has trouble staying between the lines when coloring or when writing					

COMMENTS:

Taste/Smell	Always	Frequently	Occasionally	Seldom	Never
1. Deliberately smells objects					
2. Shows preference for certain smells (List:)					
3. Shows preference for certain tastes (List:)					
4. Chews/licks on non-food objects					
5. Craves certain foods (List:)					

COMMENTS:

Figure 3-13. Sample Sensory History form.

Movement	Always	Frequently	Occasionally	Seldom	Never
1. Becomes anxious or distressed when feet leave ground					
2. Fears falling or heights					
3. Dislikes activities where head is upside down (i.e. somersaults) or rough-housing					
4. Avoids climbing, jumping, bumpy or uneven ground					
5. Avoids playground equipment or moving toys					
6. Rocks unconsciously during other activities (i.e. while watching television)					
7. Seeks out all kinds of movement activities (i.e., being whirled by adult, merry-go-rounds, play-ground equipment, moving toys)					
8. Takes risks during play (i.e., climbs high into a tree, jumps off tall furniture, etc.)					
9. Dislikes riding in a car					

COMMENTS:

Body Position (proprioception)	Always	Frequently	Occasionally	Seldom	Never
1. Hangs on other people, furniture, objects					
2. Seems to have weak muscles					
3. Tires easily, especially when standing or holding a particular body position					
4. Locks joints (e.g. elbows, knees) for stability					
5. Walk on toes					

COMMENTS:

Touch	Always	Frequently	Occasionally	Seldom	Never
1. Avoids getting hands "messy" (i.e. in paste, sand, finger paint)					
2. Becomes upset when face is washed					
3. Expresses distress over having hair cut, combed or washed					
4. Expresses distress over being bathed or groomed (i.e., cut finger nails)					
5. Prefers long sleeve clothing, sweaters, or jacket even when it's warm					
6. Expresses discomfort when people touch; even in friendly hug or pat					
7. Expresses discomfort at dental work					
8. Displays unusual need for touching certain toys, surfaces or textures					
9. Is sensitive to certain fabrics; avoids wearing clothes made of them					
10. Avoids going bare foot, especially in sand or grass					
11. Avoids wearing shoes, loves to be barefoot					

COMMENTS:

Figure 3-13. *Continued.*

Emotional/Social	Always	Frequently	Occasionally	Seldom	Never
1. Uses inefficient ways of doing things					
2. Seems to like him/herself					
3. Needs more protection from life than other children					
4. Has trouble "growing up"					
5. Is affectionate with others					
6. Is sensitive to criticisms					
7. Has definite fears					
8. Seems anxious					
9. Seems accident-prone					
10. Has difficulty tolerating changes in plans and expectations					
11. Is stubborn or uncooperative					
12. Has temper tantrums					
13. Has nightmares					

COMMENTS:

Activity Level	Always	Frequently	Occasionally	Seldom	Never
1. Always "on the go"					
2. Prefers quiet, sedentary play (i.e. watching television, books, computers)					
3. Enjoys other children					

COMMENTS:

DGC, 1989

Figure 3-13. *Continued.*

requisite information for many functional skills (i.e., eye-hand coordination).

Although *auditory* assessment is not the primary domain for occupational therapists, skilled observation can contribute to a total picture of the child. For example, does auditory stimuli distract the child, or does a particular type of auditory stimuli, such as soft rhythmic music, help a child to calm?

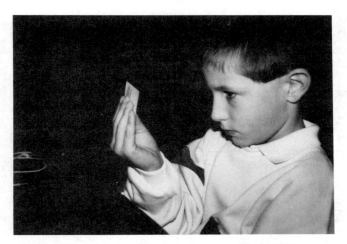

Figure 3-14. Nicholas demonstrates a modified pincer grasping pattern to hold the card and examine it: proprioceptive feedback supports this hand position.

Gustatory (taste) and *olfactory* (smell) processing must also be considered in evaluating the whole child. Besides the obvious impact that gustatory and olfactory processing have on oral-motor skills, they also impact a child's resting state and level of arousal.

Perceptual Skills. Perception is the ability to understand and interpret sensory input. All aspects of perception are considered when designing an assessment: stereognosis, kinesthesia, body scheme, right-left discrimination, form constancy, position in space, visual closure, figure ground, depth perception, and topographical orientation. Since processing of all of these components is necessary for a child to function in everyday life environments, it is essential that the occupational therapist's assessment include not only test data, but skilled observations on how perceptual skills or deficits impact the child's life. For example, low or suspect test scores on the *Test of Visual Perception* would help to validate why a child has difficulty reading left to right and copying from the board. Perceptual deficits are only relevant if they relate to a functional limitation in the child's life skills. An example of how common perceptual terms are related to functional skills can be found in Table 3-3.

Perceptual abilities are observed during task performance. Figures 3-15 and 3-16 provide a comparison of visual perception, body scheme, and motor skills being used by two-year-old Jake and six-year-old Jamie as they work with a pair

TABLE 3-3. Functional Application of Common Perceptual Terms

Word	Definition	Example
Discrimination	The ability to identify the similarities and differences among stimuli.	Recognizing a pencil from a pen. Hearing the differences between similar words (e.g. bat and pat).
Sequencing	The ability to place stimuli in their proper order.	Completing task in specified order. Writing letters of one's name in correct order.
Memory	The ability to recall stimuli.	Remembering phone number. Remembering what someone has asked you to do.
Closure	The ability to recognize existence of the whole form with only a portion of the stimulus available.	Knowing that it is a shoe and the rest of it is under the bed.
Figure-Ground	The ability to focus on the important stimuli and screen out unimportant background.	Finding an item in the junk drawer. FInding something in a busy picture. Focusing on boarding call and screening out the other airport noises.
Matching	The ability to identify the critical features of stimuli and categorize them by these characteristics.	Coordinating an outfit to wear. Picking out all the black jelly beans.
Visual-Motor/Auditory-Motor	The ability to coordinate the stimulus with the corresponding motor actions.	Tracing a picture. Following an oral direction. Stringing popcorn for the tree.
Spatial Relationships	The ability to recognize the proper relationships among stimuli.	Placing picture puzzle pieces in their proper orientation. Putting appliances in their proper place on the place on the shelf.
Form Constancy	The ability to recognize the critical features of stimuli.	Sorting the laundry. Collecting all the cups from around the house after a party.

Dunn, 1988

of scissors. Jake displays good visual attention and has a general awareness of the mobility of the two parts of the scissors. He uses both hands to open and close the parts, and therefore would have difficulty using the scissors for cutting. Jamie has developed more advanced perceptual and

motor skills; she uses her two hands in complementary tasks, visually guides the movement of the right hand to cut along the edge of the paper. Both children demonstrate adequate background postural control to support the manipulative task, and each child demonstrates age-appropriate skills. Jake's

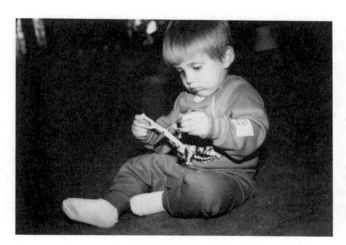

Figure 3-15. Jake (2-year-old) understands the use of scissors but can not orient them properly for use.

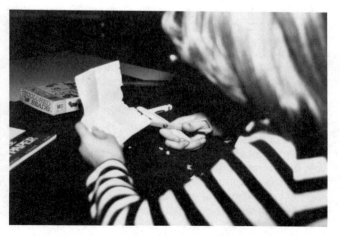

Figure 3-16. Jamie (6-year-old) has mastered both motor and perceptual performance components to use the scissors.

experimentation will facilitate development of improved perceptual and motor performance, so that he can cut a design like Jamie when he is six years old.

Neuromuscular. Neuromuscular development is comprised of those abilities which give us movement and control. Assessment of neuromuscular abilities are made up of reflexes, range of motion, muscle tone, strength, endurance, postural control, and soft tissue integrity.

Reflexes. There are a variety of ways to evaluate reflexes. Sometimes the therapist will test central nervous system (CNS) reflexes by attempting to elicit them and observing the response. This strategy provides limited, preliminary information about the basic integrity of the child's nervous system, but it provides no information about the effects of reflexive activity on the child's ability to function.

It is usually more desirable to include observation of reflex integrity during purposeful activity which requires movement and postural control. The therapist notes the presence, strength, or absence of reflexive activity, as well as asymmetry of reflexive behavior during performance. The therapist is especially concerned with reflexive behavior which compromises functional performance, or which may interfere with skill development. For example, a child may be unable to crawl on all fours due to residual persistence of the tonic labyrinthine reflex. Barnes, Crutchfield, & Heriza (1977) provide an excellent presentation of reflexes seen in children.

Range of Motion. Functional range of motion is addressed in regard to all major joints. Specific joint measurement are taken if that particular information is appropriate, requested, and relevant. For children, range of motion is most often assessed during functional work or play activities. Since muscle tone and sensory processing directly affect the amount of functional range of motion a child will display, these components of performance are frequently evaluated together.

Muscle Tone. Information is gathered regarding the child's muscle tone both at rest and during activities. Tone may be described as hypotonic, hypertonic, fluctuating, or within a normal range. Special attention is directed at all extremities, major joints, neck and trunk, relating the integrity of muscle tone to movement, postural control, and rest. The equality of tone across joints is important for both joint integrity and the child's ability to move about effectively.

Strength. Methods used to assess strength are often performed as part of the framework of fine and gross motor skills. In gross motor skills, the degree of resistance might include pedaling a bicycle, jumping rope, or climbing stairs. Structured observations of task performance are most commonly used, as opposed to individual or group muscle testing or dynamometer testing. Attention should be given to the degree of resistance that is inherent to the task.

Endurance. The level of endurance is always measured in terms of time. How long a child is able to participate in a task before becoming fatigued or distracted are clues to evaluating endurance. Therapists must be careful that they do not confuse endurance with activity tolerance. Measures of endurance assume that there is some level of tolerance. Endurance measures how long that tolerance lasts. For example, a child may be able to independently tie his shoes (activity tolerance), but it takes him ten minutes (endurance) to carry out the task.

Postural Control. Postural control is basic to all areas of performance. The degree of postural control necessary to engage independently in all areas of performance varies greatly. For example, a lesser degree of postural control is necessary to eat if you are seated in a chair with built up sides and lap tray. Determination of postural control in dynamic and static positions are directly related to the level of CNS reflex integration, range of motion, muscle tone, strength, and endurance. Postural control provides the stability out of which purposeful movement can occur.

Note the trunk and head control Jake exhibits in Figure 3-15; he is very intent on manipulating the scissors, yet he is able to maintain the upright sitting position during this task. His trunk control provides background support for this exploratory play. The same pattern of postural stability supporting active movement is depicted in Figure 3-17, in which Jake is demonstrating postural control at the lower trunk to enable the reaching action of the arms and hands.

Soft Tissue Integrity. Evaluating the integrity of soft tissue is typically described in conjunction with muscle tone, and is usually related to specific disease processes or trauma. Disease process such as muscular dystrophy or juvenile arthritis and trauma, such as burns, warrant skilled observation of muscle mass, joint tenderness, and temperature. The tissue integrity is always interpreted in relation to possible functional limitations.

Motor. The motor components include activity tolerance, gross motor coordination, crossing the midline laterality, bilateral integration, praxis, fine motor coordination, visual-motor integration and oral motor skills.

Activity Tolerance. Judgment of a child's activity tolerance is based upon the choices made during structured and unstructured play, and the length of time spent during play. For infants, activity tolerance is observed in motoric or autonomic reactions to particular stimuli. If the child chooses activities that require physical exertion and a high degree of sensory integration, the therapist can deduce that the child's tolerance for activity is quite high. Careful attention is directed to all sensory, perceptual, neuromuscular, and motor components when making statements about activity tolerance.

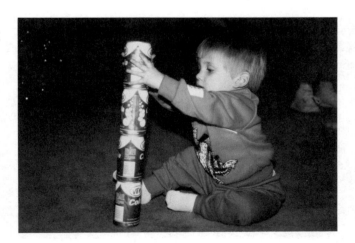

Figure 3-17. Jake demonstrates adequate postural control to interact with objects.

Each component must be identified and measured in terms of time and intensity. For example, how much visual and tactile processing is needed for a child to complete the task of dressing? The methods used for gathering data on activity tolerance are usually from structured observations. The therapist uses skilled observation to record the child's activity choice, duration and context, which can indicate what level of activity is tolerated under what conditions. This type of data is essential for occupational therapists, because it helps form the basis of recommendations for how a task or activity can be adapted. For example, the child in a classroom who is continually distracted by noise in the room, hall, and out the window, might demonstrate a low tolerance for auditory input. Adaptations to reduce auditory distractions can be made, so that the child can then be free to focus his attention on the performance area of schoolwork.

Gross Motor Coordination. As with fine motor skill assessment, qualitative descriptors of gross motor performance are as important to include in a report, as is a standardized test score, or the developmental age in contrast to the chronological age. The qualitative aspects of gross motor coordination include bilateral coordination, the use of mobility, stability and postural control, eye-foot dominance, strength and endurance, motor planning and control. Two norm-referenced tests which offer assessment of the components of gross motor coordination are the *Bruininks-Ostersky Test of Motor Proficiency* (1978), and the *Peabody Developmental Motor Scales* (1974).

Crossing the Midline. The midline is that imaginary line that therapists draw down the middle of a child. Therapists want to know if a child can perform tasks on both sides of that line. Methods used to gather this information can be more formal in nature (i.e., SIPT), or be less formal in nature (structured observation during drawing). Attention is directed not only to whether a child crosses or not, but also to the degree of accuracy and control the child displays on both sides. Crossing the midline is not confined to fine motor tasks, but are also apparent during gross motor tasks.

Laterality. The level of skill demonstrated when performing tasks on the dominant and nondominant sides of the body are interpreted as the degree of laterality. A child who is well lateralized can perform unilateral, bilateral, and reciprocal tasks with ease and accuracy. Disturbances in laterality are typically due to poorly established dominance. Methods of assessing laterality include structured observations of eye and foot dominance, and also the degree of reciprocal and bilateral skill used for task completion. de Quiros & Schrager (1978), provide an excellent discussion of lateralization assessment and intervention.

Bilateral Integration. Bilateral integration means that both sides of the body can work together in a coordinated manner to perform functional tasks that are non-cognitive and automatic. Attention is directed at observing the components of bilateral integration: manipulation and stabilization in the upper extremities, and stability and mobility in the lower extremities. The therapist can gather such data through formal measures, such as the *Bruininks-Oseretsky Test of Motor Proficiency* and/or through structured observations such as sharpening a pencil or riding a bicycle.

Jake and Dani demonstrate different bilateral integration skills in Figures 3-17 and 3-18. Jake is utilizing a symmetrical

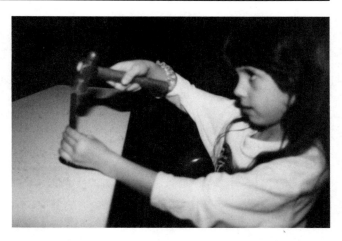

Figure 3-18. Dani demonstrates reciprocal bilateral integration as she hammers.

bilateral movement with his arms, while his lower trunk and legs provide stability. Both arms are engaging in the same movement pattern to complete the stacking task. Dani is utilizing a reciprocal movement pattern, by holding the peg with one hand and moving the hammer with the other hand; this is a more mature bilateral integration task. Children demonstrate their level of bilateral integration in many life tasks such as these.

Praxis. Praxis is the ability to conceive of and plan new motor acts. Occupational therapists are concerned with evaluating praxis in oral motor, fine motor and gross motor areas. In order to have adequate praxis, one must have an adequate hierarchy of those foundations which form the basis of praxis: sensory processing, neuromuscular, and motor components. Praxis can be observed through formal measures, such as the SIPT, and/or through structured observation, such as dressing or preparing a meal. The therapist focuses special attention on the constructional aspect of praxis, such as in putting a puzzle together so that all the pieces fit, and more sequential praxis, such as catching and throwing a ball or unwrapping a piece of candy.

Jessica demonstrates her praxis ability by combining sensorimotor and cognitive components of performance in Figure 3-19. She is using: a) visual perception skills to watch the liquid in the straw, b) oral motor skills, and somatosensory and proprioceptive feedback to produce an adequate seal around the straw, c) fine motor dexterity to position her left hand to stabilize the straw and provide an air valve at the tip, d) postural control to stabilize the head, neck, and upper arm and, e) oral motor, fine motor, visual motor, and somatomotor praxis and problem-solving skills to obtain liquid from the container, hold it in the straw, bring it to her mouth, release it from the straw and swallow it. Complex tasks, such as this one, are routinely accomplished by typical children, but are extremely difficult for children with special needs. Skilled observation of children's natural exploratory and experimental activities can provide a wealth of information. For example, a child could have difficulty with the task Jessica demonstrates, for any of the reasons listed above. An artful evaluator will be able to isolate the components of performance which interfere with age-appropriate task performance.

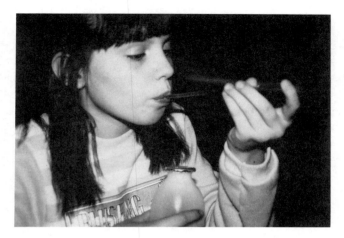

Figure 3-19.   Jessica demonstrates the complexities of praxis ability.

Fine Motor Coordination/Dexterity.   Usually, an initial goal in fine motor assessment is to determine the child's fine motor developmental age, in contrast to the chronological age. The therapist must then also provide additional information about the qualitative aspects of the child's fine motor development. Hand dominance, bilateral and reciprocal use, and prehension patterns are reported. Dexterity, accuracy, and a comparison between bilateral and bi-manual use of materials and tools are relevant to a child's functional performance, and are also described. Attention is directed towards the child's fine motor planning, motor control, and coordination of visually guided fine motor tasks (visual motor integration). Formal tests of fine motor development are listed in Table 3-1.

In Figure 3-20 Michael demonstrates an immature palmar grasping pattern to hold his cracker; he is using the fingertips and palm to secure the cracker, and holds the thumb to the side. This limits his access to the cracker when he tries to take a bite, because it is in an enclosed space in his palm. He would have greater success if he used a pincer grasp, which involve use of the thumb and fingertips to hold objects, because his fingers would taper away from the cracker so he could bite it.

Visual-Motor Integration.   Visual-motor integration is the ability to process visual information and create an accurate motor response. The response may be in the gross motor domain (such as kicking a moving ball), or in the fine motor domain (such as in reproducing geometric shapes, letters or numbers). Attention is focused during assessment on the visual field being used (far, near, table top, floor) and on the degree of motor planning and control (accuracy) that is necessary for successful completion. Methods used to assess visual-motor integration can be in the form of norm- and criterion-referenced tests, such as the *Test of Visual Motor Skills* (TVMS) and the *Brigance Diagnostic Inventory of Early Development*, respectively. It is important for the therapist to remember that the level of integration is the focus of the assessment, when looking at visual-motor skills. In order to address the level of visual-motor skills, it is wise to separate the visual and motor aspect, so that a clearer contrast can be made when vision and motor responses are combined. For example, two children who receive the same scores on

the *Beery Test of Visual Motor Integration*, may demonstrate different behaviors that affect their visual-motor skills. One child may reverse or incorrectly arrange the forms (problem with visual component); while the other child understands the direction and arrangement of the form, but reproduces it with fragmented lines that do not connect (problem with the motor component). Both children received the same score, but for very different reasons.

Examples of the skilled observations that might be made regarding visual-motor integration are provided in Figures 3-21 and 3-22. Jake watches his hand making marks on the page, and the marks are age-appropriate, but several other observations enrich these findings. He provides himself with a wide base of support by spreading his legs apart while sitting, and by propping himself with his left hand to learn forward over the paper. He uses a gross grasp on the pen, limiting his control over the writing instrument. Jamie, in Figure 3-22, utilizes a pincer grasp, increasing control of the pen, enabling her to create a more detailed drawing. She demonstrates reciprocal arm actions, with her left hand stabilizing the paper as she draws. Trunk control is an unconscious effort as she sits at the table to write; visual monitoring of the drawing task facilitates inclusion of more accurate detail.

Oral-Motor Skills.   Eating and communication are outcomes that are dependent on oral-motor skills. The child must

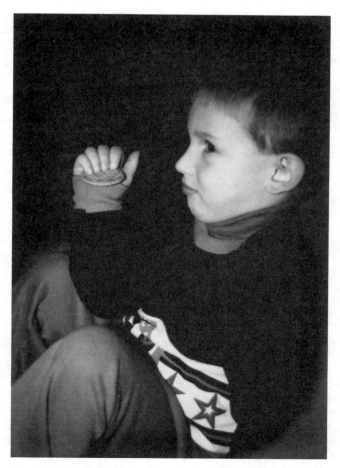

Figure 3-20.   Michael demonstrates a palmar grasp, which is an ineffective strategy for eating a cracker.

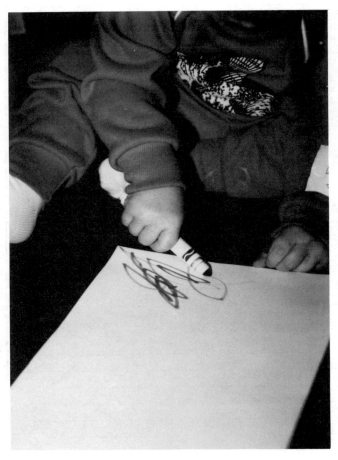

Figure 3-21. Jake demonstrates a gross grasp and emerging visual-motor integration for coloring.

be able to use the oral-motor mechanism efficiently to ingest liquids and foods of various textures, and to use eating utensils. The child must also use oral-motor mechanisms to make consistent and predictable sounds for oral communication. Assessment consists of an analysis of the responsiveness to sensory input (e.g., different textures, temperatures), motor

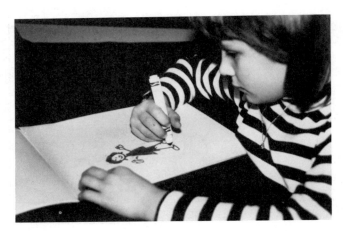

Figure 3-22. Jamie demonstrates age-appropriate visual-motor skills for drawing.

performance (e.g., sucking, chewing, swallowing, self-feeding, and behavioral reactions (e.g., pleasure, aversion) during oral-motor tasks. Norm-referenced assessments are typically not available to assess oral-motor skills. Some criterion-referenced assessment tools, such as *Developmental Programming for Infants and Young Children*, include self-help sections which incorporate feeding and eating skills. Most often, oral-motor skills are assessed by the occupational therapist through quantified observation along with other team members (e.g., *Vulpe Assessment Battery*), and structured functional tasks (e.g., a child eating the noontime meal). Figure 3-23 contains an example of a team-oriented feeding clinic evaluation summary form.

Cognitive and Psychosocial Components

In pediatric assessment, it is most common for the occupational therapist to contribute supportive data on the cognitive and psychosocial components of performance. Other professionals, such as the special educators and psychologists, provide the primary data in these areas; intelligence and achievement tests and behavioral checklists are the most common methods used. Refer to *A Therapist's Guide to Pediatric Assessment* by King-Thomas and Hacker (1987), for a review of the major tests. Chapter 16 of this text introduces the primary psychoeducational tests used by these other professionals. The occupational therapist primarily uses skilled observation, interview, and history data to assess functional skills and sensorimotor components which assist in formulating a cognitive and psychosocial impression of the individual. These data are reported to the team for consideration in diagnosis and intervention planning.

In order for the occupational therapist to contribute to the data base of a child's cognitive abilities, a framework of structured observations is necessary. These observations may include how a child learns a novel activity, and the choices made during play.

Level of Arousal/Orientation/Recognition. A child's level of arousal is monitored by internal (central nervous system responsivity) and external variables (stimuli in the environment). Occupational therapists give careful attention to internal and external variables, and the child's response to changes in both or either. A child's ability to orient and recognize environmental stimuli will have a large impact on the assessment outcomes.

Special consideration is given to assessing the state or arousal level of the child during the particular assessment session. Whether the assessment occurs in a one-time situation, or over a period of days, the child's alertness, compliance, ability to participate and cooperate, are all given careful consideration when interpreting the results of any test or evaluation procedures. The kind of behavior the child demonstrated during the assessment is described in the written report. The types of reinforcement and prompts, that might have been necessary to enable the child to complete the tasks are noted. Ultimately, the performance outcome and validity of the test results are weighed in relation to the behavior demonstrated during the assessment. Test scores and performance on specific tasks can be both positively and negatively influenced by a child's behavior on a particular

FEEDING CLINIC EVALUATION

Patient Name _____

Patient Number _____

Testing Date: _____

Birth Date _____

Chronological Age _____

Presenting Problem:
_____

Findings   Recommendations
_____

I.   GROWTH

____   Weight: %

____   Height: %

____   Weight/Height   %

____   Head Circumference: %

____   Previous Growth

____   Data (plotted on)

____   attached growth chart

II.   NUTRITIONAL STATUS

____   Analysis of 4 Day Food Record

____   Caloric Intake:

____   Protein Intake:

____   Identified marginal or

____   deficient intake of

____   specific vitamin(s)

____   and/or mineral(s).

____   Specify:

____   Pertinent Laboratory Findings.

____   Specify:

III.   POSITIONING

____   Head Control:

____   Trunk Control:

____   Extensor or Flexor Pattern:

____   Current Position Utilized for

____   Eating/Feeding

IV.   ORAL MOTOR SKILLS

____   Tactile Sensitivity:

____   Oral Reflexes Present:

____   Oral Structure:

____   Lip Control:

____   Tongue Control:

____   Swallowing:

____   Biting:

____   Chewing:

____   Assessed Oral Developmental Level:

Figure 3-23. Sample feeding evaluation form.

V. SELF-FEEDING SKILLS
_____ Readiness/Ability to Finger Feed:
_____ Readiness/Ability to Use Utensils:
_____ Cup Drinking:

VI. BEHAVIOR
_____ Cues to Indicate Hunger and/or
            Satiation:
_____ Problem Behaviors:

                                    Signatures:

Figure 3-23. *Continued.* Adapted from: *Children's Rehabilitation Unit Feeding Clinic Evaluation Form, University of Kansas Medical Center.*

day. In an evaluation setting relatively free of distractions, where there is exclusive one-on-one interaction with a child, test results may be inflated as compared to performance of similar tasks in a more natural setting. Likewise, a child's apprehensiveness and fears may adversely affect ability to relax and attend to the tasks presented. It is helpful to seek validation from someone who knows the child, such as a parent, caregiver, or teacher, to determine if the behavior that the child exhibited was truly representative of general, overall behavior.

Attention Span. Expectations for adequate attention span for task completion and exploratory play are directly related to the developmental age vs. the chronological age of the child and the environmental opportunities. Attention span is reported for both structured and unstructured situations.

Memory. Data regarding memory can be derived by verbal and motor responses from the child. If the child is incapable of both types of responses, due to a handicapping condition, then accurate reporting of memory is not possible. The therapist considers the various types of memory: short-term, long-term, remote, and recent.

Sequencing. How well a child sequences can be gathered through structured observations of activity and through task analysis. For example, in an imaginative play situation where a child is playing house, the therapist's attention could focus on which tasks precede others, and how the child organizes the progression of interactions. Breaking down the components of shoe-tying through tasks analysis, requiring a child to follow a pre-ordered series of steps to reach successful completion of the task, is an example of a structured observation opportunity.

Categorization/Concept Formation. A child's ability to categorize information and form concepts directly relates to developmental/chronological age. For example, the concept of time is not understandable to a two-year old, while it is to a five-year old. Likewise, categorizing all four-legged animals as dogs, directly relates to the complexity of a child's mental actions.

Intellectional Operations in Space. This refers to a child's ability to reverse and conserve. For example, a child's ability to understand that $3 + 2 = 5$, and that $5 - 2 = 3$, is the reverse or the same, is dependent upon the developmental age. The therapist observes this skill during tasks in which the directions or demand shift. For example, the child may be *under* the table and not understood that the table is *over* her.

Problem-Solving. Each child displays unique strategies for solving problems. Cause and effect have direct bearing on these strategies, whatever the developmental age. The strategies a child uses to solve functional life problems is valuable in understanding how a child organizes stimuli, and his own particular learning styles.

Jake demonstrates problem-solving skills along with many sensorimotor components of performance in Figure 3-24. He has figured out how to pick up the beads from the floor and place them in the jar. Although he is concentrating on this task, one can also observe his automatic use of a number of other performance components to support his carrying out of the task. He provides himself with a wide base of support for sitting stability; he uses visual perception, visual motor skills, and fine motor dexterity to pick up the beads and release them into the jar. Overflow movements in his right hand may indicate that this is a difficult movement pattern for Jake at this time. Problem-solving skill enables Jake to orchestrate all of these components to tackle this challenging task.

Generalization of Learning. Occupational therapists must never assume that, because a child demonstrated a particular skill in one environment, that the same level of accomplishment will be apparent in another setting or even at another

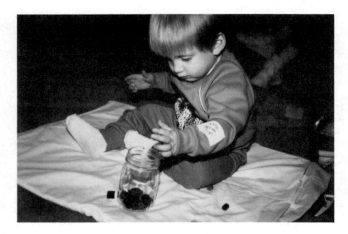

Figure 3-24. Jake demonstrates cognitive abilities during the motor task of placing objects in a container.

time. Attention must be given to environmental cues and prompts which might affect learning. For example, a child may be able to self-feed at school, but at home does not show the same level of self-feeding. Identification of all the parameters which affect skill acquisition and demonstration are considered.

Integration and Synthesis of Learning. This involves how a child applies strategies learned previously to solve future learning experiences. For example, a child progresses from rote recall of the alphabet, to visual identification and sound reproduction of the letters, to combining the letters to form words and read. The hierarchy necessary for integration and synthesis of learning to occur is integral in predicting appropriate future levels of expectations of learning.

Psychosocial Skills and Psychological Components

The pediatric occupational therapist also contributes information about the integrity of the psychosocial systems. The therapist uses skilled observation, history taking, interviewing and functional skills assessment in context to obtain this data.

Roles, Values, Interests. The roles a child is exposed to and directly experiences affect, not only the values and interests that are demonstrated, but also the degree of normal development. Different cultures, creeds, and religions influence such formation and are considered as important contexts for behaviors observed during the evaluation. For example, independence in self feeding for a toddler may not be important in some cultures, thus the toddler does not have the opportunity to demonstrate that skill.

Initiation and Termination of Activity. This is directly related to the child's motivational level and self control. Intrinsic as well as extrinsic motivation are addressed in the data gathering process. Children who have a difficult time initiating activities may have poor arousal or may display signs of depression.

Self Concept. If a child's self concept is impaired, the entire functional ability to perform in all areas of work, play,

leisure, and self care is impacted. Assessment includes overt and subtle expressions of self concept. The *Piers-Harris Assessment of Self Concept* (1984), is one rating scale that offers quantified measures of self concept.

Social Conduct/Conversation/Self-Expression. Social conduct, conversation, and self-expression are all relevant to a particular environment, and are judged in a particular environmental context. Acting out behaviors, as well as behaviors that represent compliance are noted. A child's conversation will often reflect a level of self concept. Additionally, conversation may be used as an escape from task performance. For example, a child who has significant motor planning difficulties may use conversation as an alternative coping strategy, in order to avoid the constructional tasks.

Self Management Coping Skills/Time Management/Self Control. Management of stress, conflict, joy, attention, and affection will add to the total picture of a child. Time management skills across a child's various life environments provide valuable data that correspond with self control and coping skills.

Additional Assessment Factors

Assessment of Contextual Variables

Functional performance takes place within an environmental context which includes the setting, environmental and age level demand, pertinent history, objects, and people. The occupational therapist recognizes that these variables can have a significant impact on performance outcomes, and so addresses these variables in the comprehensive assessment. Skilled observation, interviews, and history taking provide data about the context of performance.

History

Information regarding a child's history is typically obtained by parental, caregiver, or teacher reports; reviews of records from a medical or school file may also be included. Depending upon the age of the child, birth histories regarding prenatal, perinatal and postnatal status are helpful in adding to a database. Knowledge of family characteristics can also be useful in completing the history. This background information helps to establish a baseline from which recommendations can be built. A developmental history regarding the child's acquisition of major milestones, temperament, interactional skills, and play behaviors are considered. If the child is in a school system, information regarding academic performance, as it relates to functional skills and organizational behavior, are carefully considered. A sample history form is depicted in Figure 3-7.

Environmental/Ecological Assessment

Components to consider, when focusing on assessment of the environment, include accessibility and expectations for function in a particular environment. For example, if a child with cerebral palsy is to be mainstreamed into the regular classroom, adaptations for wheelchair space and placement of materials may be needed, in order for this child to participate in classroom activities.

Both the testing environment itself and the environment in which the child resides are assessed as having an affect on the child's performance. This may include the family home, or the home of an extended family member, or caregiver in a day care setting. *The Home Observation for Measurement of the Environment (HOME)* (Caldwell & Bradley, 1978) measures the content, quality and responsiveness of home environments. The relationship of the child with the other members in the various environments are considered, as expectations for performance and behavior environments vary greatly. For example, expectations and resulting behavior of the child who is at a day care center could be completely different in the family home. The family and/or caregiver of the child are assessed in terms of the inability to provide social, emotional, physical, and financial resources. Additionally, the values and ethics of a particular family must always be considered and respected. An adequate family and environmental assessment cannot be overlooked, as this information is relevant to the philosophical base of occupational therapy: function is adaptive and relative. This type of assessment may sometimes be called an ecological assessment. Ecological assessment is defined as viewing the environment and the child as a single entity (Milliken & Buckley, 1983). This concept has merit, however, it should not be oversimplified, as the interplay between a child and the many environments that are encountered during a single day, or single week, are dynamic in nature, and change over time. This must be considered in the assessment process so that the true impact of performance can be more realistically measured. A sample ecological assessment for a preschooler at snack time is provided in Figure 3-25.

ASSESSMENT STRATEGIES FOR EVALUATIONG DIFFERENT DIAGNOSTIC CATEGORIES

Even though each child is a different, unique individual, there are particular characteristics that are helpful to consider when evaluating a child with a particular diagnosis. The following text illustrates some basic considerations.

Developmental Delay

Often a referral for a child described as "developmentally delayed," is for a child of preschool age and younger. The diagnostic category of developmental delay is generic in nature, and really only tells the examiner that the child is developing in a way that is either different, or slower than most children. Regardless of the reason, the assessment is likely to be with a child who is a baby, toddler, or preschooler. Approaching a young child with confidence is essential. Young children are fearful or shy of strangers, and may need additional coaxing to make them comfortable while establishing rapport. It is important that you not only tell young children what you want them to do, but also show them. Because their attention span is usually very short, it is likely that you will be repeating items. It is beneficial to engage the parent or caregiver in demonstrating or assisting with test items when assessing infants who cannot respond to verbal in-

structions or demonstrations. Because younger children have a shorter attention span, and fatigue easier, it is wise to limit whatever tools that you use to approximately 20–30 minutes; or if this is not possible, to break the testing up over a period of sessions. Children in this age and diagnostic category usually will respond to a high contrast approach. For example, use a different tone of voice so that directions are given more in the nature of play.

Learning Disability

A child classified as learning disabled will very often either be impulsive in responses, or be very slow to respond, perhaps because of uncertainty about the directions or the answer. Additional time may be allotted during a testing session to help alleviate some inherent difficulties that this type of child may have. Additionally, learning disabled children may have motor control or sensory processing difficulties that interfere with task completion. Observations are made during the assessment process as to the particular difficulty that the child is experiencing. For example, if a child who has motor planning difficulties has a great deal of difficulty completing test items that require motor planning, it may be useful to rearrange the test so that these items are given toward the end of the session. This would lessen fatigue and frustration levels. If the child has auditory processing difficulties, and many verbal directions are required, it may be helpful to combine gestural cues with a minimal amount of verbal instruction. Often it is helpful to observe a child with learning disabilities in other environments, rather than in an isolated testing session, to ascertain some of the functional life tasks that interfere with function.

Behavior Disorder

Children who are classified as behavior disordered, or emotionally disturbed, require different kinds of assessment strategies. These children tend to be difficult to motivate or may be non-compliant. Extra patience on the part of the examiner helps to set the tone for the assessment. Many children with these diagnostic classifications do not perform well in an evaluation setting where they perceive the examiner to be an authority figure. A useful strategy might be to select performance activities where fewer interactions between the therapist and child are required. This child needs to perceive the therapist as an information gatherer rather than an authority figure.

Autism

Children with autism present inherent challenges to examiners because of their difficulty in establishing social relationships and communication skills. These children cannot focus on relevant or meaningful stimuli such as particular testing items. The usual methods of positive reinforcement, such as eye contact, smiling, and hand holding, may not be interpreted by the autistic child as effective reinforcement measures. It is necessary to gain information, prior to evaluating any child diagnosed as autistic, regarding a preferred mode of communication; however, if that information is unavailable, it is useful to use a combination of short, slow,

Ecologically Based Individualized Adaptation Inventory

Environment: Classroom snack time area   **Activity:** Eating snack, drinking juice

Plan				Observation		
A Nonhandicapped Toddler Inventory	An Inventory of Beth	Skills Beth Probably Acquire	Skills Beth May Not Acquire	Adaptation Possibilities	Assessment	Daily Plan
Move to snack area	Cannot get to table by self	Can learn to walk		Adult can assist by using facilitation	Beth walked well when facilitation at hips was used.	Teacher will fade assistance as demonstrated by therapist. Aim for walking well with one hand held within a month
Position self at table	Cannot get chair out to sit down	Can learn to get chair out; rotate to sit		Adult can assist with pulling chair out & facilitating rotation to sit	She pulled out chair with hand over hand; rotated & sat with facilitation from trunk.	Fade assistance in hand over hand for pulling chair; aim for pulling w/o increased tone in arms; teacher will fade facilitation for rotating to sit as demonstrated by therapist.
Take utensils when passed out	Can grasp large items					Beth will take utensils by self
Take food when passed out	Can grasp large items (cookies) but not small pieces		May not learn to grasp very small items	Try small toddler fork for small pieces or only give large finger foods.	Fork worked with "stabbable" foods.	Use toddler fork
Hold cup for liquid to be poured into	Cup is held sideways	Can learn to hold cup straight		Use cup with two handles	Beth held cup sides with hands through handles	Use two-handled cup.
Eat food	Can finger feed					Beth will finger feed by self
Drink liquid	Can drink but not hold cup to mouth	Can learn to hold cup		Adult assistance to facilitate cup to mouth pattern	Minimal help was needed to raise cup to mouth	Fade assistance to verbal cues "pick up cup" to no cues.
Request more if desired	Vocalizes for more		May not learn to talk	Use picture communication board during snack	A picture board with cup & correct food was used when prompted "Do you want more?" She vocalized at same time	Teacher will make picture board each day to include cup and correct food. Place board in front of Beth and watch for her to use spontaneously. If she does not indicate that she wants more, verbally prompt. Use magnetic stove board & magnet pictures. Reinforce all joint points and vocalizations.

Figure 3-25. Sample ecological assessment for a preschooler at snack time. Baumgart, D., Brown, L., Pumpian, I., Nisbet, J., Ford, A., Sweet, M., Messina, R. & Schroeder, J. (1982). Principle of partial participation and individualized adaptations in educational programs for severely handicapped students. The Journal of The Association for the Severely Handicapped, 7 (2), 17–27. Used with permission.

verbal directions with simple gestures. Therapists can become frustrated with children diagnosed as autistic, because they are not able to complete test items in the usual format. Formal, standardized assessment is not applicable to this population; the therapist may have to rely on structured observations across different environments in order to establish a data base. It is essential that functional outcomes be emphasized with these children.

Mental Retardation

Children who are classified as educably mentally retarded, typically will perform better on standardized testing that involves simple verbal instructions. It is essential that adaptive behavior be assessed in relation to various life environments. For example, the therapist would want to determine whether the child demonstrates the same limitation at school, and at home. Criterion-referenced tools are useful for this population, as they assist in program planning and provide outcome measures.

For children who are classified as trainably mentally retarded, assessment tools that are very concrete and performance-oriented are selected. Verbal directions are kept at a minimum and life skills, rather than academic skills, are emphasized. Prerequisite skills are useful, as long as they are age compatible. For example, working on shoe tying, or other bilateral manipulative skills, may be useful for a child under eight years old. However, there comes a time when that type of bilateral manipulative skill can best be met through adaptive measure such as velcro shoes, thus allowing the focus to be placed on acquiring skills in age-appropriate life tasks.

Children who are classified as severely retarded are oftentimes also severely multiply handicapped. They may or may not be ambulatory, and adaptive equipment may be a focus of assessment. Functional daily life skills are the priority for assessment and intervention.

SUMMARY

The purpose of an assessment is to gather information on a child which reflects best performance. The process for gathering this information is a challenging task that requires an examiner skilled in interpersonal relationships and testing mechanics. A broad based knowledge of available instruments is important in selecting the appropriate tool to fit the particular characteristics of a child. A format for inclusion of various areas to assess can be outlined in Occupational Therapy Uniform Terminology. Tests can enrich a therapist's understanding of a child, and help to plan a starting point for intervention, but are only one source of information for therapists. Person, environment and activity assessment create a total picture of the child within appropriate contexts.

EXPAND YOUR NEWLY ACQUIRED KNOWLEDGE

1. Design a form which would allow you to assess the contextual variables in a family's home. Be sure to remember space, person and object variables as you design your form.

2. Formulate an assessment plan for a six-year-old child who demonstrates perceptual difficulties in school and on his ball team. Include formal evaluations, informal evaluations, skilled observational techniques and interview strategies to ensure that you have completed a comprehensive assessment.

3. Compare and contrast the assessment strategies that you would design for a three year and an eight year old who both come to the occupational therapist with referral complaints of hyperactivity, distractibility, low impulse control and short attention span.

References

American Occupational Therapy Association, Inc. (1986). *Reference manual of the official documents of the American Occupational Therapy Association, Inc.* Rockville, MD: Author.

American Occupational Therapy Association, Inc. (1987). *Guidelines for occupational therapy services in school systems.* Rockville, MD: Author.

American Occupational Therapy Association, Inc. (1989). *Guidelines for occupational therapy in school systems* (2nd Ed.). Rockville, MD: Author.

Ames, L. B., Gillespie, C., Haines, J., & Ilg, F. L. (1986). *Gesell preschool test for evaluating motor, adaptive, language, and personal-social behavior in children ages 2½ to 6.* Rosemont, NJ: Programs for Education, Inc.

Arends, T. & Clark, G. (1989). *Iowa Pediatric Special Interest Group Needs Survey.* Iowa Pediatric Special Interest Group Newsletter.

Ayres, A. J. (1980). *Southern California Sensory Integration Tests, Revised.* Los Angeles: Western Psychological.

Ayres, A. J. (1987). *Sensory integration and the child.* Los Angeles: Western Psychological.

Ayres, A. J. (1988). *Sensory Integration and Praxis Test.* Los Angeles: Western Psychological.

Barnes, M., Crutchfield, C., & Heriza, C. (1977). *The neurophysiological basis of patient treatment, Volume II: Reflexes in motor development.* Atlanta: Stokesville Publishing Company.

Baumgart, D., Brown, L., Pumpian, I., Nisbet, J., Ford, A., Sweet, M., Messina, R., & Schroeder, J. (1982). Principle of partial participation and individualized adaptations in educational programs for severely handicapped students. *The Journal of the Association for the Severely Handicapped, 7*(2), 17–27.

Bayley, N. (1969). *Bayley scales of infant development: Birth to two years.* New York: Psychological.

Beery, K. & Buktenica, N. (1967). *Beery-Buktenica developmental test of visual-motor integration.* Cleveland, OH: Modern Curriculum Press.

Berk, R. A. & DeGangi, G. A. (1983). *Degangi-Berk test of sensory integration.* Los Angeles: Western Psychological Services.

Bernstein, L. & Bernstein, R. S. (1985). *Interviewing: A guide for health professionals, 4th edition.* East Norwalk, CN: Prentice-Hall.

Brazelton, T. B. (1984). *Neonatal behavior assessment scale, 2nd Edition.* Philadelphia: J. B. Lippincott Co.

Brigance, A. H. (1978). *Brigance diagnostic inventory of early development.* MA, Curriculum Associates.

Bruininks, R. H. (1978). *Bruininks-Oseretsky test of motor proficiency.* Circle Pines, MN: American Guidance Service.

Bruininks, R., Woodcock, R., Weatherman, R., & Hill, B. (1984). *Scales of Independent Behavior: Woodcock-Johnson psychoeducational battery, Part 4.* Allen, TX: DLM Teaching Resources.

Caldwell, B. M. & Bradley, R. H. (1978). Home Observation for Measurement of the Environment. Little Rock: University of Arkansas, Center for Child Development & Education.

Campbell, S. K. (1985). Measurement in developmental therapy: Past, present, and future. *Physical and Occupational Therapy in Pediatrics, 9*(1), 1–10.

Carver, R. P. (1972). Reading tests in 1970 versus 1980: Psychometric versus edumetric. *Reading Teacher, 26,* 299–302.

Chandler, L. S., Andrews, M. S. & Swanson, M. W. (1980). *Movement assessment of infants.* Rolling Bay, WA: Movement Assessment of Infants Publisher.

Colarusso, R. P. & Hammill, D. d. (1972). *Motor free visual perception test (MVPT)*. San Rafael, CA: Academic Therapy Publications.

de Quiros, J. B. & Schrager, O. L. (1978). *Neuropsychological fundamentals in learning disabilities*. San Rafael, CA: Academic Therapy Publications.

D'Eugenio, D. & Moersch, M. (Ed.) (1981). *Developmental Programming for Infants and Young Children*. (Vols 4 & 5) Ann Arbor, MI: The University of Michigan Press.

Deitz, J. C. (1989). Reliability. *Physical and Occupational Therapy in Pediatrics, 9*(1), 125–147.

Dunn, W. W. (1989). Validity. *Physical and Occupational Therapy in Pediatrics, 9*(1), 149–168.

Dunn, W. & Gray, B. (1988). Managing occupational therapy in rural education (M.O.R.E.) initial findings. *Proceedings of the Eighth Annual ACRES National Rural Special Education Conference*.

Erhardt, R. P. (1982). *Developmental Hand Dysfunction*. Laurel, MD: RAMSCO Publishing Co.

Folio, R. & Dubose, R. F. (1974). *Peabody developmental motor scales (Revised Experimental Edition)*. Nashville, TN: George Peabody College for Teachers.

Furuno, S., O'Reilly, L., Hosaka, C. M., Inatsuka, T. T., Allman, T. L. & Zeisloft, B. (1979). *Hawaii early learning profile*. Palo Alto, CA: VORT Corp.

Gardner, M. F. (1982). *Test of visual-perceptual skills (non-motor)*. Seattle, WA: Special Child Publications.

Gardner, M. F. (1986). *Test of visual-motor skills*. San Francisco: Children's Hospital of San Francisco.

Gilfoyle, E. M. (1981). *Training: Occupational therapy educational management in schools*. Rockville, MD: American Occupational Therapy Association.

Golin, A. K. & Ducanis, A. J. (1981). *The Interdisciplinary Team*. Rockville, MD: Aspen Publishers.

King-Thomas, L. & Hacker, B. J. (1987). *A therapist's guide to pediatric assessment*. Boston, MA: Little Brown and Co.

LeMay, D. W., Griffin, P. M. & Sanford, A. R. (1977). *Learning accomplishment profile-diagnostic edition (LAPD)*. Winston-Salem, NC: Kaplan Press.

Lewko, J. H. (1976). Current practices in evaluating motor behavior of disabled children. *American Journal of Occupational Therapy, 30*(7), 413–419.

Maurer, P., Barris, R., Bonder, B. & Gillette, N. (1984). Hierarchy of competencies relating to the use of standardized instruments and evaluation techniques by occupational therapists. *American Journal of Occupational Therapy, 38*(12), 803–804.

McGourty, L., Foto, M., Marvin, J., Smith, N., Smith, R., & Kronsnoble, S. (1989). *Uniform terminology for occupational therapy—Second edition*. Rockville, MD: American Occupational Therapy Association.

Montgomery, P. & Connolly, B. (1987). Norm-referenced and criterion-referenced tests used in Pediatrics and application to task analysis of motor skill. *Physical Therapy, 67*(12), 1873–1876.

Milliken, R. K. & Buckley, J. J. (1983). *Assessment of multi-handicapped and developmentally disabled children*. Rockville, MD: Aspen Systems.

Nihira, K., Foster, R., Shellhaas, M., & Leland, H. (1974). *American Association on Mental Deficiency Adaptive Behavior Scale, Revised Edition*. Washington, DC: American Association on Mental Deficiency.

Phares, E. J. (1984). *Clinical psychology: Concepts methods and profession (Revised edition)*. Homewood, IL: Dorsey Press.

Piers, E. V. (1984). *Piers-Harris children's self-concept scale. Revised Manual*. Los Angeles: Western Psychological Services.

Sanford, A. R. & Zelman, J. G. (1981). *Learning accomplishment profile, revised edition (LAP-R)*. Salem-Winston, NC: Kaplan Press.

Sattler, J. M. (1988). *Assessment of children*. (3rd Ed.) San Diego, CA: Jerome M. Sattler.

Sattler, J. M. (1982). *Assessment of children's intelligence and special abilities, 2nd ed*. Boston, MA: Allyn and Bacon.

Schafer, D. S. & Moresch, M. S. (Eds.) (1981). *Developmental programming for infants and young children*. (Vols 1–3). Ann Arbor, MI: University of Michigan Press.

Sparrow, S., Balla, D. & Ciechetti, D. (1984). *Vineland adaptive behavior scales*. Circle Pine, MN: American Guidance Service.

Thorndike, R. L. & Hagen, E. P. (1977). *Measurement and evaluation in psychology and education, 4th edition*. New York: Wiley Publishing.

Vulpe, S. (1977). *Vulpe assessment battery (2nd Edition)*. Dawnsview, Ontario: National Institute on Mental Retardation.

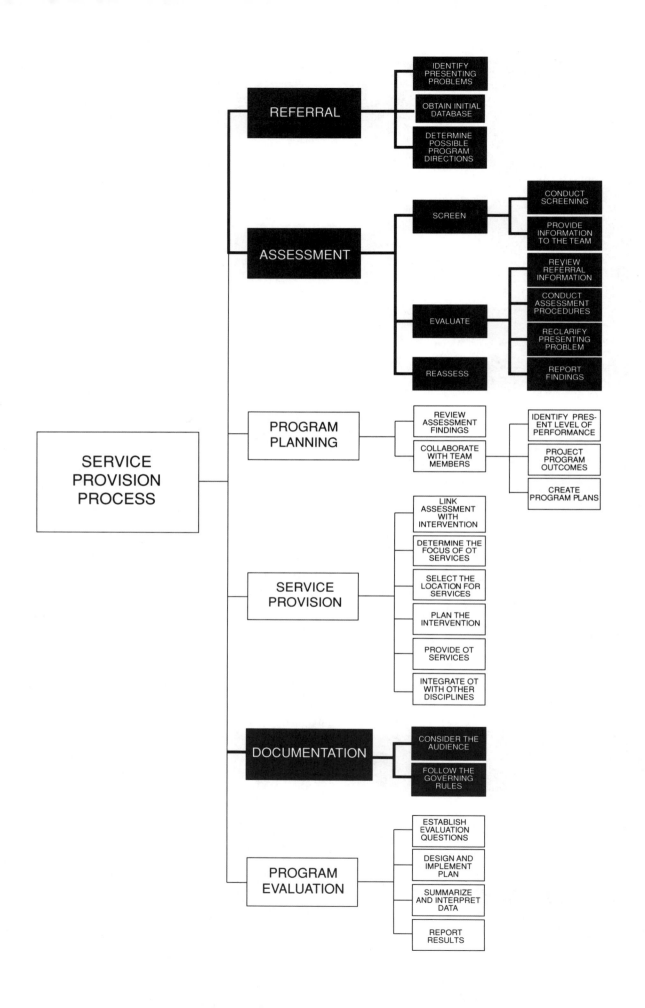

CHAPTER 4

Application of Assessment Principles

Winnie Dunn, PhD, OTR, FAOTA
Patti Oetter, MA, OTR/L, FAOTA

"The results of the assessment need to be closely interrelated, whenever possible, with treatment and reme-diation programs designed to meet the needs of the developing child. Our evaluations need to go beyond the mere presentation of test data. Data are important, but without interpretation they remain cold, sterile figures lying about like a corpse. The findings must be given a living body by including interpretations, diagnoses, and, where possible, suggestions for treatment and remediation." Sattler, 1982

The assessment process enables professionals to deter-mine a child's and family's needs. The specific kind of as-sessment is derived from the needs expressed by the referral source. The referral sources (e.g., family, physician, teacher, speech or language pathologist, physical therapist, psychol-ogist, social worker, counselor, public health nurse, attorney) are as varied as the questions prompting the referral. Chapter One discusses the referral process in depth.

Prior to conducting an assessment, it is important to gain access to relevant information from those people who have the most contact with the child. Parents, foster parents, day care workers, extended family members, baby sitters, and teachers often have the most realistic picture of the child's abilities. There are a number of formats for obtaining this information; Chapter Three provides several good examples (Figures 3-3, 3-4, 3-7, and 3-12). In many settings, primary caretakers and others are encouraged to be an integral part of the assessment, interpretation, and program planning process. Their comments can be extremely helpful in deter-mining a general focus for the assessment, and can also validate or refute performance during the assessment. The process of matching assessment data with other observa-tions prevents misdiagnosis, builds trust and confidence be-tween families and professionals, and results in programming that balances emphasis on strengths and needs.

The therapist's work setting (hospital, private practice, pub-lic or private school or program) will dictate specific guidelines regarding what evaluation tools may be used, and/or what questions may be addressed by the occupational therapist. For example, in some cases the physical therapist may as-sess gross motor development, muscle strength, joint range of motion and/or the need for making, revising, or adjusting ankle foot orthoses (AFO's), inhibitive casts, crutches, walk-ers, braces, and wheelchairs. The speech/language pathol-ogist may assess oral motor skills, feeding, and/or respiratory function related to eating and speech. The cognitive assess-ment may include tests of visual perception, visual motor skills, adaptive behavior/self help skills, developmental his-tory and/or gross and fine motor development. The physician may take a complete developmental history, including an adaptive behavior scale, and may assess muscle tone, re-

flexes, subtle neurological signs and general motor devel-opment. Although the occupational therapist is also qualified to evaluate many of these areas, it is important to determine the expectations of one's specific agency.

This chapter provides several case examples which illus-trate six different therapists' methods of approaching the oc-cupational therapy assessment process. Each case has a unique referral source, referral problems, and needs, which must be addressed in individualized ways. Furthermore, the variety of therapist styles illustrate that there are many ways to apply effective occupational therapy assessment princi-ples. Table 4-1 summarizes the case information; the children are generally presented in chronological order by their ages, when they were initially referred for occupational therapy services. Chapter seven provides the program plans and sample intervention strategies on these same cases.

CASE#1—DAVID

Pre-assessment process

Referral. David was referred to a private practice occupational therapist by the pediatrician at four months of age because of unexplained chronic irritability.

This particular private practice group included occupational therapy, physical therapy and speech/language pathology. The case was assigned to an occupational therapist with expertise in sensory integration. Following a medical release from the parents, the therapist contacted the pediatrician for more detailed referral information. The pediatrician provided a brief synopsis of the baby's history.

History. David was born at term, weighing six pounds, eight ounces with no apparent complications during the labor, pregnancy or delivery. David is the first child of two college graduates who are both involved in their careers. The mother is currently on a one year leave of absence from her professional position. The parents appear to have a healthy and supportive relationship. David's mother first became concerned when he was two to three weeks old. He was "screaming" several hours a day, was inconsolable most of the time and was unable to enjoy or complete feedings. Changes

TABLE 4-1.   Summary of Cases*

Name and Age	Diagnosis	Referral	Setting	Assessment Strategies
David 4 months	Chronic Irritability	Pediatrician	Private practice	History, observation, handling
Clifford 4 weeks	Down Syndrome	Parent group	Public 0–3	History, observation, handling
Andrea 5 mos–7 yrs	Severe cerebral palsy	Orthopedist	Easter Seal	History, clinical observation, referral, developmental skills
Ted 14 mos–13 yrs	Mental retardation/Spastic quadraplegic	Public Health Nurse	Public early intervention to schools	Clinical observation, referral, developmental skills
Jason 22 mos–3 yrs	Premie/Brain damage	Attorney, NICU follow-up	UAF Program	Clinical observation, referral, developmental skills
Richard 27 months	Dyspraxia	Speech/Language pathologist	Private practice	History, sensory motor, developmental skills
James 30 mos–5 yrs	Mild cerebral palsy	Parents	Birth to 5 program	History, clinical observation, referral, developmental skills
Randy 5 yrs 1 mo	Meningitis/Shunt/Seizure	Neurologist	School evaluation	Clinical observation, referral, developmental skills
Peter 6 yrs–8 yrs	Learning disability behavior problem	Regular education teacher	School therapist	Sensory integration, perceptual motor, tests & skilled observations
Joel 6 yrs–13 yrs	Moderate mental retardation/ low tone	Occupational therapist	Private practice	History, clinical observation, referral developmental skills
Ellen 9 yrs	Socioemotional difficulties	Psychologist	University Evaluation Program	Sensory integration, clinical observation, perceptual motor
Tammy 19 years	Moderate mental retardation	Special Education	Community Work Proj.	History, clinical observation, developmental skills, perceptual motor

* The core materials which formed the basis for these case studies were provided by master clinicians. Particular details of some cases have been altered to maintain anonymity for families, to clearly illustrate important points & to provide a wide range of examples for the reader. Please refer to the *Introduction to Contributing Authors* for the therapist's names.

in formula did not help. Subsequent laboratory tests and x-rays suggested no physical reason for David's irritability. There is growing concern on the part of David's father and the physician regarding the stress on David's mother as a result of lack of sleep and little time away from the baby.

Pre-assessment Hypothesis

Chronic irritability and feeding difficulties in the absence of medical problems could indicate poor modulation of sensory input. Since David's irritability was affecting the entire family unit, the therapist determined that both parents should be an integral part of the evaluation process. Since the parents' concern centered around feeding problems, the decision was made that David be seen at the clinic at a regularly scheduled feeding time. One of the goals would be to enhance the feelings of competence on the part of the parents and facilitate positive interactions within the family unit.

Assessment Plan

When the therapist completes a review of the initial data base, then a plan for the assessment can be designed. In David's case, the pediatrician provided significant historical information and discussed family concerns with the therapist in a telephone conversation. The therapist decided to employ several methods to investigate the reasons for irritability, in-

cluding an extensive sensory history, observation of responses to handling, feeding and movement, as well as determination of developmental level in postural and motor skills. David's age (four months), and unpredictable state, necessitated that much of the data would have to be gathered from parent interview and observation of family member interaction.

When taking sensory histories, the following format is suggested: a questionnaire with clear, concise questions, requiring a single answer from multiple options followed by an interview (See Figure 3-12). The questionnaire can be filled out by the parent(s)/primary caretakers, and then the same questionnaire, utilizing open-ended questions, is employed as an interviewing guide. Quality interviewing skills need to be employed when taking a sensory history. This ensures that answers are not defined in the question, parents are not led into inappropriate areas of concern, and spontaneity is not lost. An example might be opening with a general question such as: "Can you describe a typical feeding?"; "How does your baby like you to play with him?"; "What can you do to calm you baby?"; "What kinds of things do you think your baby likes or dislikes?"; etc. As the parent(s) begin to describe typical behaviors, more specific questions may be generated.

It is also important to investigate the perceptions of all parent(s) and primary caretakers, since viewpoints may differ. This may generate positive interaction between the parents,

SENSORY HISTORY
Checklist

Child's Name _____ **David** _____   Person Completing Form _____ **Parents** _____

Date of Birth _____   Referral Source _____ **Pediatrician** _____

Date form completed _____   Therapist _____

CA 4 months

Instructions: Please check the response that best describes your child's behavior. Add any additional comments in the space after each category. If you are unable to comment because you have not observed the behavior, or feel that it's not applicable to your child, please draw a line through all the responses (—). Please do not leave any spaces blank. Use the following key in determining your response.

Key to responses:

1. *always:* when presented with the opportunity, the child responds in this manner every time, 100%.
2. *frequently:* when presented with the opportunity, the child usually responds in this manner, at least 75% of the time.
3. *occasionally:* when presented with the opportunity, the child sometimes responds in this manner, approximately 50% of the time.
4. *seldom:* when presented with the opportunity, the child usually does *not* respond in this manner, less than 25% of the time.
5. *never:* when presented with the opportunity, the child never responds in this fashion; 0% of the time.

Auditory	Always	Frequently	Occasionally	Seldom	Never
1. Responds negatively to unexpected or loud noises (i.e., vacuum cleaner, dog barking)	X				
2. Is distracted or has trouble functioning if there is a lot of noise around	X				
3. Enjoys strange noises/seeks to make noise for noise sake					X
4. Enjoys music				X	
5. Appears to not hear what you say		X			

COMMENTS:

Visual	Always	Frequently	Occasionally	Seldom	Never
1. Expresses discomfort at bright lights (i.e. sunlight through window in car)			X		
2. Happy to be in the dark		X			
3. Looks carefully or intently at objects/people			X		
4. Puts puzzles together easily					NA
5. Hesitates going up or down curbs or steps					NA
6. Gets lost easily					NA
7. Has a hard time finding objects in competing backgrounds (i.e., shoes in a messy room, favorite toy in the "junk drawer")					NA
8. Has trouble staying between the lines when coloring or when writing					NA

COMMENTS:

Figure 4-1. David's sensory history.

Taste/Smell	Always	Frequently	Occasionally	Seldom	Never
1. Deliberately smells objects					X
2. Shows preference for certain smells (List:)				X	
3. Shows preference for certain tastes (List:)			X		
4. Chews/licks on non-food objects					X
5. Craves certain foods (List:)					X

COMMENTS:

Movement	Always	Frequently	Occasionally	Seldom	Never
1. Becomes anxious or distressed when body leaves ground		X			
2. Fears falling or heights		X			
3. Dislikes activities where head is upside down (i.e., somersaults) or rough-housing			X		
4. Avoids climbing, jumping, bumpy or uneven ground					NA
5. Avoids playground equipment or moving toys					NA
6. Rocks unconsciously during other activities (i.e., while watching television)					NA
7. Seeks out all kinds of movement activities (i.e., being whirled by adult, merry-go-rounds, playground equipment, moving toys)					X
8. Takes risks during play (i.e., climbs high into a tree, jumps off tall furniture, etc.)					X
9. Dislikes riding in a car		X			

COMMENTS: Dad thinks Danny enjoys roughhousing—calms him. Mom thinks this has a delayed effect; causing Danny to be more irritible later. Only tolerates upright position-very intolerant of prone.

Body Position (proprioception)	Always	Frequently	Occasionally	Seldom	Never
1. Hangs on other people, furniture, objects		X			
2. Seems to have weak muscles					X
3. Tires easily, especially when standing or holding a particular body position				X	
4. Locks joints (e.g., elbows, knees) for stability			X		
5. Walk on toes					NA

COMMENTS:

Figure 4-1. *Continued.*

Touch	Always	Frequently	Occasionally	Seldom	Never
1. Avoids getting hands "messy" (i.e., in paste, sand, finger paint)					NA
2. Becomes upset when face is washed	X				
3. Expresses distress over having hair cut, combed or washed	X				
4. Expresses distress over being bathed or groomed (i.e., cut finger nails)	X				
5. Prefers long sleeve clothing, sweaters, or jacket even when it's warm				X	
6. Expresses discomfort when people touch; even in friendly hug or pat	X				
7. Expresses discomfort at dental work					NA
8. Displays unusual need for touching certain toys, surfaces or textures					X
9. Is sensitive to certain fabrics; avoids wearing clothes made of them		X			
10. Avoids going bare foot, especially in sand or grass					NA
11. Avoids wearing shoes, loves to be bare-foot		X			

COMMENTS: Hates being cuddled. Hard to hold, even during breast feeding. Can sometimes pat him firmly to calm him down.

Emotional/Social	Always	Frequently	Occasionally	Seldom	Never
1. Uses inefficient ways of doing things		X			
2. Seems to like him/herself				X	
3. Needs more protection from life than other children	X				
4. Has trouble "growing up"					NA
5. Is affectionate with others				X	
6. Is sensitive to criticisms					NA
7. Has definite fears	X				
8. Seems anxious	X				
9. Seems accident-prone					NA
10. Has difficulty tolerating changes in plans and expectations	X				
11. Is stubborn or uncooperative		X			
12. Has temper tantrums	X				
13. Has nightmares (don't know)					

Figure 4-1. *Continued.*

COMMENTS:

Activity Level	Always	Frequently	Occasionally	Seldom	Never
1. Always "on the go"		X			
2. Prefers quiet, sedentary play (i.e., watching television, books, computers)					X
3. Enjoys other children				X	

COMMENTS:

DGC. 1989

Figure 4-1. *Continued.*

thus reducing the anxiety, guilt, or blame surrounding a painful situation. If an objective discussion can be maintained, the process of gathering pertinent information can be therapeutic. A possible result of the objective discussion can be that both parents have a clearer, more common understanding of their child and his needs.

Observations of responses to handling, feeding and movement, from both the therapist and the parent(s)/primary caretakers, are recorded. These observations will include changes in state (ranging from calm to irritable), changes in emotional responses (ranging from joy to fright), changes in postural responses (ranging from decreased to increased tone; flexion to extension; approach to avoidance, etc.), and also what techniques the child utilizes to alter his own state when he finds himself at one or more of these extremes.

Determination of the developmental level includes standardized testing, as well as input from parent(s)/primary caretakers. Due to time limitations, the infant's biobehavioral state, and possible negative response to a stranger, a complete sample of motor behavior may not be obtainable in David's case. It is important to remember that all children respond to and interact with multiple environments in several different ways. The variations in their responses, and the quality of their interaction, lends valuable information to determination of performance variables.

Findings and Interpretation

The evaluation data obtained on David was informal in nature in order to maximize opportunities for David to demonstrate both his best skills and his vulnerabilities to natural stimuli in his environment. A formal evaluation with a child such as David is likely to tap only his vulnerabilities, since the stimuli and the tester would be unfamiliar to him and would, therefore, be threatening. The informal environment also placed David's parents at ease, allowing them to feel comfortable providing ongoing information about their experiences with David, and their knowledge about David's skills and abilities. Multiple sources of information (observations and reports) add validity to the results obtained.

The parents' impression as summarized in the sensory history (Figure 4-1), indicates that David's biobehavioral state is most often very highly aroused, and he is vulnerable to frequent episodes of sensory overload. Sudden touch or movement, position changes, or any noise seem to result in startle responses and intense crying. He is extremely difficult to calm and has few strategies to calm himself (e.g., He does not suck on his fingers, hand or a pacifier). During the observation he made several attempts to get his hands to his mouth but each attempt resulted in a total extension pattern which reflexively moved his hands away from rather than towards his face and mouth. Once calm, the parents know of no specific clues as to how to maintain that calm, or what might "set him off" the next time.

The family's impressions are very important considerations in this case. Although it would be easy for the therapist to verify their observations by providing threatening sensory input, this strategy would not be in the family's best interest. The therapist listens carefully for validation of these behaviors across events reported by the caretakers. It is highly likely that an irritable child such as David will demonstrate these behaviors in the natural course of the time spent with him and his family. You will recall that the evaluation was scheduled at normal feeding time because this was a particularly difficult time for the family. Feeding time did prove to be difficult, and thus provided an opportunity to discuss methods for interrupting the cycle of escalating irritability and for calming him. For example, as David became more irritable, the parents became more tense; as they relived this stressful situation, they were able to recall all the strategies they have tried to calm David. An interview question outside of this context was not a successful strategy to gather this important information. This provided an excellent opportunity for the therapist to gather more information and to point out to the parents that their strategies are not the cause of the problem.

David does not seem to enjoy cuddling, even during breast feeding. He initially settles, begins to squirm, and then arches his back and begins crying. The crying quickly escalates to what the parents describe as "panic screaming." David does quiet, although he remains partially stiff, when held vertically over either parent's

PERFORMANCE AREAS

David — 4 months — PERFORMANCE COMPONENTS	ACTIVITIES OF DAILY LIVING Grooming	Oral Hygiene	Bathing	Toilet Hygiene	Dressing	Feeding and Eating	Medication Routine	Socialization	Functional Communication	Functional Mobility	Sexual Expression	WORK ACTIVITIES Home Management	Care of Others	Educational Activities	Vocational Activities	PLAY OR LEISURE ACTIVITIES Play or Leisure Exploration	Play or Leisure Performance
A. SENSORIMOTOR COMPONENT																	
1. Sensory Integration																	
a. Sensory Awareness						–		–								–	
b. Sensory Processing																	
(1) Tactile						–		–								–	
(2) Proprioceptive						/		/								/	
(3) Vestibular						0		0								0	
(4) Visual																	
(5) Auditory						–		–								–	
(6) Gustatory						–		–								–	
(7) Olfactory																	
c. Perceptual Skills																	
(1) Stereognosis																	
(2) Kinesthesia																	
(3) Body Scheme																	
(4) Right-Left Discrimination																	
(5) Form Constancy																	
(6) Position in Space																	
(7) Visual-Closure																	
(8) Figure Ground																	
(9) Depth Perception																	
(10) Topographical Orientation																	
2. Neuromuscular																	
a. Reflex						–		–								–	
b. Range of Motion																	
c. Muscle Tone						–		–								–	
d. Strength																	
e. Endurance																	
f. Postural Control						–		–								–	
g. Soft Tissue Integrity																	
3. Motor																	
a. Activity Tolerance						–		–								–	
b. Gross Motor Coordination																	
c. Crossing the Midline																	
d. Laterality																	
e. Bilateral Integration																	
f. Praxis																	
g. Fine Motor Coordination/ Dexterity																	
h. Visual-Motor Integration																	
i. Oral-Motor Control																	

/ = Strength
– = Concern
0 = Both a strength and concern

Figure 4-2. Uniform terminology 2—David. *Used with permission. Dunn 1988.*

shoulder, while being bounced and walked. The parents disagree about whether or not David calms to, or enjoys minor roughhousing in the form of firm patting on the back or buttocks, knee bouncing in a supported sitting position, or linear (heel to head) rocking prone over knees. David's father feels that David enjoys these kinds of play. He also feels David maintains a more organized state following these kinds of play. David's mother feels that he has a delayed reaction to these sessions, becoming even more irritable and less consolable an hour or so later.

David objects strenuously when placed on his stomach, and prefers being held and carried with his head in a vertical position. He

PERFORMANCE AREAS

David — PERFORMANCE COMPONENTS	ACTIVITIES OF DAILY LIVING Grooming	Oral Hygiene	Bathing	Toilet Hygiene	Dressing	Feeding and Eating	Medication Routine	Socialization	Functional Communication	Functional Mobility	Sexual Expression	WORK ACTIVITIES Home Management	Care of Others	Educational Activities	Vocational Activities	PLAY OR LEISURE ACTIVITIES Play or Leisure Exploration	Play or Leisure Performance
B. COGNITIVE INTEGRATION AND COGNITIVE COMPONENTS																	
1. Level of Arousal						−		−								−	
2. Orientation						−		−								−	
3. Recognition																	
4. Attention Span						−		−								−	
5. Memory																	
a. Short-term																	
b. Long-term																	
c. Remote																	
d. Recent																	
6. Sequencing																	
7. Categorization																	
8. Concept Formation																	
9. Intellectual Operations in Space																	
10. Problem Solving																	
11. Generalization of Learning																	
12. Integration of Learning																	
13. Synthesis of Learning																	
C. PSYCHOSOCIAL SKILLS AND PSYCHOLOGICAL COMPONENTS																	
1. Psychological																	
a. Roles																	
b. Values																	
c. Interests																	
d. Initiation of Activity																	
e. Termination of Activity																	
f. Self-Concept																	
2. Social																	
a. Social Conduct																	
b. Conversation																	
c. Self-Expression																	
3. Self-Management																	
a. Coping Skills																	
b. Time Management																	
c. Self-Control																	

/ = Strength
− = Concern
0 = Both a strength and concern

Figure 4-2. *Continued.*

goes to sleep only when walked and bounced in a vertical position, but usually wakes and cries immediately when placed in any other position (prone, supine, or sidelying) in his crib. He sleeps for two or three hours when held close to the parent's chest.

Given all of the observations above, the therapist concluded that the tactile, vestibular and auditory input are most difficult for David to process. Tactile system problems are manifested in his difficulty with cuddling and poor tolerance for the nipple and food textures. Vestibular problems are manifested in his intolerance for gravitational stimuli from various body positions (prone and supine), and his rigidity about desiring only the vertical position. His extreme reactions (screaming) to unexpected sounds led to a conclusion of auditory sensitivity. David responded positively to touch-pressure and proprioception, when he calmed to firm patting and holding; he also calmed with some vestibular stimuli while in the vertical position (i.e., bouncing). Figure 4-2 summarizes the strengths and concerns in performance components related to the performance areas of feeding and eating, socialization and play exploration.

> Postural and motor development milestones appear to be within the average range for a four-month-old. However, the quality and organization of movement patterns appears significantly disordered. While David's muscle tone appears to be in the low normal range any attempt at movement results in total extension. His discomfort in prone has prevented development of age appropriate shoulder stability. As a result, his neck is usually in hyperextension, shoulders are elevated and retracted, hands remain fisted most of the time and he is rarely able to bring his hands to his midline or his mouth. David is also having difficulty using his hands to bat at objects, and is not yet looking at his hands.

Children such as David demonstrate many postural and motor signs that can be misread as only postural and motor concerns. These patterns can also be produced when the child responds abnormally to sensory stimuli. Children who are hypersensitive to sensory input frequently withdraw from the environment to minimize contact (flexed positions), or their overreaction leads to frequent and exaggerated movements to alert to each new stimulus as it becomes available (e.g., pushing away or orienting toward stimuli). This leads to an imbalance in overall movement patterns, inhibits development of co-contraction for stability in trunk and limb joints, and prevents development of rotation in both trunk and limbs. In David's case, he is orienting and pushing away so frequently that he has been unable to develop appropriate postural control. The combination of his hypersensitivity to the sensory stimuli that becomes available, and the resulting imbalance in postural reactions, prohibits David from engaging the environment in a goal-directed manner (parents, toys, etc.), which in turn keeps him from developing more advanced motoric, perceptual and cognitive skills, such as playing and eating.

CASE #2—CLIFFORD

Pre-assessment process

> *Referral.* Clifford was referred at the age of four weeks by his mother. A support group for parents of children with Down Syndrome recommended the occupational therapy referral to a publicly funded program for children birth to three years of age. The parents' basic referral question was "How can we enhance Clifford's development, making the best use of our time and continue to meet the needs of our other two children and our marriage?"

During the phone call made to schedule the home visit, a brief history was taken.

> *History.* Clifford is the third child in this family; he has one three-year-old sister and one five-year-old brother. The sister is enrolled in a regular preschool program three mornings a week. The brother is in kindergarten. Both parents are college graduates. The mother has been in the home full time since the birth of the first child. During the sixth month of her pregnancy with Clifford, amniocentesis indicated that the baby had Down Syndrome. The parents were referred to a local support group, and have since become very involved in this organization.

Pre-assessment Hypothesis

The issues raised by this family are common concerns of families. They want to provide a rich environment for the entire family while addressing Clifford's particular needs. Children with Down Syndrome are at risk for developmental delays, and so the therapist will want to focus on possible ways to prevent negative outcomes.

Assessment Plan

Because the questions centered around family as well as child issues, the initial contact was scheduled as a home visit for a Saturday when all family members could be present. The visit would be just prior to a regular feeding time so that Clifford could be observed in several predictable states of alertness, while observing oral motor function, feeding skills and patterns, and postural mechanisms. Informal observation of family interactions could also occur to begin the process of reinforcing family strengths and facilitating a sense of competency.

Findings and Interpretation

The evaluation included both formal and informal assessment. The *Milani-Comparetti Reflex Scale* and the *Peabody Motor Development Scale* were used. Informal assessment was made of passive and active muscle tone, joint stability, response to sensory input, suck/swallow/breathe synchrony and use in feeding, respiration patterns, head control in prone, supine and sitting, functional use of trunk musculature in stability and mobility patterns, visual localization, tracking attention, and convergence, and response to toys presented. Figure 4-3 summarizes the performance strengths and concerns on Clifford.

Clifford was five weeks old when he was seen at home for the evaluation prior to, during, and an hour after a regularly scheduled feeding. Both Mr. and Mrs. B were present as well as Clifford's 3 and 5 year old siblings. It was immediately apparent that the whole family was eager to learn how to play with Clifford in order to enhance his development and "make him happy."

When the therapist arrived, Clifford's diapers were being changed on the living room sofa while both siblings observed and talked to him. Mrs. B wrapped Clifford in a light weight blanket, arms free, and placed him in an infant seat in the corner of the sofa so that his siblings could continue to visit with him. They appeared comfortable in their interaction (cooing, sing-song language, and holding and kissing his hands). Both siblings were appropriately gentle with him. Clifford responded with prolonged gaze and arm movements. His responses encouraged his siblings to continue the interaction for several minutes.

The therapist wanted to be sure that she had the opportunity to observe natural family activities, and so she made no initial attempts to redirect the family upon her arrival During this period, the therapist could reinforce positive strategies, and in this way, establish rapport. Since Clifford was only one month old, it was important to nurture the bonding that was taking place within the family.

During this period, the family demonstrated several positive strategies for positioning Clifford for interaction. For example, wrapping Clifford in a blanket while leaving arms free, and

PERFORMANCE AREAS

Clifford — 4 weeks — PERFORMANCE COMPONENTS	Activities of Daily Living Grooming	Oral Hygiene	Bathing	Toilet Hygiene	Dressing	Feeding and Eating	Medication Routine	Socialization	Functional Communication	Functional Mobility	Sexual Expression	Work Activities Home Management	Care of Others	Educational Activities	Vocational Activities	Play or Leisure Activities — Play or Leisure Exploration	Play or Leisure Performance
A. SENSORIMOTOR COMPONENT																	
1. Sensory Integration																	
a. Sensory Awareness																	
b. Sensory Processing																	
(1) Tactile																	
(2) Proprioceptive						−		−								−	−
(3) Vestibular						−		−								−	−
(4) Visual						/		/								/	/
(5) Auditory						/		/								/	/
(6) Gustatory																	
(7) Olfactory																	
c. Perceptual Skills																	
(1) Stereognosis																	
(2) Kinesthesia																	
(3) Body Scheme																	
(4) Right-Left Discrimination																	
(5) Form Constancy																	
(6) Position in Space																	
(7) Visual-Closure																	
(8) Figure Ground																	
(9) Depth Perception																	
(10) Topographical Orientation																	
2. Neuromuscular																	
a. Reflex						−		−								−	−
b. Range of Motion						−		−								−	−
c. Muscle Tone						−		−								−	−
d. Strength																	
e. Endurance																	
f. Postural Control						−		−								−	−
g. Soft Tissue Integrity																	
3. Motor																	
a. Activity Tolerance						−		−								−	−
b. Gross Motor Coordination																	
c. Crossing the Midline																	
d. Laterality																	
e. Bilateral Integration																	
f. Praxis																	
g. Fine Motor Coordination/ Dexterity																	
h. Visual-Motor Integration																	
i. Oral-Motor Control																	

/ = Strength
− = Concern
0 = Both a strength and concern

Figure 4-3. **Uniform terminology 2—Clifford.** *Used with permission. Dunn, 1988.*

PERFORMANCE AREAS

Clifford / PERFORMANCE COMPONENTS	ACTIVITIES OF DAILY LIVING Grooming	Oral Hygiene	Bathing	Toilet Hygiene	Dressing	Feeding and Eating	Medication Routine	Socialization	Functional Communication	Functional Mobility	Sexual Expression	WORK ACTIVITIES Home Management	Care of Others	Educational Activities	Vocational Activities	PLAY OR LEISURE ACTIVITIES Play or Leisure Exploration	Play or Leisure Performance
B. COGNITIVE INTEGRATION AND COGNITIVE COMPONENTS																	
1. Level of Arousal						−		−								−	−
2. Orientation						/		/								/	/
3. Recognition						/		/								/	/
4. Attention Span																	
5. Memory																	
a. Short-term																	
b. Long-term																	
c. Remote																	
d. Recent																	
6. Sequencing																	
7. Categorization																	
8. Concept Formation																	
9. Intellectual Operations in Space																	
10. Problem Solving																	
11. Generalization of Learning																	
12. Integration of Learning																	
13. Synthesis of Learning																	
C. PSYCHOSOCIAL SKILLS AND PSYCHOLOGICAL COMPONENTS																	
1. Psychological																	
a. Roles																	
b. Values																	
c. Interests																	
d. Initiation of Activity																	
e. Termination of Activity																	
f. Self-Concept																	
2. Social																	
a. Social Conduct						/		/								/	/
b. Conversation																	
c. Self-Expression																	
3. Self-Management																	
a. Coping Skills						/		/								/	/
b. Time Management																	
c. Self-Control																	

/ = Strength
− = Concern
0 = Both a strength and concern

Figure 4-3. *Continued.*

placing him in a partially upright position in the infant seat, enabled Clifford to see what others were doing, and make initial attempts at socialization with siblings. Mother recognized the importance of sibling interactions with this action. Siblings interacted visually and tactually with Clifford, and he responded positively to these overtures.

Then the therapist asked the parents about their current needs. The main question centered around feeding: How long should it take to feed him?, How can we keep him awake long enough to complete feedings?, Why does his suck seem so weak?" Other questions were more general and reflected a need to know what to expect in the next several months in terms of his motor development. They also wanted an idea of what an occupational therapist could do to promote development.

It is important to reclarify the referral question with the family during the assessment. Many times there are other concerns that have not been clearly expressed in a brief statement of the problem. This allows the therapist to frame all plans and recommendations within the proper context, and at a level that the family understands. With very young children such as Clifford, the therapist may identify concerns that the family does not presently recognize. The therapist must take cues from family members' comments to determine whether it is appropriate to address additional areas of concern outside of the family's expressed needs.

The questions raised by Clifford's parents indicate that they were focused on both present and future needs. They recognized Clifford's potential to develop many appropriate life skills, and appeared ready to provide an environment that would be enriching for him and the rest of the family. They also expressed appropriate anxiety over their ability to maintain family integrity during this process.

Clifford began to fuss, indicating to the mother that he was ready to eat. Mrs. B suggested this may be his most alert time and the best time to handle and play with him for a few minutes. For the next several minutes a brief evaluation was done of muscle tone, joint stability and a variety of postural mechanisms. Clifford's muscle tone was low, joints hyperextendable, especially at the shoulders and hips. His head control was poor with little attempt being made to right or maintain head in vertical. There was little to no observable attempts to right the head or body when suspended in either supine or prone. Clifford followed a dangling red ring with his eyes but did not turn his head and search for rattle and bell sounds.

It was insightful of the mother to recognize that Clifford would be more likely to demonstrate his movement repertoire at that particular time. Waiting until after the feeding would have been difficult, since Clifford tends to fall asleep. Since the therapist had spent time developing rapport, the mother felt comfortable, allowing the therapist to play with Clifford, even though he was a little fussy.

In order to obtain optimal assessment results and continue developing rapport, the therapist first considered Clifford's level of arousal. Clifford would not be able to cooperate with postural testing if he were too aroused and became upset. Additionally, low muscle tone and poor proximal joint stability are common correlates of Down Syndrome. Poor postural stability and control interfere with the development of head and neck control, and therefore have the potential to limit the amount and type of interactions Clifford will be able to have with toys and people in his environment. Although Clifford is presently demonstrating beginning interactional skills (e.g., visual search), more complex visual and hand manipulation skills may be affected, if postural integrity is not addressed. These areas might also affect mealtime, since postural control, attention, and muscle tone are all necessary correlates of eating.

Clifford did indeed demonstrate low muscle tone, poor proximal stability in the trunk and neck regions. Although an infant Clifford's age would not be expected to sit upright independently, or have complete head control, Clifford is at-risk for problems in these areas due to his medical diagnosis of Down Syndrome.

Then the therapist and mother shifted into feeding activities.

Evaluation of strength of the suck/swallow/breathe synchrony was checked with a finger and with a pacifier. The synchrony was

adequate initially, but deteriorated rapidly. He began breathing through his mouth and started choking after five to six sucking patterns. Clifford's suck was also weak and he was unable to maintain an adequate seal. It took great effort for him to initiate a suck and he tired very quickly.

Clifford's low muscle tone is also affecting eating. His inability to suck and maintain a seal around the nipple are indicators of low muscle tone in the oral motor region; this is a common observation among children with Down Syndrome. This will affect Clifford's eating efficiency, because he won't be able to ingest liquids if he can't establish and maintain adequate pressure. Poor postural control, as noted above, is likely to affect eating as Clifford grows. He will be expected to maintain a sitting posture during eating; activity tolerance is related to low tone, because Clifford must work very hard to produce and maintain even rudimentary movements.

CASE #3—ANDREA

Pre-assessment Process

Referral. Andrea was referred at five months of age by an orthopedic surgeon following a visit at the neonatal follow-up clinic because of stiffness in her arms and legs. She was referred to a private outpatient rehabilitation center that serves children from birth to three years of age.

The outpatient rehabilitation program to which Andrea was referred, is the primary service agent for the hospital NICU followup clinic for patients with a diagnosis of cerebral palsy. The referral was made by the physician over the telephone. Referral paperwork is then completed and sent to the referring physician for a signature, and an intake form is sent to the parents that includes a brief history, a check list of concerns, and a permission-to-evaluate form for signature. In this case, because of Andrea's long hospitalization, the program requested the family's permission to obtain records from the hospital. The following history was compiled by the social worker from the above materials.

History. Andrea is the first of a set of twins born at 30 weeks gestation due to premature rupturing of the membranes. This was a cesarean section birth and Andrea's Apgar scores were one, five, and seven. Andrea remained in the intensive care unit for 12 weeks with the following complications during the hospitalization: high bilirubin, a grade 2 interventricular hemorrhage (IVH), necrotizing enterocolitis, and left metatarsus adductus.

During her five month follow-up clinic visit, the following was noted: increased flexor tone in the left upper extremity, increased extensor tone in both lower extremities, stiffness and asymmetry throughout, head-lag on pull to sit, and increased extension when supported in a standing position. During this clinic visit the orthopedic surgeon and neurologist explained the diagnoses of cerebral palsy to the family.

Pre-assessment Hypothesis

The referral and history suggest that Andrea has multiple and perhaps severe impairments. The stiffness reported with the diagnosis of cerebral palsy suggests that Andrea has spasticity in her muscles. Her early status reports indicate that she was compromised from a very early period. This evaluation will need to focus on reporting present status and documenting her approach to interaction with persons and objects in the environment. It is likely that Andrea and her family will need long term support from the various agencies within the community, so it is important for this initial team assessment to describe her performance thoroughly for future reference.

Assessment Plan

This agency conducts all assessment done for children under two and one-half years of age in an arena style. An arena style assessment includes the family, child and the entire team; all persons gather in a comfortable playroom type of environment. Prior to the evaluation, the social worker conducts a home visit in order to establish a supportive relationship with the family, explain the assessment process, and gather information about the family's current concerns and needs. The social worker then becomes the primary support person for the family throughout the assessment and interpretation processes.

In this particular situation, the occupational therapist's responsibilities are to facilitate positioning and handling, either personally or through a family member, observe the child through other portions of the evaluation, in order to report quality of movement, response to stimulation and approach to the tasks; and stimulate Andrea to perform age appropriate functional actions.

Because this family had experienced long term hospitalization for this child, they had already established a network with other families of children who had been in the NICU. They were already familiar with the implications of the diagnosis of cerebral palsy. The information that would be most important to the family would be how cerebral palsy was compromising Andrea's development, as well as what types of intervention strategies would be most useful in optimizing her development.

Findings and Interpretation

A center-based formal assessment was conducted when Andrea was seven months old. A team consisting of an occupational therapist, physical therapist, speech/language pathologist, and social worker participated in the arena style assessment. An audiologist conducted a hearing test before the formal assessment. The occupational therapy portion included the *Revised Gesell*, a brief *Bobath Assessment* and the *Erhardt Hand Assessment*. The therapist also observed quality of movement throughout the assessment. Figure 4-4 summarizes Andrea's strengths and concerns.

Andrea's postural control and movement are dominated by low muscle tone in the face, neck, and trunk, and stiffness in all four extremities. Flexor tone dominates upper extremities, while extensor tone dominates the lower extremities. Her shoulders are elevated and internally rotated; motor patterns of the arms are dominated by an asymmetrical tonic neck reflex which is more apparent on the right. Andrea's hands are fisted and she is unable to initiate reach or grasp.

The tone patterns described in this paragraph are typical for children who have a spastic type of cerebral palsy. This pattern prohibits interaction with the environment; intervention strategies will focus on managing these predominant patterns to enable Andrea to interact with her environment.

When in the supine (on the back) position, Andrea cannot flex her trunk to move against gravity as a child would to pull to the sitting position. In the prone position (on the stomach), Andrea could lift her head momentarily, but her movement was dominated by movement to the right. With the stiffness noted in Andrea's arms, she was unable to use them to assist in holding her head and upper trunk up against gravity. The legs remained in stiff extension.

When children are positioned on the mat, gravity has a very strong effect. The child must be able to overcome the power of gravity to move. The patterns of tone noted above also make it difficult for Andrea to move when she is lying in her bed, on the floor, or in one's lap. Flexed arms are positioned next to her trunk, and therefore cannot support propping on the stomach, nor playing with toys while lying on the back. Extended legs limit contact with the supporting surface, and so Andrea does not learn how to use her legs to facilitate repositioning or exploratory activity.

Andrea was unable to roll in either direction or sit independently. She was also unable to bear weight on her legs; bilateral inversion (turning inward) was noted in both feet. In a supported sitting position, head control varied from hanging forward on her chest to asymmetrical hyperextension (right side dominant) when she initiated head righting. A pattern of scapular adduction, humeral internal rotation, elbow flexion, and wrist and finger flexion was noted at rest; this pattern increased during active movement. When Andrea became irritable, extension patterns become stronger and further compromise postural and motor function.

When Andrea is placed in more upright positions, she does not have the trunk stability to hold herself up against gravity. The predominance of the tone patterns prevents her from learning how to master these new positions.

While Andrea is not yet able to manage any solid foods, she does well on strained baby foods and with a bottle. She demonstrates definite preferences for both tastes and textures, reflecting more hypersensitivity to things in her mouth, rather than poor oral motor control.

It is good that Andrea eats strained foods and can eat from a bottle; sometimes children such as Andrea are nutritionally compromised because they have poor control over oral motor sequences. Her hypersensitivity to tastes and textures in the mouth will be an important focus of early intervention so that Andrea does not restrict herself from the broadening range of foods she will need as she grows. This may also affect Andrea's ability to formulate an accurate map of her oral motor structures, which could also restrict development of vocalizations for speech.

Andrea tried to visually fix and track distant objects, especially her parents. She has a great deal of difficulty with closer visual fixation and tracking (e.g., following a toy or face directly in front of her face). Her right eye deviates from the center position, compromising her depth perception and near vision according to the ophthalmologist.

Visual monitoring of the environment provides a mechanism for stimulation of interest and inquisitiveness. If Andrea

PERFORMANCE AREAS

Andrea — 5 months — PERFORMANCE COMPONENTS	ACTIVITIES OF DAILY LIVING Grooming	Oral Hygiene	Bathing	Toilet Hygiene	Dressing	Feeding and Eating	Medication Routine	Socialization	Functional Communication	Functional Mobility	Sexual Expression	WORK ACTIVITIES Home Management	Care of Others	Educational Activities	Vocational Activities	PLAY OR LEISURE ACTIVITIES Play or Leisure Exploration	Play or Leisure Performance
A. SENSORIMOTOR COMPONENT																	
1. Sensory Integration																	
a. Sensory Awareness								/	/					/		/	
b. Sensory Processing																	
(1) Tactile								–	–					–		–	
(2) Proprioceptive								–	–					–		–	
(3) Vestibular								–	–					–		–	
(4) Visual								–	–					–		–	
(5) Auditory								/	/					/		/	
(6) Gustatory								–	–					–		–	
(7) Olfactory								/	/					/		/	
c. Perceptual Skills																	
(1) Stereognosis																	
(2) Kinesthesia																	
(3) Body Scheme								–	–					–			
(4) Right-Left Discrimination																	
(5) Form Constancy																	
(6) Position in Space																	
(7) Visual-Closure																	
(8) Figure Ground								–	–					–		–	
(9) Depth Perception								–	–					–		–	
(10) Topographical Orientation																	
2. Neuromuscular																	
a. Reflex								–	–					–		–	
b. Range of Motion								–	–					–		–	
c. Muscle Tone								–	–					–		–	
d. Strength								–	–					–		–	
e. Endurance								–	–					–		–	
f. Postural Control								–	–					–		–	
g. Soft Tissue Integrity																	
3. Motor																	
a. Activity Tolerance								–	–					–		–	
b. Gross Motor Coordination								–	–					–		–	
c. Crossing the Midline								–	–					–		–	
d. Laterality																	
e. Bilateral Integration								–	–					–		–	
f. Praxis																	
g. Fine Motor Coordination/ Dexterity								–	–					–		–	
h. Visual-Motor Integration																	
i. Oral-Motor Control								–	–					–		–	

/ = Strength
– = Concern
0 = Both a strength and concern

Figure 4-4.   Uniform terminology 2—Andrea. *Used with permission. Dunn, 1988.*

PERFORMANCE AREAS

Andrea PERFORMANCE COMPONENTS	ACTIVITIES OF DAILY LIVING Grooming	Oral Hygiene	Bathing	Toilet Hygiene	Dressing	Feeding and Eating	Medication Routine	Socialization	Functional Communication	Functional Mobility	Sexual Expression	WORK ACTIVITIES Home Management	Care of Others	Educational Activities	Vocational Activities	PLAY OR LEISURE ACTIVITIES Play or Leisure Exploration	Play or Leisure Performance
B. COGNITIVE INTEGRATION AND COGNITIVE COMPONENTS																	
1. Level of Arousal								–	–					–		–	
2. Orientation								–	–					–		–	
3. Recognition																	
4. Attention Span								–	–					–		–	
5. Memory																	
a. Short-term																	
b. Long-term																	
c. Remote																	
d. Recent																	
6. Sequencing																	
7. Categorization																	
8. Concept Formation																	
9. Intellectual Operations in Space																	
10. Problem Solving																	
11. Generalization of Learning																	
12. Integration of Learning																	
13. Synthesis of Learning																	
C. PSYCHOSOCIAL SKILLS AND PSYCHOLOGICAL COMPONENTS																	
1. Psychological																	
a. Roles																	
b. Values																	
c. Interests																	
d. Initiation of Activity																	
e. Termination of Activity																	
f. Self-Concept																	
2. Social																	
a. Social Conduct								–	–					–		–	
b. Conversation																	
c. Self-Expression																	
3. Self-Management																	
a. Coping Skills								–	–					–		–	
b. Time Management																	
c. Self-Control																	

/ = Strength
– = Concern
0 = Both a strength and concern

Figure 4-4.   Continued.

cannot fix on interesting visual objects, she will not be motivated to explore them. This area will need to be investigated further as intervention begins.

In summary, Andrea has low muscle tone centrally (trunk, neck), and increased muscle tone in all extremities. This interferes with her ability to interact with her environment. She is consequently delayed in all areas of development. Observations are consistent with the diagnosis of spastic quadriplegic cerebral palsy.

CASE #4—TED

Pre-assessment Process

Referral. Ted was referred to the occupational therapist at the County 0-3 program by the visiting public health nurse, at age 14 months. The referral was for training family members, in positioning and handling, as well as in methods to optimize Ted's development.

PERFORMANCE AREAS

Ted — 14 months — PERFORMANCE COMPONENTS	ACTIVITIES OF DAILY LIVING Grooming	Oral Hygiene	Bathing	Toilet Hygiene	Dressing	Feeding and Eating	Medication Routine	Socialization	Functional Communication	Functional Mobility	Sexual Expression	WORK ACTIVITIES Home Management	Care of Others	Educational Activities	Vocational Activities	PLAY OR LEISURE ACTIVITIES Play or Leisure Exploration	Play or Leisure Performance
A. SENSORIMOTOR COMPONENT																	
1. Sensory Integration																	
a. Sensory Awareness																	
b. Sensory Processing																	
(1) Tactile						/		/		/							/
(2) Proprioceptive						–		–		–							–
(3) Vestibular						/		/		/							/
(4) Visual						–		–		–							–
(5) Auditory						/		/		/							/
(6) Gustatory						/		/		/							/
(7) Olfactory						/		/		/							/
c. Perceptual Skills																	
(1) Stereognosis																	
(2) Kinesthesia																	
(3) Body Scheme																	
(4) Right-Left Discrimination																	
(5) Form Constancy																	
(6) Position in Space																	
(7) Visual-Closure																	
(8) Figure Ground																	
(9) Depth Perception																	
(10) Topographical Orientation																	
2. Neuromuscular																	
a. Reflex						–		–		–							–
b. Range of Motion						–		–		–							–
c. Muscle Tone						–		–		–							–
d. Strength						–		–		–							–
e. Endurance						–		–		–							–
f. Postural Control						–		–		–							–
g. Soft Tissue Integrity																	
3. Motor																	
a. Activity Tolerance						–		–									–
b. Gross Motor Coordination						–		–									–
c. Crossing the Midline																	
d. Laterality																	
e. Bilateral Integration																	
f. Praxis																	
g. Fine Motor Coordination/ Dexterity						–		–		–							–
h. Visual-Motor Integration						–		–		–							–
i. Oral-Motor Control						/		/		/							/

/ = Strength
– = Concern
0 = Both a strength and concern

Figure 4-5. Uniform terminology 2—Ted. *Used with permission. Dunn, 1988.*

The County 0-3 program in this case consisted of an occupational and physical therapist, a speech/language pathologist, an early childhood specialist, a social worker, and a part-time nurse. Because the referral was made by a pubic health nurse, the county program nurse called her, and during the conversation compiled the following history.

History. Ted was the product of an uncomplicated full term pregnancy which resulted in a long and difficult labor and delivery. At delivery it was noted that the cord was wrapped twice tightly around Ted's neck, and resuscitation was required to begin respiration. Apgar scores were one, three, and eight within 30 minutes. Ted was released from the hospital with no complications. In the first

PERFORMANCE AREAS

Ted — PERFORMANCE COMPONENTS	ACTIVITIES OF DAILY LIVING Grooming	Oral Hygiene	Bathing	Toilet Hygiene	Dressing	Feeding and Eating	Medication Routine	Socialization	Functional Communication	Functional Mobility	Sexual Expression	WORK ACTIVITIES Home Management	Care of Others	Educational Activities	Vocational Activities	PLAY OR LEISURE ACTIVITIES Play or Leisure Exploration	Play or Leisure Performance
B. COGNITIVE INTEGRATION AND COGNITIVE COMPONENTS																	
1. Level of Arousal						/		/		/							/
2. Orientation						/		/		/							/
3. Recognition																	
4. Attention Span						/		/		/							/
5. Memory																	
a. Short-term						/		/		/							/
b. Long-term																	
c. Remote																	
d. Recent																	
6. Sequencing																	
7. Categorization																	
8. Concept Formation																	
9. Intellectual Operations in Space																	
10. Problem Solving						–		–		–							–
11. Generalization of Learning						–		–		–							–
12. Integration of Learning																	
13. Synthesis of Learning																	
C. PSYCHOSOCIAL SKILLS AND PSYCHOLOGICAL COMPONENTS																	
1. Psychological																	
a. Roles																	
b. Values																	
c. Interests																	
d. Initiation of Activity																	
e. Termination of Activity																	
f. Self-Concept																	
2. Social																	
a. Social Conduct						/		/		/							/
b. Conversation																	
c. Self-Expression																	
3. Self-Management																	
a. Coping Skills						/		/		/							/
b. Time Management																	
c. Self-Control																	

/ = Strength
– = Concern
0 = Both a strength and concern

Figure 4-5. *Continued.*

three months of his life, no particular concerns arose from either the family or the pediatrician. At his four months check up, Ted's mother expressed some concern about tightness in his extremities, apparent difficulty coordinating the use of his eyes, and lack of head control. The pediatrician advised the family that there may be complications with Ted's motor development, and asked for a public health nurse to begin monthly home visits. The public health nurse began her visits when Ted was five months of age. By eight months of age, Ted was demonstrating extreme stiffness in his extremities, so the pediatrician made the diagnosis of cerebral palsy with spastic quadriplegia. Because of extenuating family circumstances, the public health nurse remained the primary professional contact. When Ted was one year of age, the parents expressed concerns about their inability to provide the kind of activities that Ted needed to enhance his motor development. The public health nurse gave them information about County 0-3 Program and the referral was subsequently approved by the parents.

Pre-assessment Hypothesis

Children who have spastic cerebral palsy often have difficulty interacting with the environment because movement is restricted. Although sensorimotor components of performance are an obvious area for further investigation, it will be more important to focus on Ted's ability to perform functional life tasks. It is likely that Ted will require adaptations in task parameters and/or environmental variables (e.g., a positioning device) to perform some functional life tasks. Assessment data must include all of these components to enable the development of a comprehensive program plan.

Assessment Plan

During the preliminary conversation with the public health nurse, it became apparent that this family was quite apprehensive about becoming involved with a county program. Two major concerns were noted here: 1) the family did not wish to accept "charity," and 2) the parents were still overwhelmed at the diagnosis of cerebral palsy. This is not an unusual pattern of concerns for families with children at any age seeking intervention from any type of program. Respect and concern for the family's perceptions always take precedence over program convenience. During a meeting with the family, the referring public health nurse suggested that she schedule a home visit for herself and one staff member from the program. The public health nurse felt that she would be able to help the family remain comfortable and assist in the transition to new services. This plan was discussed in a transitional meeting with both staffs; everyone felt that the occupational therapist had the most expertise for the assessment.

Findings and Interpretation

The assessment was conducted during a home visit by the occupational therapist and the public health nurse. The *Sewall Early Education and Developmental Program* (SEED) evaluation was used. The SEED assesses the areas of self help, speech and language, social-emotional development, gross and fine motor skills, feeding and adaptive reasoning. Clinical observation of sensorimotor and neuromotor development and reflex integration were also recorded. The therapist also interviewed the parents to obtain information about functional skills. Ted was socially responsive and appeared to enjoy the interaction with the therapist throughout the assessment period. Ted's strengths and concerns are summarized in Figure 4-5.

The SEED is an evaluation instrument used for all children in this particular infant and toddler program, and all staff have been trained in its use. It was chosen by the group because it is easy to give, assessment materials are readily available and transportable, it does not require an excessive amount of time, and can be given in a way that resembles a free play situation. It also provides information across many developmental domains, so that intervention strategies can be designed directly from the data obtained. This also provided the therapist with an opportunity to reinforce the family's knowledge about ways to facilitate Ted's interactions and performance. The fact that Ted responded so well to the evaluation also helped the parents feel more comfortable with the process. By the time it was necessary for the therapist to handle and move Ted in a more intimate way, both he and his parents were comfortable.

Ted demonstrated difficulty in all areas of assessment. Abnormal muscle tone was noted throughout the body, with increased extensor tone noted in the lower extremities and increased flexor tone in the upper extremities. Asymmetry was also noted with increased tightness on the right side. In both supine and prone posture, hyperextension of the head and trunk is present. Ted did not demonstrate functional interactions in either supine or prone postures. In a supported sitting position Ted used head control for orienting to auditory and visual input and he was able to maintain his head in a midline position. In the supported sitting position Ted attempts to reach and grasp small toys. Passive range of motion was within normal limits, active range of motion revealed tightness in hip flexion and adduction. Ted demonstrated many persistent reflex patterns including the Moro, flexor withdrawal, tonic labyrinthine, asymmetrical and symmetrical tonic neck reflexes (the right side patterns were more pronounced), and palmar grasp.

Ted's physical status was the most obviously compromised area of development, and his parents expressed the most concern about his physical capabilities. These issues needed to be addressed in a way that would emphasize Ted's strengths while planning for his needs. The therapist would make a special effort to ask the family about the strategies they were already using and model a few extra strategies they might be able to learn within the first session. Care must always be taken not to overwhelm families with too many suggestions, ones that don't match their style or that are too complicated. The therapist encourages family members to participate in creating strategies and trying them during the intervention sessions. It is helpful for families to get some basic information about terminology and the influence of the child's condition on motor behavior and functional performance. The therapist also explains why particular strategies will increase or decrease the quality of performance. It is frequently more helpful to families to get this information during functional activities, rather than during motor skill testing or evaluation of postural reflexes, because they can apply their knowledge of their child to the comments you are making. It is not helpful for many parents to see their child's skills and limitations in isolation. It is much more helpful for them to understand these factors in the context of how they might compromise performance. All of these factors are considered during verbal and written interpretation of a child's performance.

Ted enjoys all forms of motion, tactile experiences, and appears visually alert. Ted tracks and focuses on slow moving or fixed objects or toys, although occasionally his eyes cross. Ted maintains eye contact inconsistently with toys and objects, but maintains better eye contact with faces. Ted responds to auditory stimuli by orienting to and localizing the sound.

These results are reported in a way that would be easy for the family to understand in the evaluation report. These results also contribute to program planning to facilitate Ted's continued development.

The SEED activities provided a mechanism for determining Ted's skills and his methods for approaching tasks. Skill acquisition levels are presented in Table 4-2. Ted interacts with eye contact, a variety of facial expressions and laughter. Ted turns his head in response to his name. He recognizes familiar people, looks for mommy when her name is mentioned, uses vowel sounds and

TABLE 4-2. Ted's Developmental Skill Acquisition on the SEED	
Socioemotional Skills	7 mo.
Fine Motor Skills	3–4 mo.
Gross Motor Skills	4–5 mo.
Speech and Language Skills	6 mo.
Self Care Skills	3–4 mo.
Oral Motor Skills	7 mo.

the consonant sounds of K, G, B, and varies his voice in melody and pitch when making sounds. These skills are just beginning to emerge.

He appears very interested in toys and tries to get to them even if they are out of his reach. In supported sitting he was inconsistently able to reach and attempted to grasp objects presented. He was able to hold objects, although he demonstrated no voluntary release. While he was unable to get an object to his mouth in a supported sitting position, he was able to put his mouth on toys when placed in side lying position on the floor. His visual skills exceed his manipulative skills, which is a common pattern to observe in children such as Ted. He visually pursues a lost toy, turns to a fallen toy, moves a rattle towards his mouth when it's placed in his hand, and makes attempts to retrieve a toy out of reach.

Ted rolls back-to-side, demonstrates functional head control in supported sitting and when pulling to sit. Trunk control was not functional in supported sitting (he has a forward curve in the trunk), although he can do some independent propped sitting.

Ted eats solids from a spoon, opens his mouth in anticipation, demonstrates adequate lip closure on a nipple, but is not able to hold his own bottle or get finger foods to his mouth.

Any time an evaluation instrument is utilized to gain information about cognitive and developmental performance, the family members either consciously or unconsciously are concerned about retardation. In the case of a child such as Ted, who is physically challenged, concerns about intellectual development are often intense and frightening. Skill development inventories do *not* give information about innate cognitive ability. They do give information about a child's developmental skills in relation to typical expectations of other children; care must be taken in interpreting information from these kinds of instruments when components are used with children like Ted. It is important for the therapist to describe the child's approach to the tasks, as well as actual ability to complete them, in an effort to help the family understand that manifestations of cognitive ability is impaired by physical limitations. It is also important to help the family understand the variety of strategies, equipment and adaptations that are available to enhance the child's ability to demonstrate how much he knows.

In summary, Ted is demonstrating significant difficulties in all areas of skill development, consistent with the diagnosis of spastic quadriplegic cerebral palsy. Enabling components are in the areas of social awareness, visual exploration, and oral motor skills. Ted needs interventions and adaptations to deal with gross motor and fine motor development, posture development, speech and language skills, and self care.

It is often necessary to use descriptors in a summary that will ensure access to services. The concept of labels and descriptive terms necessary to access services should be carefully discussed with the family before they are written.

CASE #5—JASON

Pre-Assessment Process

Referral. Jason was referred by the physical therapist to assess chronic irritability, feeding problems, and possible need for a sensory motor treatment approach, in addition to the neurodevelopmental approach used in physical therapy.

History. The review and consultation revealed that Jason was born three months prematurely, weighing two pounds ten and one-half ounces. In the first five days of life, he suffered initial prolonged hypoxia followed by several short periods of hypoxia. No seizures, infections or intraventricular bleeds occurred during his two month intensive care unit stay. Both parents are committed to caring for Jason. Mr. A has had a difficult time bonding to Jason and understanding what role he can play in Jason's life and development. Thus far, Jason's mother has taken responsibility for most of the program planning decisions. Both parents are high school graduates. The mother is a claims representative for a health consortium and the father is a metal worker.

Jason had been evaluated on one other occasion. The evaluation occurred when he was 18 months old and was the result of a referral from a hospital NICU followup clinic screening conducted by a physician, infant educational specialist, and an occupational therapist. The referral was made to a university development disabilities evaluation program.

The referral question to the university program was to assess cognitive ability and motor disorder. Jason had been receiving physical therapy for three months in order to determine effectiveness of intervention, and to provide a mechanism for obtaining further medical information related to cause of the motor disorder. The evaluation from the university program was requested by the parents to provide a more complete picture of Jason's problems.

The university program routinely conducts an integrated evaluation on children under two years of age. An integrated evaluation includes simultaneous assessment of the child by four team members, who each address a different component of development. The cognitive component is addressed by either a developmental psychologist, or an educational diagnostician; motor development is addressed by an occupational or physical therapist; language is addressed by a speech/language pathologist; and medical aspects are addressed by a pediatrician. The rationale for this approach is to avoid duplication of assessment items which could lead to fatigue and then poor test performance. This also decreases the stress on parent(s)/primary caretakers and the child. It incorporates evaluation, interpretation, and program planning into one family-centered process. The evaluation is scheduled so that parent(s)/primary caretakers can all be present. Parent(s)/primary caretakers may also choose to invite extended family members or friends who spend a lot of time with their child.

The primary responsibility of the occupational therapist was to handle and position Jason to facilitate his best performance during cognitive testing. In order to complete her part of the evaluation, the speech/language pathologist observed and entered into the interaction periodically.

PERFORMANCE AREAS	ACTIVITIES OF DAILY LIVING Grooming	Oral Hygiene	Bathing	Toilet Hygiene	Dressing	Feeding and Eating	Medication Routine	Socialization	Functional Communication	Functional Mobility	Sexual Expression	WORK ACTIVITIES Home Management	Care of Others	Educational Activities	Vocational Activities	PLAY OR LEISURE ACTIVITIES Play or Leisure Exploration	Play or Leisure Performance
Jason — 22 months — PERFORMANCE COMPONENTS																	
A. SENSORIMOTOR COMPONENT																	
1. Sensory Integration																	
a. Sensory Awareness						/		/									/
b. Sensory Processing																	
(1) Tactile						–		–									–
(2) Proprioceptive						–		–									–
(3) Vestibular						/		/									/
(4) Visual						–		–									–
(5) Auditory						/		/									/
(6) Gustatory																	
(7) Olfactory						–		–									–
c. Perceptual Skills																	
(1) Stereognosis																	
(2) Kinesthesia																	
(3) Body Scheme						–		–									–
(4) Right-Left Discrimination																	
(5) Form Constancy						/		/									/
(6) Position in Space						/		/									/
(7) Visual-Closure																	
(8) Figure Ground																	
(9) Depth Perception						–		–									–
(10) Topographical Orientation																	
2. Neuromuscular																	
a. Reflex						–		–									–
b. Range of Motion						–		–									–
c. Muscle Tone						–		–									–
d. Strength						–		–									–
e. Endurance						–		–									–
f. Postural Control						–		–									
g. Soft Tissue Integrity																	
3. Motor																	
a. Activity Tolerance						–		–									–
b. Gross Motor Coordination						–		–									–
c. Crossing the Midline																	
d. Laterality																	
e. Bilateral Integration						–		–									
f. Praxis																	
g. Fine Motor Coordination/ Dexterity						/		/									/
h. Visual-Motor Integration						–		–									–
i. Oral-Motor Control																	

/ = Strength
– = Concern
0 = Both a strength and concern

Figure 4-6.   Uniform terminology 2—Jason. *Used with permission. Dunn, 1988.*

Following the cognitive part of the evaluation, the occupational therapist completed evaluation of the following: postural mechanisms, stability/mobility skills, motor development, more detailed hand/eye function, and feeding/eating. Both the speech/language pathologist and the occupational therapist documented observations during play. The pediatrician facilitated discussion with the parents during the entire process. This included gathering history and addressing current questions and concerns in more detail. This interdisciplinary assessment revealed that Jason was developmentally delayed and continued to need intervention. The team decided that it was appropriate for the physical therapist to continue to treat Jason, since rapport had already been established. They felt that multiple forms of intervention would

PERFORMANCE AREAS

Jason — PERFORMANCE COMPONENTS	ACTIVITIES OF DAILY LIVING — Grooming	Oral Hygiene	Bathing	Toilet Hygiene	Dressing	Feeding and Eating	Medication Routine	Socialization	Functional Communication	Functional Mobility	Sexual Expression	WORK ACTIVITIES — Home Management	Care of Others	Educational Activities	Vocational Activities	PLAY OR LEISURE ACTIVITIES — Play or Leisure Exploration	Play or Leisure Performance
B. COGNITIVE INTEGRATION AND COGNITIVE COMPONENTS																	
1. Level of Arousal						−		−									−
2. Orientation																	
3. Recognition																	
4. Attention Span						−		−									−
5. Memory a. Short-term																	
b. Long-term																	
c. Remote																	
d. Recent																	
6. Sequencing																	
7. Categorization																	
8. Concept Formation																	
9. Intellectual Operations in Space																	
10. Problem Solving						−		−									−
11. Generalization of Learning																	
12. Integration of Learning																	
13. Synthesis of Learning																	
C. PSYCHOSOCIAL SKILLS AND PSYCHOLOGICAL COMPONENTS																	
1. Psychological a. Roles																	
b. Values																	
c. Interests																	
d. Initiation of Activity																	
e. Termination of Activity																	
f. Self-Concept																	
2. Social a. Social Conduct						−		−									−
b. Conversation																	
c. Self-Expression																	
3. Self-Management a. Coping Skills						−		−									−
b. Time Management																	
c. Self-Control																	

/ = Strength
− = Concern
0 = Both a strength and concern

Figure 4-6. *Continued.*

be disruptive to the family, but would be needed as Jason grew older.

The physical therapist continued to treat Jason after the developmental disabilities team assessment. After three more months of treatment (Jason was now 21 months old), she decided to inquire about another type of assessment strategy that would address his chronic irritability, since this behavior interfered with all his life tasks, especially during handling and eating. She discussed this with the parents, and made a referral to an occupational therapist in private practice with whom she had collaborated on other children on her case-load. During the telephone call made to request this assessment, both therapists agreed it would be appropriate to incorporate a feeding specialist into this assessment.

Pre-assessment Hypothesis

The occupational therapist reviewed the available records, and decided that Jason's irritability might be due to his inability to manage sensation. He decided to evaluate the sensory components of performance. Other components had recently been evaluated by the interdisciplinary team, and so did not need to be addressed. Findings from other evaluations, and from the physical therapist, could be used to interpret the significance of the sensory findings. It is likely that Jason's physically handicapping condition led other professionals to focus on motor difficulties, without considering possible sensory involvement.

Assessment Plan

Prior to scheduling the assessment at the private practice clinic, release of information forms were mailed, signed, and returned by the parents. Evaluation and treatment records from previously provided services were reviewed, and interviews were scheduled with other professionals who had been involved with Jason and his parents.

Findings and Interpretation

Jason was seen for a team evaluation at the private practice clinic by the occupational therapist and a registered nurse who specializes in feeding problems. Both parents, the baby-sitter who cares for Jason daily, and the physical therapist, who sees him in his home three times a week, were present. Evaluation procedures included a sensory and feeding history, an evaluation of postural and motor skills related to eating and interacting with others, and an observation of responses to sensory input. Jason's performance is summarized in Figure 4-6.

Because the family's concerns centered around feeding (how can we facilitate better weight gain), and irritability, an extensive sensory history was taken. As many of Jason's primary caretakers were present, a lengthy discussion of best management strategies was possible. While the occupational therapist obtained the sensory history, the registered nurse was also able to obtain an accurate picture of Jason's eating patterns.

Jason was quite irritable throughout the session, and his irritability provided several opportunities to assess methods to calm and organize him. Effective strategies already in use included:
1. Curling his body tightly and holding him in an infant feeding position.
2. Holding him vertically over the shoulder and rocking hard forward and back, and
3. Side lying in a sheet held and swung sideways by the parents.

Jason was fussy about the foods presented to him. Avoidance and withdrawal patterns predominated his behavioral repoirtoire during this portion of the assessment. It was difficult to interpret Jason's avoidance behaviors; it seemed to be a combination of discomfort with body positioning, food in and on the mouth, food taste and texture, and the structure of the eating task.

It is clear that functional tasks such as eating are being interrupted by Jason's poor ability to modulate sensory input. An important initial step in intervention will be to decrease sensory sensitivity and increase ability to create adaptive responses to sensation, so that Jason can engage in age appropriate exploration.

CASE #6—RICHARD

Pre-Assessment Process

Referral. Richard is a two year old boy who was referred by the speech/language pathologist, because of some confusion following a previous evaluation. It was unclear to the mother whether it was necessary for Richard to receive occupational therapy intervention, and so wanted this clarified.

The referral inferred that only an occupational therapy evaluation was being requested. The intake process for this private practice clinic includes a preliminary social, developmental, and sensory history interview with the parents.

History. Richard is the middle of three children. His siblings are reported to be developing normally. The mother had some bleeding and episodes of severe pain during pregnancy, but labor and delivery were without complications. The mother describes Richard as always having been a very happy baby and child, but slower in his development than other children. She began to worry about him when he was not talking at one year of age. About the same time it appeared that even if mother "yelled and screamed," Richard did not always respond. A hearing evaluation revealed hearing sensitivity and middle ear function to be within normal limits.

A previous occupational therapy and speech/language evaluation, in an out-of-state child development center, had given Richard a diagnosis of dyspraxia. The occupational therapist reported that skills appeared developmentally appropriate with some indication of sensory integrative dysfunction. The explanation Mrs. F received left her unsure if occupational therapy intervention was being recommended. Richard has been enrolled in the university speech/language clinic since the family's move to this state. The speech/language pathologist is concerned about oral motor planning (praxis) problems, which are affecting intelligibility, as well as gross and fine motor movement quality and organization.

During the interview the mother asked the following questions: 1) Is the diagnosis for Richard's condition given in the past still appropriate? 2) Does Richard continue to demonstrate overall delay? 3) Does he need to have occupational therapy? and 4) Why the continued lack of spontaneous speech?

Pre-assessment Hypothesis

Due to the broad nature of the parents' concerns, the options of separate evaluations at various places or referral to a university multidisciplinary evaluation team were discussed. The family preferred the multidisciplinary evaluation and subsequently contacted that program.

Very often the initial referral may not completely address the family's needs. Before the evaluation is scheduled, the occupational therapist should take the time to clearly understand the purpose of the evaluation. In this manner, the therapist will be able to provide the best service for the client. At times it may mean that there is another program better suited to the family's needs. In this particular case, there was enough credibility and trust established that when occupational therapy intervention was recommended, the family wanted to follow up on this recommendation.

Followup Referral. Richard is a two-year, ten-month old boy who has previously been diagnosed as having dyspraxia. His mother, at the suggestion of a speech/language pathologist at a university communication disorders clinic, has requested another opinion about the nature of his difficulty and what services are needed for him.

Assessment Plan

This referral resulted in a full multidisciplinary evaluation. Both parents, the grandmother, and the speech/language

PERFORMANCE AREAS

Richard — 27 months — PERFORMANCE COMPONENTS	ACTIVITIES OF DAILY LIVING Grooming	Oral Hygiene	Bathing	Toilet Hygiene	Dressing	Feeding and Eating	Medication Routine	Socialization	Functional Communication	Functional Mobility	Sexual Expression	WORK ACTIVITIES Home Management	Care of Others	Educational Activities	Vocational Activities	PLAY OR LEISURE ACTIVITIES Play or Leisure Exploration	Play or Leisure Performance
A. SENSORIMOTOR COMPONENT																	
1. Sensory Integration																	
a. Sensory Awareness								–	–								–
b. Sensory Processing																	
(1) Tactile								–	–								–
(2) Proprioceptive								–	–								–
(3) Vestibular								–	–								–
(4) Visual								/	/								/
(5) Auditory								–	–								–
(6) Gustatory																	
(7) Olfactory																	
c. Perceptual Skills																	
(1) Stereognosis																	
(2) Kinesthesia																	
(3) Body Scheme								–	–								–
(4) Right-Left Discrimination																	
(5) Form Constancy																	
(6) Position in Space								–	–								–
(7) Visual-Closure																	
(8) Figure Ground																	
(9) Depth Perception																	
(10) Topographical Orientation																	
2. Neuromuscular																	
a. Reflex																	
b. Range of Motion								/	/								/
c. Muscle Tone								–	–								–
d. Strength								/	/								/
e. Endurance																	
f. Postural Control								–	–								–
g. Soft Tissue Integrity																	
3. Motor																	
a. Activity Tolerance								–	–								–
b. Gross Motor Coordination								–	–								
c. Crossing the Midline																	
d. Laterality																	
e. Bilateral Integration								–	–								–
f. Praxis								–	–								–
g. Fine Motor Coordination/ Dexterity								/	/								/
h. Visual-Motor Integration																	
i. Oral-Motor Control																	

/ = Strength
– = Concern
0 = Both a strength and concern

Figure 4-7. Uniform terminology 2—Richard. *Used with permission. Dunn, 1988.*

pathologist were present throughout the evaluation and interpretation. After consulting with the diagnostic team and visiting speech/language pathologist, the decision was made to complete the occupational therapy assessment just prior to the speech/language assesment. The decision was also made to schedule an extra thirty minutes following the occupational therapy assessment to try some therapeutic intervention techniques. It was felt that since there was current and thorough speech/language information, and that the referring speech/language pathologist would be present, it might be beneficial to determine whether occupational therapy intervention would influence performance in the speech/language assessment. The focus of the occupational therapy assessment was determined by referral information: a) the mother's

	PERFORMANCE AREAS																	
Richard PERFORMANCE COMPONENTS	ACTIVITIES OF DAILY LIVING Grooming	Oral Hygiene	Bathing	Toilet Hygiene	Dressing	Feeding and Eating	Medication Routine	Socialization	Functional Communication	Functional Mobility	Sexual Expression	WORK ACTIVITIES Home Management	Care of Others	Educational Activities	Vocational Activities	PLAY OR LEISURE ACTIVITIES Play or Leisure Exploration	Play or Leisure Performance
B. COGNITIVE INTEGRATION AND COGNITIVE COMPONENTS																	
1. Level of Arousal								–	–								–
2. Orientation								–	–								–
3. Recognition								/	/								/
4. Attention Span								–	–								–
5. Memory																	
a. Short-term								–	–								–
b. Long-term																	
c. Remote																	
d. Recent																	
6. Sequencing								–	–								–
7. Categorization																	
8. Concept Formation																	
9. Intellectual Operations in Space																	
10. Problem Solving								–	–								–
11. Generalization of Learning								–	–								–
12. Integration of Learning																	
13. Synthesis of Learning																	
C. PSYCHOSOCIAL SKILLS AND PSYCHOLOGICAL COMPONENTS																	
1. Psychological																	
a. Roles																	
b. Values																	
c. Interests																	
d. Initiation of Activity																	
e. Termination of Activity																	
f. Self-Concept								–	–								–
2. Social																	
a. Social Conduct																	
b. Conversation								–	–								–
c. Self-Expression								–	–								–
3. Self-Management																	
a. Coping Skills																	
b. Time Management																	
c. Self-Control																	

/ = Strength
– = Concern
0 = Both a strength and concern

Figure 4-7. *Continued.*

questions concerning the appropriateness of dyspraxia as a diagnosis; b) Richard's continuing developmental delay; c) the observations by the treating speech/language pathologist regarding poor quality of movement; and d) Richard's apparent lack of interest in interacting with his environment.

Findings and Interpretation

The *Bayley Scales of Infant Development* and the *Miller Assessment for Preschoolers* were used, as well as clinical assessment of sensory responsivity, postural mechanisms, postural control, and movement quality. Figure 4-7 summarizes performance component strengths and concerns in relation to Richard's desired outcomes of socialization, functional communication and play exploration.

While gross motor development was essentially within normal limits, movements lacked variety, quality, and organization. These characteristics are consistent with a diagnosis of developmental dyspraxia. Fine motor skills were somewhat immature. Postural mechanisms were immature and also lacked quality and organi-

GRID TO SUMMARIZE PERFORMANCE COMPONENT INTEGRITY

Performance Components	higher response level rate than would be expected — 8	7	6	5	functions within expected levels — 4	3	2	1	significantly lower response or no response — 0
A. SENSORIMOTOR COMPONENT									
1. Sensory Integration									
a. Sensory Awareness									
b. Sensory Processing									
(1) Tactile									
(2) Proprioceptive									
(3) Vestibular**						*			
(4) Visual									
(5) Auditory									
(6) Gustatory									
(7) Olfactory									
c. Perceptual Skills									
(1) Stereognosis									
(2) Kinesthesia									
(3) Body Scheme									
(4) Right-Left Discrimination									
(5) Form Constancy									
(6) Position in Space									
(7) Visual-Closure									
(8) Figure Ground									
(9) Depth Perception									
(10) Topographical Orientation									
2. Neuromuscular									
a. Reflex									
b. Range of Motion									
c. Muscle Tone							*		
d. Strength									
e. Endurance									
f. Postural Control							*		
g. Soft Tissue Integrity									
3. Motor									
a. Activity Tolerance									
b. Gross Motor Coordination						*			
c. Crossing the Midline									
d. Laterality									
e. Bilateral Integration							*		
f. Praxis							*		
g. Fine Motor Coordination/Dexterity								*	
h. Visual-Motor Integration								*	
i. Oral-Motor Control								*	

**Arousal shifts significantly with vestibular inputs.

Figure 4-8. Richard's performance.

GRID TO SUMMARIZE PERFORMANCE COMPONENT INTEGRITY

Performance Components	higher response level rate than would be expected 8	7	6	5	functions within expected levels 4	3	2	1	significantly lower response or no response 0
B. COGNITIVE INTEGRATION AND COGNITIVE COMPONENTS**									
1. Level of Arousal								*	
2. Orientation									
3. Recognition									
4. Attention Span									
5. Memory									
a. Short-term									
b. Long-term									
c. Remote									
d. Recent									
6. Sequencing									
7. Categorization									
8. Concept Formation									
9. Intellectual Operations in Space									
10. Problem Solving									
11. Generalization of Learning									
12. Integration of Learning									
13. Synthesis of Learning									
C. PSYCHOSOCIAL SKILLS AND PSYCHOLOGICAL COMPONENTS									
1. Psychological									
a. Roles									
b. Values									
c. Interests									
d. Initiation of Activity									
e. Termination of Activity									
f. Self-Concept									
2. Social									
a. Social Conduct									
b. Conversation									
c. Self-Expression									
3. Self-Management									
a. Coping Skills									
b. Time Management									
c. Self-Control									

**Arousal shifts significantly with vestibular inputs.

Figure 4-8. *Continued.*

zation. His muscle tone was in the low normal range, with poor joint stability both proximally and distally. He also demonstrated poor cocontraction with extensor postures predominating. Rotation was limited in upper and lower trunk, and in forearms. Breathing patterns were rapid and shallow with little support from the diaphragm or abdominal musculature. Richard's suck/swallow/breathe synchrony was poor; this, combined with poor breathing patterns, made it difficult for Richard to grade and control breath support for speech.

Richard's arousal level appeared consistently low, although it increased markedly, with swinging, bouncing, and jumping. Total scores, as well as all scale scores on the *Miller Assessment for Preschoolers*, were at or below the fifth percentile, and seemed to reflect Richard's difficulty maintaining arousal and appropriate interaction for the various activities. Throughout the evaluation, both Richard's performance, and comments made by the mother and the speech/language pathologist, indicated that Richard's arousal level greatly affects the quality of his performance.

During the thirty minutes following the evaluation, the occupational therapist tried several strategies to increase and maintain Richard's arousal level. The purpose of this activity was to identify whether or not occupational therapy techniques could enhance Richard's arousal and attention, leading to improved performance in developmental and language activities.

It is important for the occupational therapist to identify not only a child's needs, but also to make responsible decisions about the need for, and possible effects of, occupational therapy intervention. A summary of his performance component integrity is provided in Figure 4-8. It is interesting to note the affect of one component (vestibular) on another (arousal). These relationships are important for intervention planning. In this case, the family's major concerns reflected their frustrations over the variability in Richard's performance. This made them question whether or not therapy was appropriate. The grandmother had some strong feelings about the pressure being placed on Richard to talk. She also indicated that Richard may be refusing to do his best because of stubbornness, being deliberately uncooperative. Richard's father made it very clear that he didn't think there was anything unusual about Richard's performance, and that he could not afford the cost of therapy. Richard's mother demonstrated obvious frustration, because she believes strongly that there is something that needs attention; she feels that Richard does not intentionally vary in his performance or refuse to communicate, but rather cannot perform for some reason.

Given the wide array of opinions among family members, great care needs to be taken to discuss the findings of the assessment. The occupational therapist must respect and value each person's beliefs about Richard's performance. In this case, the best way to present the evaluation findings might be to acknowledge that variability in performance is difficult to understand. The family members need to understand Richard better. Richard needs to demonstrate consistent performance across settings. Once all parties are able to discuss Richard from a common framework, it will be easier to help plan a program for him and his family.

CASE #7—JAMES

Pre-assessment Process

Referral. James was referred by his parents to a local early education program which serves children from birth to five years of age. The parents' major concerns at the time of the referral were poor oral motor skills and difficulty with eye-hand coordination. Parents were also concerned about both James' lack of speech, and difficulty understanding what he was able to say. James was two and one half years old at this time.

In this case, the parents were concerned about James' development, to the extent that they began calling community agencies to find an established program where they might be able to receive some help. James' mother personally contacted the program via a telephone call. The secretary recorded the pertinent information and sent the family a set of referral forms. Once the referral forms were returned, a team was formed, consisting of an occupational therapist, speech/language pathologist, early childhood educator, and developmental psychologist. They decided it would be best for the developmental psychologist to schedule an appointment with the parents, to take a history and identify pertinent information needed to design an assessment plan suited to the family and James' needs. While this particular program serves a large number of children, they are committed to providing individualized assessment and intervention programs. The history taken at the initial interview contains helpful information.

History. The pregnancy was apparently normal and the labor was long but not significant. James was a large baby (over 10 pounds) and apparently post term by 2–3 weeks. Early developmental milestones were delayed. He sat at one year, pulled to stand at 16 months, and walked at 22 months. James' mother noted frequent choking and gagging problems when solids were introduced. The parents managed these concerns by thinning foods, making smaller bites, and taking extra time during feeding. The parents both described James as a rather clumsy child who is motivated to try anything and persists until he can accomplish the tasks.

Pre-assessment Hypothesis

Preliminary information suggests that James is delayed in his development, but there seem to be some key areas of concern that need particular attention during the assessment. James seems to be having his most significant difficulties in activities which require organization of movement, or motor planning. It will be important to record evaluation data in such a way that the team knows not only whether James can perform a task, but to carefully document the way that he approaches tasks, and how he performs. This information will help the team formulate effective strategies.

It is also important to note that the parents have demonstrated insight in relation to James. They have been able to target James' functional needs themselves, which led them to seek assistance, and have made some very clever adaptations for James already. Additional parental information should be sought throughout the assessment.

Assessment Plan

Following the screening interview, the team met to plan the assessment. Because the family's major concerns were about oral motor skills and eye-hand coordination, the speech/language pathologist, early childhood specialist, and the occupational therapist were assigned to do the assessment. It was decided that the speech/language pathologist and the occupational therapist would observe the early childhood specialist during her interactions with James. It was felt that they could both benefit from watching James' performance and not have to duplicate assessment items. Information regarding gross motor and fine motor function was gleaned through the observation, and through information the parents provided, while observing James and the early childhood specialist with the therapists. This team decided that skill levels would be recorded and reported by the early intervention specialist; the occupational therapist would provide information about quality of gross and fine motor movements and James' ability to apply those skills to functional tasks and problem solving. This strategy is efficient, and acknowledges that James is a whole child who must function within his environment, rather than an accumulation of separate skill components. It is meaningless to report developmental levels, without also reporting the child's ability to use those skills within functional life tasks. The parents would be encouraged to observe the assessment, giving both the speech/language pathologist and the occupational therapist an opportunity to interact with them, and gain further information during this time.

The oral examination was conducted jointly by the occupational therapist and speech/language pathologist. In many programs, both the speech/language pathologist and the occupational therapist are interested in oral motor functioning and include this area in their assessment plan. While tools used and results gathered often overlap, there are some portions of a thorough oral motor examination that require specialized expertise that one discipline does not have. In this particular instance, the speech/language pathologist and occupational therapist have established a relationship which enables them to conduct a joint evaluation, each contributing expertise. The occupational therapist in this situation was primarily concerned with the variability and functional use of James' suck, swallow, and breath synchrony. Frequently children who have low normal muscle tone, demonstrate difficulty coordinating the use of various body components. Poor oral motor synchrony can be a sign of problems in other areas, and can compromise development of other orchestrated movements.

Findings and Interpretation

The *Early-Learning Accomplishment Profile* (E-LAP) was used by the early childhood specialist to gather developmental data. The E-LAP provides data in the areas of gross and fine motor development, feeding, ADL, and cognitive skills. The occupational therapist and speech/language pathologist observed this administration, and recorded approach to the task and quality of movements chosen. The occupational therapist also evaluated postural reflexes, took a sensorimotor history, and collaborated with the speech/language pathologist to complete a thorough oral motor exam. James' performance is summarized in Figure 4-9.

Gross Motor. James moves through his environment with a wide base and high guard stance. He demonstrates difficulty in balance, especially when moving quickly, and demonstrates difficulty in planning and controlling skilled gross motor patterns.

Although all two and one half year old children have some difficulty negotiating movements in space, James is having

trouble even with simple patterns of movement like running and stopping. It is common for parents to seek help during this age period because their child has become more mobile, and is frequently the victim of mishaps. The children have many more scrapes, cuts, bruises, and sometimes broken bones, because of their inability to plan and organize their movements within and around their environment. Additional information such as this can be gained during history taking.

Fine Motor. James demonstrates an immature grasping pattern; he is not yet using a pincer grasp. He enjoyed playing and building with blocks and putting puzzles together, but had difficulty in both problem solving and reproducing structures. He is just beginning to use a crayon or marker, holding it with his entire hand. He accurately reproduced a horizontal and vertical line but was unable to draw a circle or cross. James did not visually monitor his hands during these fine motor tasks. James is far sighted and wears glasses to correct this; he is also intermittently patched for strabismus (cross-eyedness). These factors may be contributing to his poor visual monitoring of fine motor activities.

James is also having trouble organizing movements with his hands. An additional complication here is his poor use of visual monitoring; when children watch their hands, they obtain further information about how their hands work, and what their capabilities are. James is probably not profiting from the sensory feedback from his eyes or his hands (visual, tactile, and proprioceptive), and therefore cannot construct accurate and reliable maps of his body. His clumsiness in fine motor movement may be due to his lack of information from which to plan his approach to the task.

Oral Motor. The oral motor exam was conducted while James ate a snack of crackers, cheese, apple sauce, and juice in a cup. James had difficulty maintaining lip closure around the cup and the spoon. There was minimal lateral movement of food with his tongue and no rotary chewing was demonstrated. Reverse swallowing or gulping was noted especially while drinking. James had difficulty initiating swallowing patterns following chewing or sucking. James used breathing patterns functionally during chewing activities, but he had difficulty synchronizing breathing during drinking or sucking. Breathing difficulties were also noted during fine motor tasks. James frequently holds his breath, apparently to increase stability for distal control. James tends to get winded easily during gross motor activities which require either strength or endurance. James' verbal language has a breathy quality to it, as though he does not always have enough air to complete a sentence or string of sentences. He takes small breaths while speaking, but they are not always at the end of phrases or sentences. This contributes to his lack of intelligibility.

The problems noted in the oral motor examination also indicate difficulty with organizing movement in relation to task demands. Breathing is such an automatic task for most of us; we do not consider that it takes coordination to breathe in relation to an activity. James could not coordinate breathing with talking, eating, or fine motor tasks. Difficulty with the sequencing, timing and orchestration of movement is a primary characteristic of dyspraxia, or the inability to organize and plan new motor acts.

Postural Mechanisms. James demonstrates low normal muscle tone and has difficulty initiating and maintaining adequate joint stability (especially in the jaw, neck, shoulders, and hips). The

PERFORMANCE AREAS

James 30 months PERFORMANCE COMPONENTS	ACTIVITIES OF DAILY LIVING Grooming	Oral Hygiene	Bathing	Toilet Hygiene	Dressing	Feeding and Eating	Medication Routine	Socialization	Functional Communication	Functional Mobility	Sexual Expression	WORK ACTIVITIES Home Management	Care of Others	Educational Activities	Vocational Activities	PLAY OR LEISURE ACTIVITIES Play or Leisure Exploration	Play or Leisure Performance
A. SENSORIMOTOR COMPONENT																	
1. Sensory Integration																	
a. Sensory Awareness						–			–					–			–
b. Sensory Processing																	
(1) Tactile						–			–					–			–
(2) Proprioceptive						–			–					–			–
(3) Vestibular						–			–					–			–
(4) Visual						–			–					–			–
(5) Auditory						–			–					–			–
(6) Gustatory						–			–					–			–
(7) Olfactory						/			/					/			/
c. Perceptual Skills																	
(1) Stereognosis						–			–					–			
(2) Kinesthesia						–			–					–			
(3) Body Scheme						–			–					–			
(4) Right-Left Discrimination						–			–					–			
(5) Form Constancy						–			–					–			
(6) Position in Space						–			–					–			
(7) Visual-Closure						–			–					–			
(8) Figure Ground						–			–					–			
(9) Depth Perception						–			–					–			
(10) Topographical Orientation																	
2. Neuromuscular																	
a. Reflex						–			–					–			–
b. Range of Motion						/			/					/			/
c. Muscle Tone						–			–					–			–
d. Strength						–			–					–			–
e. Endurance						–			–					–			–
f. Postural Control						–			–					–			–
g. Soft Tissue Integrity																	
3. Motor																	
a. Activity Tolerance						–			–					–			–
b. Gross Motor Coordination						–			–					–			–
c. Crossing the Midline						–			–					–			–
d. Laterality						–			–					–			–
e. Bilateral Integration						–			–					–			–
f. Praxis						–			–					–			–
g. Fine Motor Coordination/ Dexterity						–			–					–			–
h. Visual-Motor Integration						–			–					–			–
i. Oral-Motor Control																	

/ = Strength
– = Concern
0 = Both a strength and concern

Figure 4-9. Uniform terminology 2—James. *Used with permission. Dunn, 1988.*

asymmetrical and symmetrical tonic neck patterns remain obligatory and seem to be compromising development of postural rotation, protective responses, and righting and balance reactions. The result is poor quality of movement.

The presence of primitive postural reflexes limits James' ability to mobilize body parts in isolation from the trunk or head. It is difficult to know whether the presence of these primitive patterns is a causal or effect factor. If these primitive patterns dominated James' early movement attempts, they could have limited his movement experiences, leaving him with a small movement repertoire. On the other hand, with poor motor planning skills, James may have been unable to

James PERFORMANCE COMPONENTS	PERFORMANCE AREAS																
	ACTIVITIES OF DAILY LIVING Grooming	Oral Hygiene	Bathing	Toilet Hygiene	Dressing	Feeding and Eating	Medication Routine	Socialization	Functional Communication	Functional Mobility	Sexual Expression	WORK ACTIVITIES Home Management	Care of Others	Educational Activities	Vocational Activities	PLAY OR LEISURE ACTIVITIES Play or Leisure Exploration	Play or Leisure Performance
B. COGNITIVE INTEGRATION AND COGNITIVE COMPONENTS																	
1. Level of Arousal						–			–					–			–
2. Orientation						/			/					/			/
3. Recognition						/			/					/			/
4. Attention Span						/			/					/			/
5. Memory																	
a. Short-term						–			–					–			–
b. Long-term																	
c. Remote																	
d. Recent																	
6. Sequencing						–			–					–			–
7. Categorization						–			–					–			–
8. Concept Formation																	
9. Intellectual Operations in Space						–			–					–			–
10. Problem Solving						–			–					–			–
11. Generalization of Learning																	
12. Integration of Learning																	
13. Synthesis of Learning																	
C. PSYCHOSOCIAL SKILLS AND PSYCHOLOGICAL COMPONENTS																	
1. Psychological																	
a. Roles																	
b. Values																	
c. Interests																	
d. Initiation of Activity																	
e. Termination of Activity																	
f. Self-Concept						–			–					–			–
2. Social																	
a. Social Conduct						/			/					/			/
b. Conversation						0			0					0			0
c. Self-Expression						–			–					–			–
3. Self-Management																	
a. Coping Skills																	
b. Time Management																	
c. Self-Control																	

/ = Strength
– = Concern
0 = Both a strength and concern

Figure 4-9. *Continued.*

overcome the effects of the primitive reflex patterns to develop more mature patterns of movement. It is likely that both scenarios contributed to his present condition.

In summary, James is demonstrating a mild delay in all areas of development. His poor ability to organize patterns of movement in all activities suggests that James has motor planning problems, sometimes called developmental dyspraxia. It may be helpful for James to be seen by a pediatric neurologist to either confirm or rule out other central nervous system disorders, since James' movement organization problem is so pervasive.

It is possible that James has mild cerebral palsy. A pediatric neurology consultation could help to confirm or deny this possibility for the parents. This diagnosis will not significantly alter the program planning strategies for the team, since their observations of his performance will form the basis for intervention in any case. A specific diagnosis is sometimes very important to families; sometimes a specific diagnosis makes programs or community resources available to a family. For example, if James does indeed have a mild form of cerebral palsy, his family will have access to the resources of United

Cerebral Palsy, or the state Crippled Children's services. A differential diagnosis is also useful in those cases where a family trend may be present, or when the disorder may have new or different manifestations as the child grows. Chapter fifteen discusses the reason for considering a referral to the various pediatric specialties, and summarizes the types of information one can expect from these referrals.

CASE #8—RANDY

Pre-assessment Process

Referral. Randy was referred by a pediatric neurologist to the public schools early education assessment team with concerns regarding general development including speech and cognitive skills.

History. Randy was a full term, six-pound-ten-ounce product of a pregnancy complicated by intermittent vaginal bleeding. There were no problems at the delivery. Randy and his mother left the hospital when he was two days of age. At six days of age he developed meningitis and had associated seizures. He was hospitalized for six weeks at Children's Hospital. Post meningitic hydrocephalus was noted at six months of age; a ventricular shunt was inserted. He has had some difficulties with the shunt which have required surgical interventions. Currently the shunt is said to be working well. As noted above, he had seizures associated with the meningitis and was on phenobarbitol until he was 13 months of age. Mother describes Randy's behavior as a problem, and notes that he is uncooperative with people other than herself, has difficulty separating from her, shows resistance in taking part in learning activities and generally has problems with social interactions with both children and adults. Randy apparently does well behaviorally with his father. He notes that Randy is able to listen and follows directions that he gives him. Randy is five and has a six year old sister who demonstrates no behavior problems.

Randy is generally fearful of any unfamiliar adults and new situations. He may completely "lose it" and "throw fits" that require lengthy periods of calming before he is in control. During his most recent hospitalization, the mother said his behavior was terrible and she felt he was petrified of everyone and everything. Randy's mother feels that his behavior is most manageable at home. Even his grandparents have found their visits more enjoyable and less stressful if they go to Randy's house, rather than having Randy and his family coming to their house. Randy appears to do fairly well when they have friends over. He likes to be helpful in getting things and intermittently interacting with guests. He does not enjoy interacting with other children for any length of time, and appears to prefer to play alone or with his sister when he is not at the neighbors or helping his dad.

Randy is a good eater and there are no concerns with his diet. He goes to bed with no conflict and usually goes to sleep quickly. However, he often wakes at 3 AM and wants to play and have something to eat. Apparently he has been doing this since age 2. Recently he just comes downstairs, has a snack and goes back to bed on his own.

Pre-assessment Hypothesis

In this situation, when the occupational therapist read the referral report from the pediatric neurologist, there were two areas that seemed to warrant attention during the assess-

ment. According to the history, the family's major concerns centered around Randy's ability to interact appropriately in unfamiliar environments and sleep problems. The therapist determined she should be looking for quality of movement and visual perception in eye-hand and gross motor activities.

Assessment Plan

The purpose of this assessment was to determine whether or not Randy qualified for services through the pubic school. This particular school system is a large one, and has its own assessment team for the three and four year old program. The team includes an occupational therapist, a physical therapist, a speech/language pathologist, a school psychologist, and an early childhood special education teacher.

The assessment instruments used are determined by state guidelines. Most states have a list of instruments identified for all disciplines, that may be used to qualify a child for public school service. Some states, while not having a specific instrument to be used, do have eligibility criteria by which a child may be qualified (e.g., at or below the 10th percentile, or at least two standard deviations below the mean). In most states there is also a statement regarding clinical judgment in determining risk factors for successful school performance.

Findings and Interpretation

Randy was seen in the center for sensorimotor testing using the *Miller Assessment for Preschoolers* (MAP). He arrived crying and upset. After settling down with a toy, Randy was readily engaged with the test materials, and was able to complete seventeen items. After attempting a few gross motor items, he suddenly began crying and begging to put his shoes and socks back on. In spite of getting them on and being held by his mother, Randy could not be calmed and refused to continue. His mother tried to get him to stop crying by saying she would leave the room, but that increased his agitation.

The therapist respected the fact that Randy was frightened and uncomfortable in the unfamiliar situation. Allowing a child to explore the environment, or offering him a toy, is often a way to help a child feel more comfortable. In this situation, a toy was used, and once he was comfortable, he was more interested in engaging with the test materials and activity.

When a child is unable to continue with the formal evaluation procedures, the therapist may choose one of the following strategies: 1) move on to clinical observations of posture and movement qualities, which have less demands on following specific directions, or may be conducted while the child interacts with his family or the activities of his choice; 2) take a break, leave the room to get a drink, a snack, take a walk, etc., and then return; 3) if enough information has already been gathered to meet the purposes of the assessment, there may be no need to continue; or 4) it may be necessary to schedule the completion of the evaluation for another time.

In this situation the therapist determined she had enough information for the purposes of determining qualifications for public school service and so chose to discontinue at this point.

Because Randy did not complete all the items, a total test score could not be obtained. Based on the items that Randy did attempt,

PERFORMANCE AREAS

Randy 5 years PERFORMANCE COMPONENTS	ACTIVITIES OF DAILY LIVING Grooming	Oral Hygiene	Bathing	Toilet Hygiene	Dressing	Feeding and Eating	Medication Routine	Socialization	Functional Communication	Functional Mobility	Sexual Expression	WORK ACTIVITIES Home Management	Care of Others	Educational Activities	Vocational Activities	PLAY OR LEISURE ACTIVITIES Play or Leisure Exploration	Play or Leisure Performance
A. SENSORIMOTOR COMPONENT																	
1. Sensory Integration																	
a. Sensory Awareness								/						/			
b. Sensory Processing																	
(1) Tactile								–						–			
(2) Proprioceptive								–						–			
(3) Vestibular								–						–			
(4) Visual								/						/			
(5) Auditory																	
(6) Gustatory								/						/			
(7) Olfactory								/						/			
c. Perceptual Skills																	
(1) Stereognosis								–						–			
(2) Kinesthesia								–						–			
(3) Body Scheme								–						–			
(4) Right-Left Discrimination																	
(5) Form Constancy								/						/			
(6) Position in Space								–						–			
(7) Visual-Closure																	
(8) Figure Ground								–						–			
(9) Depth Perception																	
(10) Topographical Orientation																	
2. Neuromuscular																	
a. Reflex								–						–			
b. Range of Motion								/						/			
c. Muscle Tone								–						–			
d. Strength								/						/			
e. Endurance								–						–			
f. Postural Control								–						–			
g. Soft Tissue Integrity																	
3. Motor																	
a. Activity Tolerance								–						–			
b. Gross Motor Coordination								–						–			
c. Crossing the Midline								–						–			
d. Laterality																	
e. Bilateral Integration															–			
f. Praxis															–			
g. Fine Motor Coordination/ Dexterity								–						–			
h. Visual-Motor Integration								–						–			
i. Oral-Motor Control																	

/ = Strength
– = Concern
0 = Both a strength and concern

Figure 4-10.   Uniform terminology 2—Randy. *Used with permission. Dunn, 1988.*

his performance was generally poor. Since he was cooperating nicely during portions of the test he was able to complete, it is assumed that the testing was reliable in those instances. It is evident that Randy is having significant sensory and perceptual motor delays.

Primary areas of concern include tactile awareness and discrimination, sense of position and movement, and the ability to move against gravity efficiently. He was unable to identify common objects by feeling them, and couldn't accurately localize touch on his fingers. He had trouble maintaining a stable (static) position

PERFORMANCE AREAS

Randy — PERFORMANCE COMPONENTS	ACTIVITIES OF DAILY LIVING Grooming	Oral Hygiene	Bathing	Toilet Hygiene	Dressing	Feeding and Eating	Medication Routine	Socialization	Functional Communication	Functional Mobility	Sexual Expression	WORK ACTIVITIES Home Management	Care of Others	Educational Activities	Vocational Activities	PLAY OR LEISURE ACTIVITIES Play or Leisure Exploration	Play or Leisure Performance
B. COGNITIVE INTEGRATION AND COGNITIVE COMPONENTS																	
1. Level of Arousal								–						–			
2. Orientation								/						/			
3. Recognition																	
4. Attention Span								–						–			
5. Memory																	
a. Short-term								0						0			
b. Long-term																	
c. Remote																	
d. Recent																	
6. Sequencing								–						–			
7. Categorization								/						/			
8. Concept Formation								–						–			
9. Intellectual Operations in Space																	
10. Problem Solving								–						–			
11. Generalization of Learning								–						–			
12. Integration of Learning																	
13. Synthesis of Learning																	
C. PSYCHOSOCIAL SKILLS AND PSYCHOLOGICAL COMPONENTS																	
1. Psychological																	
a. Roles																	
b. Values																	
c. Interests								–						–			
d. Initiation of Activity								–						–			
e. Termination of Activity								–						–			
f. Self-Concept								–						–			
2. Social																	
a. Social Conduct								–						–			
b. Conversation								–						–			
c. Self-Expression								–						–			
3. Self-Management																	
a. Coping Skills								–						–			
b. Time Management																	
c. Self-Control								–						–			

/ = Strength
– = Concern
0 = Both a strength and concern

Figure 4-10. *Continued.*

with his eyes closed and accurately moving his arm in space to find his nose. Randy needed to support himself with hands when rising from half kneel to stand, indicating some deficiency in diagonal weight shifting and counteracting gravity. Clinically he demonstrated significant overflow with some intention tremor on fine motor tasks. He was somewhat impulsive in his responses and lacked fine gradation (control).

Randy also had difficulty in tasks requiring combined visual perceptual and motor skills (e.g., simple puzzles, block design, draw-a-person), as well as drawing skills.

Throughout testing Randy appeared anxious and on edge. When he became upset, his inability to modulate his emotional responses was striking. He quickly became hysterical (uncontrollable) without apparent cause, could not be reassured and actually became more agitated as attempts were made to distract or redirect him. His mother reports that this is common behavior in new situations, and at home as well. Such fearfulness and such strong fight/flight/fright reactions are uncommon in children his age.

Poor performance on sensorimotor testing and clinical observations, combined with Randy's significant medical and behavioral history, leave the impression that some of his behavior may be neurologically based. Randy's performance is summarized in Figure 4-10.

It is extremely important to note the fact that this child was unable to complete all of the items on the MAP. Adhering to scoring and interpretation guides in the manual, the therapist reported her clinical impressions of Randy's performance rather than the scores. Trying to determine what scores Randy might have achieved, had he completed the items, or using partial scores would have been inappropriate, and essentially would have invalidated the interpretation of the entire formal assessment.

The therapist wisely reported what Randy was able and not able to do and the quality of his performance. Clinical judgment was used to correlate performance strengths and concerns with the family's questions about his behavior.

CASE #9—PETER

Pre-assessment Process

Referral. Peter was referred for special education services at age six by his kindergarten teacher, because of concerns surrounding

behavior in the classroom, difficulty understanding and following directions, and difficulty on playground equipment. The occupational therapy referral (see Figure 4-11) was made in conjunction with referrals for assessment of behavior and learning ability.

This particular referral was made in response to the Spring parent conference, when concerns from both the teacher and the parents were expressed about Peter's readiness for the first grade curriculum. The occupational therapist in this school generally receives a copy of the referral questions along with a request for assessment. The occupational therapist then schedules the evaluation time with the classroom teacher and coordinates scheduling of assessment activities with other members of the assessment team. One member of the team is designated responsible for gathering pertinent history, and in this case it was the occupational therapist.

After discussing referral concerns with the kindergarten teacher in person, and with Peter's mother, in a telephone conversation, the occupational therapist had a clearer picture of Peter's needs.

History. Peter is the youngest of three boys. The pregnancy, labor, and delivery was unremarkable. Peter was described by his mother

---

TEACHER QUESTIONNAIRE

Referral Form for Occupational Therapy

Child's Name _____**Peter**_____   Grade: _____**Kindergarten**_____

Date _____   Teacher: _____

School _____

Teacher making referral: _____

Teachers: Please check the following behaviors that correspond to the concerns you have regarding your student.

_____	1	Demonstrates mixed hand dominance in classroom activities
__x__	2	Grasps pencil/crayon improperly
_____	3	Does not perform desk work from left to right
_____	4	Does not know left from right on self
__x__	5	Has difficulty staying on line & spaces when writing and printing
_____	6	Has difficulty copying from board or text
_____	7	Reverses letters/shapes in writing/drawing
_____	8	Has difficulty completing activities on time
__x__	9	Has difficulty following verbal directions
_____	10	Has dificulty following written directions
__x__	11	Has difficulty maintaining self in seat for reasonable length of time
__x__	12	Is clumsy at recess, gym, or in classroom
_____	13	Avoids physical activities with peers
_____	14	Has extreme reaction to being touched
__x__	15	Has excessively high overall activity level
_____	16	Has excessively low overall activity level
_____	17	Projects poor self image

Figure 4-11. Referral on Peter. *Adapted from: Gilfoyle, E.M. (Ed) (1980). Training: Occupational Therapy Educational Management in Schools. Rockville, MD: American Occupational Therapy Association. Used with permission.*

as an alert and active baby with a mind of his own, but she had no concerns about his development, since he achieved major milestones within expected ages. Peter's mother operates a day care business in her home, and Peter participated in play with preschool activities from the age of two until he entered school. While Peter's mother had noticed some difficulty in his ability to follow directions, stay on task, and participate in gross motor activities, she did not think he would have any difficulty in a structured kindergarten program.

Information from both parents, as well as the classroom teacher, helped define the kind of sensory input and situations that lead to overarousal, and result in fight-or-flight behaviors. It appeared that unexpected light touch, moderate to intense background noise, and unpredictable movement of children in his vicinity were most likely to negatively affect his ability to maintain attention to tasks and remain in control of his own behavior. He also becomes easily upset by unfamiliar environments, the presence of many people in close proximity, or changes in schedule. When these conditions are present, Peter demonstrates his discomfort by changing to a different activity. Both the parents and the classroom teacher had observed that Peter often chose to hang back before and during transitions to new activities. Peter has also cried for no apparent reason while riding the bus to and from school, while playing on the playground, and sometimes while spending time in the mall or at a restaurant with his family. Peter frequently ignores or redefines a directed activity. He has infrequently demonstrated mild outbursts of temper at transition times, during free play on the playground, and one time on the bus. Parents noted these behaviors are more significant at home when there is a sudden change in plans or the normal routine. As the conversation progressed it became apparent that his family has understood his sensitivity to certain situations, and have for the most part taken responsibility for protecting Peter from situations which he perceives as threatening. The classroom teacher has also begun to accommodate to his special needs by giving him more time to make transitions, allowing him to stay close to her in threatening situations, and allowing him to redefine or not participate in some directed activities.

Pre-assessment Hypothesis

Both the classroom teacher and the parents provided information that suggested possible sensory sensitivities and motor planning problems. It is common for early motor milestones—such as walking—to occur within the normal age expectations; but as the child has to problem-solve using his movement abilities, his performance breaks down. Many times these children are bright enough to manipulate situations to minimize their use of motor planning. This leads family members and other care providers to believe that the child can do things that he may not be able to do. Children with motor planning problems have motor skills, and can sometimes use them in free play situations; however, the child is unable to use those same skills when they are required in directed learning or play situations which require organization and planning on the spot.

Assessment Plan

The occupational therapist decided to follow up on these hypotheses by administering standardized and criterion-referenced measures, and by recording information from her own skilled observation. Since it is common for children with motor planning problems to be inconsistent, she wanted to make sure that she observed his performance in a variety of situations to validate her results. She also decided that further information from the mother would be helpful in intervention planning, and so decided to obtain a sensory history from her; this would provide further evidence regarding Peter's sensory sensitivities. She also wanted to observe Peter in a few school situations to see how her findings may be affecting his performance in these settings. It would take several sessions to complete all of this data collection.

Findings and Interpretation

As part of the interdisciplinary assessment, the occupational therapist administered the *Sensory Integration and Praxis Tests*, the *Bruininks Oseretsky Test of Motor Proficiency*, clinical observations of postural mechanisms and recorded quality of movement patterns, and responsiveness to sensory input in several school situations. A short sensorimotor history was also obtained from the mother over the telephone. Figure 4-12 provides a summary of Peter's performance.

A summary of the constellation and pattern of scores on the *Sensory Integration and Praxis Tests* suggest strengths in the area of visual perception, and difficulties with processing of touch and movement, and organizing and executing gross and fine motor movements (motor planning).

Peter also demonstrated hypersensitivity for sensory input. Since sensory defensiveness was an unfamiliar term to the parents, extra time was taken during the interpretation to define the term and describe the ramifications of sensory defensiveness in Peter's behavior. Clinical observation suggested low normal muscle tone, increased use of extensor patterns in both stability and mobility tasks, and difficulty assuming anti-gravity postures. The *Bruininks Oseretsky Test of Motor Proficiency* results also suggest difficulty coordinating and timing both gross and fine motor movements. These findings are confirmed in the observations of Peter's movement patterns throughout the school.

It is important to remember, when using standard scores from the *Sensory Integration and Praxis Tests*, that it is the pattern of scores, rather than individual scores, in conjunction with other test data, skilled observations, and actual performance at school, home, and within the community that determines accurate diagnosis. For example, sensory defensiveness was apparent during testing, but also manifested itself on the playground and in the classroom. Making linkages between assessment data and behaviors observed by the referral parties is an important responsibility of the therapist.

Because this evaluation was being conducted as part of a comprehensive assessment in a public school, Peter's performance strengths and deficits are considered within this context. It is the responsibility of the occupational therapist in the schools to report assessment findings in relation to facilitating or compromising classroom performance. When a school-based occupational therapist identifies a problem that is not affecting classroom performance, referrals to other community resources are appropriate. This can include swimming, gymnastics or karate programs, or may include a referral to an occupational therapy program in another agency. Care must also be taken to identify these non-school related occupational therapy needs; it is not the school district's responsibility to pay for services that are not educationally re-

PERFORMANCE AREAS

Peter — 6 years — PERFORMANCE COMPONENTS	ACTIVITIES OF DAILY LIVING Grooming	Oral Hygiene	Bathing	Toilet Hygiene	Dressing	Feeding and Eating	Medication Routine	Socialization	Functional Communication	Functional Mobility	Sexual Expression	WORK ACTIVITIES Home Management	Care of Others	Educational Activities	Vocational Activities	PLAY OR LEISURE ACTIVITIES Play or Leisure Exploration	Play or Leisure Performance
A. SENSORIMOTOR COMPONENT																	
1. Sensory Integration																	
a. Sensory Awareness																	
b. Sensory Processing																	
(1) Tactile								−						−			−
(2) Proprioceptive																	
(3) Vestibular								−						−			−
(4) Visual																	
(5) Auditory								−						−			
(6) Gustatory																	
(7) Olfactory																	
c. Perceptual Skills																	
(1) Stereognosis								/						/			/
(2) Kinesthesia								/						/			/
(3) Body Scheme																	
(4) Right-Left Discrimination																	
(5) Form Constancy								/						/			/
(6) Position in Space								/						/			/
(7) Visual-Closure								/						/			
(8) Figure Ground								/						/			/
(9) Depth Perception																	
(10) Topographical Orientation																	
2. Neuromuscular																	
a. Reflex																	
b. Range of Motion																	
c. Muscle Tone								/						/			/
d. Strength																	
e. Endurance																	
f. Postural Control								−						−			−
g. Soft Tissue Integrity																	
3. Motor																	
a. Activity Tolerance																	
b. Gross Motor Coordination																	
c. Crossing the Midline																	
d. Laterality																	
e. Bilateral Integration																	
f. Praxis								−						−			−
g. Fine Motor Coordination/ Dexterity								−						−			−
h. Visual-Motor Integration								−						−			−
i. Oral-Motor Control																	

/ = Strength
− = Concern
0 = Both a strength and concern

Figure 4-12.　Uniform terminology 2—Peter. *Used with permission. Dunn, 1988.*

lated. Although the therapist has a professional responsibility to inform families about identified needs, it is also important to delineate for them school-related needs, from other needs that they may choose to act upon using family resources. For example, the issue of family counseling came up during a discussion with the mother, due to her frustration managing Peter's outbursts. The occupational therapist noted this, and reminded herself to suggest a referral to a local pediatric

PERFORMANCE AREAS

Peter — PERFORMANCE COMPONENTS	ACTIVITIES OF DAILY LIVING Grooming	Oral Hygiene	Bathing	Toilet Hygiene	Dressing	Feeding and Eating	Medication Routine	Socialization	Functional Communication	Functional Mobility	Sexual Expression	WORK ACTIVITIES Home Management	Care of Others	Educational Activities	Vocational Activities	PLAY OR LEISURE ACTIVITIES Play or Leisure Exploration	Play or Leisure Performance
B. COGNITIVE INTEGRATION AND COGNITIVE COMPONENTS																	
1. Level of Arousal								−						−			−
2. Orientation																	
3. Recognition																	
4. Attention Span								−						−			−
5. Memory																	
a. Short-term																	
b. Long-term																	
c. Remote																	
d. Recent																	
6. Sequencing																	
7. Categorization																	
8. Concept Formation																	
9. Intellectual Operations in Space																	
10. Problem Solving																	
11. Generalization of Learning																	
12. Integration of Learning																	
13. Synthesis of Learning																	
C. PSYCHOSOCIAL SKILLS AND PSYCHOLOGICAL COMPONENTS																	
1. Psychological																	
a. Roles																	
b. Values																	
c. Interests																	
d. Initiation of Activity																	
e. Termination of Activity																	
f. Self-Concept																	
2. Social																	
a. Social Conduct								−						−			−
b. Conversation																	
c. Self-Expression																	
3. Self-Management																	
a. Coping Skills								−						−			−
b. Time Management																	
c. Self-Control								−						−			−

/ = Strength
− = Concern
0 = Both a strength and concern

Figure 4-12. *Continued*.

psychologist with whom she had worked on a similar case. She would recommend this to the team as an outside recommendation.

CASE #10—JOEL

Pre-assessment Process

Referral. Joel was referred by a European therapist to a large midwestern children's center when Joel was six years old. The referral concerns were lack of independent controlled and goal directed behavior, poor attending skills, poor ADL skills, left sided weakness and low muscle tone.

History. The pregnancy was unremarkable and while the labor and delivery process were lengthy, there were no apparent complications At three years of age, he had eye surgery to correct strabismus, and has a diagnosed seizure disorder which is controlled through medication. Joel has one brother who is two years older, with no apparent special needs. The mother and father are both at home and interested in providing for Joel's needs. However, the mother is the primary caretaker and has taken it upon herself to coordinate a program for her son.

While this situation does not occur very frequently in any therapist's practice, there are several major pediatric centers in this country that frequently see children for the express purpose of devising a program plan to take back to their home communities. In some cases there will not be an occupational therapist to carry out that plan.

Pre-assessment Hypothesis

After reviewing the records that were sent prior to the assessment, the occupational therapist listed the areas that needed to be addressed during the assessment. ADL skills were apparently one of the primary concerns of the family. The left sided weakness needed to be addressed, not only in terms of ADL, but also in terms of controlled movement. The rest of the questions centered around independent and goal directed behavior and apparent lack of ability to interact with his environment.

Assessment Plan

In any assessment process involving a child coming from long distances, care must be taken to ensure that all the arrangements and materials necessary will be available at the actual assessment time. Any school records, medical records, and therapy records should be acquired and reviewed well ahead of the actual assessment. Travel arrangements and accommodations may also need to be facilitated by the occupational therapist or another worker at the facility. Care should be taken in scheduling so that the family is well rested and comfortable in their new surroundings.

Because of the medication necessary to control his seizures, it appeared appropriate to review the effects of seizure medication on behavior (see Chapter 15). Also of importance was to look at Joel's ability to use vision to monitor and direct activity.

The preliminary plan was to administer the *Sensory Integration and Praxis Tests* to assess Joel's ability to utilize different forms of sensory input. Clinical observations of postural control, movement quality and an ADL evaluation were

GRID TO SUMMARIZE PERFORMANCE IN APPROPRIATE LIFE TASKS

PERFORMANCE AREAS	Not applicable/not age appropriate	Performs task independently	Performs task independently with adaptations	Partially performs tasks, or requires assistance to complete	Performs isolated components of task incomplete even with assistance	Unable to perform task
ACTIVITIES OF DAILY LIVING						
1. Grooming				x		
2. Oral Hygiene					x	
3. Bathing				x		
4. Toilet Hygiene		x				
5. Dressing			x			
6. Feeding and Eating				x		
7. Medication Routine	x					
8. Socialization					x	
9. Functional Communication				x		
10. Functional Mobility	x					
11. Sexual Expression	x					
WORK						
1. Home Management	x					
2. Care of Others	x					
3. Educational Activities					x	
4. Vocational Activities	x					
PLAY/LEISURE						
1. Play or Leisure Exploration				x		
2. Play or Leisure Performance				x		

Figure 4-13. Joel's ADL assessment.

PERFORMANCE AREAS

Joel — 6 years — PERFORMANCE COMPONENTS	ACTIVITIES OF DAILY LIVING Grooming	Oral Hygiene	Bathing	Toilet Hygiene	Dressing	Feeding and Eating	Medication Routine	Socialization	Functional Communication	Functional Mobility	Sexual Expression	WORK ACTIVITIES Home Management	Care of Others	Educational Activities	Vocational Activities	PLAY OR LEISURE ACTIVITIES Play or Leisure Exploration	Play or Leisure Performance
A. SENSORIMOTOR COMPONENT														*			
1. Sensory Integration														*			
a. Sensory Awareness					−								−	*			
b. Sensory Processing																	
(1) Tactile					−								−				
(2) Proprioceptive					−								−				
(3) Vestibular					−								−				
(4) Visual					−								−				
(5) Auditory					/								/				
(6) Gustatory					/								/				
(7) Olfactory					/								/				
c. Perceptual Skills																	
(1) Stereognosis																	
(2) Kinesthesia					−								−				
(3) Body Scheme					−								−				
(4) Right-Left Discrimination																	
(5) Form Constancy					−								−				
(6) Position in Space					−								−				
(7) Visual-Closure																	
(8) Figure Ground					−								−				
(9) Depth Perception																	
(10) Topographical Orientation																	
2. Neuromuscular																	
a. Reflex					−								−				
b. Range of Motion					/								/				
c. Muscle Tone					−								−				
d. Strength					−								−				
e. Endurance					−								−				
f. Postural Control					−								−				
g. Soft Tissue Integrity																	
3. Motor																	
a. Activity Tolerance					−								−				
b. Gross Motor Coordination					−								−				
c. Crossing the Midline					−								−				
d. Laterality																	
e. Bilateral Integration					−								−				
f. Praxis																	
g. Fine Motor Coordination/ Dexterity					−								−				
h. Visual-Motor Integration					−								−				
i. Oral-Motor Control																	

/ = Strength
− = Concern
0 = Both a strength and concern

Figure 4-14. Uniform terminology 2—Joel. *Used with permission. Dunn, 1988.*

also to be included. The therapist obtained thorough developmental history from the parents. Because there were so many areas needing to be assessed, three separate appointments were made to make sure that both Joel and his parents would not become overwhelmed with the process.

Findings and Interpretation

Evaluation. Joel was six and a half years old at the time of the assessment. The *Sensory Integration and Praxis Tests* were attempted, but due to extremely poor attending, high distractibility,

PERFORMANCE AREAS

Joel PERFORMANCE COMPONENTS	Grooming	Oral Hygiene	Bathing	Toilet Hygiene	Dressing	Feeding and Eating	Medication Routine	Socialization	Functional Communication	Functional Mobility	Sexual Expression	Home Management	Care of Others	Educational Activities	Vocational Activities	Play or Leisure Exploration	Play or Leisure Performance
B. COGNITIVE INTEGRATION AND COGNITIVE COMPONENTS																	
1. Level of Arousal					−								−				
2. Orientation																	
3. Recognition																	
4. Attention Span					−								−				
5. Memory																	
a. Short-term					−								−				
b. Long-term																	
c. Remote																	
d. Recent																	
6. Sequencing																	
7. Categorization																	
8. Concept Formation																	
9. Intellectual Operations in Space					−								−				
10. Problem Solving					−								−				
11. Generalization of Learning					/								/				
12. Integration of Learning																	
13. Synthesis of Learning																	
C. PSYCHOSOCIAL SKILLS AND PSYCHOLOGICAL COMPONENTS																	
1. Psychological																	
a. Roles																	
b. Values																	
c. Interests																	
d. Initiation of Activity																	
e. Termination of Activity																	
f. Self-Concept																	
2. Social																	
a. Social Conduct					−								−				
b. Conversation					/								/				
c. Self-Expression																	
3. Self-Management																	
a. Coping Skills					−								−				
b. Time Management																	
c. Self-Control					−								−				

/ = Strength
− = Concern
0 = Both a strength and concern

Figure 4-14. *Continued.*

and difficulty understanding the tasks, the results were not considered valid. Consequently, the *Peabody Developmental Motor Scale* was utilized, as well as clinical observations of sensory responsivity, development of postural mechanisms, postural control, and movement quality. A thorough developmental history was also obtained from the parents.

Once the therapist began the SIPT, she realized that several factors were interfering, thus compromising Joel's performance. These factors invalidated the results of the instrument and the therapist wisely decided to utilize a different assessment strategy.

The results of the ADL assessment are summarized on Figure 4-13. Joel was able to independently toilet himself, dress himself in elastic pull-up shorts and a loose pullover top only. Everything else required assistance for completion, including bathing, feeding and dressing throughout the day. At no time was he able, or has he been able, to be left alone to complete any of these tasks. Also noted through the ADL assessment was a moderate to severe lack of sensory awareness of the entire left body side. The left side was not used spontaneously and Joel did not cross into left body space during activities. The results of the clinical observation suggested low muscle tone throughout the body, very poor responses in prone and supine against gravity, and weak cocontraction throughout his body. Equilibrium reactions were sluggish. Symmetrical tonic neck reflex and asymmetrical tonic neck reflex were present and obligatory.

The results of the *Peabody Developmental Motor Scale* placed Joel at approximately the two and a half year age level. There were large discrepancies in his abilities, and the quality of his performance was compromised by the lack of use of his left body side. Observation of performance suggests more left body side neglect rather than a true hemiparesis. Joel's performance is summarized in Figure 4-14.

When one uses a developmental skill assessment, it is important to talk about the variability in performance, rather than to report only age level scores. In this situation, while the score suggested that Joel was at the two-and-one-half-year age level, there were many discrepancies in his abilities. Joel demonstrated a left sided weakness, which distorts the picture of developmental age. Were the therapist to plan intervention based solely on the developmental age score, the program plan would look considerably different than if the program plan is aimed at his asymmetrical performance. The therapist must also discriminate between a true left hemiparesis, which would reflect actual muscle weakness, and neglect of the left body side. The therapist determined that it was neglect of left body side, rather than true muscle asymmetry, that influenced Joel's performance. This will also have an impact on the way the program plan is designed.

Throughout the assessment period, Joel's lack of emotional stability was very apparent. He frequently demonstrated extreme mood swings, ranging from anger and resistive behavior to joy bordering on hysteria and frequently demonstrated fright. The emotional lability appeared to correspond to shifts in sensory input, as well as inability to meet the attentional and gross or fine motor demands of the task.

In this case it's extremely important for the therapist to note and incorporate the information about Joel's emotional stability and arousal state, and the fact that it appeared to correlate to the kind of sensory input he was receiving at the time. This will become extremely important information, not only in designing the program planning, but also in designing strategies to interact with Joel, both in therapy and in his home environment.

CASE #11—ELLEN

Pre-assessment Process

Referral. Ellen was referred at nine years of age to a university pediatric psychiatric program by her psychologist because of possible sensory integrative dysfunction. After consulting the local psychiatrist experienced with sensory integration theory and treatment, the psychologist felt sensory integrative dysfunction might be contributing to her difficulties in language and emotional development. Ellen's parents' main concerns centered around her social and emotional development.

This particular university program provides both inpatient and outpatient pediatric psychiatric services. This is a 60-bed residential center with its own public school approved classrooms. It also offers day school programs and after school therapy in a variety of areas. There are three occupational therapists on staff. The referring psychologist works for another university facility, which offers family and individual counseling services. The standard procedure for referrals and subsequent evaluations is a team review of referral questions, followed by planning and conducting a full assessment. Because Ellen had recently completed psychoeducational testing at her school, these areas did not need to be tested again. The primary area of need, as described in the referral, was for further information about Ellen's sensory integrative development. The occupational therapist would provide this area of expertise for the team. The occupational therapist contacted the referring psychologist and scheduled a meeting to review the records and compile the following history.

History. Ellen is a nine-year-old girl who had bacterial meningitis at the age of six weeks. Ellen walked at age 17 months, began speaking at two years, and was toilet trained at age three; her mother feels that these developmental milestones are within normal limits.

At age five, Ellen underwent comprehensive testing through the public schools, and was found to have behavioral, motoric, speech , and perceptual deficits which qualified her for a variety of special education and related services through the public schools.

Ellen has participated in a variety of physical and occupational therapy programs to improve motor skills and balance from the age of 18 months. She has also received adaptive physical education and speech/language therapy in kindergarten. In first grade she was placed in a self-contained classroom for children with learning disabilities. At the end of her third grade year, it was felt that she would be able to manage a regular education fourth grade classroom. She continues to receive speech therapy at school.

She is enrolled in a dance class to continue working on motor coordination. Her dance instructor notes that her abdomen tends to protrude a little, and that she is not as well coordinated as other children in the class. Recent evaluation by an orthopedic surgeon noted mild neuromotor involvement and slight hip flexion contractures, as well as a slight convex thoracic scoliosis. The scoliosis is being monitored.

In the middle of Ellen's third grade year, the family felt that the teacher's concern about limited peer interaction in the classroom warranted psychological intervention. A private psychologist evaluated Ellen and found hearing, vision and intelligence all well within normal limits. Ellen was performing in the above average range in classroom work, but her teacher felt she had a difficult time making friends, was often extremely withdrawn, and appeared to be in a world of her own. Individual play therapy was initiated in the spring of her third grade year. The hesitancy and coordination problems Ellen demonstrated while playing with large and small toys and games, prompted the consultation to the University psychiatric clinic and subsequent occupational therapy referral. The occupational therapist referral completed by the teacher is provided in Figure 4-15.

Pre-assessment Hypothesis

While reviewing records and discussing current function with the psychologist, her emotional ability, difficulty estab-

---

REFERRAL FOR ASSESSMENT
BY OCCUPATIONAL THERAPIST

Name _____ **Ellen** _____ School _____ Grade _____
D.O.B. _____ Teacher _____ Date _____

Gross Motor

___x___ Seems weaker than others same age
_____ Difficulty with hop, jump, skip or run
___x___ Appears stiff and awkward in movements
___x___ Clumsy, seems not to know how to move body, bumps into things, falls out of chair
_____ Tendency to confuse right and left

Fine Motor

___x___ Poor desk posture (slumps, leans on arm, head too close to work, other hand does not assist)
___x___ Difficulty drawing, coloring, copying, cutting; avoidance of these activities
_____ Poor pencil grasp, drops pencil frequently
_____ Hand dominance
_____ Quality of written work—too faint, too hard; breaks pencil often

Tactile Sensation

___x___ Seems to withdraw from touch
_____ Has trouble keeping hands to self
_____ Apt to touch everything she sees
___x___ Dislikes being hugged

Vestibular Sensation

_____ Fearful of activities moving through space (swing, teeter totter)
___x___ Avoids activities that challenge balance
_____ Excessive craving for swinging, bouncing, slides, etc.

Visual Perception

_____ Difficulty discriminating colors, shapes, doing puzzles
_____ Letter reversals after first grade
_____ Difficulty tracking—following objects with eyes holding head still
_____ Difficulty copying designs, numbers, or letters

ADDITIONAL CONCERNS OR COMMENTS:

Ellen has trouble developing peer relationships

Figure 4-15.   Ellen's referral.

lishing relationships with adults or peers, and difficulty organizing and planning and executing motor skills and language skills, appeared to be a pattern throughout Ellen's development. The occupational therapist suspected possible sensory defensiveness, developmental dyspraxia and/or vestibular dysfunction as possible contributing factors. The following assessment was designed to gather information relative to referral questions and current concerns of the family psychologist and classroom teacher.

Assessment Plan

Although the therapist will be conducting specific evaluation procedures in this case, there are many other sources of information that will have an impact on the interpretation and intervention planning processes. There is an extensive

history on Ellen which contains a wealth of information both about Ellen's functional abilities, and strategies that have been used to deal with issues as she grew. Ellen is old enough to report her own impressions of her experiences, and participate in the planning process. Formal test data from the occupational therapy evaluation will only form a part of the picture. The therapist will remain in contact with these other sources of information as she proceeds.

Findings and Interpretation

Evaluation. The occupational therapist administered the *Sensory Integration and Praxis Tests* and the *Southern California Post-Rotary Nystagmus Test*. She also conducted a clinical assessment of sensory sensitivity and responsivity, postural and ocular control, quality and endurance in gross and fine motor tasks, and problem

PERFORMANCE AREAS

Ellen 9 years PERFORMANCE COMPONENTS	ACTIVITIES OF DAILY LIVING Grooming	Oral Hygiene	Bathing	Toilet Hygiene	Dressing	Feeding and Eating	Medication Routine	Socialization	Functional Communication	Functional Mobility	Sexual Expression	WORK ACTIVITIES Home Management	Care of Others	Educational Activities	Vocational Activities	PLAY OR LEISURE ACTIVITIES Play or Leisure Exploration	Play or Leisure Performance
A. SENSORIMOTOR COMPONENT																	
1. Sensory Integration																	
a. Sensory Awareness																	
b. Sensory Processing																	
(1) Tactile								0									
(2) Proprioceptive								/									
(3) Vestibular								−									
(4) Visual																	
(5) Auditory																	
(6) Gustatory																	
(7) Olfactory																	
c. Perceptual Skills																	
(1) Stereognosis								/									
(2) Kinesthesia								/									
(3) Body Scheme																	
(4) Right-Left Discrimination																	
(5) Form Constancy								/									
(6) Position in Space								/									
(7) Visual-Closure								/									
(8) Figure Ground								/									
(9) Depth Perception																	
(10) Topographical Orientation																	
2. Neuromuscular																	
a. Reflex																	
b. Range of Motion								−									
c. Muscle Tone								−									
d. Strength																	
e. Endurance																	
f. Postural Control								−									
g. Soft Tissue Integrity																	
3. Motor																	
a. Activity Tolerance																	
b. Gross Motor Coordination																	
c. Crossing the Midline																	
d. Laterality																	
e. Bilateral Integration								−									
f. Praxis								−									
g. Fine Motor Coordination/ Dexterity								−									
h. Visual-Motor Integration								−									
i. Oral-Motor Control																	

/ = Strength
− = Concern
0 = Both a strength and concern

Figure 4-16.   Uniform terminology 2—Ellen. *Used with permission. Dunn, 1988.*

solving skills. A sensory history was also taken from both parents and Ellen. Figure 4-16 summarizes Ellen's performance.

Patterns of scores suggest strengths in the areas of visual perception and tactile discrimination. Ellen is able to accurately copy designs, although she requires more time than would be expected of a child her age. While her tactile discrimination was well within

normal limits, she had a difficult time maintaining attention to the tasks, and became increasingly more irritable and restless as the series of tactile tests proceeded.

The sensory history, as well as performance during the rest of the evaluation, suggested mild to moderate hypersensitivity to light touch, rotary movement and upside down and backward space

PERFORMANCE AREAS

Ellen — PERFORMANCE COMPONENTS	Grooming	Oral Hygiene	Bathing	Toilet Hygiene	Dressing	Feeding and Eating	Medication Routine	Socialization	Functional Communication	Functional Mobility	Sexual Expression	Home Management	Care of Others	Educational Activities	Vocational Activities	Play or Leisure Exploration	Play or Leisure Performance
B. COGNITIVE INTEGRATION AND COGNITIVE COMPONENTS																	
1. Level of Arousal								−									
2. Orientation																	
3. Recognition																	
4. Attention Span																	
5. Memory																	
a. Short-term																	
b. Long-term																	
c. Remote																	
d. Recent																	
6. Sequencing																	
7. Categorization																	
8. Concept Formation																	
9. Intellectual Operations in Space																	
10. Problem Solving																	
11. Generalization of Learning																	
12. Integration of Learning																	
13. Synthesis of Learning																	
C. PSYCHOSOCIAL SKILLS AND PSYCHOLOGICAL COMPONENTS																	
1. Psychological																	
a. Roles																	
b. Values																	
c. Interests																	
d. Initiation of Activity																	
e. Termination of Activity																	
f. Self-Concept																	
2. Social																	
a. Social Conduct								−									
b. Conversation								−									
c. Self-Expression								−									
3. Self-Management																	
a. Coping Skills								−									
b. Time Management								−									
c. Self-Control								−									

/ = Strength
− = Concern
0 = Both a strength and concern

Figure 4-16. *Continued.*

activities. Hypersensitivity to movement and gravity are reflected in postural tension when she is held or moves on her own. Ellen has always disliked playful wrestling, carnival rides that spin, and demonstrates fearfulness in heights and stairs. Hypersensitivity to touch is reflected in variability in response to everyday forms of touch, becoming easily irritated or enraged when touched by her sibling or playmates, and avoidance of play in sand, fingerpaint, or clay.

Assessment of problem solving skills suggests Ellen spends an excessive amount of time trying to maintain appropriate arousal levels and postural support. She tenses her whole body, hyper-extends her neck, shoulders, and hips and frequently holds her breath, and clenches her teeth and fists. These strategies appear only marginally helpful for very short periods of time and have probably contributed to her tight hip flexors and scoliosis. Because these strategies are so expensive in terms of energy required, Ellen frequently looks tired and on the verge of tears. The parents feel Ellen's frequent outbursts at home reflect her frustration and exhaustion in working so hard to produce schoolwork and maintain peer relationships.

Ellen has developed several strategies to protect her nervous system from becoming overwhelmed. She avoids new or crowded situations, keeps to herself, daydreams in class, and insists on predictable routines at home and school.

Extreme difficulty initiating movement patterns was noted during bilateral motor coordination and imitation of unfamiliar postures. Her fearfulness, tension and difficulty initiating movement patterns, gave a quality of hesitation and poor coordination to all fine and gross motor movement patterns. Her strength appears to be in repetition of a motor act (use of feedback from muscles and joints). As she repeats the same motor act, she is able to increase both the speed and quality of her performance.

It was also noted that while she made attempts to use language to organize motor activities (both her own and others as they responded to her questions), it does not always help her reorganize and produce quality movement patterns. According to the speech and language tests reports, Ellen has had difficulty organizing language since her preschool years. Her fourth grade teacher notes her written language is often disorganized and disjointed.

In summary, Ellen is demonstrating significant sensory integrative dysfunction in the form of sensory defensiveness, difficulty processing and using information from movement and gravity, and developmental dyspraxia (motor planning). This pattern of dysfunction appears to be a major contributing factor in the areas of social emotional development, general coordination, and use of language.

The occupational therapist confirmed the psychologist's hypothesis that Ellen has sensory integrative dysfunction. She combined information from the history, other reports, observations and test data to report her findings. This confirms that the problems are long-standing and that the occupational therapy findings are compatible with other reports and stategies. This forms the basis for an interdisciplinary intervention plan.

CASE #12—TAMMY

Pre-assessment Process

Referral. Tammy was referred by her parents and her public school program to a University-based supported employment program one month prior to her completion of high school. The supported employment program further connected Tammy to the State Division for Rehabilitation and the Division for Developmental Disabilities which were able to pool resources to pay for Tammy's post school employment services. The primary concern expressed by the referring parties was that Tammy lacked definite plans for the future and without timely intervention, it was likely that she would be spending unproductive time at home or in a sheltered workshop. These two options were unacceptable to Tammy and her family.

Supported employment is defined in federal statute as a highly individualized approach for assisting individuals with significant disabilities to obtain and maintain employment. Supported employment includes three essential components:
1. paid work,
2. employment in integrated community settings, and
3. the availability of on-going support and training as needed to assure job retention or subsequent job placement.

Figure 4-17 illustrates the critical components of the supported employment decision-making process used by the University-based program that served Tammy.

Tammy's case illustrates her "transition" from school to a productive adult worker role. Her timely referral to post secondary services (supported employment program) prevented an unnecessary waiting period while adult service systems located Tammy and identified her needs. Without a timely referral, it is likely that a significant delay or gap in services would have occurred and possibly resulted in Tammy losing valuable skills and confidence. Many school programs are now initiating the transition process at a much earlier stage to assure continuity of service after high school. It is not uncommon for secondary students to be engaged in community employment prior to their exit from public schools.

History. Tammy was in self-contained special education classes throughout her public school career due to her primary disability of moderate mental retardation. Her high school education included basic academics, some school-based training in independent living activities, and vocational preparation activities which included primarily in-class simulations of work tasks. During her last year of high school, Tammy spent a limited amount of time in a work-study position at a local nursing home. At the time of referral, Tammy had never held a job and could not identify job interests.

Tammy lived with her parents who were very supportive and desired to see Tammy assume a worker role in the community. They also expressed anxiety about Tammy traveling independently in the community. Tammy's home was on the public bus route which provided access to needed transportation although Tammy did not know how to use the bus system. Food preparation, shopping, house maintenance were all responsibilities assumed by Tammy's family although she did assist with house cleaning. Tammy had a history of some incoordination and judgement limitations when handling cleaning equipment and materials. This interfered with her ability to perform maximally in this area. Tammy performs self-care activities independently with occasional reminders from her mother. Tammy's recreational activities were almost always family centered and family initiated.

Pre-assessment Hypothesis

The information gathered from the referral sources and Tammy indicated that employment was the primary concern. School personnel and Tammy's parents also felt that she would need significant help in finding, learning, and retaining a job thus the referral for supported employment services. Although Tammy could not identify specific job-related interests, she expressed a strong desire to work and to earn money. Tammy's dependence on her parents for transportation along with her difficulty with judgment and handling materials in a coordinated manner required further investigation.

Assessment Plan

A supported employment service team was comprised of two occupational therapists, a job developer, a job coach, Tammy and her parents. To gain needed information that would assist the team in placing Tammy in a paid community job, it was decided that some in depth interviews with Tammy,

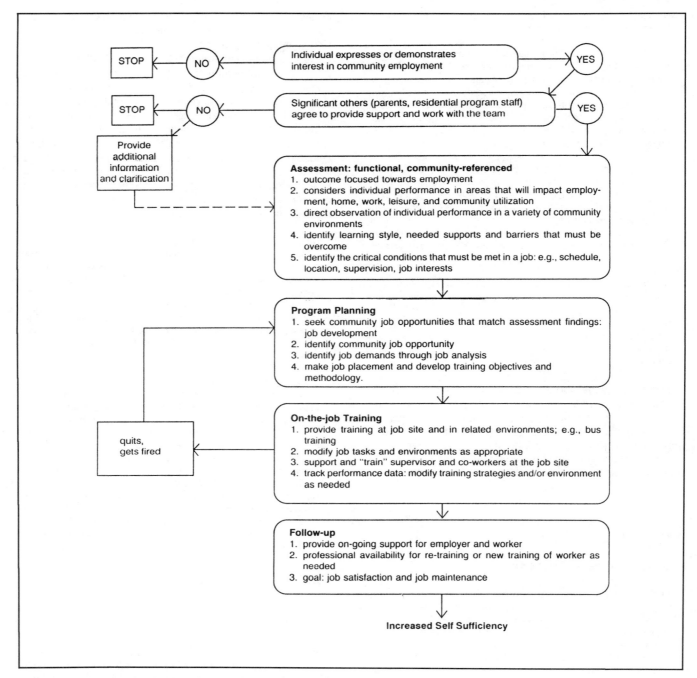

Figure 4-17.   Decision-making process for supported employment services.

her parents, and school personnel would be needed. The interviews would help the team identify Tammy's interests and abilities as they might apply to a job. The team decided that it would be important to assess not only job-related interests and abilities, but also her specific abilities at home, in the community, and recreationally. Needs or abilities in these areas can directly impact employment.

In addition to interviews, the team needed to gain information about what Tammy was able to do, how she learned, and how she operated in a variety of community environ-

ments. This would require situational observation of Tammy's performance in a variety of relevant situations such as on the city bus, at a downtown restaurant, crossing streets, and using city services. During this observation process, team members planned to identify Tammy's strengths and interests while noting any supports that were required to ensure successful performance (e.g. types of cueing needed to take the appropriate bus). Barriers to performance would also be identified (e.g. inability to plan needed time to get to appointments) along with strategies to overcome these barriers.

PERFORMANCE AREAS

Tammy — 19 years PERFORMANCE COMPONENTS	ACTIVITIES OF DAILY LIVING Grooming	Oral Hygiene	Bathing	Toilet Hygiene	Dressing	Feeding and Eating	Medication Routine	Socialization	Functional Communication	Functional Mobility	Sexual Expression	WORK ACTIVITIES Home Management	Care of Others	Educational Activities	Vocational Activities	PLAY OR LEISURE ACTIVITIES Play or Leisure Exploration	Play or Leisure Performance
A. SENSORIMOTOR COMPONENT																	
1. Sensory Integration																	
a. Sensory Awareness																	
b. Sensory Processing																	
(1) Tactile																	
(2) Proprioceptive																	
(3) Vestibular																	
(4) Visual																	
(5) Auditory																	
(6) Gustatory																	
(7) Olfactory																	
c. Perceptual Skills																	
(1) Stereognosis																	
(2) Kinesthesia																	
(3) Body Scheme																	
(4) Right-Left Discrimination																	
(5) Form Constancy																	
(6) Position in Space																	
(7) Visual-Closure																	
(8) Figure Ground																	
(9) Depth Perception																	
(10) Topographical Orientation																	
2. Neuromuscular																	
a. Reflex																	
b. Range of Motion																	
c. Muscle Tone																	
d. Strength																	
e. Endurance																	
f. Postural Control																	
g. Soft Tissue Integrity																	
3. Motor																	
a. Activity Tolerance																	
b. Gross Motor Coordination												0		0			0
c. Crossing the Midline																	
d. Laterality																	
e. Bilateral Integration																	
f. Praxis																	
g. Fine Motor Coordination/ Dexterity																	
h. Visual-Motor Integration																	
i. Oral-Motor Control																	

/ = Strength
– = Concern
0 = Both a strength and concern

Figure 4-18.   Uniform terminology 2—Tammy. *Used with permission. Dunn, 1988.*

Findings and Interpretations

The general results of Tammy's assessment have been summarized in Figure 4-18.

Tammy was found to be highly skilled in many areas and able to learn new skills effectively (e.g., identifying the correct bus, placing order in restaurant, crossing streets safely) when given the opportunity to follow a model and to practice. Tammy learned quickly in the actual community environment that required a specific skill (e.g., a store, restaurant, city bus, bank). She was unable to readily generalize learning across environments or situations. Tammy appeared to enjoy spending time in the community with people other

PERFORMANCE AREAS

Tammy — PERFORMANCE COMPONENTS	Activities of Daily Living — Grooming	Oral Hygiene	Bathing	Toilet Hygiene	Dressing	Feeding and Eating	Medication Routine	Socialization	Functional Communication	Functional Mobility	Sexual Expression	Work Activities — Home Management	Care of Others	Educational Activities	Vocational Activities	Play or Leisure Activities — Play or Leisure Exploration	Play or Leisure Performance
B. COGNITIVE INTEGRATION AND COGNITIVE COMPONENTS																	
1. Level of Arousal																	
2. Orientation												/			/		
3. Recognition																	
4. Attention Span												/			/		
5. Memory																	
a. Short-term												/			/		
b. Long-term																	
c. Remote																	
d. Recent															0		
6. Sequencing												/			/		
7. Categorization																	
8. Concept Formation																	
9. Intellectual Operations in Space																	
10. Problem Solving	0				0							0			0		
11. Generalization of Learning												–			–		
12. Integration of Learning	0				0							–			–		
13. Synthesis of Learning												–			–		
C. PSYCHOSOCIAL SKILLS AND PSYCHOLOGICAL COMPONENTS																	
1. Psychological																	
a. Roles																	
b. Values																	
c. Interests																	
d. Initiation of Activity																	
e. Termination of Activity																	
f. Self-Concept												/			/		
2. Social																	
a. Social Conduct												/			/		
b. Conversation												–			–		
c. Self-Expression												–			–		
3. Self-Management																	
a. Coping Skills												–			–		
b. Time Management												–			–		
c. Self-Control																	

/ = Strength
– = Concern
0 = Both a strength and concern

Figure 4-18. *Continued.*

than her family however she lacked confidence to do this without some sort of support and assistance. In the self care area, Tammy required cueing from her mother to shower and wash her hair on a regular basis. She also had some difficulty selecting matching clothes from her closet. Tammy's coordination was observed in a variety of functional contexts (carrying a food tray in a restaurant, walking over uneven surfaces, running to catch a bus, climbing the stairs of the bus, walking to her seat on a moving bus) and it was determined that coordination was largely functional and safe. In situations where coordination and judgement were both needed (e.g. walking across a newly mopped floor), Tammy had more difficulty. With explicit instruction and demonstration, she was able to learn to walk around (compensation) the wet area even if this took her out of her way.

When a functional situational assessment process is used it is important for the therapist to observe and record skills and needs within context. It cannot be assumed, for example, that an individual's ability to safely cross a street with a crossing light means that they can also cross safely at an unmarked intersection. A functional assessment allows the team to focus on an individual's strengths (vs. liabilities) in a variety of relevant situations. Family members generally understand and can actively contribute to such an assessment process which builds cooperation and a sense of shared planning and problem-solving.

Based on the extensive observations and interviews used to assess Tammy's work-related interests and needs, the team was able to identify the critical conditions that would need to be present in a job for Tammy. Tammy would require a job where supervision was always close-by, and a setting where co-workers would be able to redirect or instruct Tammy when she ran into difficulty. It was clear, based on the assessment, that Tammy would not do well working independently or working without frequent contact with others. Assessment of Tammy's ability to learn new tasks (e.g. riding the public bus) led the team to recommend that she have on-the-job "coaching" available in order to learn a job via explicit demonstration, practice, and feedback. It was felt that an employer would not be able to assume total responsibility for training Tammy given her unique learning needs.

The assessment process also allowed team members to identify Tammy's job-related interests. After spending time at a local restaurant, Tammy expressed that she would like to "help" with a salad bar and to "wash" tables. She also stated that she liked the uniforms worn by restaurant workers. Among other interests, it became clear that Tammy liked spectator sports, particularly professional football. The team was then able to incorporate her interests into a job search effort.

Tammy's performance is summarized in relation to home management, work, leisure performance, the targeted goals set by the team (see Figure 4-17).

EXPAND YOUR NEWLY ACQUIRED KNOWLEDGE

1. Explain why the therapists chose an in-home strategy for evaluating David and Clifford. What data may you not have obtained on each child if you had evaluated the children in an OT clinic? Explain how this might have altered the program planning process; how might these alterations have affected outcomes?
2. Review Chapter 3. Select a case from this chapter and design an alternate assessment plan that would also allow you to gain pertinent information about the child. Justify your selections.

Reference

Sattler, J. M. (1982). *Assessment of children's intelligence and special abilities*, (2nd ed.), (p. 3). Boston: Allyn and Bacon, Inc.

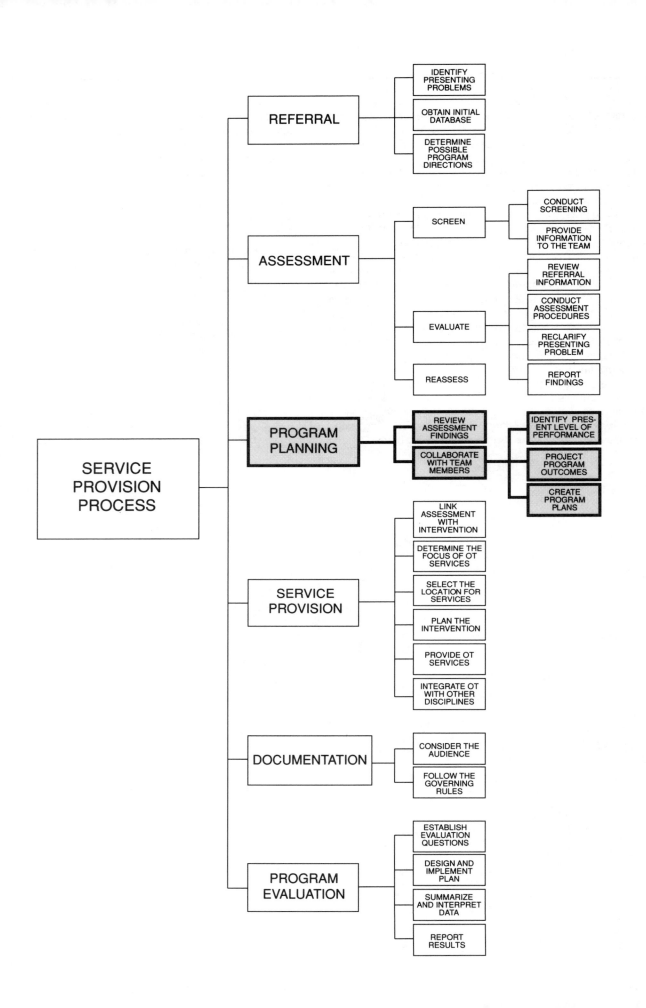

CHAPTER 5

Components of the Program Planning Process

Mary Muhlenhaupt, OTR

"Prescriptive treatment that teaches academic or important life skills, and ultimately makes the child less handicapped, is the foremost goal of assessment." Wodrich, 1986.

PROGRAM PLANNING PROCESS

Introduction

The pediatric program planning objective—to design and monitor an individualized therapeutic environment and program, which prepares a child for the transition to work and community living, is complex. Medical and healthcare costs increase, yet programs must be planned within budgetary constraints. Specialties evolve within pediatrics, creating an increasing number of persons involved in the management of individual cases. Sophisticated technologies address the survival needs of premature and high risk infants, opening new avenues in therapeutic care and long-term life management. Federal and state education laws are amended, and programs based on government funding and regulation emerge to meet the educational needs of children with all degrees of disability. Children with atypical development have a variety of needs stemming from parental, medical, educational, financial, social and cultural concerns, to name but a few. Effective program planning for these needs incorporates an understanding of family dynamics, and typical and atypical childhood development. Professionals consider processes affecting health, cognitive, physical and social-emotional growth and knowledge of learning characteristics and components of educational and vocational achievement.

Expertise from persons of varied backgrounds and experiences, with different orientations and concerns for aspects of the child's total development, is required for proper assessment and intervention. Services to meet these needs exist within homes, schools, health care, medical and community agencies. Coordinating these resources in our mobile and fast-paced society is a formidable task. Team planning (Bailey, 1984; Losen & Losen, 1985) has been recognized as an efficient means to combine the different knowledge, skills and attitudes necessary to plan services which realize the pediatric program planning goal. The pediatric team, representing a variety of disciplines and perspectives focused toward a common interest in the child's development, provides a multi-faceted in-depth assessment. Ideas are generated as members interact with each other to review and analyze impressions gained from working with the child and family. The "how's and why's" of programs planned from this approach reflect a methodology beyond what one professional or one discipline can provide. Fleming and Fleming (1983) discuss the importance of effective team decision-making on the quality of programs designed for children and their families. When members of the service team work together with the family, consistency between home, therapy, and educational programs is facilitated (Winton, Turnball, & Blacher, 1984).

The program planning process can be organized into four phases: review of assessment findings, collaboration between persons involved with the child to design a program, implementation of the program, and monitoring of results. These phases form a continuous cycle of planning and service provision activities. Initial assessment results are compared and interpreted in relation to the unique life environment and development needs of the child. The necessary remedial services are identified, coordinated and implemented. Monitoring the child's responses to the program provides feedback which the team uses to reassess the plan, and the cycle begins again.

Composition of the Pediatric Planning Team

Members of the pediatric planning team are determined in various ways. The child's needs, and resources within the agency, influence which disciplines are represented on the team. In rural areas, geography and actual human resources within the region determine the team's composition. Teams within a service system sometimes depend upon legal requirements, as in the case of special education programs. School districts are mandated to develop planning teams which include representatives from certain disciplines (for example, psychology, speech therapy and special education) and positions (parent of a child with an educational handicap who resides in the district). Specialists are involved on a periodic or ongoing basis, depending on the need for their expertise during stages of the child's development. For example, the speech pathologist will examine Carlos, a two-month-old with Down Syndrome, every six weeks and consult with the occupational therapist regarding oral-motor stimulation and pre-language concepts, which may be incorporated into early developmental play and sensory experiences. This periodic reassessment provides additional information used in planning specific programs goals and intervention activities.

The child's primary physician and medical specialists are important members of the planning team, whether it is a hospital or community-based program. In some states, physician involvement in occupational therapy programs is mandatory under licensure statutes. Physician participation during planning meetings occurs more readily when the services are provided within an agency where the doctor is employed, rather than when an educational planning team meets to develop a child's program. In this latter case, the team does not rely on the physician as a leader of the team, but rather as a peer, contributing to team decisions regarding the child's education program. Telephone contacts, copies of written evaluations, and progress reports are useful methods to share information when the physician cannot attend the educational planning meeting. Communication from the team regarding the child's program and progress is particularly valuable just prior to the child's scheduled visits with the doctor.

Parents are vital members of the pediatric planning team. Both their innate and acquired knowledge contribute to the planning process. Parental concerns, goals, and resources (Dickman, 1985; Featherstone, 1980; Zins, Graden, & Ponti, 1988) are critical to the child's development and involvement in a pediatric intervention program. For example, when a preschool program is based on the philosophy that parents are the primary teachers of their children, it is important for the planning team to know how the parents view the service agency. They may view the agency as a substitute family who manages the child the way the parents see fit, may feel they are not the child's teachers, and leave all the planning and programming to the agency staff, or may hold some combination of positions within these viewpoints. The Education for All Handicapped Children Act of 1975 (Federal Register, 1977) provides parents with the legal right to be an integral part of the educational planning teams for their children. Training materials and advocacy efforts (Deppe & Shareman, 1981; Harrison, 1983; Winton et al., 1984) encourage parents to become more knowledgeable and active in decisions regarding therapeutic and educational programs for their children.

The planning team includes involvement from other family members and the child, when appropriate. Siblings are an important part of the child's life, and in some cases, are responsible for aspects of the child's at-home care and management. Certain family traditions or situations may necessitate that extended family members are the child's primary care-givers. Children with acute or chronic medical conditions may have nurses, or other health care workers, who attend to their needs at home. These persons have the potential to play an important role in planning and implementing the child's therapeutic and educational programs. Their willingness and abilities as service providers are important considerations before specific programming recommendations are finalized.

Team Approaches

Several types of team approaches have been defined in pediatric health and education programs (Conner, Williamson, & Siep, 1978; Orelove & Sobsey, 1987; Van Dyke, Lang, Heide, & van Duyne, 1986). These approaches are categorized according to the coordination of team members' expertise in assessment, design, and implementation of the child's program. Each approach focuses on developing programs to meet the child's need for challenge and mastery in his or her unique life environment. The selection and use of a particular team planning approach, within a system or agency, depends upon legal requirements, program philosophies, traditions, experience, or preference of staff members.

Multidisciplinary Team

The multidisciplinary team members' responsibilities are clearly defined. Each professional evaluates the child and determines priorities, goals, and intervention strategies for the services he or she provides. These persons do not come together to review initial assessment reports, or summarize the services recommended for the child. Their interventions tend to be implemented in isolation from each other (Bailey, 1984). Sparling (1980) describes the multidisciplinary team as one in which disciplines "co-exist". Assessments and services are generally provided in specialized environments, such as the doctor's office or the "therapy treatment room"; however, the child's natural environment may be used, as in home-based services. Programs using this model involve a number of persons working with one child. For example, Pam visits the outpatient clinic each week for individual occupational and physical therapy sessions. Speech therapy is provided by a private therapist who visits Pam's home. While the speech therapist knows that Pam receives additional therapies, he may be unaware of their goals and intervention plans. Periodic appointments are scheduled for neurological and orthopedic re-evaluations at a regional children's rehabilitation hospital, while Pam's routine medical care is provided by the local pediatrician.

The multidisciplinary model provides therapists and other team members with ample opportunity to plan and implement interventions which reflect their own perspectives, and the philosophies of their chosen professions. While the child receives a significant amount of individualized contact with the service providers, this model is costly, time consuming, and inefficient in certain cases. When there is overlap between services, as with many young infants' programs, efforts may be needlessly duplicated. Since coordination between plans is not inherent in the model, interventions used by service providers sometimes contradict each other. For example, the occupational therapist recommends instruction in cursive writing as a strategy to improve a student's writing performance in the classroom, since cursive writing requires less starting and stopping of strokes drawn to form letters, while the teacher opposes this plan because it conflicts with classroom curriculum design. Parents, as the primary caregivers, have the responsibility to coordinate the goals and plans of the many services their child receives in the multidisciplinary model. They may feel confused by the various approaches, and receive mixed messages from the conflicting goals between services. When the confusion becomes more than the parent can manage, he or she may retreat from the challenge, and the child loses a primary source of advocacy.

Since planning meetings are not a part of their approach, team members have limited opportunities to give or receive peer support, or learn about goals and the child's response in other areas of programming. Time and travel restrictions further limit the possibility of contact when services are provided within different agencies. Written progress reports, brief impromptu meetings, and telephone conferences become the primary means of team communication. Because of the nature of these contacts, superficial information frequently becomes the focus of discussion. When the occupational therapist and teacher meet in the hallway, one reports, "Johnny did really well today and earned two stars on his feeding progress chart!". Multidisciplinary team members do not have the opportunity to assure that collaboration includes more than a comparison of the child's behavior during sessions, or a review of acquired developmental milestones and quantitative achievements made in areas of programming.

Interdisciplinary Team

While evaluations of the child are carried out in isolation, the interdisciplinary team meets to review assessment results, and reach a consensus as to appropriate goals and program plans for the child. The child and family work with several persons, since remedial activities are implemented by professionals representing each discipline included in the child's total service plan. However, collaboration during both the planing stage, and ongoing program review, facilitates interdisciplinary sharing, and coordination of the interventions provided for the child and family.

Each discipline's assessment findings are presented and team members collaborate to develop programs, which include an organized synthesis of the various expertise from those disciplines represented. The ability to translate occupational therapy assessment results, and coordinate professional perspectives with those of other team members, are important skills for the therapist on an interdisciplinary team. Unless the therapist presents findings and insights in ways that are useful across disciplines, valuable expertise cannot be integrated into the service plan developed through the interdisciplinary model.

Interdisciplinary team collaboration provides an opportunity for all staff persons to learn about the supportive services the child receives, and how they relate to the total program plan. This is particularly helpful when new services are introduced within a child's program. Furthermore, this model encourages each staff member to support the activities carried out by another, as each intervention provided reflects combined goals, and reinforces the total program plan. Planning activities and communication between team members are carried on throughout the program, since goals developed through the interdisciplinary process can be achieved only when team members continue to work together in an interactive and coordinated manner (Bailey, 1984). For this reason, the interdisciplinary model is difficult to manage when a program includes services provided by an itinerant staff. These persons tend to visit the building only when direct services with children are scheduled, thus limiting the opportunity for ongoing formal and informal collaboration with center-based staff members. Without continued collaboration, the team begins to function in a multidisciplinary manner as described earlier. Persons working within the interdisciplinary model must be alert to this concern, so that team goals are not lost as ongoing intervention activities are implemented.

As an interdisciplinary program example, Melanie's special education teacher has planned classroom goals which reflect the combined knowledge gained from the psychological, social work, educational, occupational and speech therapy evaluations. An itinerant occupational therapist works with a combined service approach, incorporating specific goals established through initial team planning. The teacher assistant reinforces Melanie's developing visual-motor abilities through classroom activities, using strategies developed by the occupational therapist and special education teacher. Speech goals are incorporated into both the classroom routine and occupational therapy sessions. Melanie also participates in weekly speech therapy group sessions outside of her classroom. The speech therapist reinforces aspects of the classroom curriculum during speech lessons, by emphasizing academic concepts, and incorporates occupational therapy goals by placing manipulative materials in designated locations, which encourage Melanie to develop visually-directed reaching and accuracy.

Transdisciplinary Team

Transdisciplinary teams work together throughout assessment, diagnostic, planning, and implementation phases of pediatric programs. Orelove and Sobsey (1987) advocate the use of this approach with children who are multiply disabled. Ottenbacher (1983), noting that transdisciplinary teams are most frequently associated with early childhood programs, suggests the use of this approach in programs where professionals train parents in the management and handling of their children. A noticeable feature of programming using the transdisciplinary approach, is the limited number of persons who implement direct services with the child and family (Conner, et al. 1978; Sparling, 1980). Each discipline contributes information to the team assessment and goal setting process, then one person implements the program, becoming the child's primary service provider or "program facilitator" (Sparling, 1980). In some cases, the parent is recommended for this role with a young infant. The primary service provider reports progress to the team, which meets to review and revise the program plan, as appropriate. Team members may observe the primary service provider working with the child to gain additional reassessment data. While support services are used for consultation, and other indirect services to the primary service provider, this approach does not exclude the use of periodic direct services by any team member (Orelove and Sobsey, 1987).

In the example of Matt, a seven-year-old boy with athetoid cerebral palsy, his teacher is the primary service provider. Matt attends a self-contained class for children with learning difficulties secondary to orthopedic impairments. The school's occupational and physical therapists provide the teaching staff with ongoing inservice training, related to handling and positioning children with cerebral palsy, during various school activities. They collaborate with each other, and with Matt's teacher, throughout the school year, developing classroom interventions to facilitate Matt's performance during daily classroom and special subject activities. Specific interventions include training in toilet transfer techniques, and the use of adaptive equipment for snack and lunch periods. The speech therapist and school psychologist provide similar consultation, enabling the teacher to integrate the strategies of various disciplines into all aspects of Matt's classroom programming. Matt's achievement of specific goals is reinforced through consistency, and ample experience during activities within the natural school environment and class routine.

The transdisciplinary approach requires administrative support, parent and staff training (Sparling, 1980), which depend upon agency and program philosophies, parent and staff commitment, time, and financial resources. Professionals working within a transdisciplinary team have the opportunity to learn more about the child, and about different remedial approaches, through the cross-disciplinary sharing that is essential in the model. However, the resulting role-blurring (Conner et al., 1978) is not advantageous to the new practitioner who is developing a professional role identity.

Building rapport and developing working relationships between parent, child, and service providers is streamlined, and consistency is increased in this model, as only one person implements the intervention activities. While transdisciplinary programming has obvious advantages for young infants, the team must realistically assess the child's needs, and the parent's willingness and ability to assume the role of the primary service provider.

Ottenbacher (1983) and Bennett (1982) cite obstacles in implementing this approach. Both include the differing philosophical beliefs held by team members from various disciplines, and the isolated nature of education and training within professions, which does not prepare graduates for the cross-disciplinary interaction of the transdisciplinary approach. The issue of professional liability, when one trains another to implement specific techniques, is also a source of concern when using this approach (Ottenbacher, 1983).

One effect of the limited number of persons working with the child on an ongoing basis, is the associated reduction in staff time required for direct service provision. The transdisciplinary approach should not be implemented in an effort to provide services in the face of reduced staff availability. When this occurs, there is a likelihood that necessary staff training has not occurred, and that important professional expertise and perspective are missing from the evaluation and planning phases. The resulting program reflects this absence and can lead to unsafe practices.

Team Process

All group members contribute to the planning team's operation (Lacoursiere, 1980). Their personal values, commitment, sense of professional identity and comfort within the particular system, influence the roles adopted by each member and the dynamics used within the group. Effective team communication facilitates members' understanding of their roles and functions (Losen and Losen, 1985). Formal and informal communications that take place during both group meetings, and casual contacts between members, are important influences for an atmosphere of understanding and commitment toward program planning activities. At times it is difficult for team members with diverse backgrounds to communicate effectively with each other and with parents. Clear language and descriptors of behaviors observed, rather than technical jargon, aid the communication process. The ability to interact and communicate effectively with center-

TABLE 5-1. Coordination of Members' Expertise in Phases of Selected Team Approaches

	Assessment	Diagnosis/ planning	Program Implementation
Multidisciplinary	isolated	isolated	isolated
Interdisciplinary	isolated	shared	isolated & shared
Transdisciplinary	shared	shared	shared

based staff is an important skill for the itinerant staff member who is present in the program on a sporadic schedule.

Some teams function with rotating roles and responsibilities. A teacher, therapist, social worker, or other staff member, may lead the team in planning meetings, and take responsibility for coordinating the necessary procedures required for the team to develop and implement the program. This approach allows members to experience different responsibilities in planning the child's program, broadening their understanding of various team member roles in the program planning process.

When a team experiences difficulty in working together to plan a child's program, the source of the problem should be assessed and resolved. Team function can be impeded by problems with the team's evolution as a group, composition, or group process used (Bailey, 1984). In discussing factors which influence team function, Bennett (1982) has raised the issue of territoriality and "protection of turf" in relation to the increasing specialization in childhood services. It is important for team members to avoid competition, and recognize and respect the varied backgrounds which are the resources used in developing the child's service plan. When expertise from diverse backgrounds is brought into play, the resulting plan is enhanced, and members share an ownership and commitment toward the common goals and programs which have been developed (Maher & Bennett, 1984). Inservice training programs can be useful for the team to develop the group process skills, which are essential to effective team planning (Crisler, 1979).

PLANNING PROCESS COMPONENTS AND OUTCOMES

Introduction

Once assessment results are reviewed, the collaboration phase of program planning begins. The team reaches consensus as to the child's current performance level, projects appropriate outcomes for the child and family, and determines the services required to achieve those goals. At the onset of program implementation, service providers develop specific intervention plans, which are coordinated with the overall goals for the child. Once the program is implemented the child's responses and progress are observed. These results provide new data which are used to measure the success of the original plan.

Identifying Present Level of Performance

Assessment results generate the information needed to identify the child's current level of performance, a picture of function which reflects the interaction of social-emotional, physical and cognitive components with the child's learning characteristics. The child's present level of performance is the foundation upon which the program is built, and the baseline against which program response is measured. In addition to test scores and grade equivalent performances, professionals describe strengths, weaknesses, and acquired adaptive behaviors across environments. It is necessary to determine the manifestations and functional significance of clinical findings observed during assessment, since each child's own unique constitution produces varying pictures of ability from a particular condition. Furthermore, individual priorities and goals necessitate that differing relative values are placed on specific performances.

Occupational therapists, focusing on human performance abilities and acquired adaptive behaviors, have a particular skill which is useful to the team in developing this part of the child's program plan. Performance descriptors need to be objective, so that the child's future status is compared to a constantly defined standard. "Andrea writes her name in two inch manuscript lettering," clearly defines a performance, while "Andrea's printing is immature," does not. Stating these indices in positive terms helps the team focus on what the child can do, and on increasing performance; a negative focus highlights deficiencies, and guides programming toward reducing dysfunction. Instead of saying "Johnny can't walk down the hall to the cafeteria independently," the statement can be rephrased: "Johnny walks down the hall to the cafeteria when an adult holds his hand."

Projecting Program Outcomes

Program outcomes are anticipated long-term functional performances the child needs for function in a realistic future environment. These performances are based on the child's own capacities and limitations, and are influenced by system goals and objectives, family goals, cultural, political, and legal factors. Pediatric programming teams are challenged to approximate usual childhood experiences, when setting goals for the child with special needs. In this light, transitions from school to work and community life, for children with handicaps, have received considerable attention in recent years (Goodall & Bruder, 1986; Rusch & Phelps, 1987; Brown, Halpern, Hasazi, & Wehman, 1987). Programs plan for this concern, when long-term life goals are considered as the child enters the service system. Family situations are an important factor in this aspect of planning. The future life environment for a child with a physical disability, with older parents experiencing personal health restrictions, will be very different from that of a child who has many siblings and a large extended family willing to assume supervisory care in the future.

The child's age and developmental history give the planning team information regarding rates of growth and progress which may be anticipated. Medical diagnosis and the acquired, versus innate nature of the child's condition, provides information regarding the potential outcome. Goals to develop athletic skills are not appropriate for Debby, since her physical activity is restricted by juvenile rheumatoid arthritis. Furthermore, characteristics of Debby's status during the course of programming, can be inferred from the diagnosis, influencing program design and implementation. For exam-

ple, certain accommodations are necessary for her during cold and rainy seasons when her joints swell and become more painful. Again, the occupational therapist has important insight into this area of program planning, and can relay the functional implications of various medical conditions during activities and performances expected of the child, within the educational program, and within the home and family environment.

Creating the Program Plan

A team determines the specific plan recommended for a child, building on the projected performance outcomes, program goals, and resources. Knowledge of previous involvement in programs, and a child's response to that intervention, are helpful so that successful strategies are emphasized and inappropriate interventions avoided. When specific information is missing, or questions exist that require further clarification, the team may need to defer the planning decisions, or note that the projected program requires review once the additional information is secured.

A quality service plan which features integrated learning in a natural and consistent environment, is the goal of the program planning process. A program that includes only a number of isolated support services may lead to fragmented intervention.

Public Law 94-142 guarantees access to mainstreamed programs for children with educational handicaps. This does not mean that every program is designed to prepare children for participation in the general education program with non-handicapped peers. Programs are planned to enable children to remain in the natural learning environment to the maximum extent possible, with justification for placements in a specialized program (Federal Register, 1977). Some students with special needs prosper from placement in a mainstreamed class setting, aspiring to the accomplishments of nonhandicapped peers and thriving on the challenge to succeed.

When developing service recommendations, the team considers available options, as well as potentially available options. Team members must always be ready to develop new alternatives for unique situations. The team may include more than one service option in its recommendations. This is an efficient use of valuable team planning time, and is particularly helpful when there are questions as to how the child may respond to a given program plan. This also provides alternatives if a particular program design is not immediately available. An estimate as to how long the child may need the service is helpful to staff in assessing the child's response, and can be useful to aid parents in developing realistic expectations for their child's development. A time-limited intervention plan also helps to facilitate change in an expeditious manner in some cases. The team considers the effective use of resources, and plans programs which acknowledge the unique abilities of team members. For example, the occupational therapist who has specialized training in neurodevelopmental treatment, may be the best team member to design positioning and handling strategies for the team.

Short-term behavioral objectives define the long term program goals. Short-term objectives are measurable statements defining child-centered behaviors which are expected from enrollment in the program. In addition to communicating the intent of the program, short-term objectives are used to monitor progress toward the anticipated outcome. Goals and strategies of all specialists involved in the service plan are incorporated and coordinated within the behavioral objectives, in order to reflect expected outcomes. This approach focuses team members on the interrelation of all disciplines in pediatric services, and facilitates consistency between remedial and instructional activities implemented in the child's program.

Developing the Intervention Plan

Once the team recommends the types of services which enable the child to achieve the projected performance outcomes, persons implementing the services develop the intervention plan, recognizing that the ultimate goal when planning programs is change in performance. Recognizing this goal, Thomas (1984) cites the importance of generalization of the change, and includes guidelines for developing effective intervention methods:

1) address multiple targets: the problem behavior; behaviors which are incompatible with the problem behavior (antagonist behaviors); the cause, or factors controlling the dysfunction; the environment
2) use the natural rather than artificial environment
3) plan intervention to be implemented by persons inherent to the natural environment.

Therapists using these principles broaden their scope to a total management approach, and consider additional intervention methods beyond the traditional direct service therapy model. Intervention is simultaneously directed into more than one facet of the child's daily activity, increasing the opportunity for exposure, experimentation, and development of specific skills or performances.

Therapy intervention is developed in relation to overall program goals, priorities, and available resources. When one school visit per month is included in Linda's education program, the therapist must capitalize on that time and be effective within the total program. In this case, the short and long-term benefits of therapist-directed procedures, provided within the empty cafeteria or "itinerant services room," must be objectively analyzed. While the therapist implements quality treatment which effects noticeable changes in Linda's visual-motor coordination during the session, carryover of the performance is not assured. Using an integrated therapy model, the therapist uses the visit to consult with Linda's teacher, and develop interdisciplinary strategies and solutions to problems Linda experiences each day while copying boardwork. The teacher implements the plan on a daily basis, providing greater opportunity for reinforcement and change, which affects Linda's functional performance abilities.

Many children with special learning needs have difficulty integrating and applying numerous learning strategies, employed in frequent isolated sessions, which are not incorporated within the total service plan. This is dramatically exemplified in Jimmy's program. He has a daily schedule of special services taped to the desktop, a notebook, homework papers and a hall pass to carry each time he leaves the classroom. Jimmy watches the clock during mathematics class, so that he is not late for his speech session. When he returns to the classroom after the speech session, he realizes that he should have gone to lunch. He checks the schedule on his desk, grabs his lunchbox, and hurries to join his classmates. Jimmy has only ten minutes to play during recess before the social worker arrives to escort him to his counseling session. At the end of the day Jimmy has difficulty remembering homework assignments from his various teachers, and doesn't have time to gather the proper notebooks, before the hall monitor announces that his bus is in the parking lot. His school day is relatively easy, when compared to the challenge he faces that evening, as he tries to complete his homework assignments in preparation for the next day!

Information from the present level of performance is useful, so that intervention activities to address areas of limitation are planned around the child's strengths. Purposeful, goal-directed tasks which are appropriate to the child's developmental stage and abilities, and respect the child's chronological age as well, are the foundation of the pediatric occupational therapist's intervention. Appropriate intervention activities reinforce the child's role within the environment, and include opportunities which approximate normal childhood developmental experiences. These conditions present a challenging task for the therapist serving a child with a profound disability. The anticipated rate of progress, along with assessment of the child's ongoing responses, influence how the activities and interventions are adapted or graded within the framework of the total program.

The child's initiation and active involvement in therapeutic interventions are important considerations. Behaviors which result only from direct participation depend upon specific stimuli in order to occur. In a situation such as this one, the child cannot express the desired behavior without the established prompt or cueing sequence, so the skill cannot be elicited during spontaneous activity, and is not useful across environments. Enabling maximum degrees of self-directed performance across environments is the ultimate objective.

Evaluating Progress

The child's behaviors are evaluated as the intervention program progresses, providing new information which is compared to the original performance level, reflecting change or maintenance in status. This reassessment occurs both formally and informally, providing continuous feedback, which indicates the need to continue, modify or replace the original program plan. At times, additional referrals within or outside of the agency may be suggested.

Information gathered in this phase is less extensive than initial assessment, and is directed more towards qualitative aspects of function (Thomas, 1984). Rather than re-administer standardized tests which were used for initial diagnostic purposes, the therapist may use criterion-referenced measurement, or observation of functional performances to gain this re-assessment data. The important concern at this stage is to assure that the child is progressing from involvement in the intervention program. When progress is not observed, or the rate of change is not satisfactory, a modification may be necessary. Alternate intervention methods and alternate or additional services are considered by the team. Figure 5-1

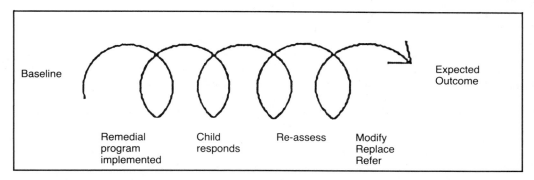

Baseline

Remedial   Child   Re-assess   Modify
program   responds   Replace
implemented   Refer

Expected
Outcome

Figure 5-1.   Evolution of the Program Planning Process.

(Muhlenhaupt, 1988) illustrates the program planning process as presented in this section.

Providing Follow-up and Discontinuing Services

A goal of occupational therapy intervention services is to develop behaviors and functional performances which eliminate the need for continued service. Team involvement is recommended when termination from therapy services within the child's program is considered. Individual programs rate a child's eligibility for support services, with entrance based on the child's need for the unique skills and knowledge of the specialist in the support field. Once the child has achieved service goals and is able to maintain the desired level of performance independently or on the basis of involvement in other required services within the program, the team reviews the need for continued service. When a service no longer effects changes that lead to improved functional performance, or the child's life role has changed, a recommendation for a team review to consider program modifications is indicated. In certain instances, the development of compensatory behaviors which enable the child to participate in appropriate activities and instruction signal a need for team review.

The functional status and the performance abilities which the child has mastered, are a focus when the team considers discontinuation of a service. Gliedman and Roth (1980) assert that societal and professional attitudes place persons with disabilities in a disadvantaged role, because of their attention to the dysfunction, rather than the ability which characterizes the person. Occupational therapists are in an ideal position to help the team recognize each child's functional performance abilities, despite the presence of a medical diagnosis, or a temporary or long-term handicapping condition, thus contributing an essential element to this phase of program planning.

Children with special needs will likely be involved with a variety of social, educational and medical services throughout some parts of their continued childhood and adult lives. Planning followup action, after a change in some aspect of the service plan, is an important responsibility. Human and non-human resources within the total environment are assessed to assure continued maintenance of performance levels. Re-assessment by members of individual disciplines may be indicated to monitor the child's status, and assure continued

maintenance or growth, as appropriate. Future programming addressing later developmental needs may be indicated.

FACTORS/ISSUES INFLUENCING THE PEDIATRIC PLANNING PROCESS

Introduction

The development of special services for children within any system is influenced by numerous internal and external factors. Understanding and working with these influences, their interactions and interrelations, is critical for the overall program plan. While certain issues are inherent within a specific system, additional unanticipated situations may occur, which will require the team's attention for action, or a strategy unique to the circumstances.

Legal

Perhaps the greatest influence on pediatric program planning in recent history is the enactment of Public Law 94-142, The Education for All Handicapped Children Act of 1975. This legislation requires that local school districts provide publicly funded education programs for all children, regardless of the nature or severity of their disability (Federal Register, 1977). Implementation of the mandate has caused school districts to establish specialized planning teams, enter into new areas of evaluation, and provide programs that include services from a variety of support personnel, who have not been traditionally associated with the delivery of public education.

Each child with special educational needs is guaranteed an Individualized Education Program or IEP, (Federal Register, 1977) under PL 94-142. The IEP includes both a planning meeting, and a document which summarizes the child's educational strengths, weaknesses, handicapping condition, projected program, and goals.

Specific components of the IEP process, and guidelines for its completion, vary between states. School therapists have an opportunity to make important contributions to the student's IEP through effective assessment and program planning skills.

Along with the additional monies and options available for children with special needs, the due process guaranteed under this legislation has influenced program planning. In order to assure student entitlement and parent participation throughout the development and implementation phases of programming, procedural guidelines for time requirements, meetings, and documentation must be followed. Due process court proceedings (Osborne, 1984) may become a part of the program planning process, reviewing and modifying recommendations made by the educational planning team. School therapists face new roles and functions in relation to this legal mandate and its requirements. Each therapist's ability to accept and respond to these challenges influences the planning process in programs designed to meet special education objectives.

PL 94-142 amendments are changing special education in some states by lowering the age at which children are eligible for public education. PL 99-457, The Education for All Handicapped Children Amendments of 1986, requires that all states provide special education programs for children ages three to twenty-one years, by the 1990–1991 school year. In states where this legislation necessitates a change in current practice, therapists in preschool special education programs will face new procedural requirements, so that services are integrated among community agencies and qualify for funding.

New early intervention services under this legislation (Federal Register, 1987) feature services to the family unit, with the development of an "Individualized Family Service Plan" (IFSP) to define the intervention. Occupational therapy is included as an intervention service. As providers of primary intervention services, occupational therapists will be challenged to develop new roles in dealing with families of infants with confirmed disabilities, or those at risk for developmental dysfunction. Specific training and experiences will be necessary for therapists to manage this new role in the early stages of program development.

Recent legislation (PL 99-372, The Handicapped Children's Protection Act of 1986) states that parents who are successful in their claims against the school district, are entitled to reimbursement for the cost of their attorney's fees (Federal Register, 1986). This has provided another alternative for parents who disagree with the school's recommendations, but avoid using their due process rights for financial reasons. Undoubtedly, this regulation will influence the types of programs planned in certain cases. Court proceedings are time consuming, expensive, and often a strain on the parties involved. School districts may make compromises and adjustments in children's programs, rather than risk the expense (not only in financial terms) of a court case, and possible reimbursement of the petitioner's legal fees.

Other legal and ethical factors, which influence program planning and implementation, include professional licensing and supervision guidelines. Therapists without specified certification and credentials are unable to practice in certain environments, thereby limiting the resources available to pediatric programs. Requirements for an occupational therapist's supervision of the occupational therapy assistant, necessitate a certain staffing pattern which may influence program planning and service provision. Therapists need to consult resources within individual states in order to become knowledgeable regarding these regulations.

Manpower

Administrative roles in establishing and defining the program's philosophy, goals and objectives, and facilitating the

team's activity, are essential (Campbell, 1987). The team depends upon these foundations for its direction and unity when assessing children's needs and designing programs. Team members' individual backgrounds and experiences have been discussed as a factor contributing to the roles and responsibilities each assumes in the program planning process, and as an influence upon the service plan which is developed.

Shortages or surpluses of pediatric therapists within a region influence program planning. In either situation, therapists are challenged to develop priorities in relation to the types of services provided, and needs addressed by occupational therapy within a program or agency. In the face of staff shortages, agencies consider alternatives to provide the needed expertise within the service system. Without regular involvement by an occupational therapist, a program may opt for consulting services from a self-employed therapist, an area hospital or, other health-care agency. The types of therapy intervention incorporated within this program differ from those provided by the staff therapist who is routinely available to consult with building staff, attend meetings, and provide intervention services. Both administration and other service personnel working within these situations, need to realize the impact that such staffing patterns will have upon the types of service provided within the program.

Therapists' ethical responsibilities prevent them from assuming caseload numbers and varieties which are beyond their ability to effectively manage and serve. While attractive employment opportunities and incentives may be available, both new graduates and experienced therapists entering the pediatric practice area, need to assure the availability of appropriate professional supervision and specific training opportunities, for the specialized work role they assume.

Financial

Available pediatric services depend on funding resources. Public spending for health and education programs has decreased in recent years. Private funding agencies often have complex procedures for reimbursement, with restrictions on eligibility or spending caps. Closely aligned with the public funding issue are local and regional political climates. Pediatric programs which are funded by government monies reflect the current political priorities within the geographic area. Since state laws and available financial resources vary, the unique service options found within communities reflect differing mandates and degrees of regulation. Cooperative funding efforts through third-party payment, grant monies, charities, and donations lead to greater resources for children with special needs. Sorting out the intricacies of funding procedures is a complex and time consuming process. Professional networks are helpful for therapists to gain additional support in this area.

Family Concerns and Perceptions

While harmonious working relationships with parents, and efforts to involve them in the design and implementation of their child's program have been stressed, individual beliefs, preferences, and resources influence their actual involvement (Winton et al., 1984; Featherstone, 1980). Parents' reactions and responses to their child are additional factors which may impede or facilitate participation in the program, and actually influence the structure and focus of the therapist's intervention (Anderson and Hinojosa, 1984). Therapists need to acknowledge their own experiences and comfort, when interpreting parental attitudes as an interference or support for the child's development.

How the team adapts to either anticipated or unexpected parent participation, as well as the lack of parent involvement in the development of a child's intervention program, plays an important role in the final outcome of the program plan. Therapists need to communicate consistently, clearly, and completely with parents, and give them the opportunity to be closely involved in decisions regarding their children's therapy program. This type of open communication provides information the therapist can use to plan intervention which is realistic, and practical within each unique family situation.

Standards of Quality

Ideal pediatric intervention programs suggest that the best possible staffing pattern is secured and maintained, with readily available consulting services from any specialist, as needed. There is no restriction to the financial base for such a program, just as there is no limitation to the building facilities, supplies, and materials made available. All staff members have previous experiences with children, are aware of all of the current theoretical and practical knowledge related to planning and implementing pediatric programs, and they have immediate access to new knowledge as it develops. The children enrolled in the programs do not experience any unexpected events which negatively influence their ability to benefit from the instructional activities presented. They are never absent, and each day they are able to gain maximum benefit from their participation in the program. They all function and progress according to a well defined expectation, so that the teachers and support service staff know exactly how to design and structure the daily program activities. Furthermore, all persons providing services in the program share the same standards of "ideal services," and agree that they are upheld in their agency. Clearly this is **not** a realistic situation! There are too many unknowns in the behavior and development of children with special needs, too many variables in service plans, too many human factors affecting both providers and receivers of the services, for such a controlled, predictable, and planned strategy to exist. Programs to meet children's special needs are based on the reality of current knowledge, reflecting available resources and experiences. These factors change over time, enabling the development of new plans and strategies to more effectively meet individual children's and families' needs. Pediatric practitioners need to recognize these realities when designing, recommending and implementing services.

Research

Program design and implementation are affected by research and technological advances as well. An agency involved in a research project focuses on a particular model or curriculum design during a test period. Treatment efficacy studies both support and refute various approaches and practice methods, and alter the instructional strategies used in programs. Augmentative communication systems, and environmental control devices, open new avenues for occupational therapy involvement in education programs for children with severe disabilities. Biomechanical advances are changing the course of therapies which traditionally address these students' motor development needs.

Therapists working with children need to consider generating research data related to the use of specific approaches and intervention methods with certain populations and developmental problems. In addition to considering causal relationships between intervention and outcome behavior, issues of cost-effectiveness and efficiency in service provision need to be addressed. Descriptive studies, clinical trials, case studies, and other research methods (Partridge and Barnett, 1986) are available to therapists planning and implementing pediatric service programs. Local study groups, or regional research consultants in affiliation with university programs, and state or regional professional associations, can be helpful resources in this area.

ISSUES OF PRACTICE ARENAS

Introduction

Specialization within professions has led to subspecialties and practitioners with expertise to work with certain populations, within specific systems, and using certain practice models or environments. Specialization equips therapists with unique knowledge, skills, and attitudes necessary for effective practice within their area of concern. Since each specialist is adept at dealing with a defined area of the child's overall development, the need for coordinated planning between specialists is critical in our current world of health care service. Therapists need to recognize the overall goal of such team planning, so as not to perceive the involvement of other persons as a threat to their autonomy.

Rural vs. Urban Practice Environments

The varying resources, needs, and priorities of rural and urban populations are reflected in the program plans used in pediatric services. Cultural and social mores place differing relative values on certain areas of human performance, causing the team to emphasize different aspects of the child's total development and function. Human resources in rural areas prompt planning teams to consider alternative methods of implementing programs for children. Geographical considerations may make regular travel to outlying homes or agencies an unrealistic option. When travel is possible in rural areas, logistics often play a role in determining which children will be seen by the therapist, and how frequently those visits will occur. Similarly, travel within the public transportation systems of urban areas is problematic for a therapist with large pieces of equipment used for certain interventions. These factors influence the options available and specific interventions chosen by individual service providers working with children. Therapists in these service systems frequently depend upon their skills and abilities as consultants, who facilitate the primary care-giver's or teacher's daily interaction with the child. When therapists and other team members consider these factors in making program recommendations, their efforts are focused on developing options which are both practical and realistic for the child and family within their environment. These plans are not viewed as negative alternatives, but rather as creative solutions to the real problems which are inherent within the specific situations facing the team.

Use of Program Model Unique to System/Environment

Pediatric practice environments include specialty areas such as public school practice, neonatal intensive care, terminal care, long term and acute rehabilitation. Specific resources and experiences are necessary for the clinician to make the transition between practice environments, and provide programming which meets the needs of the child and family seeking services. A limited background, and lack of familiarity with the goals and objectives of a service system, will impact upon the therapist's participation in the program planning process. Differing amounts of peer role-modeling and support, inservice training, past practice, and tradition are characteristics within various practice environments. At times therapists have to consult education resources outside of the agency or program in which they work, to help them develop the knowledge, skills, and attitudes unique to each practice area and service system.

Therapists working in public schools are developing a program model which is unique to the education system. "Related service" therapy programs are planned in accordance with the philosophies and objectives of the local school district, and are influenced by both state and federal government regulations. The education system's administrative model is quite different from that found in a hospital or health-care agency. School therapists work with a different level of autonomy, and with students who come into the system for reasons that contrast with those of patients seeking services in a traditional medical model. School districts, their students, and families are consumers of aspects of the pediatric occupational therapist's total knowledge and expertise.

Occupational therapists in schools face challenges associated with the profession's roots in the medical model. Bennett (1982) suggests that both doctors and other members of the educational team may experience difficulty, since the traditional medical hierarchy places the physician in the team's leadership role. Securing appropriate physician involvement within an educational program in a state which requires medical referral or prescription for the provision of therapy evaluations or services, can be a challenge to the planning team and to the therapist carrying out a related service program. Even though a physician provides a referral for an occupational therapy evaluation, the educational planning team must determine whether the evaluation is an appropriate part of the child's school program, otherwise the evaluation is conducted outside of the school context. The school therapist often becomes the mediator between school, family, and physician in this situation. Communicating the results of the therapy evaluation, and clarifying the objectives of the school therapy program in individual cases, is helpful in educating both families and community physicians about the roles and objectives of school-based therapy services.

Specialized education and advanced clinical training are prerequisites for the therapist in neonatology (Sweeney, 1986).

As scientific advances enable younger premature infants to survive, new techniques in management and care of these infants develop, requiring that therapists actively pursue ongoing education and training to keep abreast of new findings and practices in this area. Integrated teamwork between numerous developmental specialists, in an efficient and ongoing manner, is a critical component of program planning on the neonatal intensive care unit.

The therapist in a solo practice functions as program developer, administrator, clerical support staff, service provider, financial officer, and marketing manager. On-site expertise from other persons involved in the child's care is not available when the clinician is working with the child. While previous clinical experience is essential for the private practitioner, knowledge of administration and management principles is an important ingredient for the successful practice (refer to Chapters eleven & twelve for more detailed information). Guidance from both professional and business consultants can assist with the financial, legal and practical aspects of initial set-up.

Cooperation Between Agencies/Programs/Providers

The use of services from educational, medical, and social agencies to meet the diverse needs of children with atypical development has been discussed in this chapter. This in itself creates a multidisciplinary team composed of persons and teams from all the agencies working with the child and family. The disadvantages inherent in the multidisciplinary model discussed earlier are evident in this situation. Just as the pooling of resources within one agency has value for the overall program planning and implementation of services for a particular child, cooperative efforts which bring together regional resources have a valuable effect on the service options available within the area. Elder and Magrab (1980) discuss the concept of interagency collaboration, so that available resources are used efficiently, and effective programs are planned to meet children's needs. Collaborative efforts between persons working with the child, including family members, and health, medical, educational and social professionals, are a valuable means to assure communication and continuity in planning a child's program.

A case coordinator or case manager (Allen, Holm, & Schiefelbusch, 1978) functions as a communicator between and within agencies for coordination in program planning. The case manager facilitates the transfer of information and material relevant to the child's case, to coordinate potential areas of overlap and prevent duplication of services. In this manner, an effective total program is developed and implemented for the child's benefit. All persons working with the child have access to the overall program goals through communication with the case manager.

Cooperative efforts are necessary as children transfer between programs, or as families seek consultation services from one agency while their child attends another. Because of the multitude of service options that exist to meet the special needs of children with disabilities, families can easily become confused and mistrustful of the information they receive (Featherstone, 1980). Another area of concern in the transition process relates to the transfer of therapy service recommendations between programs and agencies. Service frequencies and intervention plans utilized in one agency are useful to subsequent planning teams when they are included in a summary report. However, recognizing that service plans are based on the unique needs of the child, in combination with agency priorities and the resources available, this transition requires special consideration. The child's program needs and appropriate service options within another agency may be different. For example, Beth is moving from the school district where she attends a self-contained class for children with learning disabilities. In her new district, she will attend a general education program; an occupational therapy evaluation and consultation to aid in planning classroom visual-motor training activities will be included in her education program.

There are times when transitions become particularly difficult for parents and children. One example is the transition from a home-based infant program to a school-based preschool program. The service alternatives in a center-based program are quite different from those provided at home, and clearly the parent is less involved in the actual daily intervention provided once the child attends classes at the school building. These considerations, along with the anxieties a parent may have in acknowledging the child's new level of independence, or in separating from the child who remains dependent upon adult care to meet all survival needs, require steps to insure coordination between the programs before the transition is made. One example is a school-based occupational therapist, from the preschool staff, who makes a home visit during the time the infant program therapist is working with Jeffrey. Both parents and staff discuss goals, progress, and particular concerns related to Jeffrey's future school-based program. Following the home visit, the preschool therapist returns to the building team, and helps develop Jeffrey's future service plan.

New programs for infants and toddlers with special needs (PL 99-457), will require attention toward cooperative program planning. As primary intervention service providers in this program, occupational therapists will have a new responsibility to develop specialized programs for the unique needs of the population in this family-oriented service model. Evolving transition issues will confront practitioners when children progress from early intervention to preschool programs, from preschools to the public schools, and from the public school to work and independent living.

SUMMARY

The pediatric program planning process begins with the assessment results. With that data, the team plans a program which addresses the interrelated concerns of childhood health care, and social-emotional, cognitive and physical growth. The diverse expertise which is needed for this endeavor comes from the combined knowledge of parents and other family members, along with a variety of professionals in various service systems. The coordination of their perspectives into a unified team approach influences the final program recommendation and outcome.

Once a program plan is outlined, specific interventions are designed and implemented. These plans are developed to be consistent within the framework and goals of the system which supports the intervention service. Ongoing program activities are concerned with developing specific performances and function, but are planned with respect to the child's total life environment. Accordingly, therapeutic interventions are structured to replicate appropriate childhood developmental experiences and stages. When the child no longer requires intervention within a program, discharge is planned to include appropriate follow-up from recommended services.

Remedial, compensatory and preventative interventions for children with special needs are available from a variety of disciplines, and through many service systems—each with its own unique resources. Transitions between programs can be coordinated efficiently when team members are knowledgeable regarding the options to which they have access. In this way, programs can be designed to meet the individualized and continuing needs of children with developmental dysfunction.

EXPAND YOUR NEWLY ACQUIRED KNOWLEDGE

1. Discuss the role of occupational therapy in a multidisciplinary, interdisciplinary and transdisciplinary team. Select a child performance problem (e.g., eating) and explain how services would look different in each team model. What is missed/taken advantage of in each model?

2. Discuss the benefits and difficulties of planning programs within children's natural life environments. What might the occupational therapy profession do to overcome the difficulties and enhance the benefits you identify?

3. A team projects long term outcome of augmentative communication for a ten year old girl with severe, multiple disabilities. Define the program planning contributions of the occupational therapist toward this long term outcome. How would your contributions be different if the team projected an oral language process for communication?

References

Allen, K. E., Holm, V. A., & Schiefelbusch, R. L., Eds. (1978) *Early intervention—A team approach.* Baltimore, MD: University Park Press.

Anderson, J., & Hinojosa, J. (1984). Parents and therapists in a professional partnership. *The American Journal of Occupational Therapy, 38*(7), 452–461.

Bailey, D. (1984). A triaxial model of the interdisciplinary team and group process. *Exceptional Children, 51*(1), 17–25.

Bennett, F. C. (1982). The pediatrician and the interdisciplinary process. *Exceptional Children, 48*(4), 306–314.

Brown, L., Halpern, A. S., Hasazi, S. B., & Wehman, P. (1987). From school to adult living: A forum on issues and trends. *Exceptional Children, 53*(6), 546–554.

Campbell, P. H. (1987). The integrated programming team: An approach for coordinating professionals of various disciplines in programs for students with severe and multiple handicaps. *Journal of the Association for the Severely Handicapped, 12*(2), 107–116.

Connor, F., Williamson, G., & Siep, J. (1978). *Program guide for infants and toddlers with neuromotor and other developmental disabilities.* New York: Teachers College Press.

Crisler, J. (1979). Utilization of a team approach in implementing Public Law 94-142. *Journal of Research and Development in Education, 12*(4), 101–108.

Deppe, P. & Shareman, J. (1981) *The High-Risk Child—A Guide for Parents*. New York: MacMillan Publishing Co., Inc.

Dickman, I. (1985). *One miracle at a time*. New York: Simon and Schuster.

Elder, J. O. & Magrab, P. R. (1980). *Coordinating services to handicapped children*. Baltimore, MD: Paul H. Brooks, Publishers.

Featherstone, H. (1980). *A difference in the family*. New York: Basic Books, Inc.

Federal Register, vol. 42, no. 163. August 1977. The Education for All Handicapped Children Act.

Federal Register, August 1986. Handicapped Children's Protection Act of 1986.

Federal Register, vol. 52, no. 222. November 1987. Early Intervention Programs for Infants and Toddlers With Handicaps.

Fleming, D. C. & Fleming, E. R. (1983). Consultation with multidisciplinary teams: A program of development and improvement of team function. *Journal of School Psychology, 21*, 367–376.

Gliedman, J. & Roth, W. (1980). *The unexpected minority—handicapped children in America*. New York: Harcourt Brace Jovanovich, Inc.

Goodall, P. & Bruder, K. (1986). Parents and the transition process. *Exceptional Parent, 16*(2), 22–28.

Harrison, H. (1983). *The premature baby book: A parents' guide to coping and caring in the first years*. New York: St. Martin's Press.

Lacoursiere, R. (1980). *The life cycle of groups*. New York: Human Sciences Press.

Losen, S. & Losen, J. (1985). *The special education team*. Boston, MA: Allyn and Bacon, Inc.

Maher, C. & Bennett, R. (1984). *Planning and evaluating special education services*. Englewood, NJ: Prentice-Hall, Inc.

Muhlenhaupt, M. (1988) *FIRSTS: Foundations in Relating School Therapy Services*. Northport, NY: Pediatric Therapies.

Orelove, F. P. & Sobsey, D. (1987). *Educating children with multiple disabilities—A transdisciplinary approach*. Baltimore, MD: Paul H. Brooks, Publishers.

Osborne, A. G. (1984). How the courts have interpreted the related services mandate. *Exceptional Children, 51*(3), 249–252.

Ottenbacher, K. (1983). Transdisciplinary service delivery in the school environment: Some limitations. *Physical and Occupational Therapy in Pediatrics, 3*(4), 9–16.

Partridge, C. J. & Barnett, R. E. (1986). *Research guidelines: A handbook for therapists*. Rockville, MD: Aspen Publishers, Inc.

Rusch, F. R. & Phelps, L. A. (1987). Secondary special education and transition from school work: A national priority. *Exceptional Children, 53*(6), 487–492.

Sparling, J. W. (1980). The transdisciplinary approach with the developmentally delayed child. *Physical and Occupational Therapy in Pediatrics, 1*(2), 3–16.

Sweeney, J. K., Ed. (1986). The high-risk neonate: Developmental therapy perspectives. *Physical and Occupational Therapy in Pediatrics, 6*(3–4).

Thomas, E. J. (1984). *Designing interventions for the helping professions*. Beverly Hills, CA: SAGE Publishers.

Van Dyke, D., Lang, D. J., Heide, F. & van Duyne, S. (1986). Children with Down syndrome—a multidiscipliary approach. *The Exceptional Parent, 16*(8), 46–51.

Winton, P. J., Turnball, A. P. & Blacher, J. (1984). *Selecting a preschool—A guide for parents of handicapped children*. Baltimore, MD: University Park Press.

Wodrich, D. L. (1986). The terminology and purposes of assessment. In D. L. Wodrich & S. E. Joy (Eds.), *Multidisciplinary assessment of children with learning disabilities and mental retardation*, (p. 24). Baltimore: Paul H. Brookes Publishing Co.

Zins, J. E., Graden, J. L., & Ponti, C. R. (1988). Prereferral intervention to improve special services delivery. *Services in the Schools, 4*(3/4), 109–130.

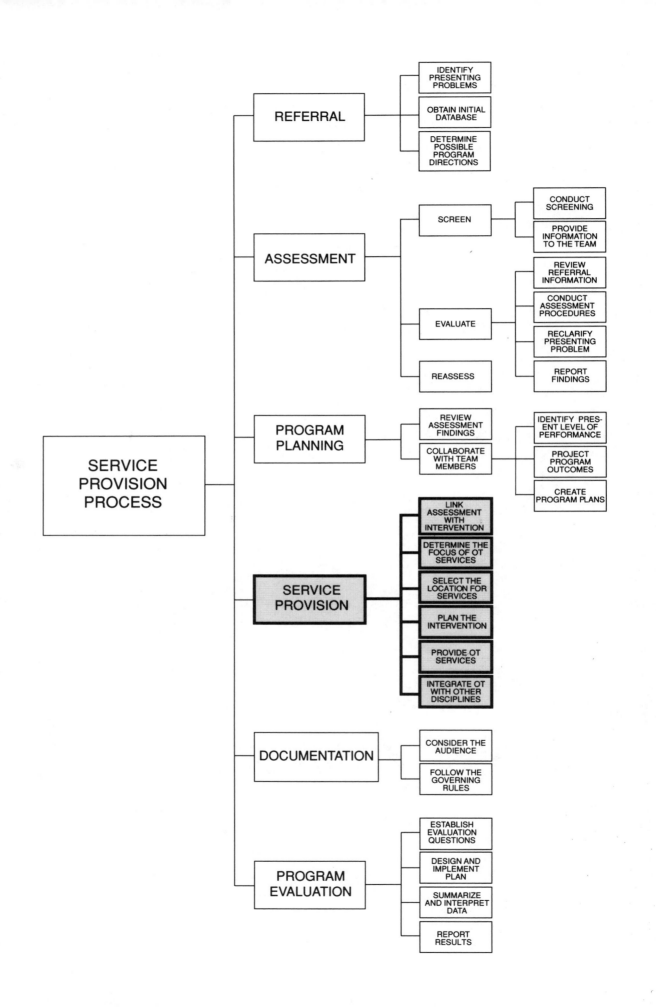

CHAPTER 6

Designing Pediatric Service Provision

Winnie Dunn, PhD, OTR, FAOTA
Philippa H. Campbell, PhD, OTR

"A willingness to learn new patterns for providing services to students will be required by specialists as they apply their expertise in new organizational models." McDonnell & Hardman, 1989

Pediatric therapy services are provided for children of different ages and with varying degrees of disability. Pediatric therapists respond to the needs of children, when providing services, by considering variables related to disability as well as environmental factors. Service provision is a fluid process that requires ongoing decision-making. This chapter outlines a framework for assisting therapists to make service provision decisions that are in the best interest of children and their families. Frameworks for decision making provide a mechanism against which decisions may be evaluated. The immediate and long-term impact of service provision decisions is determined more easily when guided by an overriding framework.

Pediatric service provision begins with an individualized plan that states desired outcomes. This plan may be an Individualized Family Service Plan (IFSP), an Individualized Education Program (IEP), an Individual Habilitation Plan (IHP), or some other similar type of service provision plan. The type of plan used to guide services is dependent upon a child's age and the agency responsible for planning and providing services.

Figure 6-1 illustrates the relationship among assessment, program planning, service provision, and evaluation. Therapists define the focus of service provision on the basis of a wide variety of data that are obtained through assessment (see Chapter Three). These data are discussed by team members to determine program outcome priorities (see Chapter Five). Therapists assist children in achieving program outcome priorities within a variety of settings, by using direct, monitoring, and consultative strategies. These services are outlined on an intervention plan that guides the provision of specific therapy services and provides the basis by which therapists document and evaluate the effects of those services.

Many children, particularly infants and toddlers, receive services through more than one agency or service provider. These services require coordination if resources are to be utilized effectively. In some cases, families perform service coordination roles for their children, while case managers may share, or totally provide coordination in other instances. Professionals contribute to the coordination process by ensuring that all services facilitate attainment of desired outcomes. Therapists who provide services through hospitals, clinics, or private practices may not have opportunities to contribute directly to early intervention or school program team decisions, but, like all other interagency team members, are responsible for ensuring that therapeutic activities support and enhance a child's acquisition of desired outcomes.

LINKING ASSESSMENT WITH INTERVENTION

Occupational therapy services are provided within age-appropriate life tasks and the environments within which those tasks are performed. Services are based on performance outcomes under the categories of: activities of daily living (ADL), work, and play/leisure. Various sensorimotor, cognitive and psychosocial performance components enable or block performance of ADL, work, or play/leisure activities. These outcome performance areas and performance components are illustrated in Figure 6-2, a grid that is based on the American Occupational Therapy Association (AOTA) *Uniform Terminology for Occupational Therapy—Second Edition* (1989). Occupational therapy assessment is directed towards identifying strengths and concerns in these performance components, and their effect on an individual's performance of ADL, work, and play/leisure outcomes. The grid is used to guide design of occupational therapy intervention programs. The performance areas are listed across the top of the grid, while the performance components are listed down the side of the grid. Areas in need of intervention emerge when the therapist identifies strengths and concerns in the performance components, as related to performance of functional life tasks. This information is used to create an intervention plan that utilizes strengths, while focusing on areas of concern. Outcomes of independence in ADL, work, and/or play/leisure are the result of intervention planning.

Functional Assessment and Program Planning

Deciding when a child requires intervention, and how that intervention will be provided, are two of the most difficult decisions in the service provision process. Table 6-1, Functional Assessment Parameters, reorganizes the components and areas of the Uniform Terminology grid, to focus on those outcome categories that are most relevant for children (Col-

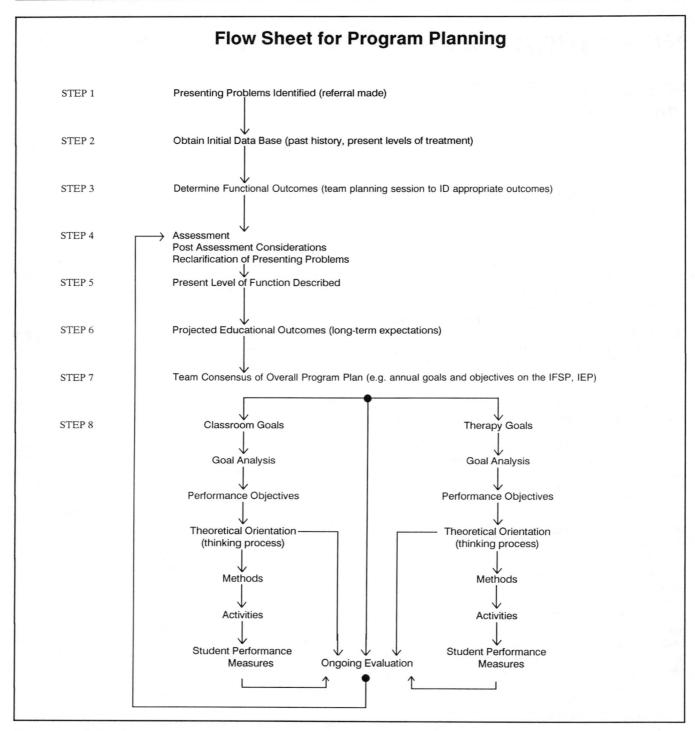

Figure 6-1. An illustrated view of the relationship between assessment, program planning, service provision, and evaluation. *Dunn, W., & Campbell, P., 1989 (adapted from Dunn, W., 1987).*

umn 1). Second, the detailed list of performance components are reorganized into functional groups (Column 2) that pertain to each outcome area. These performance components are not listings of all aspects within a particular outcome category, but include those most likely to be addressed by therapy personnel. Therapists use these parameters to synthesize assessment information and to provide information used in the team planning process to determine desired outcomes.

Performance outcome categories include: learning (skill acquisition and educational activities), work, play/leisure, communication, socialization, and activities of daily living. The outcome areas represented are those that are important for infants, toddlers, children, and youth. However, all areas are not necessarily relevant for all children at all chronological ages. In addition, other outcome areas such as mobility and positioning are represented as performance components within

PERFORMANCE AREAS

UNIFORM TERMINOLOGY GRID PERFORMANCE COMPONENTS	ACTIVITIES OF DAILY LIVING Grooming	Oral Hygiene	Bathing	Toilet Hygiene	Dressing	Feeding and Eating	Medication Routine	Socialization	Functional Communication	Functional Mobility	Sexual Expression	WORK ACTIVITIES Home Management	Care of Others	Educational Activities	Vocational Activities	PLAY OR LEISURE ACTIVITIES Play or Leisure Exploration	Play or Leisure Performance
A. SENSORIMOTOR COMPONENT																	
1. Sensory Integration																	
a. Sensory Awareness																	
b. Sensory Processing																	
(1) Tactile																	
(2) Proprioceptive																	
(3) Vestibular																	
(4) Visual																	
(5) Auditory																	
(6) Gustatory																	
(7) Olfactory																	
c. Perceptual Skills																	
(1) Stereognosis																	
(2) Kinesthesia																	
(3) Body Scheme																	
(4) Right-Left Discrimination																	
(5) Form Constancy																	
(6) Position in Space																	
(7) Visual-Closure																	
(8) Figure Ground																	
(9) Depth Perception																	
(10) Topographical Orientation																	
2. Neuromuscular																	
a. Reflex																	
b. Range of Motion																	
c. Muscle Tone																	
d. Strength																	
e. Endurance																	
f. Postural Control																	
g. Soft Tissue Integrity																	
3. Motor																	
a. Activity Tolerance																	
b. Gross Motor Coordination																	
c. Crossing the Midline																	
d. Laterality																	
e. Bilateral Integration																	
f. Praxis																	
g. Fine Motor Coordination/ Dexterity																	
h. Visual-Motor Integration																	
i. Oral-Motor Control																	

Figure 6-2. **Uniform terminology (2d ed.) grid of outcome performance areas and performance components.** *Reprinted with permission, Dunn 1988.*

outcome areas. For example, postural control and positioning are included in relation to individual outcome areas to focus not just on positioning, but on management of body position for a specific functional outcome, such as communication. Similarly, mobility skills are targeted within outcome areas to emphasize the importance of mobility within particular performance environments.

Occupational and physical therapists provide primary information to the team regarding sensorimotor components of performance. Occupational therapists also provide information about the cognitive and psychosocial components of performance, but may not be the only professionals contributing intervention strategies to resolve concerns in these areas. A goal of occupational therapy is to enable performance of

PERFORMANCE AREAS

UNIFORM TERMINOLOGY GRID PERFORMANCE COMPONENTS	ACTIVITIES OF DAILY LIVING Grooming	Oral Hygiene	Bathing	Toilet Hygiene	Dressing	Feeding and Eating	Medication Routine	Socialization	Functional Communication	Functional Mobility	Sexual Expression	WORK ACTIVITIES Home Management	Care of Others	Educational Activities	Vocational Activities	PLAY OR LEISURE ACTIVITIES Play or Leisure Exploration	Play or Leisure Performance
B. COGNITIVE INTEGRATION AND COGNITIVE COMPONENTS																	
1. Level of Arousal																	
2. Orientation																	
3. Recognition																	
4. Attention Span																	
5. Memory																	
a. Short-term																	
b. Long-term																	
c. Remote																	
d. Recent																	
6. Sequencing																	
7. Categorization																	
8. Concept Formation																	
9. Intellectual Operations in Space																	
10. Problem Solving																	
11. Generalization of Learning																	
12. Integration of Learning																	
13. Synthesis of Learning																	
C. PSYCHOSOCIAL SKILLS AND PSYCHOLOGICAL COMPONENTS																	
1. Psychological																	
a. Roles																	
b. Values																	
c. Interests																	
d. Initiation of Activity																	
e. Termination of Activity																	
f. Self-Concept																	
2. Social																	
a. Social Conduct																	
b. Conversation																	
c. Self-Expression																	
3. Self-Management																	
a. Coping Skills																	
b. Time Management																	
c. Self-Control																	

Figure 6-2. *Continued.*

functional outcomes rather than to improve isolated skills. Pediatric therapists have an obligation to ensure that their service provision is designed to have an effect on desired program outcomes. Team members collaborate to determine which program outcome(s) are appropriate for an individual child, so that everyone is working towards identical outcomes. Individual team members may offer their points of view, but decisions about overall outcomes are made collectively by team members. The outcome categories and performance components outlined on this table make the unique contributions of therapy clear to all team members, and also direct a therapist's focus toward team-determined program outcome(s) (column 1 of Table 6-1).

Functional Skills Assessment Grid

Figure 6-3 illustrates a grid that is used to make decisions about service provision in pediatric settings. Children's abilities in each performance component are graded using a five-level scale that reflects the degree of influence of performance on program outcomes. Therapists use assessment information to assign rating scores to children's performance

---

TABLE 6-1. Functional Assessment Parameters

Occupational therapists address the student's needs within program goals. Therapists do not address program goals in isolation nor do they address *all* components of a goal. Rather, they contribute expertise to enable the individual to benefit from the over-all program and achieve the program goals. For example, occupational therapists do not achieve communication outcomes alone, but rather contribute specific skills which enable the individual to gain access to communication possibilities. The individual needs addressed by occupational therapists in each area are listed below.

Program Goals	Performance Components

Learning: Skill acquisition and academics	1. manipulation/hand use
	2. interpretation of body senses
	3. perceptual skills
	    e.g.: organization of space and time
	         interpretation of visual stimuli
	4. cognitive skills
	    e.g.: problem solving
	         generalization of learning
	5. attending skills
	6. use of assistive and adaptive devices
	7. management of body position during learning
	8. management of body position during transitions
	9. movement within individual's learning environment

Work*	1. management of body position during work 2. management of body position during transitions 3. movement within individual's work environment 4. manipulation/hand use 5. use of assistive and adaptive devices
Play/Leisure*	1. management of body position during play/leisure 2. management of body position during transitions 3. movement within play/leisure environment 4. manipulation/hand use 5. use of assistive and adaptive devices
Communication*	1. oral motor movements 2. communication access 3. manipulation/hand use 4. management of body position during communication 5. movement w/in individual's communication environment 6. attending skills 7. perceptual skills 8. use of assistive and adaptive devices
Socialization*	1. self esteem 2. recognition and use of nonverbal cues 3. management of body position during socialization 4. movement within individual's social environment 5. attending skills 6. perceptual skills 7. cognitive skills
Activities of daily living*	1. oral motor movements 2. management of body position during ADL 3. movement within daily living environment 4. attending skills 5. manipulation/hand use

*When acquiring a new skill, learning components apply to the task.

Dunn, W. & Campbell, P. (1988).

of components within each outcome category area. The levels allow therapists to classify children's performance on a continuum, ranging from no evidence of difficulty ("NA") to severe difficulties which prevent performance of program outcomes ("3"). The second level ("0") is used when a therapist has identified a deficiency in a performance component which is not interfering presently with the desired program outcome(s). A score of "1" defines an identified deficiency which *influences* a child's successful performance of a program outcome(s), where "2" is used to describe a deficiency which

interferes with performance. A score of "3" is used when deficiencies *prevent* performance in one or more program outcomes. Specific programs operationalize these phrases for their settings.

The grid illustrated in Figure 6-4 was completed for a child for whom the team targeted program outcome categories of communication and ADL. Toby, a seven-year-old child with cerebral palsy, who attends second grade in a regular elementary school, eats lunch in the cafeteria. Oral motor movements are not influencing his ability to communicate, because

FUNCTIONAL SKILLS ASSESSMENT GRID
for Occupational and Physical Therapy Services

PROGRAM OUTCOME	PERFORMANCE COMPONENTS	NA	0	1	2	3	COMMENTS
Learning* skill acquisition and academics	1 Manipulation/hand use						
	2 Interpretation of body senses						
	3 Perceptual skills organization of space and time						
	interpretation of visual stimuli						
	4 Cognitive skills problem solving						
	generalization of learning						
	5 Attending skills						
	6 Use of assistive and adaptive devices						
	7 Mgmt of body positions during learning						
	8 Mgmt body positions during transitions						
	9 Mvmt w/in learning environment						
Work*	1 Mgmt of body positions during work						
	2 Mgmt of body positions during transitions						
	3 Mgmt w/in work environment						
	4 Manipulation/hand use						
	5 Use of assistive and adaptive devices						
Play/Leisure*	1 Mgmt body position during play/leisure						
	2 Mgmt body position during transitions						
	3 Mvmt w/in play/leisure environment						
	4 Manipulation/hand use						
	5 Use of assistive and adaptive devices						
Communication*	1 Oral motor movements						
	2 Communication access						
	3 Manipulation/hand use						
	4 Mgmt body pos. during communication						
	5 Mvmt w/in communication environment						
	6 Attending skills						
	7 Perceptual skills						
	8 Use of assistive and adaptive devices						
Socialization*	1 Self esteem						
	2 Recognition and use of nonverbal cues						
	3 Mgmt. body position during socialization						
	4 Mvmt w/in social environment						
	5 Attending skills						
	6 Perceptual skills						
	7 Cognitive skills						
Activities of daily living*	1 Oral motor movements						
	2 Mgmt of body position during ADL						
	3 Mvmt w/in daily living environment						
	4 Attending skills						
	5 Manipulation/hand use						

*When acquiring new skills, use the learning: skill acquisition section of this grid.

NA—No problems are identified in therapy evaluation.
0—Although a problem has been identified through evaluation, it is not presently interfering with program outcome(s). Needs may
   be met by self, parents, or professionals in other programs or agencies.
1—The problem *influences* successful program outcome(s); simple instructional or environmental changes are likely to result in
   functional performance.
2—The problem *interferes* with specific program outcome(s); specific strategies are necessary to enable functional performance.
3—The problem *prevents* successful program outcome(s), multifaceted strategies are necessary to reach functional performance.

Figure 6-3. An example of a grid that is used to make decisions about service provision in pediatric settings. *Dunn, W. & Campbell, P. (1988).*

he uses an augmentative communication system. He has difficulty chewing and swallowing his food as a result of oral motor movement dysfunction. The therapist translated assessment information onto the Functional Skills Assessment Grid (Figure 6-4) and rated performance in oral motor movements under Communication as "0" and under ADL as "2."

Therapists may identify concerns regarding performance components that do not influence, interfere with, or prevent performance of program outcomes (scores of "0"). In these instances, therapists inform both the family and the school district or agency responsible for services. The family has the right to know that a concern has been identified and to be

FUNCTIONAL SKILLS ASSESSMENT GRID
for Occupational and Physical Therapy Services

PROGRAM OUTCOME	PERFORMANCE COMPONENTS	NA	0	1	2	3	COMMENTS
Communication	1 Oral motor movements		X				
	2 Communication access						
	3 Manipulation/hand use						
	4 Mgmt body pos. during communication						
	5 Mvmt w/in communication environment						
	6 Attending skills						
	7 Perceptual skills						
	8 Use of assistive and adaptive devices						
Activities of daily living	1 Oral motor movements				X		
	2 Mgmt of body position during ADL						
	3 Mvmt w/in daily living environment						
	4 Attending skills						
	5 Manipulation/hand use						

Figure 6-4.   Functional Skills Assessment grid completed for a seven-year-old child with cerebral palsy who has oral-motor problems that are affecting eating but not communication outcomes.

given guidance about their options for addressing the concern. If the problem is not affecting a child's performance of a program outcome within a school district program, the school does not have responsibility for addressing the area of concern. When an occupational therapist is working on behalf of a school district, (s)he must work within the parameters of that agency in providing therapy services. Statements made to the family must make it clear that the identified concern may be addressed at the parent's discretion, since attainment of educational program goals is not affected. It is appropriate to offer suggestions of community resources to deal with the concern. These suggestions may be simple (e.g., karate, gymnastics or swimming lessons for a child with incoordination) or more complex (e.g., referral to a community therapist). Many school districts and other agencies have designed policies for situations such as this one. It is important to know the policies of the agency before discussing concerns with families.

Any of the performance components that are rated "1", "2", or "3" on the grid are addressed in the service provision process. Three interrelated issues concerning service provision for children are incorporated into the decision-making that guides implementation of services. The first issue centers around the overall purpose and focus of service provision. Services may be provided to prevent the development of future and/or secondary disabilities, remediate identified deficiencies, or compensate for deficiencies that cannot be addressed adequately through remedial intervention. The second issue concerns the model of service provision that will be used to address child needs, including direct service, monitoring, and consultation models. The third issue involves decisions about the locations in which services will be provided. Each of these issues are interrelated in that decisions made about one aspect of service provision impact on other aspects. For example, a compensatory approach is the most likely service provision option to facilitate access of a teenager with severe disabilities to a work program. These particular services are best provided through consultation at the work site. By observing the teenager's performance in the work environment, the therapist is more likely to design ap-

propriate compensatory strategies that can be taught to job site personnel to facilitate the teenager's performance of the work task.

DETERMINING THE FOCUS OF OCCUPATIONAL THERAPY SERVICES

Pediatric therapists collaborate with family and professional team members to determine the overall focus of services, and to select the focus that will be most effective for a child. Therapists may choose a remedial, compensatory, or prevention-intervention focus (Campbell, 1989; Campbell, in press; Dunn, Campbell, Oetter, Hall, Berger, & Strickland, 1989). A prevention-intervention focus is used when services are designed to prevent or alleviate the effects of biological or environmental factors on the developmental process. This approach recognizes the interdependency of the various areas of development on each other and on the integrity of the system as a functional unit. For example, early intervention team members decided to use a prevention-intervention approach with a 10-month-old with extremely low tone, that resulted in poor antigravity control of the head and trunk. In order to prevent delayed cognitive development, adaptive seating equipment was designed to hold the infant's head and trunk up against gravity so that the arms could be used to manipulate objects.

A remedially focused approach is implemented when the purpose of intervention is to improve functional abilities in areas of dysfunction. If the early intervention team had selected a remedial, rather than a prevention-intervention, approach for the 10-month-old described above, emphasis would have been placed totally on improving the infant's head and trunk control, without specific regard for the impact of delays in postural control on other areas of functioning. Use of a remedial approach assumes that the targeted weakness or area of concern may be made "normal" through intervention. A therapist who uses a range-of-motion intervention to lengthen shortened muscles has selected a remedial approach for intervention.

A compensatory focus is chosen when the problem area cannot be substantially changed, regardless of the interven-

TABLE 6-2. Service Provision Approaches

Variable	Remedial	Compensatory	Prevention Intervention
Does child function within chronological age zone?	yes (CA +/− 9 mo)	no (CA > age zone)	no (CA < age zone)
How *essential* is the skill component for functional outcomes?	essential (e.g., reaching)	enhancing (e.g., walking)	essential (e.g., manipulation)
How *necessary* is the outcome for overall life function?	broadens life function (e.g., playing)	critical to life function (e.g., eating)	critical (e.g., communication)
At what levels do the identified problems interfere with performance	intermittently or partially interfere	greatly (blindness)	greatly (projected) (low muscle tone)

tion strategies that are used. Compensatory approaches minimize the effect of the disabling condition, to allow a child to participate in other life experiences that may otherwise not be possible. Assistive and adaptive devices are frequently used to compensate for physical inabilities that are unlikely to be fully remediated through existing therapeutic strategies. A compensatory focus may be used by itself or as a means of preventing the development of secondary problems. A child, for example, may be provided with adaptive eating devices to become independent in self-feeding, despite the existence of inability to perform performance component skills, such as grasping or pronation/supination.

Determining when prevention-intervention, remedial, or compensatory focuses are in the best interests of the child may be difficult to judge. Prevention-intervention or promotion approaches are used most often in early intervention, where remedial and compensatory approaches are more often used as the basis for service provision for school-age students. Table 6-2 provides a framework for decisions concerning the use of remedial or compensatory approaches. Team members (or an individual therapist) ask four basic questions, and formulate an intervention plan that is based upon the configuration of the answers. Intervention focuses of prevention-intervention, remediation, and compensation may be used with all direct, monitoring, and consultation models of service provision. Table 6-3 provides examples of the interaction between these approaches to intervention and models of service provision.

Resource allocation is also a factor in this decision, but falls along a separate continuum. Both remedial and compensatory approaches may be inexpensive or costly in terms of use of resources, such as professional time and effort or finances. A compensatory focus, which requires the purchase of expensive equipment and takes extensive professional time to set up, is costly initially, but may be less expensive in the long run if the equipment allows greater independence, or prevents development of secondary physical problems such as contractures or orthopedic deformities. A remedial approach that facilitates independent reaching and hand-to-mouth patterns decreases the need for one-on-one attention during mealtime and conserves professional resources. Creative ways to identify and allocate resources are required to ensure that each child's needs are addressed effectively.

PROVIDING OCCUPATIONAL THERAPY SERVICES

The ways in which services are best provided for infants and toddlers, preschoolers, and school-age students with disabilities have been debated over the past ten years, the time period during which provision of pediatric therapy services has shifted from clinical to public school and early intervention settings (e.g., Campbell, 1987a; Campbell, 1987b; Dunn, 1989a; Dunn, 1989b; Lyon & Lyon, 1980; Sternat, Messina, Nietupski, Lyon, & Brown, 1977). Team-based service provision has been of greater interest than have the mechanisms

TABLE 6-3. Combined Use of Service Provision Models and Approaches

	Direct	Monitor	Consult
Remedial	Improve head control for looking.	Supervise all adults to facilitate tone for reaching.	Provide strategies to incorporate necessary input during play.
Compensatory	Fabricate a splint to enable grasp.	Supervise feeding program which minimizes time required to eat so student can socialize with peers.	Cut seatwork pages in half so child can be successful in completing task.
Prevention intervention	Facilitate upright postures during infancy to prevent delays in standing and walking.	Supervise parent in use of oral facilitation techniques when feeding the baby, to prevent difficulties in lip closure during eating and talking.	Teach parent a range of motion program to prevent deformities.

of providing services by individual professionals or team members. Various types of team structures have been debated and defined in terms of their major features. Of primary concern has been the extent to which therapy services are provided in isolation from the comprehensive program of education and related services being provided for a child, or in physical isolation from a child's natural life environment (Campbell, 1987a; Dunn, 1990).

Isolated Versus Integrated Service Provision

Isolated therapy services have been characterized as an approach where a therapist identifies specific child needs and designs an individualized intervention plan to address those needs. Intervention is implemented by removing the child from the natural life environment to a separate environment, such as a therapy room, and providing individualized one-on-one or small group services. Three underlying assumptions of an isolated service provision model are that: a) skills observed in an isolated therapy environment will occur in the child's other life settings; b) intermittent intervention (e.g., once or twice a week) will have a significant effect on skill acquisition and performance; and c) children with disabilities acquire developmental skills in the same sequence, and in the same patterns, as children without handicaps (Sternat, et al., 1977).

Many factors have prolonged the use of isolated therapy models. First of all, programs for children with special needs too often are located in isolated buildings or agencies that are separate from programs for typical children. Second, programming provided in isolated and segregated settings often is based on a remedially focused approach, where services are designed to facilitate acquisition of developmental milestone skills, even when these skills are not functional for the individual child or applicable to life independence as a child grows older. In this model the extent to which an individual child will have access to normal life environments is determined by professionals by examining developmental milestone acquisition (Baumgart, Brown, Pumpian, Nisbet, Ford, Sweet, Messina, & Schroeder, 1982).

More recent approaches to programming for children with disabilities demonstrate that assumptions concerning isolated and remedially-based programming are unfounded. Rather, as therapists approach the final decade of the 20th century, a more proactive position regarding isolated therapy approaches is necessary. Isolated approaches to intervention, such as use of a direct service provision model in a separated setting, may be necessary to address the needs of a limited number of children. Use of this service model requires justification by explaining why the isolated setting is necessary for the therapeutic outcome. This proactive position enables children to profit from the expertise of occupational therapy throughout their living, learning, and working day (i.e., the therapist functions within these settings), thus increasing the potential impact of occupational therapy on children's lives.

Taylor (1988) suggests that effective intervention decisions will be based on the demands of the individual's life settings. He reminds us of the constant and ongoing evolution of ideas in the human service professions:

". . . concepts and principles can help us get from one place to another, to move closer to a vision of society based on enduring human values like freedom, community, equality, dignity, and autonomy. Yet they must be viewed in historical context. The concepts that guide us today can mislead us tomorrow . . . [When one concept] is achieved we must be prepared to find new ideas and principles to guide us through the challenges and dilemmas we will undoubtedly face . . ." (p. 51).

The American Occupational Therapy Association has defined models of service provision for the school-based therapy and early intervention (AOTA, 1987, 1989; Dunn et al., 1989). A continuum model of service provision is outlined which allows therapists to design a comprehensive set of services for all children in various types of settings. The continuum includes direct service, monitoring, and consultation service provision models.

Direct Therapy

Direct therapy refers to those intervention activities that are individually designed, and are carried out by the therapist and one child, or the therapist and a small group of children. The focus of direct therapy is to meet children's individualized needs through very specialized therapeutic strategies. A key factor in choosing direct therapy as the intervention model of choice, is to identify procedures that cannot be safely carried out by other personnel within the child's natural environment. Neurobiologically-based treatment paradigms most commonly fall into this category. For example, many sensory integration and neurodevelopmental treatment strategies can only safely be carried out under the on-site supervision of a therapist. Those theoretical frameworks require constant and ongoing monitoring of the autonomic nervous system mechanisms, the sensory processing mechanisms, and the postural and motor output systems. A therapist with an extensive background in the neurobiological systems is able to monitor changes that occur within these systems, and alter the treatment intervention very quickly to accommodate for changes that occur.

Direct therapy may occur within natural environments; it is still considered an isolated form of intervention if strategies are not incorporated into routines. For example, many of the postural weight shifts that occur as part of the normal sequences of neurodevelopmental treatment, may be easily incorporated into a young child's classroom routine. The proactive position for the future is that direct therapy integrated into a child's natural environment is more appropriate than isolated service provision. Isolated direct therapy is chosen only when the therapeutic task interferes with a child's natural life environment. For example, a therapist would interfere with a junior high student's socialization if s/he provided a neurodevelopmental treatment activity during the physical education class. In this case, if neurodevelopmental treatment was essential, providing consultation regarding age-appropriate adaptations in PE class, and conducting NDT activities in a more private environment, would be more responsive to the student's age-appropriate needs. Therapists must consider creative ways to incorporate the theoretical frameworks of occupational therapy into daily life tasks as much as possible, even when a direct intervention approach is appropriate. Incorporating the expertise of the occupational therapist into daily routines increases the opportunities for a child to practice the task and therefore acquire the functional skill.

Monitoring

Monitoring is the second service provision category. The importance of occupational therapy expertise for the natural life environments of the individual is addressed through monitoring. The importance of consistency in the implementation of strategies across all environments is also recognized through monitoring. Use of monitoring for service provision requires that the therapist conduct an assessment to identify the strengths and needs of the individual child. The therapist designs an intervention plan to meet individual needs and remains responsible for the outcome of the plan. Another person within the child's natural environment is trained by the therapist to carry out the plan, so that procedures will be implemented on a consistent basis and therefore have greater chance for generalization. The therapist remains in regular contact with the person who carries out the monitored program, so that necessary alterations in the program can be implemented in a timely manner. Three criteria are met in order to successfully choose a monitoring service provision model (AOTA, 1987, 1989). First, the health and safety of the child must be protected when the plan and procedures are carried out by the trained individual. Second, the implementor must be able to demonstrate the procedures without error and without cues from the therapist. Third, the implementor must be able to name the precautions, or the signs of risk or failure within the procedure, without cues from the therapist. Clearly the second and third criteria are measures to meet the first criterion of protecting the health and safety of the child. A monitoring program should not be given to an individual for regular implementation, if the therapist cannot ensure that these criteria are met. Failure to meet these criteria would put the child at risk and therefore put the therapist in a position of defending a program that is not being carried out in the designed manner. Ongoing contact between the therapist and the implementor is essential to ensure that high quality program implementation is assured and that adaptations are made in a timely manner.

Monitoring is a viable service provision alternative in many situations. Parents incorporate monitored programs within daily life routines such as bathing, diaper-changing, eating, and dressing. Teachers and teacher-aides provide monitored programs within the daily school routine in areas such as positioning and handling, eating, functional mobility and functional communication. Supervisors in a work environment provide monitored programs which adapt tasks to facilitate the worker's timely task completion. Monitored programs provide a means for occupational therapists to address the best fit between the individual's skills and needs, and demands of the environment, by providing more opportunities for generalization and practice than would be possible through a direct service model.

Consultation

Consultation is the third form of service provision and one which differs from direct therapy and monitoring in one sig-

nificant way: the therapist is using his or her expertise to enable another person to address issues and outcomes identified by that person. The therapist is not directly responsible for the outcomes of the individual in the consultation model. Rather, the consultee is responsible for the outcomes with the individual child, but the therapist is responsible for the collaborative efforts with the adult who is carrying out the program. Three types of consultation are important in pediatric therapy: a) case consultation, an approach that focuses on the needs of individuals; b) colleague consultation where the needs of peers within a service environment are targeted; and c) system consultation which focuses on improvements of the system within which services are provided. In case consultation, the therapist and teacher might meet to discuss the ways in which the teacher might facilitate greater participation of a particular student in the reading group. A therapist collaborates with the teacher to design methods for the teacher to effectively calm the children down after recess in colleague consultation. Participation in a system-wide curriculum committee, or serving as a speaker in a pre-school Parents' Information Night, are examples of system consultation, where the objective is to improve how the system works so that all children will benefit.

A collaborative style of consultation acknowledges the specialized expertise of both the consultant and the consultee (Idol, Paolucci—Whitcomb & Nevin, 1987). For example, in a school situation, the occupational therapist and the classroom teacher each contribute specialized expertise from their own professions to work together to solve specific problems. When professionals collaborate, they share responsibility for identifying the problem, creating possible solutions, trying the solutions, and then altering them as necessary for greater effectiveness. The unique skills of the occupational therapist lend themselves very nicely to a collaborative style of consultation. Occupational therapists have backgrounds in behavior across the life span of individuals and understand the context of performance. These skills are easily translated into collaborative consultation. Dunn (in press) found that a collaborative consultation approach with preschoolers yielded an equivalent number of achieved IEP goals (approximately 70%). However, teachers who participated in a collaborative consultation reported that the therapists contributed to goal attainment in 24% more instances than teachers whose children received isolated direct services. Other professionals have different focuses that contribute to the collaborative relationship in different ways. Classroom teachers, for example, focus on the products of learning such as written work, verbal responses, staying on task to complete assignments, and attaining outcome competencies in subject areas.

Selecting the Service Provision Model

The range of service provision choices available to occupational therapists are outlined on Figure 6-5. The chart matches the severity rating from the Functional Skills Assessment Grid (Figure 6-3) with a range of intervention models that include direct treatment, monitoring, and consultation. Definitions and examples for each of the intervention models are provided in Table 6-4. Consultation involves use of several strategies, including adaptations to the child's environment, and teaching adults, such as teachers or family members, to implement intervention methods within daily life

SEVERITY OF PROBLEMS AND THEIR RELATIONSHIP TO INTERVENTION OPTIONS								

Through interview and observation, the therapist will create a hypothesis about how the problem is interfering with program outcomes and will determine an assessment plan to confirm this hypothesis.
In collaboration with the team, the therapist will determine which level of interference is created by the problem(s). If documented evidence is available that the individual's behavior is currently interfering with his/her ability to benefit from intervention, the team reconvenes to reestablish priorities and create a new plan.

Rating	Parameter definition	No interv.*	Make recommendations*	Consultation			Monitor	Direct Service
				Adapt task matls environ.*	Adapt posture mvmt.*	Tch adult*	Spvs adult*	Use therapist admin. strategies*
NA	No problems are identified in therapy evaluation.	X						
0	Although a problem has been identified through evaluation, it is not presently interfering with the program outcomes. Needs may be met by self, parents, or professionals in other programs or agencies.		X					
1	The problem *influences* successful program outcomes; simple instructional or environmental changes are likely to result in functional performance.			X	X	X	X	
2	The problem *interferes* with specific program outcomes; specific strategies are necessary to enable functional performance.			X	X	X	X	**
3	The problem *prevents* successful program outcomes; multi-faceted strategies are necessary to reach functional performance.			X	X	X	X	**

* See Table 6-4 for definitions and examples.
** This level of service is
    1. Only provided in conjunction with other levels of service (e.g., adaptation, supervision).
    2. Only chosen if ONLY the therapist can provide the intervention safely.
    3. Provided as part of the life environment unless the intervention interferes with age appropriate tasks.

Figure 6-5. Service provision choices available to occupational therapists.

routines. Therapists monitor implementation of strategies that require ongoing supervision as they are carried out by others. Direct service is provided when therapists administer intervention strategies themselves. Many of the problems demonstrated by children are addressed ideally through use of several service provision models. More than one type of service provision is preferable, because the chances for generalization of learning to many environments are increased.

SELECTING THE LOCATION FOR SERVICES

The location where services are provided is determined by a therapist on the basis of individual child needs. Services may be provided, in the community at a job training site, in classrooms, or in homes. Consultation and monitoring are more likely to be provided in homes, classrooms, or other similar locations, because the purpose of these service provision models is to improve a child's ability to function in natural environments. Direct services are designed also to improve functional skills and may be provided in natural environments such as homes and community work sites. More often direct services are provided separately from the natural environments of the child, due to the types of intervention techniques that are being used. The natural environments

where the outcomes desired for a child are actually going to be used, are the preferred locations for services. For this reason, provision of direct services is always paired with consultation or monitoring to ensure use of newly learned skills in natural environments.

INTEGRATING OCCUPATIONAL THERAPY WITH OTHER DISCIPLINES

Direct, monitoring, and consultation models of service provision are implemented within a team structure. The primary team structure used within schools and early intervention programs is one of integrated services (e.g., Campbell, 1987a; Campbell, 1987b; Dunn, 1989; Dunn, 1990 Rainforth & York, 1986; Giangreco, 1986a, Giangreco, 1986b). Integration is a term that is used widely to describe service systems for individuals with disabilities. Figure 6-6 diagrams a model of comprehensive integration that differentiates among three distinct types of integration (Dunn, 1990). Many children with disabilities attend school and community programs that include children who are not disabled. Infants and preschoolers may attend day care programs or be enrolled in community preschool programs. Older children may participate in community sports activities. Young adults may work in commu-

TABLE 6-4. Definitions and Examples of Severity of Problems Categories

	Interventions	Definitions	Examples
	No intervention	There is not a need for therapy intervention	
	Make Recommendations	The problem(s) which has been identified by the therapist is/are not related to targeted life task performance. The therapist makes appropriate recommendations to parents or other professional to enable them to take care of the problem.	Provide parent with information regarding community resources for recreational opportunities.
Consultation	Adapt task materials or environment	The therapist alters materials and objects in the environment to accommodate the individual's needs.	The therapist gets the handouts made with larger print for the individual.
	Adapt posture/movement	The therapist designs alternate strategies to facilitate good position and movement patterns.	The therapist constructs a well fitting seat for the individual.
	Teach Adult	The therapist shows another individual how to handle a situation. Ongoing contact may not be necessary.	The therapist shows the teacher how to position a child on the sidelyer.
Monitor	Supervise Adult	The therapist monitors a program designed by the therapist but carried out by another individual. There is ongoing contact.	The therapist supervises the child's feeding program.
Direct Service	Use Therapist Administered Strategies	The therapist provides direct service.	The therapist provides intervention using neurodevelopmental & sensory integrative techniques.

nity-based competitive jobs while living in supervised apartments. These situations, characterized by their inclusion of individuals without disabilities, are described as *peer integration*.

The term integration also describes the use of therapeutic expertise to address children's needs within natural life environments. Therapists adapt tasks, materials, environments, or the posture and movement patterns of an individual, to achieve *functional integration*. Therapeutic objectives and strategies that enable children to achieve outcomes that are identified by all team members are examples of functional integration. In contrast, functional integration has not been achieved when therapy objectives are separate and isolated from the overall purpose of a child's program of early intervention or special education and related services.

A third use of the term integration relates to the combined use of intervention strategies that typically are associated with education and therapeutic practices. A therapist, teacher, and speech pathologist who design a switch activation task for a child, where switch closure results in different responses to teacher requests, have collaborated in *practice integration*. In this instance, the intervention strategies selected combine the expertise of more than one team member, rather than reflect the perspective of one discipline in isolation.

Optimal services for children with disabilities include all three components of comprehensive integration: a) peer integration; b) functional integration; and c) practice integration. However, any one or two types of integration can be present in a particular situation. The arrows marked "A," "B," and "C" on Figure 6–6 indicates the combinations of two types

of integration. Arrow "A" represents peer and functional integration, or situations in which the child participates with typical peers and the therapist creates adaptations within that environment. Arrow "B" represents the combination of peer and practice integration, or the therapist and teacher collaborating to create a plan for a regular education classroom. Arrow "C" represents the combination of functional and practice integration; this occurs when therapists work within self contained special education classrooms.

The types and amounts of integration that occur for children with whom a therapist interacts, are a critical factor in determining where therapy services will be provided. Underlying an integrated therapy approach to service provision are assumptions that therapeutic assessment and intervention are most useful when undertaken within natural life environments. Further, the greatest number of opportunities for generalization of functional skills occur when services are provided in natural life environments. Occupational therapists identify those performance components that are interfering with natural life outcomes by focusing on the performance outcomes of learning, work, play/leisure, communication, socialization, and activities of daily living.

PLANNING INTERVENTION

Planned interventions are more likely to lead to attainment of the desired outcomes established for children, than are interventions that are provided without accommodation for individual children's strengths and needs. Thoughtful interventions result from a planning process used by therapists

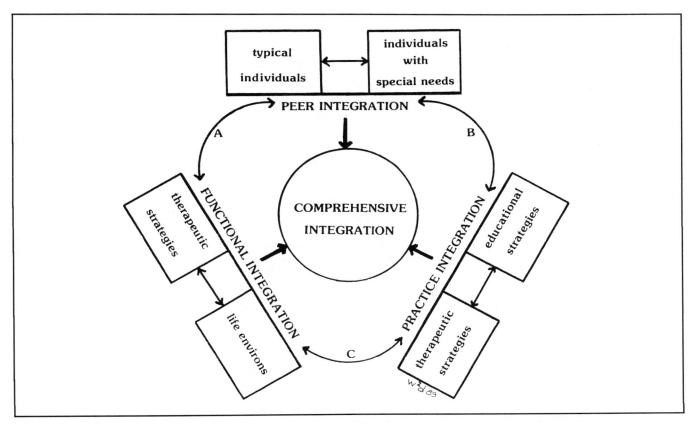

Figure 6-6. Model of the components of comprehensive integration. *Dunn, W. (1991). Integrated related services. In L. Meyer, C. A. Peck, & L. Brown (Eds.), Critical issues in the lives of people with severe disabilities. Baltimore: Paul H. Brookes. Reprinted with permission.*

to determine parameters of service provision. A format designed to guide the process of planning for occupational therapy intervention is outlined on Figure 6-7. Therapists account for all aspects of planning by completing information on the form in collaboration with other team members or, in some instances, without input from other team members. The written form, in turn, documents the decisions made during the planning process.

All occupational therapy interventions provided for children are designed to enhance attainment of desired outcomes stated on a formal planning document, such as the IEP or IFSP. Therapists establish separate objectives for occupational therapy services, including those implemented through direct service, monitoring, or consultation. This target objective defines the specific purpose and emphasis of therapy service provision by defining an objective that is related directly to achievement of the overall outcome. A therapist designed a consultation intervention program to facilitate a child's ability to play independently, an outcome that was identified by the child's parent and by team members as a whole. The occupational therapy target objective required the child to use reach and touch skills to manipulate large toys that had been modified to facilitate the child's ability to interact with objects independently. Team members established an

outcome for a seven-year-old student to communicate with others in his school environment. The occupational therapist provided direct therapy twice weekly within the child's classroom, with the objective of improving the efficiency of reach and pointing skills for access, and use of a direct selection communication device. In addition, the therapist also developed a monitoring program where the speech pathologist and teacher used specific facilitation and inhibition procedures whenever the child communicated, using the device with the objective of improving efficiency of reach and pointing skills.

Intervention planning provides a means for description and documentation of: a) performance components, including those that enable performance and those that are of concern; b) service provision models that will be used; and c) specific intervention procedures within each of the service provision models selected for use.

Enabling Components and Concerns

The positive and negative impacts of sensorimotor performance components on the stated outcome are transferred from the Functional Skills Assessment Grid (see Figure 6-3) and become the basis for intervention that will use a child's enabling performance components to address areas of con-

INTERVENTION PLAN

Child's name: _____   Date: _____
                                                 Birthdate: _____
Agency name: _____   Chron. Age: _____ yrs. _____ mo.
Outcome Statement: _____
Outcome Category: _____ Learning   _____ Work
                           _____ Play/Leisure   _____ Communication
                           _____ Socialization   _____ ADL
Performance Components:
     ENABLING COMPONENTS: CONCERNS:
     _____   _____
     _____   _____
     _____   _____
     _____   _____

Service Provision Models:
_____ Direct*   _____ Monitoring   _____ Consultation
                             _____ supervise adult _____ teach adult
                                                       _____ adapt posture/mvmt
                                                       _____ adapt task/matls
                                                       _____ adapt environ

*provided in conjunction with one or more other service models
_____ **DIRECT**   _____ n.a.
Target Objective: _____
_____
Intervention Approach: _____ remed. _____ compens. _____ prevent-interv.
     Describe: _____
_____
Location of Services: _____
Intervention Procedures: _____
_____
Method for Documentation of Performance:
     behavior to be observed: _____
     natural environment for observation: _____
     measurement/data to be collected: _____
     criterion for successful performance: _____
_____ **MONITORING**   _____ n.a.
Target Objective: _____
_____
Intervention Approach: _____ remed. _____ compens. _____ prevent-interv.
     Describe: _____
_____
Location of Services: _____
Intervention Procedures: _____
_____
Implementor: _____ teacher _____ family _____ aide _____ other: _____
Training and Verification Strategies: _____
_____
Proposed Meeting Schedule: _____ weekly _____ bimonthly _____ monthly
Location of meeting: _____
Method for Documentation of Performance:
     behavior to be observed: _____
     natural environment for observation: _____
     measurement/data to be collected: _____
     criterion for successful performance: _____
_____ **CONSULTATION**   _____ n.a.
Area of Concern: _____
Identified by: _____ role: _____

Figure 6-7.   Format designed to guide the process of planning for occupational therapy intervention.

Statement of Area to be Addressed: _____

Location of Services: _____
Strategies: _____

Proposed Meeting Schedule: _____ weekly _____ bimonthly _____ monthly
Location of meeting: _____
Method for Documentation of Performance:
  behavior to be observed: _____
  natural environment for observation: _____
  measurement/data to be collected: _____
  criterion for successful performance: _____

Figure 6-7. *Continued.*

cern. Enabling components are those performance components that have been rated on the Functional Skills Assessment Grid as "NA," no problems are identified in therapy assessment. Scores of "1," "2," and "3" indicate performance components that are influencing, interfering, or preventing performance of a specific component, and are listed as areas of concern that will be addressed through intervention. The ways in which both enabling components and concerns are accommodated within a specific intervention program derives directly from the overall intervention approach selected for use. Enabling performance components become a means to bypass areas of concern when a compensatory approach is selected. These same enabling components provide a vehicle by which concerns are addressed directly when remedially focused intervention is provided. For example, a therapist identified all performance components under the outcome area of socialization as "NA," with the exception of attending skills which was rated as "3." The therapist used the child's existing performance components as a means to enable and develop attending skills during social activities.

Service Provision Models and Intervention Strategies

The plan for the model of service provision is stated for each outcome that will be addressed through occupational therapy services. The format allows a therapist to indicate both the service provision model and the strategies that are planned for use.

The specific or target objective addressed by each model of service provision selected for use is indicated on the Intervention Plan. Descriptions of the service provision approach, and the location where services will be provided, are also stated. A brief description of the intervention procedures to be used, and statements of the methods for documenting performance complete the plan.

Altering the Intervention Plan

Many of the parameters that are included on the Intervention Plan are also contained in legal planning documents such as the IEP or IFSP. Both of these documents require statements of the services that will be provided, their frequency,

and duration. Legal requirements in particular states establish other parameters of the service provision process that also must be included on official planning documents. Any changes made in the Intervention Plan that are also included on legal documents, may only be made under the conditions established for changing IEPs, IFSPs, or other types of plans. Federal and most state legal requirements concerning plans of these types require formal review mechanisms, including conferences with parents and school administrators, before changes may be made in the types of early intervention or related services being provided, the frequency at which those services occur, and their duration. Families of children with disabilities are key members of programming teams. Changes in the service provision model(s) being used, frequency of contact between the therapist and child, duration of service, or termination from services, are first discussed with the child's family. No changes are made in occupational therapy Intervention Plans, or more formal documents, without first providing families with an explanation and rationale for proposed changes, so that parents have the opportunity to contribute to these decisions and they can be shared with professional team members.

Some parameters of intervention planning may be changed by therapists, and documented in progress notes or other records that are kept as an ongoing record of services being provided. The intervention procedures that a therapist plans to use to enable a child to achieve a target objective may be changed on the basis of objective clinical judgement or documentation data. A therapist, for example, planned to use jaw control procedures to facilitate coordinated mouth opening and closing during eating, with a child with low tone in the oral musculature and difficulty closing the mouth. Clinical observation indicated that the child did not tolerate jaw control and attempted consistently to remove the therapist's hand. Intervention procedures were changed so that a program of touch pressure stimulation was provided before eating, in order to allow the child to accommodate eventually to the touch pressure stimuli provided through jaw control.

Use of the Intervention Plan

Occupational therapy Intervention Plans are outlined in Figures 6-8 and 6-9 to illustrate the outcome of the intervention

INTERVENTION PLAN

Child's name: **Jared**   Date: **Jan. 25, 1989**

Birthdate: **Sept. 14, 1980**

Agency name: **Washington School**   Chron. Age: _____**8**_____ yrs. _____**4**_____ mo.

Outcome Statement: **Jared will complete his seatwork legibly**

Outcome Category: __**xx**__ Learning   _____ Work

                                        _____ Play/Leisure   _____ Communication

                                        _____ Socialization   _____ ADL

Performance Components:

    ENABLING COMPONENTS: CONCERNS:

      perceptual skills   **manipulation/hand use**

      cognitive abilities   **mgmt. of body position**

      attending skills

Service Provision Models:

_____ Direct*   __**xx**__ Monitoring   __**xx**__ Consultation

                                            __**xx**__ supervise adult   __**xx**__ teach adult

                                                                                    __**xx**__ adapt posture/mvmt

                                                                                    __**xx**__ adapt task/matls

                                                                                    _____ adapt environ

*provided in conjunction with one or more other service models

_____ **DIRECT**   __**xx**__ n.a.

Target Objective: _____

_____

Intervention Approach: _____ remed. _____ compens. _____ prevent-interv.

    Describe: _____

_____

Location of Services: _____

Intervention Procedures: _____

_____

Method for Documentation of Performance:

    behavior to be observed: _____

    natural environment for observation: _____

    measurement/data to be collected: _____

    criterion for successful performance: _____

__**xx**__ **MONITORING**   _____ n.a.

Target Objective: **(a) Jared will remain in his chair throughout the seatwork period. (b) Jared will complete a workbook page legibly**

Intervention Approach: __**xx**__ remed. _____ compens. _____ prevent-interv.

    Describe: **(a) experiences to increase balance and postural control; (b) activities to improve hand use**

Location of Services: **(a) gym   (b) special education classroom**

Intervention Procedures: **(a) movement exploration; experimentation with body movement. (b) manipulation tasks**

Implementor: __**xx**__ teacher _____ family _____ aide _____ other: _____

(a) physical educator; (b) special educator

Training and Verification Strategies: **teachers will demonstrate techniques to therapist; therapist and teacher will record data on same activities and compare results**

Proposed Meeting Schedule: _____ weekly __**xx**__ bimonthly _____ monthly

Location of meeting: **(a) gym   (b) special education classroom**

Method for Documentation of Performance: **(postural control; hand use)***

*Note: Measurement addresses classroom performance because this is the desired outcome from the interventions that will be provided in special education and PE).

    Behavior to be observed: **sitting at desk and working during seatwork period**

    Natural environment for observation: **regular classroom**

Figure 6-8. Occupational therapy intervention plan.

Measurement/data to be collected: **time spent without hanging on chair back or lying on desktop; amt. of work**

Criterion for successful performance: **remains in chair for 30 min. and completes at least two pages of work**

__xx__ CONSULTATION _____ n.a.

Area of Concern: **Learning**

Identified by: **Abigale Jennings** role: **classrm. tchr.**

Statement of Area to be Addressed: **Jared's ability too complete seatwork in a legible manner**

Location of Services: **regular classroom**

Strategies: **adapt pencil, adapt ruler, find alternate body positions, allow taping of harder work, provide more space to write**

Proposed Meeting Schedule: _____ weekly __xx__ bimonthly _____ monthly

Location of meeting: **Washington School Conference Room**

Method for Documentation of Performance:
Behavior to be observed: **completion of legible seatwork**

Natural environment for observation: **regular classroom**

Measurement/data to be collected: **seatwork pages that have been completed within a thirty minute seatwork period**

Criterion for successful performance: **completion of two pages of seatwork with 90% legibility in a 30 minute seatwork period. (legibility criterion set by teacher and therapist**

Figure 6-8. *Continued.*

planning process for two children. Figure 6-8 outlines the plan developed for Jared, an eight-year-old child with slightly diminished muscle tone, poor balance and postural control, and fine motor difficulties, who was originally labeled as developmentally delayed at the age of three years. Jared is enrolled in a regular education second grade class. His teacher referred him to the school district's diagnostic team due to concerns about his difficulties in completing legible seatwork. The team decided that Jared's areas of concern were best addressed by itinerant special education and occupational therapy services. The occupational therapist planned services that utilized monitoring of the special educator and physical educator and consultation with the classroom teacher.

Figure 6-9 illustrates the plan developed for Rebecca, a 14-month-old with Down syndrome, whose mother identified an outcome of desiring Rebecca to eat independently. The infant educator requested assistance from the program's occupational therapist who, in turn, determined that direct services and consultation with the mother were needed to assist Rebecca in achieving the desired outcome. She arranged to accompany the infant educator once weekly on a visit to Rebecca's home during lunchtime. The therapist provided direct intervention during this time period and also reviewed Rebecca's performance and the strategies used at home with the mother.

ADDRESSING MANAGEMENT ISSUES

Determination of Caseload

An important aspect of the service provision process is the determination of an appropriate caseload. Too many children on a caseload interferes with effective service provision, because sufficient time is not available to give proper attention to individual needs. Therapists establish caseloads that acknowledge the variety of tasks that are required within the

service provision process, and provide a mechanism for interacting with significant individuals such as family members, other team members, referral sources and administrators.

There are three task categories in the determination of caseload. The first category is comprised of the non-service provision tasks. This includes activities such as travel, lunch, and supervisory responsibilities. The time needed in this category is calculated by adding the actual time spent in each of these tasks. The second category is comprised of associated service provision tasks, such as team meetings and assessments. These tasks contribute to the service provision process by providing time for interaction and data gathering. An exact amount of time for these tasks is difficult to determine, due to variance from week to week or by time of year (e.g., more assessments at the beginning or end of the school year for school based therapists). An average amount of time spent per week is estimated. The time spent in these two categories is added and the total subtracted from the total time available in the work week. (see Figure 6-10 for an example).

Total time available per week: **40 hours**

−total of categories one and two: **x hours**

Time available for service provision: **hours**

The third category is comprised of actual service provision tasks. Service provision includes both the time spent with the individual, and the time needed to prepare for the intervention and document those interactions properly. Documentation provides a written record of the actions taken and decisions made on behalf of the individual. Chapter Eight provides an informative discussion about effective documentation strategies. An 80/20 ratio between time spent providing services, and time spent in related preparation and documentation has been suggested (AOTA, 1987). Use of this ratio means that

INTERVENTION PLAN

Child's name: **Rebecca**

Date: **March 24, 1989**

Birthdate: **Jan. 11, 1988**

Agency name: **Midstate Regional Ctr.**

Chron. Age: _____ **1** _____ yrs. _____ **2** _____ mo.

Outcome Statement: **Rebecca will eat independently**

Outcome Category:

    xx Learning   _____ Work

    _____ Play/Leisure   _____ Communication

    _____ Socialization   **xx** ADL

Performance Components:

ENABLING COMPONENTS: CONCERNS:

   mgmt. of body position   **utensil use**

   mvmts. for eating   **oral motor movements**

   perceptual skills

   likes textures of foods

Service Provision Models:

_____ **xx** Direct*

        _____ Monitoring   **xx** Consultation

        _____ supervise adult   **xx** teach adult

                                    _____ adapt posture/mvmt

                                      _____ adapt task/matls

                                      _____ adapt environ

*provided in conjunction with one or more other service models

_____ **xx** **DIRECT**   _____ n.a.

Target Objective: **Rebecca will eat a meal independently**

Intervention Approach: _____ **xx** remed. _____ compens. _____ prevent-interv.

   Describe: **provide developmentally appropriate tasks, provide support for development of eating skills, use enabling skills**

Location of Services: **the Velcoper home**

Intervention Procedures: **provide oral motor facilitation; provide verbal and physical cues for utensil use; incorporate object manipulation and oral motor skills into other play activities**

Method for Documentation of Performance:

   behavior to be observed: **eating during snack or mealtime**

   natural environment for observation: **Rebecca's home**

   measurement/data to be collected: **amount of liquid drunk from straw; number of spoonsful eaten**

   criterion for successful performance: **(a) drinking 4 ounces of liquid through a straw and (b) eating 6 spoonsful of food by bringing the spoonful to her mouth and scraping the food from the spoon with her lips.**

_____ **MONITORING**   **xx** n.a.

Target Objective: _____

Intervention Approach: _____ remed. _____ compens. _____ prevent-interv.

   Describe: _____

Location of Services: _____

Intervention Procedures: _____

Implementor: _____ teacher _____ family _____ aide _____ other: _____

Training and Verification Strategies: _____

Proposed Meeting Schedule: _____ weekly _____ bimonthly _____ monthly

Location of meeting: _____

Method for Documentation of Performance:

   behavior to be observed: _____

   natural environment for observation: _____

   measurement/data to be collected: _____

   criterion for successful performance: _____

Figure 6-9. Occupational therapy intervention plan for Rebecca.

___xx___ **CONSULTATION**   _____ n.a.

Area of Concern: **Activities of Daily Living: Eating**

Identified by: **Pat Velcoper**   role: **parent**

Statement of Area to be Addressed: **Rebecca's ability to eat by herself**

Location of Services: **the Velcoper home**

Strategies: **teach mom about oral motor control, technqiues for mouth and lip closure; provide techniques to improve utensil use**

Proposed Meeting Schedule: ___xx___ weekly _____ bimonthly _____ monthly

Location of meeting: **the Velcoper home**

Method for Documentation of Performance:

    behavior to be observed: **eating during meal or snack time**

    natural environment for observation: **Rebecca's home**

    measurement/data to be collected: **amount of liquid drunk from straw; number of spoonsful eaten**

    criterion for successful performance: **(a) drinking 4 ounces of liquid through a straw and (b) eating 6 spoonsful of food by bringing the spoonful to her mouth and scraping the food from the spoon with her lips.**

Figure 6-9. *Continued.*

for every four minutes of service provision, an additional one minute is set aside for preparation and documentation. For example,

• . . . . for 30 minutes of service provision, an additional 7.5 minutes are needed for preparation and documentation, for a total of 37.5 minutes. This translates to 0.625 of an hour (37.5 minutes/60 minutes = 00.625).

• . . . . for a 60 minute service provision session, an additional 15 minutes would be needed for preparation and documentation. This total of 75 minutes translates into 1.25 hours. (75 minutes/60 minutes = 1.25).

The therapist uses decimals such as these to determine the number of slots available for intervention:

$$\frac{\text{hours available for service provision}}{\text{decimal representing length of sessions}} = \text{no. of intervention slots available}$$

If the therapist sees children for thirty minute sessions, but sees children twice per week, then the total from the above

calculation must be divided by 2 to arrive at the number of individuals that can be served. If the therapist sees children once a week for 60 minutes, then the total obtained from this division represents both the number of slots available, and the number of individuals who can receive intervention. When children are seen in groups, the total amount of time for the group is divided among the members to keep calculations consistent, and to accurately represent the amount of therapist time that is dedicated solely to each individual. All these options are combined to produce a more realistic schedule that is responsive to individual needs (e.g., some individually addressed in direct service, monitoring, or consultation; some seen in groups; some sessions 30 minutes per week, and some sessions 60 or 90 minutes per week). Figure 6-11 provides an example of service provision calculations.

A maximum caseload of 40 is recommended by AOTA (1987) for any school-based therapist. However, this figure is too high if travel, supervision, or other duties are a regular part of the work week. Professionals must consider seriously whether children are actually receiving effective occupational therapy services when caseloads exceed recommended numbers.

SAMPLE CALCULATIONS

Service Provision Time

Mary works full time for a community-based agency. She travels two hours per week between the early intervention program and the independent living center. She spends 30 minutes per day at lunch. She spends an average of three and a half hours per week in team meetings and assessment tasks, although some times during the year are more concentrated on these tasks than others.

total time available per week:		40 hours

total of Category One:
  travel = 2 hours
  lunch = 2.5 hours
		−4.5 hours

	subtotal	35.5 hours

total of Category Two:
  team meetings
  assessments
		−3.5 hours

Time Available for Service Provision		**32.0 hours**

Figure 6-10. **Sample calculation to determine average amount of time available for service provision.**

SAMPLE SERVICE PROVISION CALCULATIONS FOR MARY
(See Figure 6-10)

Time available for service provision = 32 hours

for 30 minute sessions
(0.625)

for 60 minute sessions
(1.25)

32 hrs/0.625 = 51 sessions
available
per week*

32 hrs/1.25 = 25 sessions
available
per week

* if each child participates in two sessions per week, 25 persons can be scheduled.

SAMPLE CALCULATIONS FOR SERVICES WHICH ARE PROVIDED IN GROUPS

20 hours available for service provision

60 minute sessions (1.25)

If there are two individuals per group, each individual would have half of the time dedicated to her/him, or 0.625 hour per person (0.625 + 0.625 = 1.25)

Therefore, although 20 hours/1.25 = 16 sessions, if one considers the number of individuals who can be served, (20 hours/0.625 = 32) 32 persons receive services.

Figure 6-11. **Example of service provision calculations.**

Scheduling and Time Management

Efficient scheduling and management of time is one mechanism that allows therapists to adequately address the needs of all children on a caseload. Scheduling requires planning to increase efficiency. For example, therapists who schedule children in one special education classroom for services during a large time block, will more efficiently accommodate for scheduling problems, such as student absences, than will the therapist who schedules children for individual time slots (e.g., Campbell, 1987a & b). Scheduling all children receiving services, who are assigned to the same public school cluster group, is another way of scheduling to manage time more efficiently. Similarly, scheduling home visits for all children in the same area of the city on the same day, decreases the amount of time that may be required for travel. Therapists also consider creative plans for scheduling intervention with particular children. For example, a more intense direct service and monitoring schedule, over a shorter period of time, may enable a child to become successful more quickly in a regular education placement, than if that same child received those services spread out over the entire school year. Problems concerning scheduling and time management are challenging issues for occupational therapists. Creative solutions that are responsive to the organizational structure of the school or early intervention program, are possible when therapists consider all options for service provision and maximally utilize available resource personnel.

Use of Equipment and Materials to Enhance Intervention Outcomes

Therapists frequently use special types of equipment and materials to carry out intervention programs. The equipment and materials are chosen because of the properties necessary to achieve functional outcomes. Therapists who select equipment and materials, on the basis of the properties required to achieve intervention objectives, have many alternatives available to them from children's environments. For example, equipment that provides an unstable surface to facilitate postural weight shifts may include not only a therapy ball, but also a high density foam block (available through furniture upholsterers), the cage ball from physical education, or rocker boats and other elementary school gross motor and playground equipment. Not only is a wider range of equipment available when therapists use available resources, but also skills are more likely to generalize to functional life tasks. The objective of the intervention provided to develop postural shifting, is to enable the child to use this skill in functional situations, such as when using playground equipment. Skills are more likely to be established for functional use when natural, rather than contrived types of equipment are selected.

PROVIDING COMPREHENSIVE SERVICES

Many agencies have different purposes when providing early intervention or special education and related services. The purpose of early intervention is to provide services designed to meet the developmental needs of children and the needs of families related to enhancing their children's development. Public education programs for children with disabilities are structured to provide education and those related services necessary for children to benefit from education. Hospitals and other community agencies have as their missions to provide services for special purposes, such as medically-related health, financial assistance, work preparation and training, or mental health programs. Pediatric occupational therapists may be employed in any number of settings by a wide variety of agencies. Occupational therapy services provided under that agency's administration and financing are aligned with the purpose of the agency. For example, services provided in public education settings enable children to benefit from educational opportunities. Addressing all of the concerns identified through assessment is appropriate only when all areas of concern negatively impact on the child's participation in education. Areas of concern that do not influence a child's educational performance are addressed by other community agencies or resources.

Each occupational therapist has professional goals and purposes. It is important for therapists to define these purposes clearly for themselves so that chosen professional activities enhance goal attainment. Employment choices play a major role in either enhancing, or blocking professional goal attainment, with the best outcomes occurring when the mission of the employing agency and one's professional goals are aligned. Agency purposes often require professionals to play a variety of roles and have a wide range of responsibilities. For example, a role that occupational therapists may be required to play in early intervention programs is that of a case manager or service coordinator for specifically assigned families. Similarly, many therapists employed in school settings may be responsible for coordination of children's therapy services with those being provided by other community agencies or medical facilities. Traditional roles of occupational therapists are expanding as current practices with infants and children change to better reflect current public policy and legislation.

EXPAND YOUR NEWLY ACQUIRED KNOWLEDGE

1. Design materials for an effective monitoring program for a child with severe handicaps who requires eating intervention. Include forms which document intitial plan, regular contacts, precautions and adaptations in the plan.

2. Describe three strategies for OT intervention for a 14 year old child for whom socialization is a team priority. Presume that "recognition and use of non verbal cues" and "attending skills" are the factors that are interfering with attainment of socialization outcomes.

3. Consider a 6 year old child with cerebral palsy who has just recently been placed in a regular first grade classroom. Learning is a primary goal for the team. Outline one functional integration and one practice integration strategy you might implement.

References

American Occupational Therapy Association (1987). *Guidelines for occupational therapy services in school systems*. Rockville, MD: Author.

American Occupational Therapy Association (1989). *Guidelines for occupational therapy services in school systems—Second Edition*. Rockville, MD: Author.

American Occupational Therapy Association (1989). Uniform terminology for occupational therapy—Second Edition. *American Journal of Occupational Therapy, 43*(12), 808–815.

Baumgart, D., Brown, L., Pumpian, I., Nisbet, J., Ford, A., Sweet, M., Messina, R., & Schroeder, J. (1982). (1982). Principle of partial participation and individualized adaptations in educational programs for severely handicapped students. *The Association for Persons with Severe Handicaps, 7*, 17–27.

Campbell, P. H. (1987a). Integrated therapy and educational programming for students with severe handicaps. In L. Goetz, D. Guess, & K. Stremel-Campbell (Eds.), *Innovative program design for individuals with sensory impairments*. Baltimore: Paul H. Brookes.

Campbell, P. H. (1987b). The integrated programming team: An approach for coordinating professionals of various disciplines in programs for students with severe and muliple handicaps. *Journal of The Association for Persons with Severe Handicaps, 21*(2), 107–116.

Campbell, P. H. (1989). Posture and movement. In C. Tingey (Ed.), *Implementing early intervention*. Baltimore: Paul H. Brookes.

Campbell, P. H. (In press). Service delivery approaches. In M. J. Wilcox and P. H. Campbell (Eds.), *Community Programming from Birth to Three: A handbook for public school professionals*. San Diego: College Hill Press.

Dunn, W. (1989a). Integrated related services for preschoolers with neurological impairments: Issues and strategies. *RASE, 10*(3), 31–39.

Dunn, W. (1989b). Occupational therapy in early intervention: New perspectives create greater possibilities. *American Journal of Occupational Therapy. 43*(11), 717–721.

Dunn, W. (1990). Integrated related services. In L. Meyer, C. A. Peck, & L. Brown (Eds.), *Critical issues in the lives of people with severe disabilities*. Baltimore: Paul Brooks.

Dunn, W. (in press) A comparison of service provision models in school-based occupational therapy services. *Occupational Therapy Journal of Research*.

Dunn, W., Campbell, P. H., Oetter, P. L., Hall, S., Berger, E., & Strickland, R. (1989). *Guidelines for occupational therapy services in early intervention and preschool services*. Rockville, MD: American Occupational Therapy Association.

Giangreco, M. (1986a). Delivery of therapeutic services in special education programs for learners with severe handicaps. *Physical and Occupational Therapy in Pediatrics, 6*(1), 5–15.

Giangreco, M. (1986b). Effects of integrated therapy: A pilot study. *Journal of The Association for Persons with Severe Handicaps, 11*(3), 205–208.

Idol, L, Paolucci-Whitcomb, P & Nevin, A. *Collaborative Consultation* Austin: Pro Ed 1987.

Lyon, S., & Lyon, G. (1980). Team functioning and staff development: A role release approach to providing integrated educational services for severely handicapped students. *Journal of the Association for the Severely Handicapped, 5*(3), 250–263.

McDonnell, J. (1987). The integration of students with severe handicaps into regular public schools: An analysis of parents' perceptions of potential outcomes. *Education and Training of the Mentally Retarded, 22*(2), 98–111.

McDonnell, A. P., & M. L. Hardman (1989). The desegregation of america's special schools: Strategies for change. *Journal of the Association for Persons with Severe Handicaps, 14*(1), 68–74.

Rainforth, B., & York, J. (1986). The role of related services in community-referenced instruction. *Journal of the Association for Persons with Severe Handicaps,*

Sternat, J., Messina, R., Nietupski, J., Lyon, S., & Brown, L. (1977). Occupational and physical therapy services for severely handicapped students: Toward a naturalized public school service delivery model. In E. Sontag (Ed.), *Educational Programming for the Severely and Profoundly Handicapped*. Reston, VA: Division on Mental Retardation.

Taylor, S. J. (1988). Caught in the continuum: A critical analysis of the principle of the least restrictive environment. *Journal of the Association for Persons with Severe Handicaps, 13*(1), 41–53.

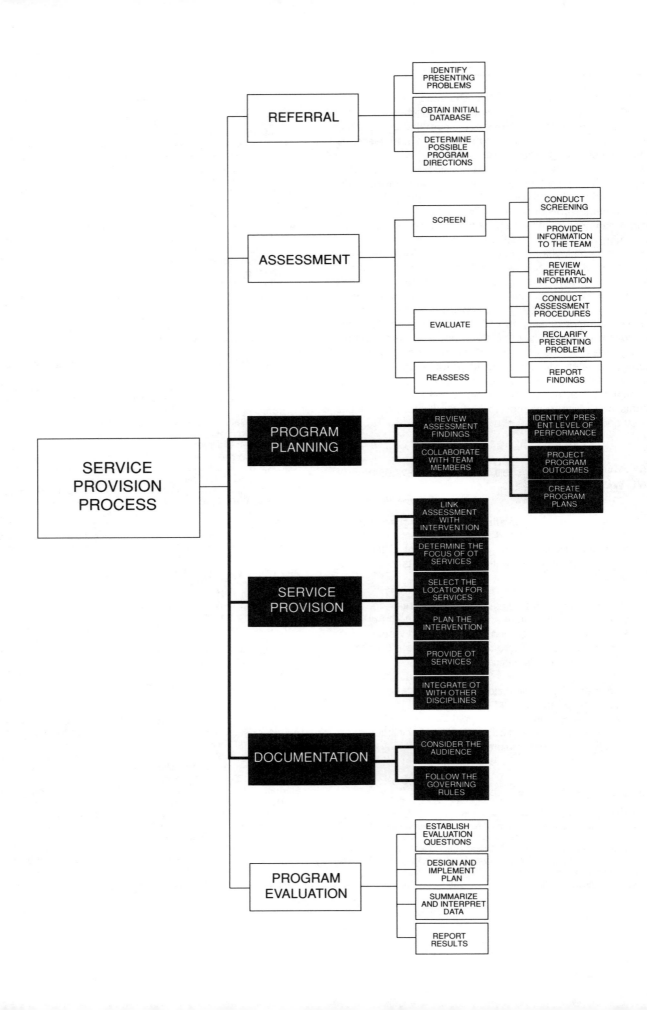

CHAPTER 7

Application of the Program Planning and Service Provision Processes

Winnie Dunn, PhD, OTR, FAOTA
Patti Oetter, MA, OTR/L, FAOTA

". . . our objective is to help the child function better physically, emotionally, and academically. We want to help him become more capable of learning any motor skill, or academic ability, or type of good behavior he needs in his life. Motor activity is valuable in that it provides the sensory input that helps to organize the learning process . . ." Ayres, 1980

Program planning is an integral part of the therapeutic process. For occupational therapists, goals reflect the **PERFORMANCE AREAS** of activities of daily living (ADL), work, and/or play and leisure. Children learn to dress, eat, and care for personal needs as activities of daily living. Work not only includes job performance for an adolescent, but also includes school work and participation in organized sports. Play is sometimes considered the work of very young children, since this is how they explore and learn about their environment. For school-aged children and adolescents, play and leisure includes dating, playing on the school playground, listening to music, and socializing at group gatherings. Program planning goals must address one or more of these performance areas.

The occupational therapy assessment process is designed to identify strengths and concerns in **PERFORMANCE COMPONENTS,** those variables that enable or compromise task completion in the performance areas. Please refer to the Appendix for a copy of the *Uniform Terminology for Occupational Therapy*, Second Edition document (AOTA, 1989) which outlines and defines performance areas and performance components. The program plan is designed to enhance strong performance components, facilitate improvement in weaker performance components, and adapt tasks and environments to accommodate individual's needs. The emphasis in a specific program will be determined by the outcomes desired, environmental demands, caregiver needs and abilities, and agency mission and guidelines.

Service provision encompasses not only intervention strategies, but also includes attending to the funding sources, scheduling, and location in which services are to be provided. Child and family needs within natural environments will be the primary consideration in all service provision decisions. When needs cannot appropriately be met within a specific agency's mission or scope of service, referrals to other community agencies are in order. The following case studies illustrate a variety of strategies used by experienced occupational therapists. (Their assessment data is contained in Chapter Four.) The emphasis in this chapter is on the process used to identify goals and intervention strategies. Specific theoretical and applied frames of reference for intervention are discussed thoroughly in other texts (e.g., Ayres, 1980; Grady, Gilfoyle & Moore, 1981).

CASE #1—DAVID

Program Planning for David

David's programming team consisted of the parents, the therapist, and the referring pediatrician, so all these points of view needed to be considered in the program plan. When considering the pattern of performance component strengths and concerns, and the expressed needs of the family, a prioritized plan of action was developed for David and his parents. The first priority was to increase the duration of night time sleeping to enable David to interact more appropriately during waking hours (play exploration); this also would allow his parents to be more rested, thus having more personal resources to invest positive energy into the family unit. The second priority focused on reducing the stress generated during mealtime and improving feeding and eating. A related priority was to enhance parental confidence in their ability to nurture and interact with David (socialization). Figure 7-1 summarizes evaluation results in relation to these priorities on the Functional Skills Assessment Grid (see chapter 6 for further explanation). Please remember that this grid is a condensed version of the Uniform Terminology for easier use in team planning. Exact details for the therapist will still be contained in more detailed evaluation data summaries.

Because the assessment included the parents, interpretation of findings occurred throughout the assessment interview and observation. Strengths were noted in both David's performance and his parents' skills. Because the feelings of incompetence as a parent are so strong in families that include a child with sensory sensitivities, it is especially important to note when any family member has initiated or responded in a way that enhanced interaction. (i.e., "When you hold him over your shoulder like that and bounce, he seems much happier and is able to look over and give mom a smile"). In order to facilitate parental confidence and increase so-

FUNCTIONAL SKILLS ASSESSMENT GRID

for Occupational and Physical Therapy Services

PROGRAM OUTCOME	PERFORMANCE COMPONENTS	NA	0	1	2	3	COMMENTS
Learning	1 Manipulation/hand use	X					check all NA's as David
Skill	2 Interpretation of body senses					X	grows and these skills
Acquisition and	3 Perceptual skills						
academics*	organization of space and time	X					would be expected in
related to	interpretation of visual stimuli	X					typical development and as
socialization, play,	4 Cognitive skills						
feeding/eating	problem solving	X					his repertoire expands.
	generalization of learning	X					
	5 Attending skills				X		
	6 Use of assistive and adaptive devices	X					
	7 Mgmt of body positions during learning				X		
	8 Mgmt of body positions during transitions	X					
	9 Mvmt within learning environment	X					
Work*	1 Mgmt of body positions during work						
	2 Mgmt of body positions during transitions						
	3 Mgmt within work environment						
	4 Manipulation/hand use						
	5 Use of assistive and adaptive devices						
Play/Leisure*	1 Mgmt body position during play/leisure				X		
	2 Mgmt body position during transitions	X					
	3 Mvmt within play/leisure environment	X					
	4 Manipulation/hand use	X					
	5 Use of assistive and adaptive devices	X					
Communication*	1 Oral motor movements						
	2 Communication access						
	3 Manipulation/hand use						
	4 Mgmt body pos. during communication						
	5 Mvmt within communication environment						
	6 Attending skills						
	7 Perceptual skills						
	8 Use of assistive and adaptive devices						
Socialization*	1 Self esteem	X					
	2 Recognition and use of nonverbal cues					X	
	3 Mgmt. body position during socialization				X		
	4 Mvmt within social environment	X					
	5 Attending skills					X	
	6 Perceptual skills	X					
	7 Cognitive skills	X					
Activities of daily living*	1 Oral motor movements				X		
(feeding/eating)	2 Mgmt of body position during ADL				X		
	3 Mvmt within daily living environment	X					
	4 Attending skills				X		
	5 Manipulation/hand use	X					

(see Chapter 6)   Dunn, W. & Campbell, P. (1988).

*When acquiring new skills, use the learning: skill acquisition section of this grid.

NA—No problems are identified in therapy evaluation.
 0—Although a problem has been identified through evaluation, it is not presently interfering with program outcome(s). Needs may be met by self, parents, or professionals in other programs or agencies.
 1—The problem *influences* successful program outcome(s); simple instructional or environmental changes are likely to result in functional performance.
 2—The problem *interferes* with specific program outcome(s); specific strategies are necessary to enable functional performance.
 3—The problem *prevents* successful program outcome(s); multifaceted strategies are necessary to reach functional performance.

Figure 7-1. Functional Skills Assessment Grid for David.

cialization, the therapist incorporates examples of alternative positioning and handling techniques which incorporate variations of sensory input that could be introduced during play and self care.

David needed to develop a larger repertoire of self regulatory strategies so that he could engage the environment more frequently in a goal directed way. The therapist decided to design an intervention approach which incorporated the sensory qualities and physical properties of objects and tasks, and the inherent characteristics of the environment. Figure 7-2 summarizes the principal parameters to be considered for this type of intervention (Intervention Planning Guide, Oetter, 1988). One must remember that sensory experiences and reactions are difficult to conceptualize, because therapists observe only reactions to stimuli, which are motoric in nature, demonstrating the intimate relationship between input and response (Dunn, 1990, a and b). Additionally, motor actions produce sensations for the individual and must be considered in this framework.

There are some general principles for using the intervention planning chart effectively. One sensory system defines each column from left to right on the chart; they are in an order which represents increasing complexity. The more complex sensory systems require a greater degree of interaction among other sensory and neuromuscular systems. The rows are characterized by components of each sensory system. One moves down on the chart within a column; the program plan incorporates the simpler components above the target component. The therapist also incorporates programming strategies from those sensory systems to the left and right of the target system. Finally, the therapist considers rhythm, intensity, frequency, and duration of sensory input, recognizing that alteration of one parameter may necessitate simplifying other parameters for a successful outcome.

In David's case, the therapist wanted to provide appropriate sensory input in order to establish and maintain an organized state for functional performance. Figure 7-3 illustrates the pattern of David's strengths, as determined from the assessment. Since proprioception and vertical bouncing are strengths, these would form the basis for the intervention plan. One would not want to begin the program plan by directing input toward poorly processing sensory channels, because goal directed behavior would then be difficult. For example, David presently reacts to the horizontal position by becoming upset and losing postural control. Use of this position as the primary form of input would immediately trigger these "fight or flight" reactions, leaving the nervous system even more poorly equipped to interact with the environment. Any introduction of an undeveloped sensory parameter must be incorporated into intense use of strongly developed parameters.

David's family's priorities are best addressed through the use of monitoring; a home program to initially decrease sensory sensitivity, and then increase functional interaction with the environment will be most useful for David. Because home programs require a significant personal commitment from the

INTERVENTION PLANNING GUIDE

Taste/ Smell	Oral Texture	Tactile	Vestibular Movement	Vestibular Gravity	Visual	Auditory
Sweet/ Vanilla	Suck/ Blow	Joint & muscle activity Cool to neutral warmth	Joint & muscle activity	Vertical	Light/ Dark Color	Vibration
Salt/ Brine	Bite/ Crunch	Deep pressure Moderate temperatures	Oscilla- tion (bouncing)	Horizontal	Form (bounda- ries)	Rhythm Music Sing-song speech Rhyme
Sour/ Citrus Spice	Chew	Touch pressure Moderate temperatures	Linear movement (swinging)	Out of straight planes (diagonals)	Place (location)	Vocaliza- tion/ speech sounds
Bitter/ Smoke	Lick	Light touch (may be unexpected) Extreme temperatures	Rotary movement (spinning or partial rotation)	Upside down/ backwards space	Movement through time and space	Language

RHYTHMIC INPUT OVER TIME - *DECREASES* AROUSAL LEVEL
ARHYTHMIC INPUT OVER TIME - *INCREASES* AROUSAL LEVEL

Rhythm   of   Input   +
Intensity   of   Input   +
Frequency   of   Input   +
Duration   of   Input   =

INTERVENTION

Figure 7-2.   Sample Intervention Planning Guide which considers the sensory components of performance. *Patti Oetter MA, OTR/L, FAOTA (1989).*

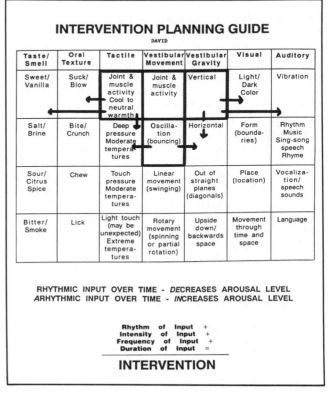

INTERVENTION PLANNING GUIDE
DAVID

Taste/ Smell	Oral Texture	Tactile	Vestibular Movement	Vestibular Gravity	Visual	Auditory
Sweet/ Vanilla	Suck/ Blow	Joint & muscle activity Cool to neutral warmth	Joint & muscle activity	Vertical	Light/ Dark Color	Vibration
Salt/ Brine	Bite/ Crunch	Deep pressure Moderate temperatures	Oscilla- tion (bouncing)	Horizontal	Form (bounda- ries)	Rhythm Music Sing-song speech Rhyme
Sour/ Citrus Spice	Chew	Touch pressure Moderate temperatures	Linear movement (swinging)	Out of straight planes (diagonals)	Place (location)	Vocaliza- tion/ speech sounds
Bitter/ Smoke	Lick	Light touch (may be unexpected) Extreme temperatures	Rotary movement (spinning or partial rotation)	Upside down/ backwards space	Movement through time and space	Language

RHYTHMIC INPUT OVER TIME - *DECREASES* AROUSAL LEVEL
ARHYTHMIC INPUT OVER TIME - *INCREASES* AROUSAL LEVEL

Rhythm   of   Input   +
Intensity   of   Input   +
Frequency   of   Input   +
Duration   of   Input   =

INTERVENTION

Figure 7-3.   Intervention Planning Guide for David.

parents, the therapist assists the parents in choosing the best time for them to begin the program. Variables to consider include: a non-stressful time for the family; a time when concentrated attention can be devoted to the program so that there is not pressure to perform for any family member.

Target Objective 1

David will remain quiet and calm during parental interactions.

Intervention Approach

Activities to decrease over-responsiveness to sensory input.

Intervention Procedures (Examples which prepare the system for functional tasks in other target objectives)

a. Use joint compression by stabilizing the body and limbs proximal and distal to the limb joints and pressing the joints together for 3–5 seconds.
b. Introduce tactile sensations while David is being bounced in a vertical position; this pairs an acceptable stimulus with one that is more difficult for David to process.
c. Prepare mouth before each feeding. Rub roof of mouth and gums with light pressure. Use finger or nipple; do it quickly before David can react negatively.

Figure 7-4 provides an example of a completed Intervention Plan form, using this first Target Objective. All of the Target Objectives would be fleshed out in this same manner on David's complete Intervention Plan. (See Chapter Six, Figure 6-7).

Since David spends most of his time in a highly aroused state, rhythmic input is preferred because it is more calming. Pairing of rhythmic input with a well functioning sensory component will be a good place to start (e.g., level 1 tactile, movement and gravity, and level 2 movement, see Figure 7-3). Secondly, one would want to increase intensity of a strong sensory component, and begin pairing that input, either with a less functional component at the same level (e.g., two level 1 components), or a level 2 component in a sensory channel that has a strength already (e.g., move from level 1 vertical toward level 2 horizontal in the vestibular area). For David, the choices would include (see Figure 7-3): level 1 taste, visual or auditory, and level 2 tactile, gravity.

Target Objective 2

David will quiet himself to interact with persons or objects in the environment.

Intervention Approach

Increase repertoire and appropriateness of self regulating behaviors.

Intervention Procedures (Examples)

a. Offer opportunities for suck, blow and bite; notice strength utilized. Observe lip, teeth, and tongue movements (e.g., biting endurance, efficiency).
b. Provide graded bouncing during play (vertical vestibular; oscillating) to help organize behavior (gentle but arhythmical to alert, hard but rhythmical to calm). Observe David's participation in, or use of, similar activities (e.g., use of hard rocking, bouncing, shaking hands, rhythmic noises).
c. Provide deep hugs through shoulders and/or hips (tactile levels 1 and 2). Observe negative (clenching jaw, arching back, arms away from midline, taking a deep breath and holding it) and positive (moving towards person, snuggling) responses.
d. Provide opportunities to bear weight on hands through shoulders, hands and knees, and in kneel stand. Provide toys, pictures and other colorful objects for David to look at while he is bearing weight. He may need external support through head, tummy, hips, and shoulders. Observe pushing with hands, leaning into hands, or pulling up.

Although an important area of focus with David is improvement of postural control, this area has been compromised because of the sensory processing problems noted above. It is not likely that this system will spontaneously develop as the sensory concerns are addressed, and therefore will also require direct intervention. It is important to remember that all of the postural activities will simultaneously provide David with organizing sensory input, which will facilitate additional improvements in regulation of state (Target Objectives 1 and 2). In order for this plan to be effective, David's state must constantly be monitored to ensure that he will be able to accept and integrate the sensations that become available through the activity.

Target Objective 3

David will play with persons and objects in his immediate environment.

Intervention Approach

Increase use and variety of postural mechanisms.

Intervention Procedures (Examples)

Strategies that would be incorporated into David's life routines are to:

a. Provide frequent opportunities to play and socialize in semi-supine (upper trunk, head, and pelvis supported in neutral to partially flexed as in an infant seat) and supported prone positions.

  1. Activities suggested in previous sections would also facilitate this target objective.
  2. Provide linear movement and joint compression opportunities during play that can be initiated and man-

INTERVENTION PLAN

Child's name: _____**David**_____   Date: _____

Birthdate: _____

Agency name: _____   Chron. Age: _____ yrs. _____ mo.

Outcome Statement: **David will interact positively and appropriately with his parents and**
other environmental stimuli.

Outcome Category: _____Learning   _____Work
                                 __*___Play/Leisure   _____Communication
                                 _____Socialization   __*___ADL

Performance Components:
  ENABLING COMPONENTS: CONCERNS:
  proprioception _____   **sensory awareness** _____
  vertical, linear vestibular _____   **tactile, auditory, visual** _____
                                                    other vestibular _____
  _____   **reflex, tone, postural control** _____
                                                    activity tolerance, arousal, _____
                                                    orientation, attention _____

Service Provision Models:
  _____Direct*   __*___Monitoring   _____Consultation
                               __*___ supervise adult   _____teach adult
                                                             _____adapt posture/mvmt
                                                             _____adapt task/matls
                                                             _____adapt environ

*provided in conjunction with one or more other service models
  __*___**MONITORING**   _____n.a.

Target Objective: **Danny will remain quiet and calm during parental interactions** _____

Intervention Approach: __*___remed.   _____compens.   _____prevent-interv.

  Describe: **Activities to decrease overresponsiveness to sensory input** _____

Location of Services: **family home** _____

Intervention Procedures: **Use joint compression by stabilizing the body and limbs proximal**
and distal to the limb joints and pressing the joints together for 3–5 seconds.
Introduce tactile sensations while bouncing David vertically.
Prepare mouth before each feeding. Rub roof of mouth and gums with light pressing. Use
finger or nipple; do it quickly before David can react negatively.

Implementor: _____teacher ____*___family_____aide _____other: _____

Training and Verification Strategies: **Therapist will demonstrate procedures, then observe**
and prompt parents; therapist and parents will discuss observed behaviors.

Proposed Meeting Schedule: __*___weekly   _____bimonthly   _____monthly

Location of meeting: **family home** _____

Method for Documentation of Performance:
  behavior to be observed: **quietness & attentiveness during parental interaction** _____
  natural environment for observation: **family home** _____
  measurement/data to be collected: **number of consecutive and cumulative seconds** _____
    David is quiet (sucking, looking, cooing); no screaming. _____
  criterion for successful performance: **10 consecutive minutes of quiet behavior.** _____

Figure 7-4. Occupational Therapy Intervention Plan for David.

aged by the child (i.e., on all fours over a foam roll, small therapy or playground ball, or through a suspended innertube).

3. Provide input to proximal joints (e.g., pushing/pulling, cocontraction and weight bearing); target jaw, neck, shoulders, hips. This facilitates stability.
4. Create smooth movement patterns to extend functional use of rotation. Note: David is not yet ready for these activities, but the therapist must be ready to facilitate functional movements when opportunities present themselves. The following movements can be facilitated when David is motivated to move in a purposeful way
   —Moving body separately from head movements
   —Moving head separately from neck movements
   —Moving shoulders separately from neck movements
   —Moving arms separately from shoulders movements
   —Moving thumbs separately from finger movements
   —Moving upper trunk separately from lower trunk

As David is more able to consider input useful to him, he will become more aware of his own body and its potential abilities. This natural curiosity reinforces self regulation and a sense of competence to deal with the environment on new terms. Activities which foster this curiosity while controlling state, will allow David to gather information to form an accurate and reliable map of his body.

Target Objective 4

David will actively participate in mealtime activities. (Note: remember, the exact parameters of this target objective would be defined in the "Method for Documentation of Performance" section of the Intervention Plan.)

Intervention Approach

Increase interest in, and knowledge of, body parts for use in functional activities.

Intervention Procedures (Examples)

a. Prepare mouth before each feeding. Rub roof of mouth and gums with light pressure. Use finger or nipple (do it quickly, before David can resist).
b. Provide gentle, firm massage of face, arms, legs, and back.
c. Offer opportunities for suck, blow, and bite; notice strength utilized. Observe lip, teeth, and tongue movements.
d. Provide frequent opportunities for suck, blow, lick, crunch, chew, bite, noise-making, and prolonged phonation (blow toys, rubber textures and shapes, imitating the hiss sounds with variance in length and volume).
e. Provide low frequence vibration around mouth and jaw; allow David to regulate amount with his responses.
f. Provide support and/or intermittent pressure or tapping to abdomen or rib cage, to affect respiratory pattern.

Communication includes nonverbal reactions, vocalizations, muscle tone, eye contact, etc. David is communicating with persons, but his messages are predominantly of the avoidance type. This program plan must also address the parents' ability to recognize David's communication, and to be able to provide safe input that will enable him to communicate more positive messages about their interactions.

Target Objective 5

David will interact with parents effectively.

Intervention Approach

Increase effectiveness of David's socialization.

Intervention Procedures

a. Watch for David's clues while engaging in the initiating activities from other target objectives (e.g., looking, quieting); respond by continuing the activity (e.g., bouncing during postural task) or by copying his action. Wait for corresponding socialization responses to continue activity.
b. Use suck, blow, and chest/tummy tapping to facilitate oral motor skills, and noise making with eye contact. Imitate his activity, then imitate skills you want him to learn.

OUTCOME

David and his parents were initially scheduled to meet with the therapist three times per week. Health insurance covered 100% of the costs of occupational therapy for six months. After this period, they would cover 80% of the costs, as long as the therapist could document continued improvements in David's condition.

David's parents began the home program emphasizing target objectives 1 and 2. Within the first week, David was sleeping five to six hours at a stretch during the night, and taking two 2-hour naps, one in the morning and one in the afternoon. By focusing on providing David with organizing sensory input, he was able to calm and get rest.

The mother reported an immediate change in feeding patterns. David was able to remain calm and enjoy up to ten minutes of nursing before fussing. At that point, his mother was able to quickly calm him by holding him vertically, patting his back firmly a few times, and returning him to the other breast. She learned how to use organizing sensation to increase his functional performance.

The therapist talked with the parents on several occasions to lend support and answer questions. David participated in occupational therapy intervention three times a week for the first six months, twice a week for the next ten months and once a week for the last two months (total of 18 months). The speech/language pathologist recommended another evaluation when he reached four years of age. When David was released from occupational therapy, the therapist recommended that the parents follow a home program which provided a variety of experiences and peer interaction opportunities. It was also recommended that unless they had particular concerns, David would not need to be seen until his reevaluation at four years of age.

CASE #2—CLIFFORD

Program Planning for Clifford

The family and the therapist determined three primary areas to be addressed in the intervention plan. The family was very concerned about eating, and so this became the first focus of attention. In order to address this area successfully, the therapist included supportive activities to improve muscle tone and postural control. The parents also expressed their desire to facilitate normal family interactions, and so socialization and play were also targeted as initial outcomes. Figure 7-5 summarizes the data obtained from the assessment with these targetted outcomes.

Throughout the assessment, the therapist and the parents discussed the information being gathered and possible strategies for dealing with problems. Several feeding and handling strategies were demonstrated, then tried by both parents. The last half hour of the visit was spent creating a collaborative short term plan for a home-based intervention program.

Because of his age, the parents preferred to have therapy in the home until they felt more comfortable about his level of susceptibility to infections. They also requested that therapy be scheduled late in the afternoon so that Mr. B could take little time off his job and still be present.

Target Objective 1

Clifford will actively participate in eating at mealtime.

Intervention Approach

Increase oral motor control and activity tolerance for eating.

Intervention Procedures (Examples)

a. 15 to 20 minutes before meals provide sensory input to increase arousal and prepare mouth and body for eating tasks. Use playful interactions with Clifford. Bounce Clifford, while providing external postural support. Stimulate the face and mouth regions with one's fingers or with a cloth or sponge.
b. During eating, provide playful interactions which facilitate oral motor control. Tug on the nipple while he is sucking to provide resistance. Encourage eye contact. Tap jaw, chin and mouth region.

Since Clifford is not hypersensitive to sensory input, the family may use strong or weak sensory channels to establish the appropriate level of arousal for eating. They may use high intensity level 1 and 2 parameters from the Intervention Planning Guide (see Figure 7-6); the family might also introduce lower intensity level 3 input within a sensory system already being activated. For example, the family might play with Clifford in a partially upright position by humming, laughing, and using eye contact (level 1 and 2 visual and auditory input) and then introduce language as in a song or chant (level 3

auditory input). This series of interactions will raise Clifford's level of arousal and attention to the environment, and will make it easier for him to maintain this alert state during eating. (This example actually occurred during the therapist's visit, and so reinforced the family's feelings of competence for dealing with Clifford.)

Initially Clifford will be very hungry. His desire to satiate his hunger will override his interest in play. The parents will need to address hunger first, and then will be able to successfully introduce playful interactions into the eating task. Since all family members wanted to work on this area, and mother was breast-feeding, these activities were also carried out by using the pacifier. Both sensory and motor components are addressed in these activities. Taste and smell are primitive sensations that facilitate the eating process; tactile input occurs with facial and mouth contact. Oral motor movements occur as a result of, and in conjunction with, these sensations (e.g., rooting reflex in newborns-tactile stimulus yields a motor response), and so are listed in the taste/smell column of the intervention chart (Figure 7-6). Other sensory channels can be incorporated into eating tasks, even though they are not inherent properties of eating itself. Family members might initially gently pull on the pacifier to encourage Clifford to hold onto it by sucking. This reinforces muscle tone and provides sensory feedback to skin and muscle receptors. Later, they might begin to pop the pacifier out of Clifford's mouth, which forces him to reestablish the seal, and triggers amusement or other social interactions.

Target Objective 2

Clifford will initiate play behaviors.

Intervention Approach

Facilitate postural and righting reactions which support the body for interaction with the environment.

Intervention Procedures (Examples)

a. Rock Clifford while holding him in various positions (prone, supine, vertical).
b. Place visually or auditorially interesting toys in various positions and encourage Clifford to look at them.

This is another goal that combines sensory and motor activity. The chosen activities must be structured to maintain Clifford's attention to the environment. For example, rocking can become a soothing form of input that reduces one's ability to attend, and facilitates rest rather than interaction. This would not improve postural control mechanisms. Auditory and visual input can be altered so rapidly that the child either cannot keep track of them, or becomes overly excited. In either case, his ability to interact with the toy would diminish. The therapist must clearly explain to family members how to watch Clifford's reactions to determine his responsivity to the task. Because he has low muscle tone, activity tolerance must also be considered. If Clifford is placed completely prone or supine on a stable surface, he will quickly tire as he tries to work against the force of gravity. Supported positions on

FUNCTIONAL SKILLS ASSESSMENT GRID
for Occupational and Physical Therapy Services

PROGRAM OUTCOME	PERFORMANCE COMPONENTS	NA	0	1	2	3	COMMENTS
Learning	1 Manipulation/hand use	X					check all NA's as Clifford
Skill	2 Interpretation of body senses			X			grows and these
Acquisition and	3 Perceptual skills						
academics*	organization of space and time	X					
related to	interpretation of visual stimuli	X					performance components
socialization, play,	4 Cognitive skills						are developmentally
feeding/eating	problem solving	X					appropriate to consider.
	generalization of learning	X					
	5 Attending skills				X		
	6 Use of assistive and adaptive devices	X					
	7 Mgmt of body positions during learning				X		
	8 Mgmt body positions during transitions	X					
	9 Mvmt within learning environment	X					
Work*	1 Mgmt of body positions during work						
	2 Mgmt of body positions during transitions						
	3 Mgmt within work environment						
	4 Manipulation/hand use						
	5 Use of assistive and adaptive devices						
Play/Leisure*	1 Mgmt body position during play/leisure				X		
	2 Mgmt body position during transitions	X					
	3 Mvmt within play/leisure environment	X					
	4 Manipulation/hand use	X					
	5 Use of assistive and adaptive devices	X					
Communication*	1 Oral motor movements						
	2 Communication access						
	3 Manipulation/hand use						
	4 Mgmt body pos. during communication						
	5 Mvmt within communication environment						
	6 Attending skills						
	7 Perceptual skills						
	8 Use of assistive and adaptive devices						
Socialization*	1 Self esteem	X					
	2 Recognition and use of nonverbal cues			X			
	3 Mgmt. body position during socialization				X		
	4 Mvmt within social environment	X					
	5 Attending skills			X			
	6 Perceptual skills	X					
	7 Cognitive skills	X					
Activities of daily living* (feeding/eating)	1 Oral motor movements				X		
	2 Mgmt of body position during ADL				X		
	3 Mvmt within daily living environment	X					
	4 Attending skills				X		
	5 Manipulation/hand use	X					

(see Chapter 6)
Dunn, W. & Campbell, P. (1988).

*When acquiring new skills, use the learning: skill acquisition section of this grid.

NA—No problems are identified in therapy evaluation.
0—Although a problem has been identified through evaluation, it is not presently interfering with program outcome(s). Needs may be met by self, parents, or professionals in other programs or agencies.
1—The problem *influences* successful program outcome(s); simple instructional or environmental changes are likely to result in functional performance.
2—The problem *interferes* with specific program outcome(s); specific strategies are necessary to enable functional performance.
3—The problem *prevents* successful program outcome(s); multifaceted strategies are necessary to reach functional performance.

Figure 7-5. **Functional Skills Assessment Grid for Clifford.**

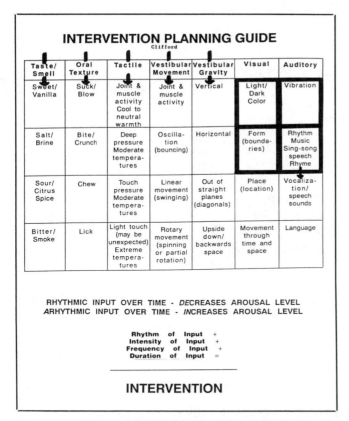

INTERVENTION PLANNING GUIDE

Clifford

Taste/ Smell	Oral Texture	Tactile	Vestibular Movement	Vestibular Gravity	Visual	Auditory
Sweet/ Vanilla	Suck/ Blow	Joint & muscle activity Cool to neutral warmth	Joint & muscle activity	Vertical	Light/ Dark Color	Vibration
Salt/ Brine	Bite/ Crunch	Deep pressure Moderate temperatures	Oscillation (bouncing)	Horizontal	Form (boundaries)	Rhythm Music Sing-song speech Rhyme
Sour/ Citrus Spice	Chew	Touch pressure Moderate temperatures	Linear movement (swinging)	Out of straight planes (diagonals)	Place (location)	Vocalization/ speech sounds
Bitter/ Smoke	Lick	Light touch (may be unexpected) Extreme temperatures	Rotary movement (spinning or partial rotation)	Upside down/ backwards space	Movement through time and space	Language

RHYTHMIC INPUT OVER TIME - *DECREASES* AROUSAL LEVEL
ARHYTHMIC INPUT OVER TIME - *INCREASES* AROUSAL LEVEL

Rhythm   of   Input   +
Intensity   of   Input   +
Frequency   of   Input   +
Duration   of   Input   =

INTERVENTION

Figure 7-6. Intervention Planning Guide for Clifford.

partially unstable surfaces (e.g., over one's leg or shoulder, on a bolster or innertube, etc.) decrease the force of gravity, and increase the feedback about his own attempts to shift posture.

Target Objective 3

Clifford will interact appropriately with family members.

Intervention Approach

Facilitate socialization and communication among family members.

Intervention Procedures (Examples)

a. Use the semisupine position frequently to play with Clifford.
b. Incorporate visual and vocal plays into family interactions.
c. Exaggerate and maintain facial expressions when interacting with Clifford.

The semisupine posture is the social posture for infants. It is less challenging posturally, and therefore frees the child to engage the environment. It controls the available visual field, and so interactions must take place within that range. Generally, 8-12 inches from the infant's face is an optimal distance for interaction. Visual and auditory input together

produce a map of the external environment and provide a base of knowledge for the communication process. Facial expressions are very early forms of nonverbal communication, and are easily provided within the context described above. Vocalizations frequently emerge from successful facial play. A sample partial intervention plan for this target area is presented in Figure 7-7.

Children with Down Syndrome are frequently at risk for language delays. The concerns and goals for Clifford point out several possible reasons for this occurrence. Poor control of the oral motor mechanisms makes it difficult for these children to produce the movement patterns that are precursors to speech sounds. Postural control, which supports the head in an upright position, and facilitates respiratory support for speech, is frequently poorly developed. Nonverbal communication is dependent on specific motor skill development (e.g., facial muscles, hands). Delays in motor interactions can interfere with this form of communication. All factors must be considered when planning for long term outcomes.

OUTCOME

Because of his age, the parents preferred to have home-based intervention until they felt more comfortable about Clifford's immunity to infections, and until they felt that intervention priorities would better be served in a community-based program. The therapist respected the family's need to have intervention in the home, recognizing that the family was focused on the impact of their of their situation with Clifford within their family. Home provides a familiar territory for these early attempts to facilitate his development and their roles as family members with Clifford. The parents requested that therapy be scheduled late in the afternoon so that the father could take as little time off from his job as possible, and still be present.

The therapist met with Clifford and his family once a week for the first six months; family members provided excellent support and followup throughout the weeks. After that time, Clifford and his parents came to an outpatient clinic for services; the therapist continued to visit their home every two months to instruct the siblings in new play strategies. At 18 months, Clifford entered a center-based early intervention program, so that he would also have peer interactions in addition to other developmental intervention. The occupational therapist facilitated the transition by consulting with the early intervention staff to set up a successful environment for Clifford, and to ensure that therapeutic goals would be incorporated into his curricular activities. During the period that Clifford attended this early intervention program, the occupational therapist also continued to see Clifford twice a week, using direct service provision with goals in self care, play and pre-academic areas such as tool use (e.g., writing utensils). Because the early intervention program was using sign language, the occupational therapist also incorporated signing into intervention activities.

When Clifford turned three years old, he entered a public school preschool program. By this time Clifford was independent in mobility, although signs of low muscle tone were still present. He demonstrated age appropriate eating, dressing, and personal hygiene, although he was still a bit slower than other children to perform these tasks. Clifford used a lot

INTERVENTION PLAN

Child's name: **Clifford**

Date: _____

Birthdate: _____

Agency name: _____

Chron. Age: _____ yrs. _____ mo.

Outcome Statement: **Clifford will interact with family members.**

Outcome Category:
_____Learning	_____Work
_____Play/Leisure	_____Communication
* Socialization	_____ADL

Performance Components:
ENABLING COMPONENTS: CONCERNS:

orientation/recognition   **activity tolerance**

visual processing   **level of arousal**

auditory processing   **postural control**

social conduct

Service Provision Models:

_____Direct*   *___Monitoring   *___Consultation

                              _____ supervise adult   *___teach adult

                                                              *___adapt posture/mvmt

                                                              _____adapt task/matls

                                                              _____adapt environ

*provided in conjunction with one or more other service models

___*___**MONITORING**   _____n.a.

Target Objective: **Clifford will initiate and respond to family member's attempts to play.**

Intervention Approach: _____remed.   _____compens.   *___prevent-interv.

  Describe: **Experiences to capitalize on enabling components; experiences which reinforce family members**

Location of Services: **family home**

Intervention Procedures: **1. play peek-a-boo 2. make facial expressions with noises that Clifford enjoys and may repeat (e.g., "raspberries").**

Implementor: _____teacher   *___family   _____aide   _____other: _____

Training and Verification Strategies: **family members will watch demonstration from therapist initially, then will demonstrate their interactions for the therapist.**

Proposed Meeting Schedule: _____ weekly   *___bimonthly   _____monthly

Location of meeting: **the family home**

Method for Documentation of Performance:

  behavior to be observed: **family member interactions w/Clifford**

  natural environment for observation: **the family home**

  measurement/data to be collected: **number of Clifford's initiations/responses**

  criterion for successful performance: **Clifford demonstrates at least 10 initiations/responses in 2 minutes.**

___*___ **CONSULTATION**   _____ n.a.

Area of Concern: **Activities of Daily Living: Socialization**

Identified by: _____   role: **parents**

Statement of Area to be Addressed: **Clifford's ability to interact with family members**

Location of Services: **the family home**

Figure 7-7. **Occupational Therapy Intervention Plan for Clifford.**

Strategies: **teach parents age appropriate activities; design & teach parents semi-supine position for Clifford**

Proposed Meeting Schedule: __*__ weekly   _____ bimonthly   _____ monthly

Location of meeting: **the family home**

Method for Documentation of Performance:
  behavior to be observed: **Clifford's initiation and response and family member interactions**
  natural environment for observation: **home**
  measurement/data to be collected: **no. of Clifford's initiations/responses**
  criterion for successful performance: **Clifford demonstrates at least 10 initiations/responses in 2 minutes**

Figure 7-7. *Continued.*

of vocalized words, but supplemented his talking with gestures, facial expressions, and signs learned throughout the school day. Clifford demonstrated good social skills with peers, but had a tendency to be overly sensitive to emotionally charged situations. Clifford continued to have a short attention span for school-related tasks, shifting frequently from one place to another, perhaps to compensate for poor trunk stability. He used pencils, crayons, and scissors during school activities, but still struggled with accuracy. The occupational therapist was able to provide the school team with a lot of valuable information, since she had served Clifford and his family since he was an infant. She assisted in the development of the IEP and related program plans.

The occupational therapist also assisted with the transition from the preschool program to the elementary school. She met with the school personnel to facilitate the placement decision, and offer suggestions regarding environmental and curricular adaptations that would support Clifford's needs. By school age, additional support and adaptations are frequently needed for children such as Clifford, to ensure continued progress throughout the developmental period.

This case illustrates the ongoing and evolving role of the occupational therapist as children grow up and change programs. It is not always the same occupational therapist making all of these transitions, but each transition requires the support of the professionals involved with the child and family. For Clifford, the therapist shifted her role, service provision models, and approaches as needs and demands changed. These professional demands go well beyond knowledge and skill in direct service intervention techniques, toward an understanding and appreciation of the system within which services are provided.

CASE #3—ANDREA

Program Planning for Andrea

Findings were discussed with the family members throughout the evaluation. Their comments regarding effective strategies were utilized to optimize Andrea's performance. A program plan was constructed from this data. The Functional Skills Assessment Grid summarizing evaluation findings is presented on Figure 7-8.

In this particular program, team members meet for approximately 30 minutes following the evaluation. While they are meeting, the social worker meets with family members to discuss questions that have come up during the assessment, and issues related to program planning. The entire group then meets together to design program strategies to best suit the needs of the child and family.

This rehabilitation program offers center-based individual and small group occupational therapy, physical therapy, and speech therapy, with family followup and support. While there is not a formal classroom program, an early childhood specialist is on the staff to act as a liaison between early childhood programs, elementary, and secondary public school programs. Because Andrea had a twin sister who was not eligible for the public school early childhood program, and the family wanted Andrea to have as many experiences with normal peers as possible, the decision was made to find a private community preschool program that could address Andrea's special needs. The family was able to find such a program and the center staff (the early childhood specialist and therapists) arranged to provide support to the preschool teacher, in addition to the direct services that would be provided at the rehabilitation program.

The occupational therapist targeted four areas of emphasis for Andrea's program:

1. Provide sensory input directed at improving Andrea's ability to accept handling and interaction with others;
2. Combine use of head control and visual orientation to get Andrea engaged in her environment;
3. Facilitate postural control and beginning movement patterns in supported sitting; and
4. Facilitate reach and grasp.

An Intervention Planning Guide and a partial intervention plan is provided in Figures 7-9 and 7-10.

Target Objective

Andrea will remain calm while being handled by an adult.

Intervention Approach

Provide high intensity, calming sensory input (e.g., touch pressure and proprioception); pair sensory input with positioning that minimizes the effects of her spasticity.

FUNCTIONAL SKILLS ASSESSMENT GRID

for Occupational and Physical Therapy Services

PROGRAM OUTCOME	PERFORMANCE COMPONENTS	NA	0	1	2	3	COMMENTS
Learning	1 Manipulation/hand use					X	
Skill	2 Interpretation of body senses				X		
Acquisition and academics*	3 Perceptual skills						
	organization of space and time	X					check later
	interpretation of visual stimuli				X		
	4 Cognitive skills						
	problem solving	X					
	generalization of learning	X					
	5 Attending skills				X		sensorimotor factors
	6 Use of assistive and adaptive devices	X					
	7 Mgmt of body positions during learning					X	
	8 Mgmt body positions during transitions	X					
	9 Mvmt within learning environment					X	
Work*	1 Mgmt of body positions during work						
	2 Mgmt of body positions during transitions						
	3 Mgmt within work environment						
	4 Manipulation/hand use						
	5 Use of assistive and adaptive devices						
Play/Leisure*	1 Mgmt body position during play/leisure					X	
	2 Mgmt body position during transitions	X					
	3 Mvmt within play/leisure environment				X		
	4 Manipulation/hand use					X	
	5 Use of assistive and adaptive devices	X					obj. positioned for Andrea
Communication*	1 Oral motor movements					X	consider aug. comm.
	2 Communication access	X					
	3 Manipulation/hand use	X					
	4 Mgmt body pos. during communication				X		
	5 Mvmt within communication environment				X		
	6 Attending skills				X		
	7 Perceptual skills				X		
	8 Use of assistive and adaptive devices	X					will need later
Socialization*	1 Self esteem	X					
	2 Recognition and use of nonverbal cues			X			
	3 Mgmt. body position during socialization				X		
	4 Mvmt within social environment				X		persons come to Andrea
	5 Attending skills				X		sensorimotor factors
	6 Perceptual skills				X		
	7 Cognitive skills	X					
Activities of daily living*	1 Oral motor movements						
	2 Mgmt of body position during ADL						
	3 Mvmt within daily living environment						
	4 Attending skills						
	5 Manipulation/hand use						

(see Chapter 6)   Dunn, W. & Campbell, P. (1988).

*When acquiring new skills, use the learning: skill acquisition section of this grid.

NA—No problems are identified in therapy evaluation.

0—Although a problem has been identified through evaluation, it is not presently interfering with program outcome(s). Needs may be met by self, parents, or professionals in other programs or agencies.

1—The problem *influences* successful program outcome(s); simple instructional or environmental changes are likely to result in functional performance.

2—The problem *interferes* with specific program outcome(s); specific strategies are necessary to enable functional performance.

3—The problem *prevents* successful program outcome(s); multifaceted strategies are necessary to reach functional performance.

Figure 7-8. Functional Skills Assessment Grid for Andrea.

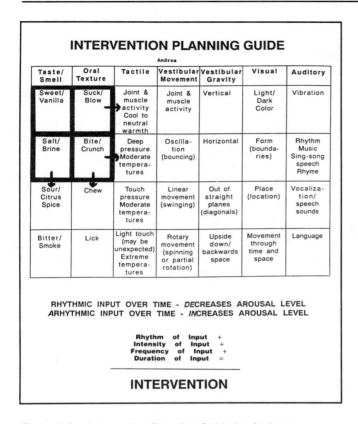

Figure 7-9.   Intervention Planning Guide for Andrea.

Intervention Procedures

The mother provided information regarding successful handling techniques. She reported that Andrea remains calm when they wrap her and hold her tightly in a fully flexed position, while rhythmically bouncing lightly. The family uses this strategy before they begin to play with Andrea. The parents would then slowly unwrap Andrea while maintaining the flexed position and provide pressure to shoulders and hips. This sequence provides Andrea with constant sensory input of touch pressure and proprioception, allowing Andrea to get organized before having to tolerate additional handling and movement. The therapist demonstrated an effective way to slowly move Andrea from prone to supine, supine to sidelying then prone to the therapist's lap.

Massage with lotion is another strategy that provides Andrea with touch pressure input over her entire body. Massage can also precede other handling activities as a preparatory experience. Light to moderate joint compression and traction through the jaw, neck, shoulders, and hips was used frequently during handling activities to provide proprioceptive input, help Andrea inhibit reflexive patterns, and maintain a comfortable state of arousal.

Target Objective 2

Andrea will watch her family members as they talk to her.

Intervention Approach

Position Andrea to facilitate recognition and use of visual input; provide high contrast and interesting visual stimuli; introduce cause-effect actions with visual play.

Intervention Procedures

The school staff and family were instructed to use brightly colored toys with moveable parts or lights during handling activities to facilitate visual attention. The therapist encouraged Andrea's twin and parents to play with Andrea directly in front of her visual field, using highly animated facial expressions and sounds to encourage Andrea to watch them. The school was encouraged to suspend or stabilize interesting visual and auditory toys for those times that Andrea was positioned in sitting or on the mat.

Target Objective 3

Andrea will initiate interaction with objects in the environment.

Intervention Approach

Provide positioning to support motor interactions; provide physical support and prompting to initiate movements.

Intervention Procedures

The semisupine position provides support for the trunk and legs, while allowing a variety of movement options for the head, neck, shoulder, arms, and hands. This position can be combined with visual stimulation to produce beginning adaptive responses for Andrea. Prone and supine positions are more difficult for Andrea to manage; the transitional patterns from prone to sidelying to supine to sitting are a more functional set of movements to stimulate Andrea. Static positions do not encourage movement and postural adaptation, especially in children who must cope with spasticity.

Adults can also position Andrea in prone with the legs flexed (e.g., over the lap), facilitating her ability to bear weight on the forearms. This will facilitate endurance, head control, and provides proprioceptive input to the upper extremities.

Target Objective 4

Andrea will hold and visually inspect a toy.

Intervention Approach

Encourage arm and hand movement to the front; provide positions to encourage use of the hands; provide sensory input to support reach and grasp.

Intervention Procedures

Utilization of strategies previously discussed, as well as positioning in semisupine postures, facilitates bilateral reach, and unilateral and bilateral grasp of objects. For example, placing Andrea's hands in a forward position and encouraging

INTERVENTION PLAN

Child's name: _____**Andrea**_____   Date: _____

Birthdate: _____

Agency name: _____   Chron. Age: _____ yrs. _____ mo.

Outcome Statement: **Andrea will explore a toy.**_____

Outcome Category: | **x**___Learning | _____Work
_____Play/Leisure | _____Communication
_____Socialization | _____ADL

Performance Components:
  ENABLING COMPONENTS: CONCERNS:
  sensory/awareness_____   **sensory processing**_____
  auditory processing_____   **orientation**_____
  olfactory processing_____   **muscle tone**_____
  _____   **visual motor integration**_____

Service Provision Models:
  x___Direct*   **x**___Monitoring   **x**___Consultation
                                     x_supervise adult   **x**_teach adult
                                                                     x_adapt posture/mvmt
                                                                     x_adapt task/matis
                                                                     x_adapt environ

*provided in conjunction with one or more other service models
  x___**DIRECT**   _____n.a.

Target Objective: **Andrea will reach and grasp a toy.**_____

Intervention Approach: **x**___ remed.   **x**___ compens.   _____ prevent-interv.
  Describe: **Provide postural support; provide physical prompting; provide high contrast**_____
        visual & auditory stimuli._____

Location of Services: **Rehab program**_____

Intervention Procedures: **Provide preparatory sensory input; pair postural support with**
    visual/auditory arousal, recognition; provide physical prompts to initiate movement.

Method for Documentation of Performance:
  behavior to be observed: **exploring a toy**_____
  natural environment for observation: **play with parent**_____
  measurement/data to be collected: **contact with toy. Movement of toy in hands.**_____
  criterion for successful performance: **grasping the toy with palmar surface and one**
      move of toy within or between hands in two minutes.

  x___ **MONITORING**   _____ n.a.

Target Objective: **Andrea will visually inspect a toy.**_____

Intervention Approach: **x**___ remed.   _____ compens.   _____ prevent-interv.
  Describe: **Provide preliminary sensory stimulation to arouse Andrea; provide a variety**_____
      of stimuli throughout the day._____

Location of Services: **Classroom**_____

Intervention Procedures: **Use proprioception and touch-pressure input; suspend toys from ceiling in front**
    of seat; attach toys to tables, chairs that are within vision field; provide auditory cues.

Implementor: **x**___teacher   _____ family   _____ aide   _____ other: _____

Figure 7-10. Occupational Therapy Intervention Plan for Andrea.

Training and Verification Strategies: **teacher will demonstrate activities from previous**
   week and will review precautions verbally; written cue sheets will be provided.

Proposed Meeting Schedule: _____ weekly   __x__ bimonthly   _____ monthly

Location of meeting: **day care/preschool**

Method for Documentation of Performance:
   behavior to be observed: **visual attention to the toy**
   natural environment for observation: **classroom**
   measurement/data to be collected: **Length of time to fix on object; length of time to inspect object.**
   criterion for successful performance: **Less than 30 sec. to look at object after it is**
      presented; at least 20 sec. of visual contact in next minute

__x__ **CONSULTATION**   _____ n.a.

Area of Concern: **Learning**

Identified by: **family & team**   role: _____

Statement of Area to be Addressed: **Andrea's ability to explore and interact with objects.**

Location of Services: **Home**

Strategies: **Teach parents about optimal positions, about arousal techniques; about how**
   to analyze objects for their optimum characteristics.

Proposed Meeting Schedule: __x__ weekly   _____ bimonthly   _____ monthly

Location of meeting: **rehab center**

Method for Documentation of Performance:
   behavior to be observed: **Exploring a toy**
   natural environment for observation: **play with parents**
   measurement/data to be collected: **contact with toy; movement of toy in hands.**
   criterion for successful performance: **Grasping the toy with palmar surface and one**
      move of toy within or between hands in two minutes.

Figure 7-10. *Continued.*

her to knock over a stack of blocks is a game she can both enjoy and accomplish with minimal assistance. The therapist showed the school staff and family how to support Andrea's arms and hands to the side to promote weight bearing; this also provides opportunities for weight shift and proximal stability for reach and grasp, as well as upper trunk rotation.

OUTCOME

Occupational therapy was provided twice weekly in coordination with physical therapy and speech/language therapy. All three disciplines coordinated their strategies and frequently served Andrea together. The team also scheduled time to address home and school needs such as positioning, transportation, splinting, and the provision of other adaptive equipment.

At age three surgery was carried out to release muscles in the legs. The physical therapist constructed bilateral ankle foot orthoses (AFO) and the occupational therapist fabricated wrist cock-up splints. A modified spoon was designed so Andrea could feed herself. A stroller was purchased and a tri-wall insert was made for lateral trunk support. A prone stander was purchased to provide Andrea with weight-bearing experiences.

As Andrea approached kindergarten age, it was apparent that she would be able to manage in a regular kindergarten classroom with assistance and adaptations. An electric wheelchair was purchased prior to kindergarten; the orthotist made an insert of upholstered wood and foam to support a functional sitting position. Additionally, the chair was equipped with a right-sided joy stick, foot rests with foot straps, and a strap across her hips to inhibit extensor thrusts. Andrea also participated in a dressing group with four other children and their parents, to design effective strategies in which the children could assist during dressing activities.

Andrea was placed in a regular kindergarten with her twin sister; she continued to receive occupational therapy, physical therapy, and speech therapy from the same team that had seen her in the early intervention program. The public school therapists also serve Andrea in her classroom, collaborating closely with the community therapists and the educational team members.

By first grade, Andrea was using her right hand for grasp and release in eating and simple tool use, assisting in upper extremity dressing, operating her own wheelchair, and was beginning to use a computer with her right hand. Andrea used a head pointer to hit the keys for typing. Although her language was labored, it was adequate to communicate with peers, ask questions in class, and provide simple information.

While continuing to work on general posture and motor control, classroom performance is also being addressed. Frequent consultation is provided in collaboration with the public school therapist to the family and public school personnel in terms of positioning, mobility at school, and ways of modifying classroom work to fit her motor needs. Options for positioning in the classroom include sitting on a bench during group activities, using a walker for short distances, rolling during floor play, and positioning in a prone posture on extended arms during listening activities. Options for classroom work include the utilization of a keyboard, use of multiple choice papers where Andrea needs only make a mark on the correct answer, and utilizing a tape recorder for assignments requiring more extensive language.

CASE #4—TED

Program Planning for Ted

With the addition of a new baby to Ted's family, the family's needs are for respite care, positioning and transporting. As a result, weekly home visits are being scheduled to help the parents find ways of positioning and transporting Ted. A consultation model of service provision will be used to meet these needs. After an initial visit to the center-based program, family members will be invited to participate in the center program as their schedules permit. They are invited to use that time for respite care as they feel the need to have this support. During the times that Ted attends the center-based program, a direct service model of service provision will be employed.

This particular family was feeling overwhelmed at the point that the center became involved. Therapists and other professionals sometimes try to "fix" or "relieve" the family of some of their concerns. Families do not always respond positively over time to this kind of an approach. Families want to manage their own needs and solve their own problems. Our responsibility as professionals is to provide the family with information from which they can make informed decisions, and then to respect and support the decisions they make. It would be extremely inappropriate in this case to teach the parents remedial exercises or activity routines to be done several times a day. Their main concern at this point in time is providing adequate parenting, love, and support to Ted, as well as their new baby. When parents ask for suggestions about home activities, they usually want suggestions that will meet their own personal in-home concerns, rather than those which address particular concerns of the program staff. Program staff can inadvertently convey messages that imply expectations that a "super-parent" is needed to make any progress. When we ask parents questions regarding their concerns and their needs, we need to listen for information that will help us design strategies that fit into their life styles.

Another issue that might arise in the future is the parent's concern about their second child's development. Therapists want to watch for cues, such as suggestive or leading questions, which might indicate this concern so it can be dealt with at that time.

Two areas of concern would be addressed in the consultation component of service provision. These areas are to:

1. Identify strategies for effective positioning throughout the day; and to
2. Apply these strategies to various transporting needs as the family moves about with Ted in the house and in the community.

The therapist will use data collected from the home visits to identify positions already being used, and will reinforce those positions that are useful, employing appropriate adaptations when necessary. Through discussion with the parents, they will identify problem times during the day, and the therapist will design options for the parents to try. All strategies will be demonstrated, and paired with opportunities for the parents to try the positioning techniques under the therapist's guidance. Effective positioning principles will then be applied to the family's transporting needs throughout the day and week. The therapist will accompany the family on an errand to provide support for effective transporting techniques into and out of the car, buildings, etc. A log of discussions, suggestions, and strategies will be kept as a reference, along with comments on the usefulness of each position for the tasks. This will enable the therapist to evaluate the effectiveness of the consultative program.

Four primary areas are targeted for the direct service component of occupational therapy intervention at the center. These areas are to:

1. Increase social skills for play and interaction with people;
2. Increase active muscle tone to allow balanced movement in all positions;
3. Develop skills in reach-grasp-release and object manipulation for play and self care; and
4. Increase eating skills and independence in eating.

A summary of the enabling components (those marked with a * in the comments section) and areas of concern is provided in Figure 7-11. A partial intervention plan is provided in Figures 7-12. Since Ted is processing many types of sensory input successfully, this can be seen as a strength to support other areas of need. (Levels one, two and three on the intervention planning guide, see Figure 7-2).

Target Objective 1

Ted will interact with toys and people in an appropriate manner.

Intervention Approach

Provide age appropriate tasks with necessary adaptations to enable Ted access to the activities; provide high intensity feedback for all attempts to interact with toys and people, to establish patterns of interaction.

Intervention Procedures

Whether Ted is held or positioned in a bean bag or with pillows, the semisupine posture will maximize Ted's functional ability to interact with objects or people. Visually interesting toys suspended or stabilized within Ted's easy reach,

FUNCTIONAL SKILLS ASSESSMENT GRID
for Occupational and Physical Therapy Services

PROGRAM OUTCOME	PERFORMANCE COMPONENTS	NA	0	1	2	3	COMMENTS
Learning	1 Manipulation/hand use				X		
Skill	2 Interpretation of body senses	X					*strength for Ted
Acquisition and	3 Perceptual skills						
academics*	organization of space and time	X					
in regard to	interpretation of visual stimuli	X					*strength for Ted
play, socialization	4 Cognitive skills						
and ADL	problem solving	X					
	generalization of learning	X					
	5 Attending skills	X					
	6 Use of assistive and adaptive devices	X					positioning facilitates
	7 Mgmt of body positions during learning				X		interaction w/persons, obj.
	8 Mgmt body positions during transitions	X					
	9 Mvmt within learning environment				X		
Work*	1 Mgmt of body positions during work						
	2 Mgmt of body positions during transitions						
	3 Mgmt within work environment						
	4 Manipulation/hand use						
	5 Use of assistive and adaptive devices						
Play/Leisure*	1 Mgmt body position during play/leisure				X		
	2 Mgmt body position during transitions	X					positioning used
	3 Mvmt within play/leisure environment				X		
	4 Manipulation/hand use				X		
	5 Use of assistive and adaptive devices	X					positioning helps
Communication*	1 Oral motor movements						
	2 Communication access						
	3 Manipulation/hand use						
	4 Mgmt body pos. during communication						
	5 Mvmt within communication environment						
	6 Attending skills						
	7 Perceptual skills						
	8 Use of assistive and adaptive devices						
Socialization*	1 Self esteem	X					
	2 Recognition and use of nonverbal cues	X					*strength for Ted
	3 Mgmt. body position during socialization				X		family moves to Ted
	4 Mvmt within social environment	X					
	5 Attending skills	X					
	6 Perceptual skills	X					
	7 Cognitive skills	X					
Activities of daily living*	1 Oral motor movements			X			
	2 Mgmt of body position during ADL				X		positioning devices
	3 Mvmt within daily living environment				X		to support Ted
	4 Attending skills	X					
	5 Manipulation/hand use				X		select adaptive devices

(see Chapter 6)   Dunn, W. & Campbell, P. (1988).

*When acquiring new skills, use the learning: skill acquisition section of this grid.

NA—No problems are identified in therapy evaluation.
  0—Although a problem has been identified through evaluation, it is not presently interfering with program outcome(s). Needs may
     be met by self, parents, or professionals in other programs or agencies.
  1—The problem *influences* successful program outcome(s); simple instructional or environmental changes are likely to result in
     functional performance.
  2—The problem *interferes* with specific program outcome(s); specific strategies are necessary to enable functional performance.
  3—The problem *prevents* successful program outcome(s); multifaceted strategies are necessary to reach functional performance.

Figure 7-11. Functional Skills Assessment Grid for Ted.

INTERVENTION PLAN

Child's name: **Ted**   Date: _____

                                                                    Birthdate: _____

Agency name: _____   Chron. Age: _____ yrs. _____ mo.

Outcome Statement: **Ted will eat independently**

Outcome Category: _____ Learning   _____ Work

                           _____ Play/Leisure   _____ Communication

                           _____ Socialization   __X__ ADL

Performance Components:

ENABLING COMPONENTS: CONCERNS:

   tactile processing   **muscle tone**

   gustatory processing   **endurance**

   olfactory processing   **postural control**

   oral motor control   **visual motor integration**

   level of arousal

   social conduct

Service Provision Models:

__X__ Direct*   _____ Monitoring   __X__ Consultation

                          _____ supervise adult   __X__ teach adult

                                                       __X__ adapt posture/mvmt

                                                       __X__ adapt task/matls

                                                       _____ adapt environ

* provided in conjunction with one or more other service models

__X__ **DIRECT**   _____ n.a.

Target Objective: **Ted will eat a meal independently**

_____

Intervention Approach: __X__ remed. __X__ compens. _____ prevent-interv.

   Describe: **Extend use of hands and arms for play into activities related to eating;**
   identify food textures and taste preferences identify adpative devices to support eating

Location of Services: **County 0–3 program**

Intervention Procedures: **position head & trunk to focus effort on arms & hand movement;**
   provide facilitation & physical support for reach, grasp, hand to mouth; design &
   introduce adaptive devices.

Method for Documentation of Performance:

   behavior to be observed: **use of two handed bottle**

   natural environment for observation: **lunch time in 0–3 program**

   measurement/data to be collected: **amount of time Ted holds bottle to mouth with both hands**

   criterion for successful performance: **When positioned properly Ted holds**
   bottle to mouth with both hands for 5 minutes (cumulative) during lunch.

__X__ **CONSULTATION**   _____ n.a.

Area of concern: **ADL: Eating**

Identified by: **Team members**   role: **many**

Statement of Area to be Addressed: **Ted's ability to eat by himself**

_____

Location of Services: **County 0–3 Program**

Strategies: **Teach classroom personnel about effective feeding/eating techniques; create adaptations &**
   instruct classroom staff in proper use; observe their performance to insure accuracy.

Figure 7-12. Occupational Therapy Intervention Plan for Ted.

Proposed Meeting Schedule: _____ weekly   **X** bimonthly _____ monthly

Location of meeting: **Classroom** _____

Method for Documentation of Performance:

behavior to be observed: **Use of two handed bottle** _____

natural environment for observation: **lunch time in 0–3 program** _____

measurement/data to be collected: **Amount of time Ted holds bottle with both hands.**

criterion for successful performance: **When positioned properly Ted holds bottle**

to mouth with both hands for 5 minutes (cumulative) during lunch. _____

Figure 7-12. *Continued.*

such as a mirror or a homemade mobile made out of Ted's favorite toys or objects, can provide ongoing opportunities for him to slap, grasp, bang, or knock the objects.

As Ted is already vocalizing several sounds, imitation of those sounds, as well as modeling lip and tongue sounds, will increase his use and variety of communicative abilities.

Target Objective 2

Ted will interact with the environment in an appropriate manner.

Intervention Approach

Increase active muscle tone to allow balanced movement in all positions (remedial); to facilitate play in more distant space; and to facilitate functional hand use. This approach moves Ted from vestibular-movement to vestibular-gravity and visual on the *Intervention Planning Guide* (Figure 7-13).

Intervention Procedures

Facilitating rolling from stomach to back, and back to stomach, with some stability provided at his hips and shoulders, provides experience in initiating more balanced movement patterns with maintenance of best muscle tone possible. Positioning in semisupine, sidelying, or over a roll placed under the upper trunk, decreases the influence of abnormal muscle tone and allows more functional movement. Supported sitting, circle or taylor sitting, with support on a slightly unstable surface, or movement provided by an adult's hands or lap, can provide experiences in weight shifting from side to side and front to back. Supported rocking on all fours provides the same kind of information. When Ted is helping initiate straight plane movement (side to side or front to back), one might vary the sequence by tilting or moving in a diagonal or partial postural rotation pattern. This allows for more asymmetrical movement patterns and also helps facilitate more normal muscle tone in the trunk and extremities. Bilateral reaching, especially with hands working in the midline, can be facilitated with suspended toys, with positioning in prone over a ball, or prone through a suspended to stationary innertube. Facilitating open hands might be accomplished by using weight shifting activities in a prone on elbows posture, by playing with large smooth surface toys, or by pushing on

a ball or hard surface such as a wall or floor. Once Ted's hands can be actively opened and remain open, grasp and release can be accomplished with smaller toys, water play, or intermittent use of joint traction or compression to the shoulders, elbows, wrists, and fingers.

Target Objective 3

Ted will eat a meal independently.

Intervention Approach

Extend use of hands and arms for play into activities related to eating (remedial); identify food textures and tastes that Ted

INTERVENTION PLANNING GUIDE
Ted

Taste/ Smell	Oral Texture	Tactile	Vestibular Movement	Vestibular Gravity	Visual	Auditory
Sweet/ Vanilla	Suck/ Blow	Joint & muscle activity Cool to neutral warmth	Joint & muscle activity	Vertical	Light/ Dark Color	Vibration
Salt/ Brine	Bite/ Crunch	Deep pressure Moderate temperatures	Oscillation (bouncing)	Horizontal	Form (boundaries)	Rhythm Music Sing-song speech Rhyme
Sour/ Citrus Spice	Chew	Touch pressure Moderate temperatures	Linear movement (swinging)	Out of straight planes (diagonals)	Place (location)	Vocalization/ speech sounds
Bitter/ Smoke	Lick	Light touch (may be unexpected) Extreme temperatures	Rotary movement (spinning or partial rotation)	Upside down/ backwards space	Movement through time and space	Language

RHYTHMIC INPUT OVER TIME - *DECREASES* AROUSAL LEVEL
ARHYTHMIC INPUT OVER TIME - *INCREASES* AROUSAL LEVEL

Rhythm of Input +
Intensity of Input +
Frequency of Input +
Duration of Input =

INTERVENTION

Figure 7-13.   Intervention Planning Guide for Ted.

prefers; and to identify adaptive devices that will support Ted's eating endeavors (compensatory).

Figure 7-12 illustrates sample portions of an intervention plan for Ted in this area.

Intervention Procedures

As Ted is able to move his head to observe his hands, or a toy placed in his midline directly under his head, this posture can be used to facilitate interest and motivation to get things to his mouth. A supported semisupine posture that provides stability to his shoulders will increase the likelihood that Ted will be able to bring his hands to his mouth. Utilization of objects or food items with pleasing textures could be used to spark his interest. Use of a two-handed bottle may provide the shape required for Ted to begin participating in bottle feeding. The semisupine posture with stabilization provided at the shoulders should be provided during this activity, to minimize the amount of effort that Ted must expend to hold his trunk and head in position. This enables him to focus on the reach and grasp pattern to bring the bottle to his mouth and hold it there.

Adaptive equipment options are identified, considering the family's needs and desires. Families want their children to look as much like their peers as possible. While they may be willing to use adaptive equipment in their home, they may be reluctant to use adaptive equipment in a school setting or in the community. Another issue to consider is the cost of the adaptive equipment. Some families prefer not to accept assistance from state or county facilities, even if it means that they will have to wait a longer period of time before they can afford to personally purchase the equipment. This choice should be respected and, if possible, another form of equipment should be devised. In some situations, family members may prefer to design and make their own equipment, and this choice should also be respected. The therapist provides information, diagrams, or other support to assist the family in this regard. Many times family members have extremely good ideas for adapting existing materials, or designing new forms of adaptive equipment, that are more functional for their own particular child than anything available in catalogues. Some insurance policies cover the cost of adaptive equipment; the therapist also provides assistance to obtain funding when this is a possibility.

OUTCOME

Occupational therapy services were provided during each of the in-center programming sessions, and during the weekly home visits. Most of the center-based intervention was implemented in the classroom, which provided an opportunity to model positioning and handing techniques, as well as strategies to present classroom activities and interactions in a way that would facilitate Ted's participation. Consultation was also provided to the classroom staff.

A standard car seat provided Ted with enough support for transport in either a car or a school bus. A Tumble Form feeder seat was provided for eating and playing with toys and family members. At age two and a half Ted was fitted for an electric wheelchair utilizing a joy stick on the left hand side; a carved form foam insert, a neck support, a wedge

seat, and harness straps and two foot rests, with foot straps, were added to support a useful position in the chair.

Respite care options were explored in a cooperative fashion with other families in the local area. Respite care is frequently difficult for families and program personnel to address. As professionals we should be willing to acknowledge, or help families acknowledge, their right to some "time off." In this case, the family's need for respite care was verbalized as one of their main needs. It is the responsibility of the professionals involved to give parents information about formal and informal respite opportunities. In this particular situation, there were other families in the program with the same needs and the family chose to become involved in a cooperative respite arrangement with three other families. This not only provided them with respite care but also increased their support network.

As transition to the public school three- to four-year-old programs approached, public school personnel were able to visit the county program, observe Ted in the classroom setting, and meet with the family and 0–3 program staff to plan future goals and programming strategies. The goals, as Ted enters the 3 and 4-year-old program, include: increasing self care skills, expanding Ted's repoirtoire of manipulation and mobility skills for learning and exploring his environment, and increasing speech and language abilities. The preschool program acknowledged that communication would obviously be an area of strength for Ted in his interactions. They wanted to initiate adaptations immediately to maximize Ted's communication abilities, so they considered preparing Ted for keyboarding and the use of tape recorders as part of the program plan. Adaptations such as these can facilitate Ted's placement in peer integration settings.

CASE #5—JASON

Program Planning for Jason

Discussion and interpretation of responses occurred throughout the assessment. The performance component strengths and concerns identified during Jason's assessment are summarized on Figure 7-14. Intervention techniques were discussed and demonstrated and then tried by both parents and the attending therapist.

The family, the therapists, and the nurse determined five areas to be addressed in the program plan. Since the family was primarily concerned with Jason's irritability, this became the first focus of attention for planning. The parents also expressed their concern about Jason's eating habits and lack of expected weight gain and growth. Jason's babysitter was primarily concerned with ways to enhance Jason's interaction with people and objects in his environment. The physical therapist was also concerned that the irritability was interfering with her therapeutic attempts at establishing better postural control for Jason. Developing positioning strategies, so that Jason would be able to interact with better quality and endurance with toys, was a concern for everyone.

Target Objective 1

Decrease over-responsivity to sensory input.

FUNCTIONAL SKILLS ASSESSMENT GRID

for Occupational and Physical Therapy Services

PROGRAM OUTCOME	PERFORMANCE COMPONENTS	NA	0	1	2	3	COMMENTS
Learning	1 Manipulation/hand use				X		adapt posture to facilitate
Skill	2 Interpretation of body senses				X		hand use
Acquisition and academics*	3 Perceptual skills						
	organization of space and time	X					
	interpretation of visual stimuli	X					
	4 Cognitive skills						
	problem solving	X					check these as irritability
	generalization of learning	X					decreases
	5 Attending skills				X		related to poor sensory
	6 Use of assistive and adaptive devices	X					
	7 Mgmt of body positions during learning				X		
	8 Mgmt body positions during transitions				X		
	9 Mvmt within learning environment				X		
Work*	1 Mgmt of body positions during work						
	2 Mgmt of body positions during transitions						
	3 Mgmt within work environment						
	4 Manipulation/hand use						
	5 Use of assistive and adaptive devices						
Play/Leisure*	1 Mgmt body position during play/leisure				X		combine remedial and
	2 Mgmt body position during transitions				X		compensatory strategies
	3 Mvmt within play/leisure environment				X		
	4 Manipulation/hand use				X		
	5 Use of assistive and adaptive devices	X					
Communication*	1 Oral motor movements						
	2 Communication access						
	3 Manipulation/hand use						
	4 Mgmt body pos. during communication						
	5 Mvmt within communication environment						
	6 Attending skills						
	7 Perceptual skills						
	8 Use of assistive and adaptive devices						
Socialization*	1 Self esteem	X					
	2 Recognition and use of nonverbal cues	X					check later
	3 Mgmt. body position during socialization				X		
	4 Mvmt within social environment				X		
	5 Attending skills				X		related to poor sensory
	6 Perceptual skills	X					
	7 Cognitive skills	X					
Activities of daily living*	1 Oral motor movements			X			
eating	2 Mgmt of body position during ADL				X		
	3 Mvmt within daily living environment				X		
	4 Attending skills				X		related to poor sensory
	5 Manipulation/hand use				X		related to posture/position

(see Chapter 6)   Dunn, W. & Campbell, P. (1988).

*When acquiring new skills, use the learning: skill acquisition section of this grid.

NA—No problems are identified in therapy evaluation.

  0—Although a problem has been identified through evaluation, it is not presently interfering with program outcome(s). Needs may be met by self, parents, or professionals in other programs or agencies.

  1—The problem *influences* successful program outcome(s); simple instructional or environmental changes are likely to result in functional performance.

  2—The problem *interferes* with specific program outcome(s); specific strategies are necessary to enable functional performance.

  3—The problem *prevents* successful program outcome(s); multifaceted strategies are necessary to reach functional performance.

Figure 7-14. Functional Skills Assessment Grid for Jason.

Intervention Procedures

The sensory sensitivity program designed for David would be appropriate here, but would be adapted for an older child.

Planning an intervention program to decrease sensory sensitivity for Jason became an important tool for all of those dealing with Jason. Between all members present, it was possible to determine those kinds of activities and those sensory components that helped Jason organize and maintain a level of arousal appropriate to a variety of situations. Those that seemed most appropriate initially, were level one and two tactile, level one and two movement and gravity, level one, two, and three visual, and levels one through four in auditory components. (Refer to Figure 7-2.) Feedback from muscle and joint activity contributes to the maintenance of an appropriately aroused state. Jason's motor abilities are very compromised, making it difficult for Jason to provide himself with necessary joint and muscle feedback. It was determined that Jason's use of biting was probably a useful strategy for him, because it provides muscle and joint feedback to the jaw and face. Figure 7-15 summarizes the relationship among the suck/swallow patterns of eating with breathing synchrony and other self regulatory activities. Consequently, a number of chewable foods and toys were recommended for Jason. The team also recommended that caregivers use a small light, a radio, flannel sheets and pillows to surround Jason to increase the length of time Jason would be able to maintain a calmer sleep state in his own bed.

Target Objective 2

Increase positive interaction with toys and people in his environment.

Intervention Procedures (Examples)

a. Utilize toys with level one and two visual components from Figure 7-2 (e.g., natural light shaded area, use of a toy flashlight, use of primary colors), and level 1–4 in auditory components (e.g., variable speed vibrator, music and story tapes).

b. Make sure the mechanics of toys are easy enough for Jason to operate, so that he will frequently be reinforced by the action he produces.

c. Position Jason in semisupine posture in a pillow bean bag, or the adults crossed legs, for prolonged social contact.

d. When language is part of the interaction, use bouncing, the blow toys, and arhythmical firm hand patting on his chest, to increase the breath support for speech and to help him maintain appropriate arousal levels.

Target Objective 3

Increase the variety and amount of foods Jason will eat. Figure 7-16 provides a partial intervention plan for this target objective.

Intervention Procedures (Examples)

a. Utilize the components of suck, bite and crunch when planning snacks or meals.

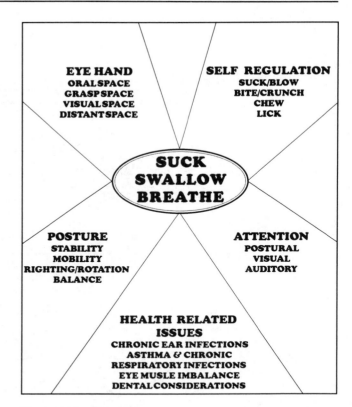

Figure 7-15.   The relationship of the suck/swallow/breathe synchrony to sensorimotor development. *Patti Oetter MA, OTR/L, FAOTA, 1989.*

b. Utilize tastes sweet, sour, citrus and spice, or a combination thereof, when planning meals and snacks.

c. Utilize straw in bottle during each meal and snack to maintain oral function and arousal state.

d. Utilize finger foods as often as possible to increase the tactile interaction with foods in order to support oral motor function.

Target Objective 4

Improve postural control.

Intervention Procedures (Examples)

a. Frequent light to moderate joint traction and compression through the jaw, neck, shoulders and hips will maintain Jason's awareness of body position and state of trunk musculature.

b. Provide firm patting and stability through the chest and abdominals to help maintain balanced cocontraction of trunk flexion and extension.

c. Frequent use of blow toys during therapy will help maintain trunk function; Jason will be motivated to continue the activity as well.

d. Utilize snacks and bottle with straw frequently during handling techniques to maintain arousal and support balanced trunk function.

INTERVENTION PLAN

Child's name: **Jason**   Date: _____

                                                                                   Birthdate: _____

Agency name: _____   Chron. Age: _____ yrs. _____ mo.

Outcome Statement: **Jason will eat a variety of foods independently** _____

Outcome Category: _____ Learning   _____ Work

                                      _____ Play/Leisure   _____ Communication

                                      _____ Socialization   **X** ADL

Performance Components:

 ENABLING COMPONENTS: CONCERNS:

  sensory awareness _____   **tactile processing** _____

  fine motor coordination _____   **olfactory processing** _____

  position in space _____   **postural control** _____

  form constancy _____   **bilateral integration** _____

                                                    arousal _____

Service Provision Models:

 X Direct*   **X** Monitoring   _____ Consultation

                          X supervise adult   _____ teach adult

                                                          _____ adapt posture/mvmt

                                                          _____ adapt task/matls

                                                          _____ adapt environ

* provided in conjunction with one or more other service models

Target Objective: **Jason will eat a variety of foods.** _____

_____

Intervention Approach: **X** remed. _____ compens. _____ prevent-interv.

 Describe: **Provide multisensory experiences in food options; incorporate organizing**

   input/feedback into activities. _____

Location of Services: **therapy room** _____

Intervention Procedures: **choose suck, bite, crunch foods; choose sweet, sour flavors; introduce straw**

   for input and feedback while sucking; provide finger foods to increase tactile input to hands.

Method for Documentation of Performance:

  behavior to be observed: **food choices Jason makes** _____

  natural environment for observation: **snack time at home** _____

  measurement/data to be collected: **number of food types eaten in a week.** _____

  criterion for successful performance: **at least five different food types per day for a week**

   (See intervention plan guide for categories). _____

 X MONITORING   _____ n.a.

Target Objective: **Jason will eat a variety of foods.** _____

_____

Intervention Approach: **X** remed. _____ compens. _____ prevent-interv.

Describe: **begin with two options and build to greater number; explain the categories**

   and their importance to parents. _____

Location of Services: **therapy room** _____

Intervention Procedures: **have parents describe characteristics of foods used in therapy;**

   describe why, review past week's history _____

Implementor: _____ teacher **X** family _____ aide _____ other: _____

Figure 7-16. Occupational Therapy Intervention Plan for Jason.

Training and Verification Strategies: **family observes therapist; family keeps log of home activity and foods eaten**

Proposed Meeting Schedule: __**X**__ weekly _____ bimonthly _____ monthly

Location of meeting: **therapy room**

Method for Documentation of Performance:
    behavior to be observed: **food choices Jason makes**
    natural environment for observation: **snack time at home**
    measurement/data to be collected: **number of food types eaten in week.**
    criterion for successful performance: **at least five different food types per day for a week**
       (See intervention plan guide for categories.)

Figure 7-16. *Continued.*

e. Utilize NDT strategies for weight shift at shoulders, head and neck, upper and lower trunk rotation and righting responses.

Therapeutic Objective 5

Utilize a variety of positions for Jason during fine motor tasks.

Intervention Procedures (Examples)

a. Facing forward between an adult's crossed legs provides support of Jason's low back, and intermittent stability for his hands or elbows to maintain a sitting posture.
b. Use a corner chair to provide lateral and rear support during sitting activities. This diminishes the effort required to control posture, so that energy can be focused on hand use.
c. Place Jason in sidelying position with head and shoulder support, when he must interact with very small objects, to decrease the demand to hold head and upper trunk in a vertical position.
d. Use a partially filled water pillow in his small rocking chair when fine motor demands are not too stressful for him. This will provide constant feedback through his lower trunk, and help maintain upper trunk and head posture for freer use of arms and hands.

OUTCOME

Since Jason was already being seen three times a week by the physical therapist, a discussion ensued about whether or not occupational therapy should be just prior to the physical therapy sessions, or whether they should be on separate occasions. Because the physical therapist was primarily concerned about Jason's irritability during handling procedures, it was decided that they would see Jason simultaneously for a few weeks and then on separate days. The family was concerned about Jason's endurance with one therapy session following the other. The joint sessions were primarily utilized to help the physical therapist find strategies that would help maintain an arousal level, within which Jason could comfortably participate with the handling strategies. This lasted approximately three weeks. The occupational therapy sessions were then conducted twice weekly for hourly sessions, on the days he was not receiving PT. Because both parents worked, it was decided to begin a notebook where information could be exchanged between the parents and the therapists. Once a month appointments were made late in the afternoon, so that the parents could be involved during the therapy session. At the same time, any questions that had arisen could be discussed.

The program and the changes in his sleep environment improved Jason's sleeping patterns markedly. Within a few weeks Jason only required personal attention once during the night, and then only two or three times per week.

With the dietary instructions from the nurse, and the attendance to both taste and texture of foods offered, Jason began expanding the repertoire of foods he would eat. Resulting weight gain and growth has been slow but steady.

The physical therapist began utilizing bouncing, chest patting, a straw in a bottle, and snacks during her treatment sessions; and felt that these additions enabled her to make adequate progress with her NDT techniques.

The family acquired a variety of blow toys and positioning options for Jason. They have also acquired a tape recorder, children's musical tapes, and children's story tapes. According to the parents and the babysitter, Jason was able to entertain himself, or interact with another person for much longer periods of time. Within three months, the initial concerns about eating and irritability had diminished to the point where the routine was well enough established that no further intervention in those areas was required. The emphasis then focused on development of endurance for sitting, fine motor and visual motor skills, and expressive language.

About a year later, Jason was enrolled in a public school preschool program for children with special needs, and began receiving occupational and physical therapy through the schools. The treating occupational therapist at the time helped the family make the transition by attending the team meeting at the school and helping develop the IEP.

CASE #6—RICHARD

Program Planning for Richard

Because of the wide variety of opinions presented by the family members during the program planning process, extra care needed to be taken in arriving at goals that each family member could support. The benefits of utilizing a speech pathologist and an occupational therapist in the same intervention session were discussed. Therapists needed to maintain Richard's arousal level, and work with him in a place which would be comfortable and motivating, so that he would use language to interact with his environment. Because Richard was in attendance at this meeting, it was possible to demonstrate a few strategies that facilitated Richard's intermittent interaction with the therapist and the family members.

A combination of occupational therapy with speech/language therapy was recommended twice weekly. The occupational therapist and speech/language pathologist collaborated when writing their goals. The occupational therapist contributed expertise about arousal, sensory processing, and neuromuscular control to support interaction and motor planning skills to the process. Figure 7-17 indicates the strengths and concerns in relation to the outcomes of socialization, functional communication and play. A partial intervention plan, using the third and fourth Intervention Approaches, is provided in Figure 7-18.

Outcome Statement

Richard will interact with people and objects in his immediate environment.

Intervention Approach

Maintain appropriate arousal for improved exploration and interaction with the environment.

Intervention Procedures (Discussion of examples)

In this situation, it is important to choose activities that incorporate graded intensity using input which is organizing to Richard. It is important to combine sensory components with activities, to prevent over arousal and enable Richard to respond with adaptive behavior patterns. For example, in order to utilize sweet and sour tastes (levels one and three in the taste column of the intervention planning guide), the therapist could place cranapple or cranraspberry juice in a plastic bottle with a straw; sucking the juice facilitates both motor and sensory components which enable Richard to establish and maintain his state of arousal while engaging in the activity. Blow toys might then be introduced as a motivating environmental task which Richard can pursue.

Intervention Approach

Improve ability to process combined forms of sensory input for more age appropriate interaction skills.

Intervention Procedures (Discussion of examples)

Keeping the strategies for managing state in mind, the therapist designs more complex sensory motor combinations incorporating multiple sensory channels. For example, the therapist might tap the auditory and vestibular components by playing a familiar and pleasing record or tape while swinging; the therapist might then stop for a moment to incorporate a speech and language task into this activity, to help Richard produce his best performance. The therapist might also assist Richard in a sequence such as popping off an air mattress onto the mat, rolling over, completing one speech and language task, and then returning to the mattress. In a third example, the therapist would assist Richard in climbing a rope ladder to the very top to get a puzzle piece for the speech and language activity, bringing it down to the speech/language pathologist, making the appropriate vocalization and then returning to the climbing activity.

Intervention Approach

Improve functional postural mechanisms which support quality interaction with toys and people.

Intervention Procedures (Discussion of examples)

Functional postural control can be stimulated through activities carried out on unstable surfaces. Suspended equipment, large pillows, or a waterbed that is partially filled with air or water, provide constantly changing stimuli that both motivate and challenge the child. Unstable surfaces also inhibit the tendency to fix proximal joints, which is often seen in children like Richard.

Intervention Approach

Increase recognition and use of facial expressions, body language and gestures.

Intervention Procedures (Discussion of examples)

When adults exaggerate and hold a variety of facial expressions, body language cues, and gestures, the child has enough time to notice, and then begin reading them and using them himself.

Intervention Approach

Improve suck/swallow/breathe synchrony and strength to support both speech production and self regulatory strategies.

Intervention Procedures (Discussion of examples)

The therapist can introduce a variety of blow toys and a straw in a plastic bottle to encourage sucking, blowing, and rhythmic breathing. Food or toys with various textures and motor requirements facilitate the use of an appropriate suck/swallow/breathe pattern. As children such as Richard develop more oral motor synchrony, speech production will also be easier. Richard can also regulate his own level of arousal through normalized breathing patterns.

FUNCTIONAL SKILLS ASSESSMENT GRID
for Occupational and Physical Therapy Services

PROGRAM OUTCOME	PERFORMANCE COMPONENTS	NA	0	1	2	3	COMMENTS
Learning Skill Acquisition and academics*	1 Manipulation/hand use	X					
	2 Interpretation of body senses				X		
	3 Perceptual skills organization of space and time				X		
	interpretation of visual stimuli	X					a strength
	4 Cognitive skills problem solving			X			may be related to dyspraxia
	generalization of learning			X			
	5 Attending skills				X		underarousel
	6 Use of assistive and adaptive devices	X					
	7 Mgmt of body positions during learning				X		
	8 Mgmt body positions during transitions				X		
	9 Mvmt within learning environment				X		dyspraxia
Work*	1 Mgmt of body positions during work						
	2 Mgmt of body positions during transitions						
	3 Mgmt within work environment						
	4 Manipulation/hand use						
	5 Use of assistive and adaptive devices						
Play/Leisure*	1 Mgmt body position during play/leisure				X		
	2 Mgmt body position during transitions				X		
	3 Mvmt within play/leisure environment				X		
	4 Manipulation/hand use	X					
	5 Use of assistive and adaptive devices	X					
Communication*	1 Oral motor movements				X		
	2 Communication access	X					
	3 Manipulation/hand use	X					
	4 Mgmt body pos. during communication			X			
	5 Mvmt within communication environment	X					
	6 Attending skills				X		
	7 Perceptual skills	X					
	8 Use of assistive and adaptive devices	X					
Socialization*	1 Self esteem				X		
	2 Recognition and use of nonverbal cues				X		miscues may be due to
	3 Mgmt. body position during socialization				X		sensorimotor difficulties
	4 Mvmt within social environment				X		
	5 Attending skills				X		
	6 Perceptual skills	X					
	7 Cognitive skills				X		
Activities of daily living*	1 Oral motor movements						
	2 Mgmt of body position during ADL						
	3 Mvmt within daily living environment						
	4 Attending skills						
	5 Manipulation/hand use						

(see Chapter 6)   Dunn, W. & Campbell, P. (1988).

*When acquiring new skills, use the learning: skill acquisition section of this grid.

NA—No problems are identified in therapy evaluation.
0—Although a problem has been identified through evaluation, it is not presently interfering with program outcome(s). Needs may be met by self, parents, or professionals in other programs or agencies.
1—The problem *influences* successful program outcome(s); simple instructional or environmental changes are likely to result in functional performance.
2—The problem *interferes* with specific program outcome(s); specific strategies are necessary to enable functional performance.
3—The problem *prevents* successful program outcome(s); multifaceted strategies are necessary to reach functional performance.

Figure 7-17. Functional Skills Assessment Grid for Richard.

Intervention Approach

Improve motor planning (praxis) in both body and oral motor regions, in order to improve problem solving skills, speech intelligibility, and organization of language production.

Intervention Procedures (Discussion of examples)

Simple two to three step activities, emphasizing internal or expressive language incorporating "wh" questions, will en-

INTERVENTION PLAN

Child's name: **Richard** _____   Date: _____
                                                             Birthdate: _____

Agency name: _____   Chron. Age: _____ yrs. _____ mo.

Outcome Statement: **Richard will interact appropriately with persons and objects** _____

Outcome Category: _____ Learning   _____ Work
                             X Play/Leisure   _____ Communication
                             X Socialization   _____ ADL

Performance Components:
  ENABLING COMPONENTS: CONCERNS:
  visual processing _____   **muscle tone** _____
  range of motion _____   **endurance** _____
  strength _____   **postural control** _____
  recognition _____   **activity tolerance** _____

Service Provision Models:
  X Direct*   _____ Monitoring   **X** Consultation
                                  _____ supervise adult   **X** teach adult
                                                          _____ adapt posture/mvmt
                                                          _____ adapt task/matls
                                                          _____ adapt environ

* provided in conjunction with one or more other service models
  X **DIRECT**   _____ n.a.

Target Objective: **Richard will spontaneously shift position during interactive play activities.** _____

Intervention Approach: **X** remed. _____ compens. _____ prevent-interv.
   Describe: **improve functional postural mechanisms which support quality interactions**
   with toys and people. _____

Location of Services: **therapy clinic** _____

Intervention Procedures: **use unstable surfaces for play and interactions; move**
   location of stimuli during play and interaction. _____

Method for Documentation of Performance:
   behavior to be observed: **postural shifts during interactions with family** _____
   natural environment for observation: **play room next to clinic** _____
   measurement/data to be collected: **number of upper trunk shifts during play activity** _____
   criterion for successful performance: **at least 10 shifts in a five minute play period.** _____

  X **CONSULTATION**   _____ n.a.

Area of concern: **Communication** _____

Identified by: **family, speech pathologist** _____   role: _____

Statement of Area to be Addressed: **Richard's ability to recognize and use body language for communication.** _____

Location of Services: **therapy clinic** _____

Strategies: **teach family how to exaggerate expressions and movements during commucation;**
   teach family how to reinforce approximations of body language in Richard. _____

Proposed Meeting Schedule: **X** weekly   _____ bimonthly   _____ monthly

Location of meeting: **therapy clinic/play room** _____

Method for Documentation of Performance:
   behavior to be observed: **eye contact and smiling during play with family member** _____
   natural environment for observation: **play room** _____
   measurement/data to be collected: **number of smiles, amount of eye contact** _____
   criterion for successful performance: **at least 4 smiles in 2 min.; at least 45 seconds of**
      eye contact in 2 minutes. _____

Figure 7-18. Occupational Therapy Intervention Plan for Richard.

hance the organizing, planning, and executing of a variety of thinking and motor performances. For example, one might ask, "How high should we hang the inner tube?," "Which foot might you want to put in first?," "How many hops on the hoppity-hop will it take us to get to the door?," or "What else would you do with this?" Once the therapist begins initiating these kinds to questions, one usually finds the child responding; perhaps with another question or an answer. The answer does not have to be verbal. It may facilitate reprogramming the motor act itself. Once the motor act is organized and predictable, the child can reliably attach language to the experience.

OUTCOME

During the program planning process, it was decided that Richard would receive combined speech/language and occupational therapy intervention twice weekly at a private practice clinic. The private practice clinic offers sliding scale fees, which enable Richard's family to have a small payment schedule, since their insurance coverage was minimal.

The implementation of strategies to increase and maintain Richard's arousal level resulted in immediate increased interaction and use of expressive language. Richard's mother accompanied him to therapy, and replicated activities and approaches to interaction at home. Rapid progress was noted for the first six months of intervention, and then it leveled off, but continued in a steady upward direction. When Richard turned three, a referral was made to the public school preschool program to see if he would qualify for their program. This referral was made in order to provide services within a more appropriate life environment (with age peers), and because they would be less costly to the family. The results of the public school assessment revealed that Richard would not qualify for the program. The therapists and family determined that a short break (three to four months) in intervention was appropriate; since the mother had been carrying through with activities at home, support for Richard's continued growth was still provided. At the end of the three months, the family reported that while Richard had maintained his skills, he had not gained at the rate that they had observed when he was receiving intervention. The therapists reinitiated intervention, but placed Richard in a group with another child to increase age appropriate socialization, and to decrease cost to family. This strategy proved successful, and provided a smooth transitional service into the public school programs the next year.

CASE #7—JAMES

Program Planning for James

The targetted program goals and the integrity of performance components are summarized on Figure 7-19 on the Functional Skills Assessment Grid.

Following the assessment, the team met with the family to discuss findings and establish a program plan. This was the parents' first experience with a service agency; concerns were addressed in relation to their referral questions. Team members discussed their findings by describing the quality of James's performance in all areas, since the quality of his performance was the cornerstone of the parents' concerns and the need for intervention. Diagnostic

labels were discussed in relation to service accessibility within the community.

James's formal diagnosis would qualify or reject him from particular community services. The team felt that James's performance warranted a label of either mild cerebral palsy or developmental dyspraxia. The diagnosis of cerebral palsy is a medical diagnosis, and is more familiar to both third party insurance companies and public school programs. Developmental dyspraxia is less familiar to payors, and therefore requires more justification to be deemed eligible for funding. The family wanted to know everything they could about James's condition, and so the decision was made to pursue the possibility of a diagnosis of mild cerebral palsy through the services of a pediatric neurologist. This referral would provide the parents with an additional source of information. In this case, James's family have insurance options available to them; he will also be entering public school in a few years, which will open up a new set of services for him. Various federally supported programs have different eligibility criteria than do local programs or public school programs. Knowledge of eligibility criteria is essential for appropriate and adequate intervention planning.

The occupational therapist would play a key role in James's service provision process. Primary areas targeted for occupational therapy include:

1. Increase the use of more mature postural control mechanisms and gross motor planning skills for effective movement within the environment;
2. Improve oral motor skills for eating and talking; and
3. Improve eye-hand coordination and manual dexterity for learning, self care and play.

Figure 7-20 presents a flow chart which shows the relationships among task demands and performance. Based on an Intervention Planning Guide in Figure 7-21, a partial Intervention Plan is provided in Figure 7-22.

Target Objective 1

James will move around efficiently in the classroom.

Intervention Approach

Provide strong proprioceptive input during activities; incorporate vestibular input into exploratory behaviors to increase adaptive input.

Intervention Procedures

James preferred running, climbing, and jumping for the sheer fun of the experience, rather than working on postural or gross motor skill. Utilizing short duration, but intense heavy work (an effective proprioceptive input), during the activities requiring skill at or just beyond James's level, will help him organize, plan, and execute gross motor activities with more quality and skill. Since James also seeks and enjoys intense movement experiences, utilizing movement with heavy work in activities that require planning a sequence of steps, will promote better performance and more interest and motivation for the activity.

FUNCTIONAL SKILLS ASSESSMENT GRID

for Occupational and Physical Therapy Services

PROGRAM OUTCOME	PERFORMANCE COMPONENTS	NA	0	1	2	3	COMMENTS
Learning	1 Manipulation/hand use				X		
Skill	2 Interpretation of body senses			X			
Acquisition and academics*	3 Perceptual skills						
	organization of space and time			X			related to motor planning
	interpretation of visual stimuli	X					
	4 Cognitive skills						
	problem solving	X					
	generalization of learning			X			? related to motor planning
	5 Attending skills	X					parents report task
	6 Use of assistive and adaptive devices	X					persistence
	7 Mgmt of body positions during learning			X			
	8 Mgmt body positions during transitions			X			
	9 Mvmt within learning environment					X	
Work*	1 Mgmt of body positions during work						
	2 Mgmt of body positions during transitions						
	3 Mgmt within work environment						
	4 Manipulation/hand use						
	5 Use of assistive and adaptive devices						
Play/Leisure*	1 Mgmt body position during play/leisure			X			
	2 Mgmt body position during transitions			X			
	3 Mvmt within play/leisure environment				X		
	4 Manipulation/hand use				X		
	5 Use of assistive and adaptive devices	X					
Communication*	1 Oral motor movements				X		suck/swallow/breathe
	2 Communication access	X					
	3 Manipulation/hand use				X		
	4 Mgmt body pos. during communication			X			
	5 Mvmt within communication environment			X			
	6 Attending skills	X					
	7 Perceptual skills			X			
	8 Use of assistive and adaptive devices	X					
Socialization*	1 Self esteem						
	2 Recognition and use of nonverbal cues						
	3 Mgmt. body position during socialization						
	4 Mvmt within social environment						
	5 Attending skills						
	6 Perceptual skills						
	7 Cognitive skills						
Activities of daily living*	1 Oral motor movements			X			suck/swallow/breathe
	2 Mgmt of body position during ADL				X		
	3 Mvmt within daily living environment				X		
	4 Attending skills	X					
	5 Manipulation/hand use				X		

(see Chapter 6)   Dunn, W. & Campbell, P. (1988).

*When acquiring new skills, use the learning: skill acquisition section of this grid.

NA—No problems are identified in therapy evaluation.
  0—Although a problem has been identified through evaluation, it is not presently interfering with program outcome(s). Needs may be met by self, parents, or professionals in other programs or agencies.
  1—The problem *influences* successful program outcome(s); simple instructional or environmental changes are likely to result in functional performance.
  2—The problem *interferes* with specific program outcome(s); specific strategies are necessary to enable functional performance.
  3—The problem *prevents* successful program outcome(s); multifaceted strategies are necessary to reach functional performance.

Figure 7-19. Functional Skills Assessment Grid for James.

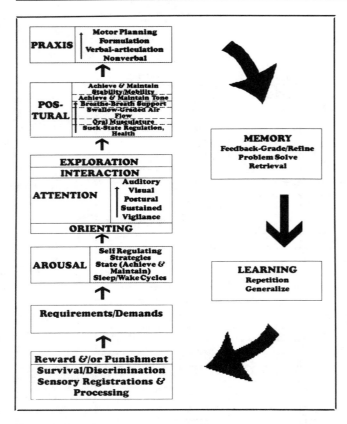

Figure 7-20.   Flow chart depicting the relationships among task demands and performance. *Patti Oetter MA, OTR/L, FAOTA, 1989.*

The use of unstable surfaces or alternate postures during visual motor and fine motor activity often promotes skill and endurance in those tasks. Options include: prone over pillows; prone through a stationary or suspended innertube; sitting or straddling a suspended or stationary innertube; sitting or sidelying on a large pillow; sitting on a therapy ball or hoppity hop; and sitting on a T-stool or a small flotation device partially filled with air or water. Each of these positions allows increased feedback from small postural movements, while the child is engaging in another activity. For postural control to be effective, it must be delegated to unconscious, automatic monitoring during other tasks. When the child must concentrate on posture, efforts toward the perceptual, cognitive, or motor tasks are diminished. These strategies often promote skill, endurance, as well as time on task.

The use of suck and/or blow activities (discussed below) within antigravity extension provides additional sensory input; the intensity of this input facilitates development of body scheme which supports the child's perception of his own movement through space.

Target Objective 2

James will interact with peers intelligibly.

Intervention Approach

Focus on suck and breathe patterns as indicators of the organization of the oral motor structure; incorporate oral mo-

tor tasks into other activities to increase synchrony of movements across systems; provide intense oral motor activities to increase sensory input and feedback to this area, and to increase endurance in the sensorimotor process. (See Figure 7-21.)

Intervention Procedures

Increasing strength and endurance of suck and blow for use in eating as well as producing speech sounds, can be accomplished with frequent use of straws, a pacifier, thumb, or nipple on a bottle if applicable, and blow toys or instruments. Children find these instruments extremely appealing; the blow toys are interesting and provide an opportunity for therapeutic free play. In this case James used his pacifier frequently, especially during fine motor tasks, liked to blow bubbles with a straw or tube in the tub, a small container of water, or his cup, and quickly became quite attached to the harmonica. This particular family had no objection to James using a pacifier. Some families have strong feelings about the use of a pacifier or thumb-sucking; if the parents are uncomfortable utilizing these strategies, the therapist designs an alternative to these therapeutic forms of input. For example, the child can be introduced to the straw, rubber tubing, toys and other instruments that provide similar input. Most children independently discard the pacifier, quit using their thumb, or the bottle, as soon as they have developed strategies that are as useful for them. The therapist must also consider the child's age, selecting activities that would be considered appropriate for that age child. It is not helpful to

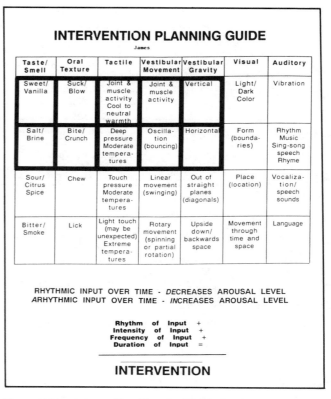

Figure 7-21.   Intervention Planning Guide for James.

INTERVENTION PLAN

Child's name: __James__   Date: _____

                                                                       Birthdate: _____

Agency name: _____   Chron. Age: _____ yrs._____ mo.

Outcome Statement: __James will write his name_____

Outcome Category: __x__ Learning   _____ Work
                            _____ Play/Leisure   _____ Communication
                            _____ Socialization   _____ ADL

Performance Components:
  ENABLING COMPONENTS: CONCERNS:
   __recognition_____   __sensory processing_____
   __attention span_____   __perceptual skills_____
   __social conduct_____   __strength & endurance_____
   _____   __postural control_____
                                                 __praxis_____
                                                 __visual motor integration_____

Service Provision Models:
  __x__ Direct*   _____ Monitoring   __x__ Consultation
                             _____ supervise adult   __x__ teach adult
                                                             _____ adapt posture/mvmt
                                                             _____ adapt task/matls
                                                             _____ adapt environ

* provided in conjunction with one or more other service models
  __x__ DIRECT   _____ n.a.

Target Objective: __James will use a writing utensil in an age appropriate manner_____

Intervention Approach: __x__ remed. _____ compens. _____ prevent-interv.
  Describe: __Provide facilitation to support increased endurance & coordination in visual__
     __motor tasks; pair visual motor activities with oral motor and postural control__
     __demands to assist in coordination of entire body during purposeful activity.__

Location of Services: __Preschool classroom_____

Intervention Procedures: __Use high intensity sensory experiences; incorporate oral motor__
     __& postural control requirements; imbed sensory intensity into visual motor tasks.__

Method for Documentation of Performance:
  behavior to be observed: __Writing his name_____
  natural environment for observation: __classroom_____
  measurement/data to be collected: __accuracy of letter formation_____
  criterion for successful performance: __all letters are correctly oriented within 40°, are identifiable to a person__
     __who has not seen James' writing, and are in correct sequence__

  __x__ CONSULTATION   _____ n.a.

Area of Concern: __Learning_____

Identified by: __parents & diagnostic team_____ role: _____

Statement of Area to be Addressed: __James' ability to use a writing utensil and other tools__

Location of Services: __classroom_____

Strategies: __teach teacher and aide how to prepare James for visual motor tasks;__
     __instruct in task analysis for activity selection__

Proposed Meeting Schedule: __x__ weekly   _____ bimonthly   _____ monthly

Location of meeting: __teacher's lounge_____

Method for Documentation of Performance:
  behavior to be observed: __writing his name_____
  natural environment for observation: __classroom_____
  measurement/data to be collected: __accuracy of letter formation_____
  criterion for successful performance: __all letters are correctly oriented within 40°, are identifiable to a__
     __person who has not seen James' writing, and are in correct sequence__

Figure 7-22. Occupational Therapy Intervention Plan for James.

give children and families activities that make the child look more different or out of place in relation to their peers.

The use of interesting and variable textures and tastes during snacks and meals, will often immediately improve both oral motor skill and endurance. James preferred crangrape juice and snacks that had the textures for crunch and bite; these items also supported oral motor performance.

As James began socializing with his peers, it became increasingly apparent that intelligibility issues were compromising his efforts to communicate with his peers. There were two other children in the classroom utilizing sign language; James became interested in this method of communicating, and began imitating signs he found useful in interaction with other classmates. As a result, a total communication program was explained to James's family; they agreed to follow up with the same communication at home. Simple signs were used, since James also had trouble using his hands for effective movements. The words were always paired with the signs used, to give James the opportunity to imitate the sounds as he could. As James became more comfortable in his ability to communicate with others, and his breathing patterns became strong enough to support fluent speech, James discontinued using signs independently and increased his use of age appropriate gestures. This strategy can be extremely helpful in a variety of cases where facial or verbal communication skills are compromised.

Target Objective 3

James will use a writing utensil in an age appropriate manner.

Intervention Approach

Provide facilitation to support increased endurance and coordination in visual motor tasks; pair visual motor activities with oral motor and postural control demands to assist in coordination of entire body during purposeful activity.

Intervention Procedures

Incorporating a variety of textures and weights (i.e., water or bean play) in actual objects or toys that James and his friends are playing with, provides intense sensory input for development of an accurate body scheme, promotes skill acquisition, and generates endurance in both fine motor and visual motor areas. Heavy to light joint traction and compression from shoulders through fingers during activity will also promote skill and endurance in fine motor and visual motor performance. This includes tasks such as stretching arms over the head, pushing down on a chair or into a table, interlocking fingers, stretching arms over head so fingers are in full to hyperextension, and pushing hands together in front of the body. Observing typical peers provides the therapist a variety of ideas of activities that can be utilized or modified for use with a child such as James.

Oral motor activities, as discussed above, can also be used to support the development of visual motor integration. The therapist can incorporate sucking, blowing, and biting into postural and visual motor activities to increase the sensory input during the task and facilitate endurance and strength throughout the system. Oral support can be used both before and during visual motor tasks. Children often seek oral input to organize visual motor tasks, and while care should be taken to observe and be prepared for choking or gagging on an item, it is unlikely that either will occur if the child chooses the kind of oral support he needs for the activity presented. Adults frequently and incorrectly assume that a child cannot move with something in his mouth without choking or gagging, because they choke or gag at rest. It is often the combination of sensory input from the oral motor task and the postural or visual motor task simultaneously, that provides adequate sensorimotor intensity to carry out the activity. Even as adults we use several oral strategies (paper clips, pen tops, erasers, gum, candy, chips, etc.) to support both endurance and performance in visual motor activity. The less mature or disordered nervous system oftentimes requires more intense, or more frequent oral support to achieve visual motor skills.

OUTCOME

James qualified for a half day, four-day-a-week center-based program. The program included early intervention programming, lunch, and occupational and speech/language therapy. Most of the time, the occupational therapist provided intervention within the classroom routine. Occasionally, she would serve James in a private room; this occurred when James was learning a new strategy which required a high level of concentration, or would cause an extreme amount of disruption to the ongoing classroom activities. Consultation was also provided to the classroom staff, and home visits were made once a month. The therapist paid special attention to include activities, media, and sensory experiences within the classroom curriculum that would enhance James's ability to increase the quality of his performance. The speech/language pathologist and occupational therapist collaborated to design an effective oral motor program, and to incorporate a total communication approach to enhance James's nonverbal communication skills.

James received direct service and consultative occupational therapy in the early childhood program until he entered kindergarten. During his kindergarten year, direct service was provided, and the therapist designed a monitoring program with the classroom teacher.

As James entered the regular classroom situation, intervention priorities focused more strongly on the components of performance related to learning. The therapist and teacher addressed improving tool use, especially writing utensils and scissors, with emphasis on visual direction of tools. They also created plans to help James improve his organizational skills for classroom work and materials. The therapist and physical education teacher focused on improving stability and organization of movement for gross, fine, and visual motor activity, and improving visual monitoring of movement through space. The occupational therapist met with the parents on a quarterly basis to assist them in organizing the home environment and planning play activities for James.

CASE #8—RANDY

Program Planning for Randy

Following the assessment, the child study group met with Randy's parents to discuss the findings and develop a plan to meet Randy's needs. The parents expressed continued concern regarding Randy's ability to interact in environments outside of his home. They were particularly concerned about his entrance into kindergarten in the fall. Team members shared testing results which indicated that Randy was developmentally behind his peers in the areas of sensorimotor development, language development, social/emotional development and possibly cognitive development. Everyone agreed that a preschool special education program would be beneficial for Randy, both in relation to learning and socialization needs. Figure 7-23 summarizes Randy's performance in relation to learning and socialization on the Functional Skills Assessment Grid.

During the meeting with the family it was apparent that the family's major concerns surrounded his fearfulness in new or unfamiliar situations. Whenever a family is introduced to the concept of sending their three or four-year-old child off to school, it is necessary to both acknowledge and respect their apprehension; frequently, families perceive that they might be losing some of their control over the child's life when school begins. Very often in our attempts to "sell" our expertise and ability to help a child, we often put the parents in a situation where they may begin feeling either inadequate or incompetent. It is important to present the professional role as consultants to the family in the process of the child's development. Of ultimate importance is the process of planning a program to meet the family's needs in regard to their goals and expectations for the child.

In this case, the family demonstrated concern about Randy's ability to be comfortable outside the home and without one of his parents. All families want their children to be comfortable and happy, and are usually unwilling to place their children in a situation where they may be unsuccessful. Team members were able to negotiate a plan that allowed one or both parents to participate in helping Randy make the transition to school. Once these issues were addressed, and the family was able to feel they were still an integral part of the program planning process, it was easier to establish the rest of the program plan. Three primary areas were targetted as special contributions to be made by the occupational therapist in the preschool program:

1. Decrease sensory sensitivity so that Randy has a better ability to interact within the environment appropriately.
2. Improve postural control in order to increase endurance and quality of gross motor, fine motor, and visual motor performance which are required for many preschool tasks.
3. Increase the repertoire of coping strategies in order to achieve and maintain appropriate behavior.

A small portion of Randy's intervention plan is provided in Figure 7-24.

Intervention Approach 1

Decrease sensory sensitivity so that Randy has a better ability to interact within the environment appropriately.

Intervention Strategies

Many of the activities described in other cases to decrease sensory sensitivity can be adapted for older children like Randy.

Other strategies to decrease sensory sensitivity include providing heavy work activities throughout his daily routine; these can be incorporated into routine family activities. Randy's father had a workshop in the basement; Randy frequently enjoyed time with his father using the tools. This was encouraged, and Randy's father was able to come up with a number of projects they could work on together. Randy also enjoyed digging in the yard and playing with the garden hose. Since his mother enjoyed working outdoors, she was able to come up with a list of activities they could do outside, regardless of the weather. The parents purchased a number of garden tools and a small plastic wheel barrel for Randy to use outside. They also purchased a chin-up bar to fit in their doorway at home, so that Randy would have the opportunity to hang and swing from it, rather than from the breakfast bar or door knobs. Randy also liked jumping on his bed, or off the furniture. The family was able to gather some old pillows and cushions and a mini-trampoline. They set these items up in their family room, and put extra pillows in Randy's room, so that he could use them when necessary. Randy also liked pushing the vacuum cleaner, and his mother suggested that she could give him the job of vacuuming the hallway and the larger portions of the rugs in their home.

What is interesting to note here, is that once the family felt themselves to be an integral part of Randy's intervention plan, and understood what Randy needed, they were able to come up with a wide variety of appropriate strategies. The professionals were empowering the family to act in Randy's best interests within their daily life routine.

Intervention Approach 2

Improve postural control in order to increase endurance and quality of gross motor, fine motor, and visual motor performance, which are required for many preschool tasks.

Intervention Procedures

Strategies that include unstable surfaces, such as a large air mattress, a water bed, large pillows, and suspended equipment, will both develop and challenge development of postural control. The use of extra pillows and mats, and suspension of equipment close to the ground allows Randy to feel more safe. When children such as Randy feel safe enough to take risks, they also receive opportunities to enjoy the challenges of gravity and movement. Fine motor and visual motor activities can be incorporated into the situations as well.

Intervention Approach 3

Increase repertoire of coping strategies in order to achieve and maintain appropriate behavior.

Intervention Procedures

The team decided that a number of strategies could be initiated at preschool to help Randy learn how to negotiate activities with his peers. They paired Randy with one other child, and they took turns pulling or pushing each other in a wagon, whenever the class was making a transition between activities, going down the hall to the bathroom, or outside to

FUNCTIONAL SKILLS ASSESSMENT GRID

for Occupational and Physical Therapy Services

PROGRAM OUTCOME	PERFORMANCE COMPONENTS	NA	0	1	2	3	COMMENTS
Learning Skill Acquisition and academics*	1 Manipulation/hand use				X		
	2 Interpretation of body senses					X	
	3 Perceptual skills						
	organization of space and time			X			
	interpretation of visual stimuli			X			
	4 Cognitive skills						
	problem solving			X			
	generalization of learning			X			
	5 Attending skills				X		
	6 Use of assistive and adaptive devices	X					
	7 Mgmt of body positions during learning				X		
	8 Mgmt body positions during transitions				X		
	9 Mvmt within learning environment					X	related to fears
Work*	1 Mgmt of body positions during work						
	2 Mgmt of body positions during transitions						
	3 Mgmt within work environment						
	4 Manipulation/hand use						
	5 Use of assistive and adaptive devices						
Play/Leisure*	1 Mgmt body position during play/leisure						
	2 Mgmt body position during transitions						
	3 Mvmt within play/leisure environment						
	4 Manipulation/hand use						
	5 Use of assistive and adaptive devices						
Communication*	1 Oral motor movements						
	2 Communication access						
	3 Manipulation/hand use						
	4 Mgmt body pos. during communication						
	5 Mvmt within communication environment						
	6 Attending skills						
	7 Perceptual skills						
	8 Use of assistive and adaptive devices						
Socialization*	1 Self esteem				X		
	2 Recognition and use of nonverbal cues					X	
	3 Mgmt. body position during socialization				X		
	4 Mvmt within social environment					X	related to fears
	5 Attending skills				X		
	6 Perceptual skills			X			
	7 Cognitive skills			X			
Activities of daily living*	1 Oral motor movements						
	2 Mgmt of body position during ADL						
	3 Mvmt within daily living environment						
	4 Attending skills						
	5 Manipulation/hand use						

(see Chapter 6)

Dunn, W. & Campbell, P. (1988).

*When acquiring new skills, use the learning: skill acquisition section of this grid.

NA—No problems are identified in therapy evaluation.

0—Although a problem has been identified through evaluation, it is not presently interfering with program outcome(s). Needs may be met by self, parents, or professionals in other programs or agencies.

1—The problem *influences* successful program outcome(s); simple instructional or environmental changes are likely to result in functional performance.

2—The problem *interferes* with specific program outcome(s); specific strategies are necessary to enable functional performance.

3—The problem *prevents* successful program outcome(s); multifaceted strategies are necessary to reach functional performance.

Figure 7-23.   Functional Skills Assessment Grid for Randy.

INTERVENTION PLAN

Child's name: **Randy** _____   Date: _____

   Birthdate: _____

Agency name: _____   Chron. Age: _____ yrs. _____ mo.

Outcome Statement: _____

Outcome Category: __x__ Learning   _____ Work

                     _____ Play/Leisure   _____ Communication

                     _____ Socialization _____ ADL

Performance Components:

   ENABLING COMPONENTS: CONCERNS:

   visual processing _____   **other sensory processing** _____

   form constancy _____   **postural control** _____

   strength _____   **bilateral integration** _____

   short term memory _____   **praxis** _____

   categorization _____   **generalization of learning** _____

Service Provision Models:

_____ Direct*   _____ Monitoring   __x__ Consultation

                        _____ supervise adult   __x__ teach adult

                                                     _____ adapt posture/mvmt

                                                      __x__ adapt task/matls

                                                     _____ adapt environ

* provided in conjunction with one or more other service models

__x__ CONSULTATION   _____ n.a.

Area of Concern: **Learning** _____

Identified by: _____   role: **family, eval. staff** _____

Statement of Area to be Addressed: **Randy's ability to respond appropriately to**

   environmental stimuli _____

Location of Services: **home, preschool** _____

Strategies: **discuss home routines with family; review school routines with team,**

   discuss Randy's special needs with family, and other team members, identify

   adaptations which are in Randy's best interest _____

Proposed Meeting Schedule: _____ weekly   _____ bimonthly   __x__ monthly

Location of meeting: **child study group conference room** _____

Method for Documentation of Performance:

   behavior to be observed: **digging in the garden** _____

   natural environment for observation: **home/yard** _____

   measurement/data to be collected: **length of time Randy continues the garden task** _____

   criterion for successful performance: **10 minutes of continuous participation in**

   garden task; (e.g., planting seeds, flowers). _____

Figure 7-24.   Occupational Therapy Intervention Plan for Randy.

the playground. Teachers gave Randy the option of sitting in someone's lap during small or large groups, gave him frequent bear hugs or asked him for hugs during the day, which incorporated touch-pressure input into activities. The occupational therapist participated in the classroom to help establish these routines.

Team members also discussed their need to respect Randy's apprehension about new environments or unfamiliar tasks. They acknowledged that there may be times Randy would need two to three more minutes than the other children to prepare for changes. They also discussed the importance of

letting Randy know what is expected of him in each task; when Randy is more familiar with routines, he can describe what he is going to do next.

OUTCOME

Because of Randy's difficulty with emotional self regulation and extreme hypersensitivity to environmental stimuli, it was decided that he be introduced to the school setting in a carefully graded manner. One of his parents brought him to the school to receive occupational therapy on an individual basis two to three times per week, at no additional cost to the family. Parental presence would gradually be reduced, and exposure to other areas of the school and to peers were gradually introduced as Randy tolerated these changes. This continued until half day programming in the classroom was occurring with the support of occupational therapy, speech therapy, and psychology.

Randy was accompanied to school initially by his father, with whom he has a warm and trusting relationship. He exhibited anxiety but did not lose emotional control. His intervention program began with a routine progression, playing with a familiar toy each session, moving to a familiar puzzle, to a non-familiar puzzle, to some sensory activities, and movement with heavy resistance in guided space exploration and interaction. Randy was insecure in space and tolerated proprioceptive activities better than vestibular-based activities. He was very dependent upon the routine, so within a routine he began to tolerate new activities as the intervention sessions progressed.

Intervention began in an isolated therapy room, moving after several sessions to the hallway outside the room, and to other school hallways. The speech therapist began attending intervention sessions, after a few sessions to avoid dependence on one adult. After several sessions, a different child was incorporated into the intervention activities and eventually both children were served together. At this time, Randy was able to visit the classroom to see his friends from therapy. After approximately six weeks, Randy joined the classroom for five half-days a week.

Randy continued to progress over the summer. Psychological testing at the end of the year placed him in the mildly mentally handicapped range. His behavioral improvement was so dramatic that the school planned for a regular kindergarten placement.

CASE #9—PETER

Program Planning for Peter

The interpretation meeting included the parents, all members of the evaluation team, and the kindergarten teacher. Performance area strength was noted in overall cognitive ability and language. Performance area concerns were noted in the social domain and learning. Figure 7-25 summarizes the component strengths and concerns related to learning and socialization. After all areas of strength and concern were fully discussed, the team went on to discuss possible placements for Peter in school the next year. Placement in a self contained learning disabilities classroom was discussed, but the family and team members agreed that the first choice would be a less restricted environment. The team members felt that a fall placement in a transitional first grade classroom, with support from the occupational therapist, the speech/language pathologist, and the learning disabilities teacher would be optimum for Peter. The occupational therapist would provide direct service within the classroom, monitoring with the physical education teacher, and consultation with the classroom teacher and parents.

The occupational therapist would provide expertise to:

1. Increase tolerance and use of sensory input (especially touch and movement) to increase attention to learning, socialization, and play tasks.

2. Increase postural control so that Peter can manage his body within the classroom environment.
3. Improve gross and fine motor planning for learning and cognitive performance.

Based on an Intervention Planning Guide in Figure 7-26, a partial intervention plan is provided in Figure 7-27.

Target Objective

Peter will attend to classroom tasks within the learning environment an appropriate length of time.

Intervention Approach

Provide environmental adaptations to accommodate problem areas during stressful activities; to provide a graded sensory program to increase Peter's ability to process input; and to provide parents and teachers with management and remedial strategies.

Intervention Procedures

The transitional first grade teacher implemented many of the strategies used by the kindergarten teacher to minimize Peter's hyperexcitability. Because the bus ride and the lunch room were two of the most difficult environments for Peter, the teacher and occupational therapist collaborated to identify some successful strategies for these particular situations. They approached the bus driver about assigning a front seat for Peter, to minimize the amount of space he would have to negotiate getting to his seat, and to decrease the amount of inadvertent bumping and shoving that he would have to cope with during the trip. The bus driver agreed that this would be a manageable plan. They decided to introduce Peter to the lunchroom in a graded manner. Initially, Peter would be allowed to eat his lunch with one or two of his classmates in the hall right outside the lunch room. Sometime during the fall, Peter and his selected friends would eat at a separate table in the corner of the lunchroom. As he tolerated it, they would add children to the able, and then begin moving the table closer to the others, until he would be fully integrated.

The family requested more information on strategies they could employ at home. The occupational therapist described Peter's needs in relation to activities that occur within the home. Bathtime was always a challenge, so they discussed why this activity was difficult for Peter, and created strategies for managing this time. For example, rubbing Peter lightly with a towel would upset him, due to his sensitivity for light touch. A better strategy would be to press the towel firmly into his skin to dry him after his bath. Other strategies were developed as the parents identified problem situations.

The occupational therapist also designed a direct service intervention program to increase Peter's tolerance for sensory input. She planned many experiences which would allow Peter to explore the nature of his own sensory input, and create adaptive responses to these stimuli. She also emphasized increasing the range and complexity of stimuli that Peter could manage, since natural life environments provide unpredictable amounts and types of stimuli. The occupational therapist joined the class during a body awareness period once a week to provide intervention, since Peter was in a

FUNCTIONAL SKILLS ASSESSMENT GRID
for Occupational and Physical Therapy Services

PROGRAM OUTCOME	PERFORMANCE COMPONENTS	NA	0	1	2	3	COMMENTS
Learning	1 Manipulation/hand use				X		
Skill	2 Interpretation of body senses					X	
Acquisition and academics*	3 Perceptual skills organization of space and time	X					
	interpretation of visual stimuli	X					
	4 Cognitive skills problem solving	X					strength
	generalization of learning	X					
	5 Attending skills			X			
	6 Use of assistive and adaptive devices	X					
	7 Mgmt of body positions during learning				X		
	8 Mgmt body positions during transitions			X			
	9 Mvmt within learning environment					X	
Work*	1 Mgmt of body positions during work						
	2 Mgmt of body positions during transitions						
	3 Mgmt within work environment						
	4 Manipulation/hand use						
	5 Use of assistive and adaptive devices						
Play/Leisure*	1 Mgmt body position during play/leisure				X		
	2 Mgmt body position during transitions			X			
	3 Mvmt within play/leisure environment				X		
	4 Manipulation/hand use				X		
	5 Use of assistive and adaptive devices	X					
Communication*	1 Oral motor movements						
	2 Communication access						
	3 Manipulation/hand use						
	4 Mgmt body pos. during communication						
	5 Mvmt within communication environment						
	6 Attending skills						
	7 Perceptual skills						
	8 Use of assistive and adaptive devices						
Socialization*	1 Self esteem				X		when he can control
	2 Recognition and use of nonverbal cues			X			situations with language,
	3 Mgmt. body position during socialization				X		does better
	4 Mvmt within social environment			X			
	5 Attending skills			X			
	6 Perceptual skills	X					
	7 Cognitive skills	X					
Activities of daily living*	1 Oral motor movements						
	2 Mgmt of body position during ADL						
	3 Mvmt within daily living environment						
	4 Attending skills						
	5 Manipulation/hand use						

(see Chapter 6)   Dunn, W. & Campbell, P. (1988).

*When acquiring new skills, use the learning: skill acquisition section of this grid.

NA—No problems are identified in therapy evaluation.
0—Although a problem has been identified through evaluation, it is not presently interfering with program outcome(s). Needs may be met by self, parents, or professionals in other programs or agencies.
1—The problem *influences* successful program outcome(s); simple instructional or environmental changes are likely to result in functional performance.
2—The problem *interferes* with specific program outcome(s); specific strategies are necessary to enable functional performance.
3—The problem *prevents* successful program outcome(s); multifaceted strategies are necessary to reach functional performance.

Figure 7-25. Functional Skills Assessment Grid for Peter.

INTERVENTION PLANNING GUIDE
Peter

Taste/ Smell	Oral Texture	Tactile	Vestibular Movement	Vestibular Gravity	Visual	Auditory
Sweet/ Vanilla	Suck/ Blow	Joint & muscle activity Cool to neutral warmth	Joint & muscle activity	Vertical	Light/ Dark Color	Vibration
Salt/ Brine	Bite/ Crunch	Deep pressure Moderate temperatures	Oscillation (bouncing)	Horizontal	Form (boundaries)	Rhythm Music Sing-song speech Rhyme
Sour/ Citrus Spice	Chew	Touch pressure Moderate temperatures	Linear movement (swinging)	Out of straight planes (diagonals)	Place (location)	Vocalization/ speech sounds
Bitter/ Smoke	Lick	Light touch (may be unexpected) Extreme temperatures	Rotary movement (spinning or partial rotation)	Upside down/ backwards space	Movement through time and space	Language

RHYTHMIC INPUT OVER TIME - *DECREASES* AROUSAL LEVEL
ARHYTHMIC INPUT OVER TIME - *INCREASES* AROUSAL LEVEL

Rhythm of Input +
Intensity of Input +
Frequency of Input +
Duration of Input =

INTERVENTION

Figure 7-26. Intervention Planning Guide for Peter.

transitional first grade which emphasized exploratory and developmental aspects of learning. Many of the strategies the therapist used were slowly incorporated into Peter's classroom day, as the teacher began to understand what Peter needed; having the therapist in the classroom providing intervention was very helpful in this process. The occupational therapist also designed a monitored program with the physical education teacher to increase Peter's tolerance for movement.

Target Objective

Peter will remain in his seat throughout a work period in the classroom.

Intervention Approach

Provide touch pressure and proprioception as a base for activity; provide alternative seating options; introduce a wide variety of activities in which Peter must challenge gravity and his postural control mechanisms in an exploratory environment.

Intervention Procedures

Many of the strategies used to address postural control also contain a very strong sensory component, (primarily touch pressure and proprioception), which is very organizing and provides input to develop an accurate and reliable body scheme. The therapist designed activities to promote strength and endurance in postural flexion and rotation, and incor-

porated heavy work patterns (proprioception), and deep pressure (touch pressure input). For example, the teacher employed bear hugs, deep back rubs, and compression to shoulders and/or hips frequently during the classroom day. Peter was also given chores in the classroom which required heavy work and postural adjustments such as moving tables, desks, or chairs, collecting or distributing books, and washing the blackboard. He was also given several seating options for completing classroom assignments. He preferred sitting on a hoppity hop at his desk or sitting in a curled position inside a stack of two innertubes, or inside of a carpeted barrel.

In the gymnasium, Peter preferred hanging by his hands and/or knees, swinging, dropping from a trapeze, playing on top of the air mattress, and constructing obstacle courses that included crawling under pillows, climbing, swinging, or jumping.

Target Objective

Peter will move about in the classroom without disrupting ongoing activities; Peter will write a legible sentence.

Intervention Approach

Provide a wide range of opportunities for Peter to plan motor acts; provide controlled opportunities at first to minimize incorrect performance or failure; enrich activities with organizing sensory input.

Intervention Procedures

Organizing and planning gross motor and fine motor acts was extremely difficult for Peter. This is due to his poor sensory processing, which provides a paucity of information from which Peter can build useful motor responses. When a child's body maps are inaccurate or unreliable, it is difficult for the child to plan well orchestrated movements. All of the activities described in the areas above will also contribute to better motor planning, because they provide Peter with dependable sensory information about his body which he can then use to plan a response. Additional strategies are added to the sequence to ensure that Peter is also having to solve problems with the information he has obtained.

Because language was a strength for Peter, utilization of "WH" questions ("Who", "What", "Why", "Where", "When", and "How"), were incorporated throughout activities to allow him to build problem solving of motor acts upon his language strength. Questions such as "How low should we hang this?," "What do we need to put around it to make it safe?," "How high are you going to climb?," "What comes next?," "Will that work?," "How can we get this done?," continually reinforce that the language-based problem solving skills can be used to direct and describe the motor acts, which helps organize Peter's overall behavior. Since Peter had developed a pattern of controlling situations with language to avoid performing acts himself, this strategy helps to make those two areas integrated rather than separated. Peter needs to sense his own physical competency and understand that he can be in control of his own behavior. This does not mean that Peter can do whatever he pleases; the adult who provides intervention must understand that controlling situations has been his coping strategy. It is helpful with children such as Peter

INTERVENTION PLAN

Child's name: **Peter**   Date: _____

Birthdate: _____

Agency name: _____   Chron. Age: _____ yrs. _____ mo.

Outcome Statement: **Peter will work successfully within a regular classroom.**

Outcome Category: __x__ Learning   _____ Work
                        _____ Play/Leisure   _____ Communication
                        _____ Socialization   _____ ADL

Performance Components:
  ENABLING COMPONENTS: CONCERNS:
   visual perception   **tactile processing**
   recognition   **vestibular processing**
   short term memory   **praxis**
   conversation   **postural control**

Service Provision Models:
  _____ Direct*   __x__ Monitoring   _____ Consultation
                                __x__ supervise adult   _____ teach adult
                                                           _____ adapt posture/mvmt
                                                           _____ adapt task/matls
                                                           _____ adapt environ

* provided in conjunction with one or more other service models
  __x__ MONITORING   _____ n.a.

Target Objective: **Peter will remain in his seat throughout the work period.**

Intervention Approach: __x__ remed. _____ compens. _____ prevent-interv.

  Describe: **Provide activities which have a strong touch pressure and/or**
        proprioception component

Location of Services: **gym**

Intervention Procedures: **use suspended equipment, air mattress, climbing equipment;**
        create obstacle courses with tough-pressure, proprioception components and
        postural shifts required.

Implementor: __x__ teacher _____ family _____ aide _____ other: _____

Training and Verification Strategies: **therapist demonstrates, then observes PE teacher;**
        PE teacher must list precautions and goals for activities verbally without cues.

Proposed Meeting Schedule: _____ weekly __x__ bimonthly _____ monthly

Location of meeting: **PE teacher's office next to gym**

Method for Documentation of Performance:
  behavior to be observed: **seated in chosen seating option**
  natural environment for observation: **classroom**
  measurement/data to be collected: **length of time Peter stays in his seat.**
  criterion for successful performance: **15 minutes in seat and one page of**
        work completed.

Figure 7-27.   Occupational Therapy Intervention Plan for Peter.

to give activity choices (in which both choices are therapeutic for him), and to design ways to complete activities that ensure successful task completion.

OUTCOME

  While Peter's behavior and attention improved during his first grade year, he continued to have difficulty with fine motor planning, and with carrying out oral directions, both of which compromised his learning. Therefore, the learning disabilities specialist became more involved so that Peter would not lose academic ground while working on other areas of need. The occupational therapist remained involved with Peter in a similar manner as in the first grade program.

  By the end of second grade, it was felt that Peter would be able to manage a regular third grade classroom with occupational therapy assistance. Occupational therapy was provided through a monitoring and consultation program in collaboration with the classroom teacher.

During his third grade year, Peter was designated as a helper in one of the special education classrooms, where he was able to participate in play sessions. These sessions served to help improve Peter's self esteem and solidify his feelings of competency in free play situations.

CASE #10—JOEL

Program Planning for Joel

Following each of the assessment sessions, some time was taken to review any issues that had come up during that session. Occupational therapy strengths and concerns are summarized in Figure 7-28. Both parents were involved during each of the assessment periods and some conversation had occurred throughout. When all of the assessment was completed and reviewed by the therapist, another meeting was scheduled with the parents. Joel was cared for by another person so that the parents could concentrate on developing a program plan for him.

The family's circumstances allowed them to consider staying in this country for a year so that initial intervention activities could begin. The family was concerned about activities of daily living and skills for learning and development. The objectives were to:

1. Facilitate body awareness.
2. Facilitate gross motor skills.
3. Facilitate fine motor skills.
4. Facilitate greater independence and skill in relevant activities of daily living.

A partial intervention plan is included in Figure 7-29.

Target Objective

Joel will care for personal needs independently.

Intervention Approach

Facilitate sensory processing and body awareness.

Intervention Procedures (Discussion)

Because of Joel's frequent variability of state, it will be necessary to design sensory input that will not only help Joel manage his state, but also provide him comfortable and pleasant input in relation to his body. The parents provided extensive information about types of input that Joel seeks at home. These strategies were employed in designing home and therapy environments. They included: frequent sucking and biting on objects and preferences for smooth or crunchy textures in foods; frequent bear hugs and short periods of playful wrestling with his parents; bouncing on the edge of his bed, a chair, or the sofa; preferences for direct sunlight in gross motor activities and shade or low lighting during visual motor activities; putting his face or hands on any vibrating object (e.g., vacuum cleaner, washing machine or dryer, the refrigerator); and seeking music from the radio or record player (Joel's preference was for light rock music). The parents also noted that Joel always seems most organized during bathing and swimming.

When considering the combination of Joel's preferences for sensory input, and the quality of his motor performance under these conditions, it became apparent that Joel understood a lot about the requirements of his own nervous system. Joel's preferences were for rhythmic, intense and frequent (although short) periods of sensory input. With this knowledge, the therapist hypothesized that decreasing the intensity of input may enable Joel to increase the duration of his exploratory behaviors, which might also lead to more opportunities for adaptive responses. Additionally, the environmental cues that the parents described would provide another way to both control Joel's situation, and cue him about the requirements of the task.

For example, the utilization of low lighting and small spaces was useful for visual motor, dressing, and social interactions, because Joel was able to focus on the details of these tasks without additional distractions. The utilization of direct daylight and a larger room with several mats, pillows, and air mattresses, and only one or two pieces of equipment, facilitated gross motor activity. The family brought some tapes of Joel's favorite music, and this enabled Joel to stay engaged in gross motor tasks a longer period of time.

Intervention Approach

Facilitate gross motor skills for life tasks.

Intervention Procedures

Once the sensory environment was established to generate longer periods of interest and interaction, activities were designed to incorporate development of skill in those experiences. He enjoyed crawling over and between the heavy pillows, jumping into the pillows and bouncing around the room on a hoppity hop, or bouncing in rhythm to the music, straddling or prone through a suspended innertube. All of these activities increased the symmetry between body sides (right, left and top, bottom), and Joel independently began creating games and sequences of motor acts with these activities. He also began to direct the therapist nonverbally to move equipment in order to accomplish his plans. Because of the nature of the equipment already discussed, Joel began taking risks and incorporating linear and rotary movement experiences, as well as three dimensional postural responses very quickly. Once a child feels safe and physically confident in his environment, he is both comfortable and motivated to begin taking risks to develop and challenge new motor skills.

Intervention Approach

Facilitate oral motor and fine motor skills for school work and activities of daily living.

Intervention Procedures

Small spaces were created with mats, foam pieces, and eventually a suspended parachute, which formed a tent for fine motor and dressing activities. Snacks of crackers, pret-

FUNCTIONAL SKILLS ASSESSMENT GRID

for Occupational and Physical Therapy Services

PROGRAM OUTCOME	PERFORMANCE COMPONENTS	NA	0	1	2	3	COMMENTS
Learning Skill Acquisition and academics*	1 Manipulation/hand use				X		
	2 Interpretation of body senses					X	
	3 Perceptual skills						
	organization of space and time			X			
	interpretation of visual stimuli	X					
	4 Cognitive skills						
	problem solving			X			
	generalization of learning			X			
	5 Attending skills				X		
	6 Use of assistive and adaptive devices	X					
	7 Mgmt of body positions during learning					X	
	8 Mgmt body positions during transitions				X		
	9 Mvmt within learning environment			X			
Work*	1 Mgmt of body positions during work						
	2 Mgmt of body positions during transitions						
	3 Mgmt within work environment						
	4 Manipulation/hand use						
	5 Use of assistive and adaptive devices						
Play/Leisure*	1 Mgmt body position during play/leisure						
	2 Mgmt body position during transitions						
	3 Mvmt within play/leisure environment						
	4 Manipulation/hand use						
	5 Use of assistive and adaptive devices						
Communication*	1 Oral motor movements						
	2 Communication access						
	3 Manipulation/hand use						
	4 Mgmt body pos. during communication						
	5 Mvmt within communication environment						
	6 Attending skills						
	7 Perceptual skills						
	8 Use of assistive and adaptive devices						
Socialization*	1 Self esteem						
	2 Recognition and use of nonverbal cues						
	3 Mgmt. body position during socialization						
	4 Mvmt within social environment						
	5 Attending skills						
	6 Perceptual skills						
	7 Cognitive skills						
Activities of daily living*	1 Oral motor movements				X		
	2 Mgmt of body position during ADL					X	
	3 Mvmt within daily living environment			X			
	4 Attending skills			X			
	5 Manipulation/hand use				X		

(see Chapter 6)

Dunn, W. & Campbell, P. (1988).

*When acquiring new skills, use the learning: skill acquisition section of this grid.

NA—No problems are identified in therapy evaluation.
  0—Although a problem has been identified through evaluation, it is not presently interfering with program outcome(s). Needs may be met by self, parents, or professionals in other programs or agencies.
  1—The problem *influences* successful program outcome(s); simple instructional or environmental changes are likely to result in functional performance.
  2—The problem *interferes* with specific program outcome(s); specific strategies are necessary to enable functional performance.
  3—The problem *prevents* successful program outcome(s); multifaceted strategies are necessary to reach functional performance.

Figure 7-28. Functional Skills Assessment Grid for Joel.

INTERVENTION PLAN

Child's name: **Joel** _____ Date: _____
Birthdate: _____
Agency name: _____ Chron. Age: __**6**__ yrs. __**7**__ mo.

Outcome Statement: **Joel will care for personal needs independently** _____

Outcome Category: _____ Learning _____ Work
_____ Play/Leisure _____ Communication
_____ Socialization __**x**__ ADL

Performance Components:
ENABLING COMPONENTS: CONCERNS:
  auditory processing **other sensory processing**
  range of motion **body scheme**
  generalization of learning **position in space**
  conversation **figure ground**
_____ **intellectual operations**
in space

Service Provision Models:
__**x**__ Direct* _____ Monitoring __**x**__ Consultation
_____ supervise adult __**x**__ teach adult
_____ adapt posture/mvmt
__**x**__ adapt task/matls
__**x**__ adapt environ

* provided in conjunction with one or more other service models
__**x**__ DIRECT _____ n.a.

Target Objective: **Joel will dress himself independently** _____

Intervention Approach: __**x**__ remed. _____ compens. _____ prevent-interv.
  Describe: **facilitate body awareness; improve gross and fine motor skills** _____

Location of Services: **private school** _____

Intervention Procedures: **provide controlled sensory environment to increase duration of purposeful behavior** _____

Method for Documentation of Performance:
  behavior to be observed: **donning shirt** _____
  natural environment for observation: **school room** _____
  measurement/data to be collected: **completion of task, including fasteners; length of time to complete** _____
  criterion for successful performance: **shirt donned in 3 min.** _____

__**x**__ CONSULTATION _____ n.a.

Area of Concern: **Activities of Daily Living** _____

Identified by: _____ role: **parents** _____

Statement of Area to be Addressed: **Joel's ability to dress himself** _____

Location of Services: **school room; home** _____

Strategies: **teach adults about Joel's sensory and environmental needs so they can** _____
  control external variables; design several small spaces for work in ADL _____

Proposed Meeting Schedule: __**x**__ weekly _____ bimonthly _____ monthly

Location of meeting: **private school** _____

Method for Documentation of Performance:
  behavior to be observed: **donning shirt** _____
  natural environment for observation: **school room** _____
  measurement/data to be collected: **completion of task, including fasteners, amount of time to complete** _____
  criterion for successful performance: **shirt donned in 3 min. or less** _____

Figure 7-29. Occupational Therapy Intervention Plan for Joel.

zels, pudding, apple sauce, and apple juice were utilized in these small spaces to help Joel maintain state while working on eating and hand skills. Whistles and blowing activities provided opportunities to work on trunk and respiratory musculature and provide immediate feedback about the oral motor movements. For example, when Joel blew through an 18″ piece of rubber tubing into a small tub of water with a few drops of dishwashing liquid, he received immediate feedback about his blowing from the bubbles that formed. Joel enjoyed these activities and wanted to take several of the blow toys home with him. The parents responded positively to his interest by purchasing a harmonica for him. This toy selection was insightful because it not only has oral motor benefits with immediate feedback, it also produces music, another preference for Joel. In fact, the parents reported that Joel began entertaining the family with his harmonica and his tapes. Joel increased his vocalizations, nonverbal communication and use of words, both during and following these activities.

Because Joel enjoyed water and blowing bubbles in the small tub of water, the therapist included some visual motor activities in these activities. Waterproof blocks, puzzle pieces, and pegs were placed in the tub, and Joel would dig to find the objects under the bubbles; then he would put the puzzle pieces, block or peg design together, matching colors and sequence, or pattern.

Joel also played with beans, peas, popcorn, and rice, learning how to pour, dump, fill, sort, and make patterns with the seeds. Activities such as these provide a great deal of sensory feedback during the activity, allowing more intense information to be processed and stored for future use.

Intervention Approach

Facilitate greater independence and skill in relevant activities of daily living.

Intervention Procedures

The environments and activities already described provided many opportunities to address ADL skills. They were incorporated as a precursor, or part of the activity, rather than being addressed directly. This allowed Joel to prepare for a new activity and for minor changes in activity, thereby allowing for generalization to broader experiences as he grows.

OUTCOME

Because the family's access to an occupational therapist in their home country and town did not exist, the family made a decision to move to the Midwest for one year to establish an ongoing intervention program that could then be transferred to someone they would hire upon returning to Europe. Fortunately, their financial situation was such that it was possible for them to management this commitment. Joel would be enrolled in a private school for children with special needs, where he could receive speech/language therapy and occupational therapy throughout the week.

When the family made their plans to return to Europe, they asked the occupational therapist to join them in the trip, and help them to locate a suitable person to carry out a home program. A man trained as a gymnastics instructor was hired,

and the occupational therapist spent several weeks intensely training this man in the techniques and observational skills that would be necessary to work effectively with Joel. The therapist must be careful, in situations such as these, that the child's health and safety are protected; it is necessary to teach safe techniques and precautions about what the child's response might be in given activities. Since this therapist had worked with Joel for a long time, she was well prepared to provide detailed information about effective and safe strategies with Joel.

In the subsequent years, the same occupational therapist has returned to Europe to spend several weeks reviewing Joel's progress and reformulating intervention goals and techniques. She has also been able to integrate Joel's needs into his school and play activities in his home environment as he grown older. Adaptations are made depending on the demands of other children who are Joel's chronological age. The latest shift for Joel's program has been to address vocational choices, examining his skills in relation to the options available in his community. The parents are committed to Joel having independent living and competitive work options available and feasible for him when he graduates from high school.

CASE #11—ELLEN

Program Planning for Ellen

The family met with the referring psychologist and the occupational therapist and psychiatrist from the university program to discuss assessment results. Interpretation included a review of the results of previous evaluations, a summary of interventions that have been used with Ellen and a report of current test data. It was important to include pertinent past history because these data were being used to make the conclusions about Ellen's needs. Occupational therapy information was a central focus of this meeting, because this was new information, and the parents were most curious about this. Figure 7-30 summarizes assessment findings.

The family and Ellen felt they would be more comfortable obtaining private therapy for Ellen. They felt that this would have less of an impact on Ellen's peer relationships at school, and would allow more privacy to explore her personal needs, without worrying if other children thought badly of her. Related service support would continue at the school, and the psychologist would continue to see Ellen, working towards a group therapy situation.

The occupational therapist identified several key areas to target during intervention (please refer to Figure 7-31 for a sample portion of her intervention plan). The objectives were to:

1. Decrease sensory sensitivity so that Ellen can interact with her peers without discomfort or fear.
2. Increase postural control mechanisms so that Ellen can stay in her seat to complete assignments at school.
3. Improve sensorimotor patterns that Ellen uses to maintain postural stability and arousal, so that she can attend in school, communicate effectively and can carry out chores and self care at home.
4. Improve Ellen's repertoire of problem solving mechanisms to support organization, planning and initiation of

FUNCTIONAL SKILLS ASSESSMENT GRID

for Occupational and Physical Therapy Services

PROGRAM OUTCOME	PERFORMANCE COMPONENTS	NA	0	1	2	3	COMMENTS
Learning	1 Manipulation/hand use						
Skill	2 Interpretation of body senses					X	
Acquisition and academics*	3 Perceptual skills						
	organization of space and time	X					
	interpretation of visual stimuli	X					
	4 Cognitive skills						
	problem solving	X					
	generalization of learning	X					
	5 Attending skills						
	6 Use of assistive and adaptive devices	X					
	7 Mgmt of body positions during learning		X		X		collaborate with
	8 Mgmt body positions during transitions	X					school therapist
	9 Mvmt within learning environment	X					
Work*	1 Mgmt of body positions during work						
	2 Mgmt of body positions during transitions						
	3 Mgmt within work environment						
	4 Manipulation/hand use						
	5 Use of assistive and adaptive devices						
Play/Leisure*	1 Mgmt body position during play/leisure						
	2 Mgmt body position during transitions						
	3 Mvmt within play/leisure environment						
	4 Manipulation/hand use						
	5 Use of assistive and adaptive devices						
Communication*	1 Oral motor movements						
	2 Communication access						
	3 Manipulation/hand use						
	4 Mgmt body pos. during communication						
	5 Mvmt within communication environment						
	6 Attending skills						
	7 Perceptual skills						
	8 Use of assistive and adaptive devices						
Socialization*	1 Self esteem					X	
	2 Recognition and use of nonverbal cues			X			
	3 Mgmt. body position during socialization				X		
	4 Mvmt within social environment	X					
	5 Attending skills						
	6 Perceptual skills	X					
	7 Cognitive skills	X					
Activities of daily living*	1 Oral motor movements						
	2 Mgmt of body position during ADL						
	3 Mvmt within daily living environment						
	4 Attending skills						
	5 Manipulation/hand use						

(see Chapter 6)   Dunn, W. & Campbell, P. (1988).

*When acquiring new skills, use the learning: skill acquisition section of this grid.

NA—No problems are identified in therapy evaluation.
0—Although a problem has been identified through evaluation, it is not presently interfering with program outcome(s). Needs may be met by self, parents, or professionals in other programs or agencies.
1—The problem *influences* successful program outcome(s); simple instructional or environmental changes are likely to result in functional performance.
2—The problem *interferes* with specific program outcome(s); specific strategies are necessary to enable functional performance.
3—The problem *prevents* successful program outcome(s); multifaceted strategies are necessary to reach functional performance.

Figure 7-30. Functional Skills Assessment Grid for Ellen.

INTERVENTION PLAN

Child's name: __Ellen__   Date: _____
                                                                 Birthdate: _____
Agency name: _____   Chron. Age: _____ yrs. _____ mo.
Outcome Statement: _____
Outcome Category: _____ Learning   _____ Work
                         _____ Play/Leisure   _____ Communication
                         __x__ Socialization   __x__ ADL

Performance Components:
  ENABLING COMPONENTS: CONCERNS:
   __visual perception_____   __tactile processing_____
   __interests_____   __vestibular processing_____
   __concept formation_____   __praxis_____
   __intellectual operations in space____   __activity tolerance_____

Service Provision Models:
  _____ Direct*   _____ Monitoring   __x__ Consultation
                                  _____ supervise adult   __x__ teach adult
                                                              _____ adapt posture/mvmt
                                                              __x__ adapt task/matls
                                                              _____ adapt environ

* provided in conjunction with one or more other service models
   __x__ CONSULTATION   _____ n.a.
Area of Concern: __Socialization_____
Identified by: __parents_____   role: _____
Statement of Area to be Addressed: __Ellen's ability to socialize with peers_____
Location of Services: __home and community_____
Strategies: __identify age appropriate oral motor tasks which provide high intensity activity;__
   __instruct parents in relationship between poor oral motor synchrony and socialization__
Proposed Meeting Schedule: _____ weekly   __x__ bimonthly _____ monthly
Location of meeting: __conference call_____
Method for Documentation of Performance:
   behavior to be observed: __peer interactions with Ellen (eye contact, verbal exchange,__
      __interactive play tasks)_____
   natural environment for observation: __free play at recess_____
   measurement/data to be collected: __length of peer contacts_____
   criterion for successful performance: __at least 10 minutes of peer contact in a fifteen__
      __minute recess__

Figure 7-31. Occupational Therapy Intervention Plan for Ellen.

skilled movement patterns for peer interactions, and getting around in school, and the community.

Target Objective 1

Decrease sensory sensitivity so that Ellen can interact with her peers without discomfort or fear.

Intervention Approach

Provide information so that the family can understand Ellen's difficulties and needs; design adaptations with Ellen's input; and provide graded touch and motion input through exploratory activities.

Intervention Procedures

Sensory defensiveness was explained to the family, and with Ellen's help, Ellen's protective patterns of "flight and fight" were listed. Behaviors include withdrawal, crying, daydreaming, or removing herself physically and/or emotionally from difficult situations, or avoiding any activity or situation she finds threatening. At home she has been known to throw infrequent, although lengthy tantrums.

Because Ellen finds movement, touch, and antigravity experiences so threatening (because she cannot process and utilize the input she does receive), care and respect is taken to identify activities that will be helpful to her. Unstable surfaces and opportunities for free three dimensional movement are the activities of choice. In order for Ellen to be able to tolerate them initially, equipment is hung close to the floor and large pillows or mats are placed under or around them. Incorporating heavy work or proprioception to proximal joints, especially the jaw, hips, and shoulders will enhance her ability to process and use sensory information for more functional postural control. Pushing, pulling, lifting, climbing, carrying, and hanging by her hands may provide the required input she needs to take the risk to try these activities. At the beginning, Ellen may need to place her head, knees, or elbows on the ground in order to feel comfortable ("grounded"). Rolling back and forth over a small therapy ball on her stomach and chest, allowing either her hands or elbows to push, then her knees or feet to push back, without any of them ever leaving the ground may be a way she finds enjoyable to begin experimenting with gravity and movement. Prone or sitting in a suspended innertube where her hands or feet can also touch the floor may be another beginning activity.

Target Objective 2

Increase postural control mechanisms so that Ellen can stay in her seat to complete assignments at school.

Intervention Approach

Utilize repetition strategy, since Ellen has demonstrated its utility for her; connect postural control/adaptive responses to sensory activities; and provide information regarding the relationship to her demand for routines.

Intervention Procedures

Repetition of a movement is a strategy Ellen has used for both learning and improving the quality of her performance. Repetition also seems to help Ellen organize and maintain postural control and comfortable arousal levels. The therapist made plans (in collaboration with the school-based therapist) to instruct the parents and the teacher about postural patterns that would be helpful for Ellen, so they could provide opportunities for repetition of these adaptive movements throughout the days.

Her preference for routine is also related to Ellen's attempts to have repetition in her life; it gives her patterns of actions that she can predict, and therefore use to plan her own responses. Initially, it will be important for both the classroom teacher and the family to prepare Ellen for unexpected changes in routine as well ahead of time as is possible. It may require reminding her of the change several times before it actually occurs, and having her verbalize the change in routine so that she can develop strategies for coping with the coming event. As Ellen develops more adaptive behaviors it will also be important to expect more flexibility from her.

The therapist planned to build on the activities described in the first section to address postural control during individualized intervention. Facilitating antigravity extension and rotation postures, as well as graded respiration, will help Ellen manage and maintain a comfortable level of postural control and overall arousal, which is discussed further below.

Target Objective 3

Improve sensorimotor patterns that Ellen uses to maintain postural stability and arousal, so that she can attend in school, communicate effectively, and carry out chores and self care at home.

Intervention Approach

Provide age appropriate activities which contain high intensity oral sensory input and oral motor control; identify activities within Ellen's natural life environment which require oral motor function to increase endurance and strength; and identify activities which require synchrony between the suck/breathe patterns and body postural control.

Intervention Procedures

Sucking with a straw requires intense oral motor action; Ellen obtained a sports bottle with the inserted straw and used it at home and on trips in the community to provide frequent opportunities for sucking throughout her day. Thicker liquids such as milk shakes or fruit slushes will help build strength and endurance for sucking. Because Ellen is nine years old, the toys and whistles one would use with younger children are inappropriate. However, blow toys that have problem solving and motor planning components are good choices. For example, some blow toys require the user to keep a ball suspended, or a string moving. These activities will also be more interesting for Ellen, and she can share them with her friends.

The team also discussed the possibility of Ellen singing or playing a musical instrument at school. Ellen was interested in both chorus and band and both were available in her school curriculum. She chose the flute, and found practicing and playing her flute an organizing activity. Flute playing encourages strength and endurance, requires graded respiratory control, and is a socially interactive task which provides Ellen with daily contact with peers who have a similar interest. Finding activities like this that are embedded into the child's social and reinforcement structure, is critical to sustaining adaptive changes in the child's life. This will be much more beneficial than oral motor exercises during therapy sessions.

Target Objective 4

Improve Ellen's repertoire of problem solving mechanisms to support organization, planning and initiation of skilled movement patterns for peer interactions, getting around in school, and the community.

Intervention Approach

Provide contextual problem solving tasks; to include other children in tasks to address socialization; and to control for complexity to ensure success.

Intervention Procedures

Because Ellen's strategies for problem solving were compromising her efforts in social, emotional, and language development, strategies were designed to incorporate interaction with a peer, and/or the therapist or parent during therapy. Activities described in the first three goals were consistently used. The therapist provided simple activities that required two or three steps, and helped Ellen plan, organize sequence, and execute the motor patterns required to complete the activities successfully. She was also encouraged to bring a classmate of her choice to therapy sessions at least once a week. In this way they could be encouraged to cooperatively plan and organize activities or games. Because the activities were designed to utilize sensory information that would enhance Ellen's performance, her sense of competency increased to the point that she was able to interact with her peer appropriately. Ellen began to translate many of these strategies to her classroom and playground during free play, and this gave her an opportunity to interact with her classmates in a positive manner. Once the speech/language pathologist began collaborating in therapy sessions, strategies to accomplish this goal included understanding and use of language, to both follow and create directions for and modifications of motor tasks.

OUTCOME

Occupational therapy was provided through the public schools and focused on classroom adaptations and consultation with Ellen's teachers. Private occupational therapy was initiated at the request of the parents, two times a week for 45 min sessions. Bimonthly consultation with the family, psychologist, school therapist, and classroom teacher was arranged in the form of conference telephone calls to provide information that would help Ellen both in the classroom and at home. The family took responsibility for organizing the telephone calls and coordinating schedules.

Ellen was extremely aware of her own sensory sensitivities, as well as her difficulty initiating skilled motor patterns. She began asking questions about how her body worked within the first few intervention sessions. She easily understood the basic principles of sensory integration and was very quickly able to utilize that cognitive information both in the classroom and at home to solve her own problems.

Her peer relationships at school improved markedly, and the psychologist moved her from individual to group play therapy. The psychologist included her in a group of three other children around her age, whom he felt had similar sensory sensitivity issues. She identified those classmates with whom she felt comfortable, and began inviting those children to her home for play and overnight visits. She was discharged within the following year.

Within a few months of the initiation of occupational therapy, Ellen's language difficulties were discussed again with the family, and joint speech/language and occupational therapy sessions were initiated. The individual sessions were discontinued and the joint sessions were scheduled twice weekly for 45 minutes. With Ellen's expanding knowledge of sensorimotor principles, the speech/language pathologist was able to help her begin to pair language and motor skills. Then

then enabled her to use more language to initiate more motor activity. The results became apparent within a few months in both her verbal and written language.

Ellen was discontinued from both speech and language and occupational therapy 17 months later, with the recommendation that she attend a summer camp for children with sensory integrative problems the following summer. This recommendation was made to provide an opportunity for Ellen to reinforce self esteem and self concept. Ellen has been to this camp twice, spending part of her time the second year assisting with younger children. When Ellen entered the 7th grade, she utilized consultative support from the occupational therapist as needed.

Ellen now calls her occupational therapist intermittently to request assistance in problem solving, and ways of managing assignments or organizing materials and schedules. She also gives the therapist tips that she can pass along to other children, so that they too can interact more effectively in their environment. This proactive behavior indicates that Ellen has taken charge of herself, understands the demands she faces, and is taking responsibility for positive outcomes. When we include children in this problem solving process early, they can become advocates for their own needs; this will enable children like Ellen to face any new situation, because they have the internal resources to identify a plan for themselves.

CASE #12—TAMMY

Program Planning for Tammy

The supported employment service team focused primary attention on the performance area of work. Activities of daily living and leisure/recreation received a secondary focus as the team felt that they would impact employment. Figure 7-32 depicts the primary areas of strength and need in relation to the desired outcome of community employment.

Community based programs utilize a team oriented effort to plan programs, and therefore resembles the individual within the environment. The contribution that the occupational therapist makes on the team is unique and vital, but is incorporated into natural life tasks along with the contributions of the other team members. Community-based programs demonstrate this important principle very well, and therefore provide a model for all program planning across the life span. Figure 4-17 illustrates the program planning process for supported employment services. Out of the assessment data, the team identifies a good match between the individual and a community job opportunity.

In Tammy's case, the team had to consider not only a work outcome, but how home life and recreation/leisure activities might impact work. The team members decided upon a five step process that would lead to the development of an appropriate program plan for Tammy. These steps are to:

1. Identify Tammy's individual strengths, interests, and her desired outcome for the service provision process.
2. Identify a Frame of Reference (e.g., a normalization philosophy, a focus on chronologically age appropriate performance vs. developmental milestone acquisition, occupational behavior, learning theory, and psychosocial theory base).

FUNCTIONAL SKILLS ASSESSMENT GRID
for Occupational and Physical Therapy Services

PROGRAM OUTCOME	PERFORMANCE COMPONENTS		NA	0	1	2	3	COMMENTS
Learning	1	Manipulation/hand use	X					
Skill	2	Interpretation of body senses	X					
Acquisition and academics*	3	Perceptual skills						
		organization of space and time			X			
		interpretation of visual stimuli			X			
in relation to work	4	Cognitive skills						
		problem solving				X		
		generalization of learning				X		
	5	Attending skills	X					
	6	Use of assistive and adaptive devices	X					
	7	Mgmt of body positions during learning			X			
	8	Mgmt body positions during transitions			X			
	9	Mvmt within learning environment			X			
Work*	1	Mgmt of body positions during work			X			related to cognitive
	2	Mgmt of body positions during transitions			X			demands of task
	3	Mgmt within work environment			X			
	4	Manipulation/hand use	X					
	5	Use of assistive and adaptive devices	X					
Play/Leisure*	1	Mgmt body position during play/leisure						
	2	Mgmt body position during transitions						
	3	Mvmt within play/leisure environment						
	4	Manipulation/hand use						
	5	Use of assistive and adaptive devices						
Communication*	1	Oral motor movements						
	2	Communication access						
	3	Manipulation/hand use						
	4	Mgmt body pos. during communication						
	5	Mvmt within communication environment						
	6	Attending skills						
	7	Perceptual skills						
	8	Use of assistive and adaptive devices						
Socialization*	1	Self esteem			X			
	2	Recognition and use of nonverbal cues			X			
	3	Mgmt. body position during socialization			X			
	4	Mvmt within social environment	X					
	5	Attending skills	X					
	6	Perceptual skills			X			
	7	Cognitive skills			X			
Activities of daily living*	1	Oral motor movements						
	2	Mgmt of body position during ADL						
	3	Mvmt within daily living environment						
	4	Attending skills						
	5	Manipulation/hand use						

(see Chapter 6)   Dunn, W. & Campbell, P. (1988).

*When acquiring new skills, use the learning: skill acquisition section of this grid.

NA—No problems are identified in therapy evaluation.
0—Although a problem has been identified through evaluation, it is not presently interfering with program outcome(s). Needs may be met by self, parents, or professionals in other programs or agencies.
1—The problem *influences* successful program outcome(s); simple instructional or environmental changes are likely to result in functional performance.
2—The problem *interferes* with specific program outcome(s); specific strategies are necessary to enable functional performance.
3—The problem *prevents* successful program outcome(s); multifaceted strategies are necessary to reach functional performance.

Figure 7-32. Functional Skills Assessment Grid for Tammy.

INTERVENTION PLAN

Child's name: _____**Tammy**_____ Date: _____

Birthdate: _____

Agency name: _____ Chron. Age: **19**___ yrs. **5**_____ mo.

Outcome Statement: **Tammy will obtain and maintain a paid community job**

Outcome Category:
_____Learning   **x**___Work
_____Play/Leisure   _____Communication
_____Socialization   _____ADL

Performance Components:
  ENABLING COMPONENTS: CONCERNS:
  interest and motivation_____   **generalization of learning**_____
  ability to learn_____   **need for help with jobs**_____
  mobility_____   **search**_____
  social skills_____   **need for explicit job training**_____

Service Provision Models:
  __**x**___Direct*   __**x**___Monitoring   _____Consultation
         __**x**_supervise adult   _____teach adult
                                          _____adapt posture/mvmt
                                          _____adapt task/matis
                                          _____adapt environ

*provided in conjunction with one or more other service models

__**x**___**DIRECT** _____n.a.

Target Objective: **Tammy will restock the salad bar at Pizza Hut.**

Intervention Approach: _____ remed. __**x**___ compens. _____ prevent-interv.
  Describe: **Modification of job tasks/environment and cueing systems to enable successful performance**

Location of Services: **Job site**

Intervention Procedures: **Direct job training based on detailed job analysis**

Method for Documentation of Performance:
  behavior to be observed: Independent stocking of salad bar
  natural environment for observation: **Pizza Hut**
  measurement/data to be collected: **Completion of task, time to complete**
  criterion for successful performance: **Refills all containers within five minutes**

__**x**___ **MONITORING** _____ n.a.

Target Objective: **Modification of job tasks/environment; cueing systems to enable successful performance**

Intervention Approach: _____ remed. __**x**___ compens. _____ prevent-interv.
  Describe: **Support provided to employer and co-worker re. type of direction/supervision Tammy needs**

Location of Services: **Job site**

Intervention Procedures: **Observation of co-workers interactions with Tammy, verbal**
  feedback and demonstration

Implementor: _____teacher _____ family _____ aide _____ other: **co-workers**

Training and Verification Strategies: **Modeling for co-workers, feedback**

Proposed Meeting Schedule: __**x**___ weekly _____ bimonthly _____ monthly

Location of meeting: **Job site**

Method for Documentation of Performance:
  behavior to be observed: **Restocking salad bar**
  natural environment for observation: **Job site**
  measurement/data to be collected: **Task completion, time to complete**
  criterion for successful performance: **Refills all containers within five minutes**

Figure 7-33. Occupational Therapy Intervention Plan for Tammy.

3. Clarify community service provision outcomes: paid employment.
4. Develop goals which reflect anticipated outcomes.
5. Develop objectives to achieve goals: **Remember**, all service providers must develop objectives and learning activities that contribute directly to goal achievement. This assures that all team members are pulling in the same direction to address performance needs in relevant environments, and are not focusing on isolated skill development.

Target Objective

Tammy will obtain and maintain a paid community job that matches her abilities and interests.

Intervention Approach

1. Supported employment.
2. On-the-job training and support with needed job modifications or adaptations.

Intervention Procedures (Examples)

Figure 7-33 provides a sample portion of an intervention plan. In order to act on this plan, the following intervention sequence will be implemented:

a. Analyze the work environment and specific job tasks to identify opportunities (e.g., a supportive co-worker, color coding on salad bar ingredients) and barriers (business use of many written notices and written instructions for workers) for Tammy.
b. Observe Tammy doing the work activities; adapt environment or teaching methods to allow Tammy to succeed.
c. Meet with employer and co-workers to discuss job adaptations needed and to provide support and direction regarding interaction with Tammy.

OUTCOME

Tammy receives supported employment services from a University based project titled "Transition to Community Employment." This supported employment project designs and provides individualized community-based services that lead to paid employment.

Occupational therapists are critical members of the team and utilize their skills in functional assessment, environmental and job analysis, and adaptation to maximize opportunities for employment success. Tammy's service environments are the environments she uses on a regular basis and include her home, the city bus system, and her job. Utilization of natural community environments for assessment and training promotes meaningful learning and retention of skills and behaviors. Enabling Tammy to operate in a variety of natural environments (vs. simulated environments) allows the team

to bypass her problems with generalization while greatly increasing the efficiency of her intervention program.

Tammy, with the help of the supported employment service team, obtained a paid job at a local Pizza Hut restaurant. She required extensive on-the-job training by a job coach (supervised by the occupational therapist) for the first few months of employment. Additionally, the job coach provided explicit training in the use of the public transportation system until Tammy was able to demonstrate independent and consistent use. Tammy's parents were very supportive in prompting Tammy to shower regularly and launder her uniform. They also prompted Tammy to get ready each morning and to catch the bus at the appropriate time. After several months of direct support by the OT and the job coach, Tammy demonstrated competence traveling and on the job which necessitated very occasional follow-up by the supported employment team. Her co-workers and employer assumed responsibility for daily support and training and reported tremendous satisfaction with Tammy's performance. The supported employment team gradually became "consultants" to the employer but remained available on an as-needed basis.

EXPAND YOUR NEWLY ACQUIRED KNOWLEDGE

1. Design materials for an effective monitoring program for a child with severe handicaps who requires eating intervention. Include forms which document initial plan, regular contacts, precautions, and adaptations in the plan.
2. Describe three strategies for OT intervention for a 14 year old child for whom socialization is a team priority. Presume that "recognition and use of nonverbal cues," and "attending skills" are the factors that are *interfering* with attainment of socialization outcomes.
3. Consider a six-year-old child with cerebral palsy who has just recently been placed in a regular first grade classroom. Learning is a primary goal for the team. Outline one functional integration and one practice integration strategy you might implement.

References

American Occupational Therapy Association (1989). Uniform Terminology for Occupational Therapy (2nd ed.). American Journal of Occupational Therapy, *43*, 808–815.

Ayres, A. J. (1980). Sensory integrative therapy. *Sensory integration and the child*, (p. 140–141). Los Angeles: Western Psychological Services.

Dunn, W. (1990a). The Sensory Components of Performance. In Christiansen, C. & Baum, C. (eds.) Human Performance Deficits. Thorofare: C. B. Slack, Inc.

Dunn, W. (1990b). Assessing the Sensory Components of Performance. In Christiansen, C. & Baum, C. (eds.) Human Performance Deficits. Thorofare: C. B. Slack, Inc.

Grady, A., Gilfoyle, E., & Moore, J. (1981). Children Adapt. Thorofare: C. B.. Slack, Inc.

Oetter, P. (1988). Intervention PLanning Guide, an unpublished figure.

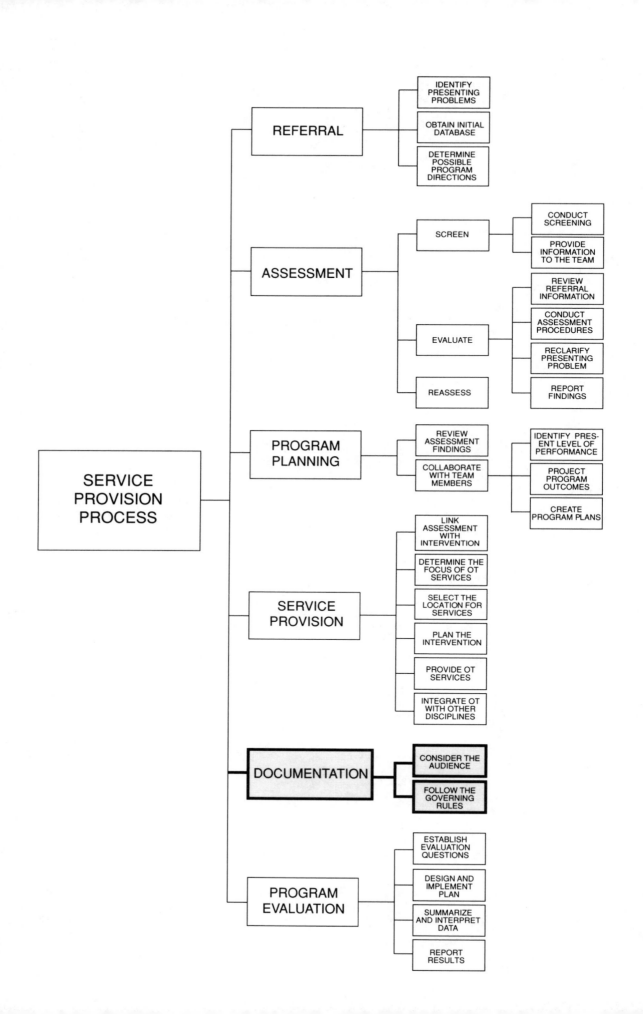

CHAPTER 8

Documentation

Linda Haney McClain, PhD, OTR, FAOTA

"Many practitioners find that in the doing, they are more concerned about the performance than the recording of what it is they do. But verbal recollections do not serve the profession (or the professional) well unless they are recorded. That is a professional's responsibility." Acquaviva & Malone, 1981

Much data crosses the mind and desk of the occupational therapist relative to each child served. Earlier chapters dealt with the key child-centered activities in pediatric settings (developing and receiving referrals, screening and assessing children, planning and implementing intervention, determining the timing for changes in service provision models or discontinuation of service, and conferring with parents and other professionals). How does the therapist manage so much information? Relevant facts must be organized and written down: **Documentation!**

Why document? The influence of occupational therapy intervention impacts the lives of children with handicaps and their families. It is therefore important! And although the occupational therapist sees interactions with the child as paramount, the documentation of facts is the only evidence of professional decision-making.

Four themes recur, when one explores the purposes for documentation. Documentation: 1) facilitates efficacious treatment, 2) provides communication among the team members and family, 3) justifies reimbursement and 4) stands as a legal record (American Occupational Therapy Association, 1986; Baum, 1983; Kuntavanish, 1987; Tiffany, 1983). Therefore, poor documentation can have ethical, financial, and legal consequences. Within this chapter, general and specific information will assist the occupational therapist to critically analyze the content and style of documentation within contemporary service provision models. Learning activities and resources are provided. Furthermore, writers will learn to approach the task of documentation from the outside in, by considering their audiences prior to writing. An appreciation for the requirements of a variety of audiences will be developed.

Occupational therapists who work with infants, toddlers, children, and adolescents serve in a variety of settings. According to data from those who completed the American Occupational Therapy Association (AOTA) 1986 *Member Data Survey*, of the occupational therapists who serve children (ages 0–18), approximately 55% are employed in school settings. Of the remaining pediatric occupational therapists, approximately 21% work in hospital settings (hospitals 6.5%, pediatric hospitals 5.5%, rehabilitation hospitals 4.2%, psychiatric hospitals 4.1%, rehabilitation units 0.5%); 18% in community settings (private practice 6.9%, voluntary agencies 3.3%, outpatient clinics 2.6%, public health agencies 1.5%, day care 1.5%, home health agencies 1.2%, and community mental health centers 0.6%); and 4% in residential

settings. Lower incidence settings account for the approximate 2% remaining: private industry, health maintenance organizations, research facilities, sheltered workshops, vocational settings, and doctors' offices (American Occupational Therapy Association, 1988).

Consider the diversity of the documentation requirements mandated by the wide variety of treatment populations, intervention teams, and regulating and reimbursing agencies in these service provision models. No wonder the task of documentation can seem overwhelming. Just as one cannot play a game fairly or with skill until the rules are understood, one cannot document skillfully until he or she has mastered the rules. The rules for documenting in any specific work setting must be built upon an appreciation for: 1) the needs of the children in the setting, 2) the team (and the teams which interface this setting), 3) the payor(s), and 4) the governmental and accreditation regulations. Attention to these audiences provides the structure for good documentation.

THE WRITER'S AUDIENCE

Effective documentation is telling a true story with a particular style. It calls for the ordinary tasks of day-to-day experience to be succinctly stated in writing. The true story about any child who has a disability is not a simple tale. Because each child's unique set of strengths and deficits within a particular family, social structure, and community generates a vast diversity of data, occupational therapists must selectively choose what to report and how to report it. In documentation, one must comprehensively address the requirements of the regulations of the particular setting, yet do so in a clear and brief manner which conveys selective communicative information.

The Child

At any one step of the referral, screening, assessment, planning, intervention, or reassessment process, the occupational therapist deals with information from a variety of sources. At any one time, a therapist is dealing with the child's family and its historical and current concerns, results of formal and informal evaluations from occupational therapy and other professions, medical issues, service provision possibilities, reimbursement or justification of service issues, accreditation standards, and the ethics of possible decisions. The complexity of these interrelated child-centered issues demands that the occupational therapist be organized. Planning is not a spontaneous activity and therefore documentation is a complex cognitive task. The children served count on the professional's ability to deal with the complex data of their lives in an organized way.

Data must be integrated, prioritized, and sequenced in conjunction with the family and other professionals. For whom does the occupational therapist write? FOR THE CHILD. Quality care is the underlying element of all documentation.

Documentation causes one to create logical categories in the mind and on paper. These ordered ideas become substantiated professional opinions and are the basis for professional decisions. As ideas become ordered and conclusions are reached, documentation becomes the culminating act of clinical reasoning.

Team Communication

With an appreciation of the data synthesizing aspect of documentation, and an emphasis on its child-centered nature, the more obvious mission of documentation is to convey ideas to others. Seldom is a child's problem isolated to deficits requiring only one team member, and never is it isolated from the family or primary care-givers. Occupational therapists' written accounts, therefore, occur most optimally in conjunction with the family and intervention team members. No matter what service team the occupational therapist has joined (school-centered program, acute hospital, home health team, mental health agency, intermediate or long term care facility, etc.), the therapist can facilitate team work with effective use of the documentation process to supplement and validate verbal communication. The team approach is reflected in writing. Team members share a serious responsibility not only to write well, but also to read other team members' documentation, as they plan complementary and non-duplicative service.

Depending upon the service provision model, the family participates in the documentation process (e.g., Individualized Education Plan or the Individualized Family Service Plan); the needs of the family may generate separate, specific documentation (i.e., written home program). In each model of service provision, therapists are urged to define the special documentation needs of the family and implement strategies so that the documentation process itself helps assure the family's place as a prominent team member.

As a means of communication, the written word produces special challenges. In verbal conversation, one has the advantage of continual feedback from the receiver of the message. The listening party provides nods of affirmation, questioning frowns, or blank stares as cues about the effectiveness of communication. Without this immediate feedback as one communicates through writing, the ideas must stand alone, leaving no question of meaning in the mind of the reader (Acquaviva and Malone, 1981).

Without immediate feedback from the message receiver, therapists must continually monitor the clarity of their story-telling. One method of self-assessment is the RUMBA test. RUMBA is a method originally developed by the Quality Assurance Division of the American Occupational Therapy Association, with Patricia Ostrow, OTR and John Williamson, MD. It was later suggested for use in the AOTA's *Guidelines for Occupational Therapy Services in School Systems, Sec-*

ond Edition (1989). The RUMBA test was originally designed to evaluate the effectiveness of intervention objectives, but here its application will be expanded to assess not only objectives, but also general documentation effectiveness. Take it one letter at a time and RUMBA:

R = Is my reporting RELEVANT?

U = Is my reporting UNDERSTANDABLE?

M = Is my reporting stated in MEASURABLE terms?

B = Am I reporting BEHAVIORAL data?

A = Are my reported plans ACHIEVABLE?

R = RELEVANT. So what? Occupational therapy documentation should be able to pass the SO WHAT test. Intervention plans ultimately deal with quality of life issues and report some aspect of function in appropriate life tasks. Occupational therapists are urged to return to reporting functional levels and activities of daily living, rather than totally relying on the report of evaluations, which have nice tidy increments associated with them (i.e., degrees of range of motion or grades on a muscle test). Although the numbers associated with evaluations certainly give one an objective measure of progress, it is more relevant to the agency, as well as the child and family, to establish functional goals and to report functional gains. As an example, it is more relevant to report that the individual can now reach his mouth with a spoon, rather than only reporting a 40 degree increase in range of motion of the elbow. It is more relevant to report that the child now has the standing tolerance to complete all grooming activities at the bathroom sink independently, rather than reporting only an increase of standing tolerance from 1 minute to 5 minutes. Numbers are meaningful only if they are given meaning by answering the SO WHAT question.

Therapists need to attend not only to the global relevance of their documentation, but also to consider whether it is relevant to this particular child with this particular set of deficits and strengths, in this particular team's setting. It is possible for a truly functional deficit to be identified, a goal established, and an objective well written, which does not meet the R criteria. Common errors include: 1) documentation of problem areas and goals which are not team priority issues, 2) documentation of goals outside the scope of occupational therapy, 3) documentation of goals which are not relevant because of the child's age, potential, socioeconomic or family expectations, etc., and 4) documentation of problem areas which are not appropriate in the particular service model (i.e., medical goals in an education setting, or educational goals in a medial setting).

U = UNDERSTANDABLE. Can another person (including family/caregivers) understand the meaning? There are a number of separate issues to be dealt with in an effort to make documentation understandable; some are basic and some are complex.

1. The words themselves must be **readable**. Handwriting must be legible. When writing, black ink is used, as it is more clearly reproduced if the report has to be copied. Copies should be checked for readability. Typewritten

or word processed reports are more easy to read than handwriting. Always proof read.

2. Consider whether **meaning** will be apparent to the average reader:

   a. Avoid medical terminology and jargon (i.e., report on problems with balance, not vestibular dysfunction; report on labored breathing during activity, not dyspnea).
   b. Break up long sentences.
   c. Eliminate unnecessary words.
   d. Focus on actions, not lengthy descriptions.
   e. Avoid awkwardness (often reading it aloud will clarify the source of the confusion; if not, ask a peer).

3. The **active voice**, is prefered over the passive voice (i.e., report that Joe put on his shirt independently and buttoned four half-inch buttons in seven minutes, rather than reporting that the shirt was donned and buttons were buttoned by Joe in seven minutes).

4. You may find this one difficult. I suggest, that you use **I statements**. (See how easy that was; I did it!) We have been taught to avoid I, we, us, etc. in professional writing. However, because of the necessity of being absolutely clear, this rule has recently been laid aside. The current health and education climate will not tolerate vagueness. We must be specific for the child's sake, as well as for issues of reimbursement and justification of services. We must stop making statements like, "it has been determined that . . . " *Who* determined it? If it was *your* determination, then *say* so! "Based on my home visit, and reports from the teacher, Jill's attention span averages two minutes." In this case my opinion is based on firsthand and secondhand information and I so stated. To state "it has been determined that Jill's attention span . . . ," leaves the reader wondering who observed this and in what situations. Take ownership and avoid vagueness. If you can't bring yourself to say "I" or "my" (or if it is not sanctioned at your agency), then at least report "this student," or "this therapist determined that . . . ."

5. A related stylistic trend, which targets vagueness in written communication, urges therapists to **stop using noncommittal language**. It is no longer acceptable to state that "It appears that . . . " It is, or it isn't, and if one can't state a professional opinion, then it shouldn't be commented upon. Instead of "It appeared that Julie was angry," report observed behavior (i.e., "When I replaced Julie's splint, she displayed anger by screaming and throwing herself off the chair and onto the floor."). If it isn't readily apparent whether Julie was angry, and this is relevant information, simply report the observed behavior, ("When I replaced the splint, Julie made no effort to communicate. She avoided eye-contact, and did not respond to questions regarding its comfort.").

6. Attend to issues of grammar and spelling. Help each other in a constructive way! There are a number of good resources available. A brief listing is provided in Appendix E. The *Goof-Proofer* (Manhard, 1987) is a must!

7. Use the AOTA (1989a) *Uniform Terminology for Oc-cupational Therapy, Second Edition*, to describe the child's strengths and deficits; this is one of the best ways to educate team members regarding occupational therapy priorities, and provides consistency in vocabulary from therapist to therapist and from center to center. Remember, your goal of good writing is understandability.

M = MEASURABLE. Have you stated your problems and goals in terms which aid in the writing of measurable objectives, so that progress can be clearly documented?

B = BEHAVIORAL. Have you clearly stated problems and goals in terms of the child's behavior?

M and B are more easily discussed together. In all child-centered documentation, it is imperative that the written report deals with the observable and measurable behaviors of the child. Therapists should read their own written work and ask, "Have I defined the goal behavior clearly enough so that my audience can observe the child and know immediately 'Yes there's one,' or 'No, he or she doesn't do it yet'?" Behaviors can be seen and counted.

There are numerous things one may be tempted to report which are vague or have individual interpretations. Avoid attitudes or labels such as happy, unhappy, friendly, cheerful, appropriate, depressed, naughty, lazy, sad, etc. These attitudes and labels are not behaviors. It is apparent that there is no consensus of "happy" or "depressed" or "appropriate." Therefore, if one charts the fact that the child is happier, the reader is left guessing, as what was observed could literally be any one of dozens of behaviors (e.g., decreased crying, decreased self-abuse, increased laughing, etc.).

Behaviors are action words (e.g., sits, slams, throws, cries, dresses, smiles, cuts, puts, writes, dons, stacks, stands, uses, makes, rolls, sucks, folds, types, ties, drives, reads, washes, creeps, reaches, turns, pushes, draws, jumps, says, lifts, follows, waves, dries, chews, points, etc.). In all documentation tasks, from formal team planning to informal notes sent home with the mother, a focus is maintained on child-centered targeted behaviors.

A series of tasks is provided to enhance basic skills leading more specifically toward the writing of measurable behavioral objectives. The goal is twofold: 1) the attainment of skills to write measurable behavioral objectives, and 2) the generalization of this skill so that all child-centered documentation becomes focused upon measurable behaviors.

First, to be able to document well, one must be an astute observer. Therapists need to document observations so that there is no doubt about the particular behavior being reported. The first task provides an exercise in recording observed behaviors (See Figure 8-1). Once the behaviors are recorded one asks whether a peer could read the observation list and be SURE he or she observed the specific behavior.

Once the therapist is able to isolate and specifically state a behavior, the next step is to develop skills in charting (counting) behaviors to determine the severity of problems. Charting behaviors is used clinically to determine problems, and to establish goals and objectives, and later to document progress. Care should be taken to select the most meaningful method of charting for each specific behavior.

Many behaviors can be charted relative to duration and frequency. Documentation of duration is simply recording how

---

OBSERVATION

Describe two specific behaviors observed under each category. Place a + in the space before each number if the behavior is age-appropriate or advanced for the child's age. Place a - in the space if the behavior is a problem (i.e. abnormal behavior or not age appropriate). At the bottom of the page, list the sources used to determine if the behavior was age appropriate. If a particular component of behavior was not observed, briefly explain the reason.

Age: ___ Setting: _____
(i.e. preschool playground, shopping mall, kitchen, classroom)

Language
__1._____

__2._____

Cognitive
__1._____

__2._____

Fine Motor
__1._____

__2._____

Gross Motor
__1._____

__2._____

Social Emotional
__1._____

__2._____

Self Help
__1._____

__2._____

Sources:

Figure 8-1. Observation and recording of specific behaviors.

long the specific behavior lasted (i.e., How long could he tolerate the splint? How long did she sit at her desk? How long did the screaming episode last? How long did he hold his head upright?). On the other hand, documentation of frequency is the recording of how many isolated times the behavior occurs within the specified recording time, (i.e., How many splint wearing sessions occurred during the school day? How many at-desk periods occurred during a school day? How many episodes of screaming occurred during the one hour therapy session? How many repetitions of holding the head upright occurred during the 30 minute therapy session?).

In each of these examples, the behavior can be recorded and reported in terms of duration and frequency. As an example, it could be reported that "Aimee's splint wearing tolerance during school hours has increased from three to four sessions per day, and the average session has increased from ten to fifteen minutes." (Of course the functional relevance of this behavior would also be reported, i.e., "Aimee has gained enough finger extension to allow her to inde-

pendently release ½ inch objects, e.g., kindergarten pencil, sandwich, etc."). It could be reported that, "During one hour occupational therapy sessions, Jonathan's screaming episodes have decreased from ten per session to three per session, with the duration of each screaming episode remaining on the average three minutes." (Again, the functional gain that this particular change in behavior elicited would also be reported, "With reduced screaming behavior, Jonathan can now be engaged in visual tracking activities for up to 20 seconds at a time, with an average of 10 tracking episodes per half hour of therapy.") Figure 8-2 provides practice opportunities for defining behaviors, defining conditions, and recording (quantifying) the duration and frequency of behaviors.

There are some behaviors which are more appropriately counted or measured using duration alone, or frequency alone. When trying to diminish a negative behavior that lasts only a second or two, the objective is to simply decrease the frequency of that behavior (i.e., spitting, hitting, pinching). It would be ridiculous to try to catch the duration of each in-

OBSERVATION

Describe two specific behaviors observed under each category. Place a
+ in the space before each number if the behavior is age-appropriate or
advanced for the child's age. Place a - in the space if the behavior
is a problem (i.e. abnormal behavior or not age appropriate). At the
bottom of the page, list the sourses used to determine if the behavior
was age appropriate. If a particular component of behavior was not
observed, briefly explain the reason.

Age: _4_   Setting: _In kitchen with mother & observer_
                (i.e. preschool playground, shopping mall, kitchen, classroom)

Language
_+_ 1. _longest sentence = 5 words_

_−_ 2. _Does not use past tense verbs - i.e. When asked "Where_
       have you been?" responds "I go store."
Cognitive
_−_ 1. _Cannot count beyond 1, 2. Repeats numbers, but cannot_
       use them actively to count past 2.
_−_ 2. _Names only the color red. When asked other colors,_
       responds "red" to all.
Fine Motor
_−_ 1. _Can cut straight line with blunt scissors but cannot_
       cut around a picture
_−_ 2. _Cannot manipulate 1" figure forms with plastic_
       ball.
Gross Motor
_+_ 1. _Can jump forward on both feet and can hop forward_
       on one foot
_+_ 2. _While standing, can catch a large bounced ball_

Social Emotional
_+_ 1. _Left mother in the kitchen with no separation problem_
       to go with a stranger (me) to the other room.
_+_ 2. _Many questions about my family constellation. i.e. "Do you_
       have a grandpa?" "Do you have a boy?" "Where's your mom?"
Self Help
_−_ 1. _Cannot button shirt_

_+_ 2. _Uses fork and spoon accurately._

Sources: 1. _Miller Assessment for Preschoolers (MAP)_
         2. _Schuster & Ashburn (1980). The Process of Human Development._
            Boston: Little, Brown, & Co.

Figure 8-1a.   An example of a completed observation worksheet.

dividual "spit" on your stop watch. But if the frequency of this behavior actually interferes with performance (i.e., may even keep the child from placement in a particular classroom which may be optimal for him), then documentation of the decreased frequency of this behavior may be vitally important. There are also positive behaviors which may be most optimally recorded as frequency alone. One may record how many meals Gary ate with no spills, how many times Sheila remembered to tie her shoes, how many buttons Cory buttoned, how many times Kristin rolled from prone to supine, etc. For instance, it might be charted and reported that "Margaret independently took care of her toiletting needs four times during the school day."

When considering one dimension of a variable, a graph is a useful visual aid to show if the behavior is increasing or decreasing. The first step is to make a horizontal line (the abscissa) for plotting the independent variable (i.e., the date). The second step is to make a vertical line (the ordinate) for plotting the dependent variable (the behavior you are counting). The third step is to number the ordinate and the abscissa. In the figures which follow, graphs are included as part of the exercises. Figure 8-3 provides opportunities for the practice of charting and graphing behaviors which are appropriately reported in frequency alone.

Some behaviors lend themselves more appropriately to duration alone. For example, if Tanya was working toward efficiency in organizing her morning work independently (defined as putting her coat and books away, checking her mailbox for an "A.M. Plan," collecting the materials listed in "A.M. Plan," and joining her group at the work table), charting could record the duration of this activity, and progress could be recorded from day-to-day as the duration moved from her current time of 20 minutes to her target of 10 minutes. Opportunities are provided in Figure 8-4 for you to chart and graph behaviors which are more appropriately reported in endurance.

RECORDING BEHAVIOR: FREQUENCY AND DURATION

Begin by briefly (5-10 minutes) observing the patient/client/
child's repertoire of behaviors. Do not interact with the child.
As you observe, list examples of behaviors you observe. Choose
one behavior to chart for a TEN minute period (or define another
time frame prior to onset).

1.   Define the behavior:

2.   Define the condition (setting, others present, level of
     independence, stimulus):

3.   Record both the <u>frequency</u> and the <u>duration</u> of the observed
     behavior (make a tally mark in the frequency column each time
     the behavior occurs, and note in the duration column how long
     each occurance lasted, in seconds or minutes):

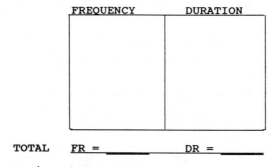

         TOTAL   <u>FR =</u>_____   DR =_____

4.   Summarize what you observed:

5.   Behavior specific enough?   ____yes ____no

     Condition specific enough?   ____yes ____no

6.   Restate the behavior and/or condition to create a more
     chartable behavior:

Figure 8-2.   Defining the behavior and the condition, and recording the behavior.

In each of the examples above, duration simply referred to sequential time units (usually reported in seconds, minutes, or hours), and frequency referred to the number of times the behavior occurred within a specified time period. In these examples, an **interval scale** was used. The behavior was defined in such a way that the units were discrete tallies and could be counted. An interval scale is used when the units are equal, so that adding them indicates magnitude. In each case above, the number eight represents a unit which is twice as many as four and four times as many as two (i.e., eight minutes is twice as many as four minutes and eight buttons is twice as many as four buttons). In other words, interval scales use real numbers.

When an interval scale is used, the tally system described above (tally of time or tally of events) is the most simple method for reporting behaviors. However, this is often inadequate, unless the conditions are understood. It is obvious that if it is reported that the behavior occurred three times,

more information may be needed. Simple tallies suffice when the condition provides guidelines which give the numbers structure (i.e., it is recognized that recording occurs during the entire school day, or each shift, or each week, etc.). This simple system also makes the assumption that the child has equal opportunity to do the behavior from one day to the next.

When the time frame for eliciting the behavior is not always the same, one of the easier ways to report behaviors is to report the number of times the behavior occurred, divided by the amount of time over which the behaviors were counted. In this case you are reporting a **rate of response**. Rate of response works well when there are no restrictions on the number of opportunities to respond within the time frame. As an example, if one counted five behaviors (e.g., a child approaches another child) during a 50 minute session on day one, six behaviors during a 48 minute session on day two, and one behavior during a 20 minute session on day three, the comparable summary score for each session would be

RECORDING BEHAVIOR: FREQUENCY AND DURATION

Begin by briefly (5-10 minutes) observing the patient/client/
child's repertoire of behaviors. Do not interact with the child.
As you observe, list examples of behaviors you observe. Choose
one behavior to chart for a TEN minute period (or define another
time frame prior to onset).

1. Define the behavior: *Hold spoon - palmar grasp*

2. Define the condition (setting, others present, level of
   independence, stimulus): *When plate is presented at mealtime in the own kitchen with the family. Holds independently 30 minutes.*

3. Record both the <u>frequency</u> and the <u>duration</u> of the observed
   behavior (make a tally mark in the frequency column each time
   the behavior occurs, and note in the duration column how long
   each occurance lasted, in seconds or minutes):

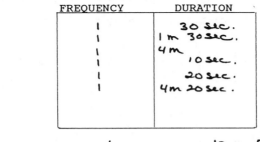

FREQUENCY	DURATION
I	30 sec.
I	1 m 30 sec.
I	4 m
I	10 sec.
I	20 sec.
I	4 m 20 sec.

TOTAL   FR = *6*   DR = *10 m. 50 sec.*

4. Summarize what you observed: *Concentrated well. Determined. Low muscle tone.*

5. Behavior specific enough? _____ yes   ✔ no
   Didn't state if she had to pick it up or if ok for mom to place it.
   Condition specific enough? ✔ yes _____ no

6. Restate the behavior and/or condition to create a more
   chartable behavior: *Pick up and hold the spoon: palmar grasp.*

Figure 8-2a. An example of a completed worksheet.

rate per minute, and would be 5/50 = .10 for day one, 6/48 = .125 for day two, and 1/20 = .05 for day three. Comparing the rate per minute (.10, .125, and .05) is much more meaningful than comparing tallies (5, 6, and 1). Refer to Figure 8-5 for practice opportunities in charting and graphing rate of response.

In contrast, **times/trials** (or response per opportunity) can be used when the number of trials for the behavior to occur is restricted and may vary from day to day. It is obvious that a child's opportunities for hitting a home run are in direct proportion to his number of times at bat. To figure times/trials, simply divide the number of times the behavior occurred, by the total number of trials (opportunities) for that behavior to occur at each session, just like figuring a daily batting average. Therefore, the **percentage** obtained is comparable from session to session As an example, the goal for Chaundra is to increase spoon-to-mouth skill. The meal on day one may lend itself to only 10 scoops of the spoon (i.e., Monday's

lunch is a hot dog, french fries, and applesauce), whereas day two's lunch may have 30 possible scoops (i.e., Tuesday's lunch is chili and crackers, and pudding). If the child obtained a tally of 9 accurate scoops the first day and 10 accurate scoops the second day, you will get an inaccurate picture if you simply compared these tallies (9 scoops and 10 scoops). A more accurate picture would be to report the times/trials, which would be 90% (9/10) accuracy for the first day and a 33.3% (10/30) accuracy for the second day. Times/trials (reporting percent) charting and graphing can be practiced by turning to Figure 8-6.

Although most behaviors lend themselves best to one of these interval scales (reported in frequency, duration, frequency and duration, rate of response, or times/trials), two other scales are useful at times; nominal and ordinal. Nominal and ordinal scales are discrete, rather than continuous scales. A **nominal assessment scale** is the simplest scale, and is appropriate when one wants to report an either/or behavior

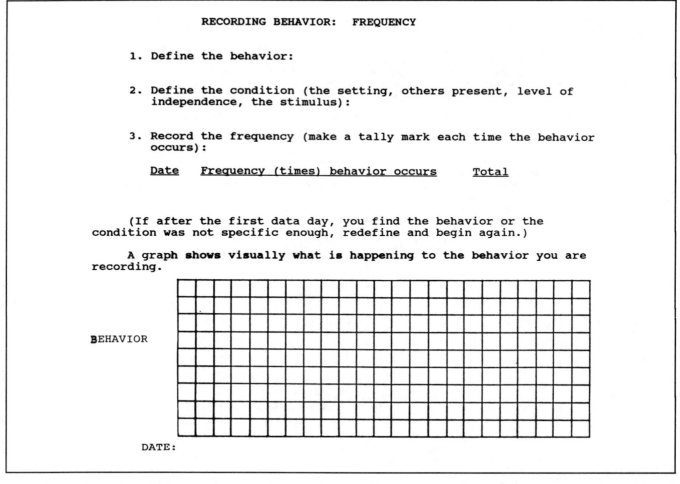

RECORDING BEHAVIOR: FREQUENCY

1. Define the behavior:

2. Define the condition (the setting, others present, level of
   independence, the stimulus):

3. Record the frequency (make a tally mark each time the behavior
   occurs):

   <u>Date</u>   <u>Frequency (times) behavior occurs</u>   <u>Total</u>

   (If after the first data day, you find the behavior or the
   condition was not specific enough, redefine and begin again.)

   A graph shows visually what is happening to the behavior you are
   recording.

BEHAVIOR

DATE:

Figure 8-3. Defining the behavior and the condition, and recording and graphing frequency across data days.

or response. The only restriction is that responses put into one group must have something in common with each other, and be different from responses in other groups. The classic examples of nominal scales are gender (the child is male or female), or blood type (a specific type is based upon certain exclusionary differences). The primary purpose of a nominal scale is for categorization (Glasnapp and Poggio, 1985). One practical use of this scale is for behaviors needing only a "yes" or a "no" count. As an example, an adolescent may be considered for a promotion in a behavioral level (as defined by the facility) on the mental health unit, if he totally refrains from swearing for a 24 hour period. In other words, the staff doesn't want to know how many times he swears, or the quality of his swearing, or even how long the swearing lasts. They just want to know at the end of the 24 hour period if he is in the group of adolescents who swore, or if he is in the group who didn't swear. Each group is exclusionary. During that time he is observed, each staff person notes swearing behavior and documents this at the end of the shift, using just "yes" or "no" categories (not counting a tally). At the end of 24 hours he is categorized as having met the criteria or not having met the criteria.

Examples of other behaviors which might be charted using

the "yes/no" application of nominal assessment, include charting: 1) an A.M. dry bed, or 2) adolescent arrived at work on time, etc. In each case the child is placed in a particular category (i.e., wet or dry, late or on time). See Figure 8-7.

An **ordinal assessment scale** involves ranking behavior on a dimension into three or more levels. There is an order in the ranking, but there is not necessarily the same interval between ranks (see Figure 8-8). As an example, a child's self help skills may be described on a rating system from 0 to 10 (or from 1 to 5, etc.), with clearly defined criteria, so that it is clear what the child must do to rate a 5 over a 4. A child's performance may be charted over days, to rate progress (or lack of it). Although 6 shows marked progress from a 3 rating, a 6 isn't necessarily twice as good as 3. The improvement from 4 to 5 may not be exactly the same amount as the improvement from 5 to 6.

Charting an increase in muscle strength from a fair to a good muscle grade is an example of an ordinal scale, whereas reporting an increase in ability from lifting two pounds to lifting five pounds is an interval scale. A Likert scale is ordinal reporting. As an example, a hostile adolescent may be asked to rank his anger daily on a scale from 0 to 10 (with definitions of the meanings of 0 through 10), to assist with clarifying

RECORDING BEHAVIOR: FREQUENCY

1. Define the behavior: *Arrive at classes on time*

2. Define the condition (the setting, others present, level of independence, the stimulus): *The change-of-class bell is the stimulus. No reminders. No directions to the next class (7 class changes daily).*

3. Record the frequency (make a tally mark each time the behavior occurs):

Date	Frequency (times) behavior occurs	Total
4-21	I I I	3
4-22	I I	2
4-23	I I I I	4
4-26	I I I I	4
4-27	⊩⊩ I	5
4-28	I I I I	4
4-29	⊩⊩ I I	7

(If after the first data day, you find the behavior or the condition was not specific enough, redefine and begin again.)

A graph shows visually what is happening to the behavior you are recording.

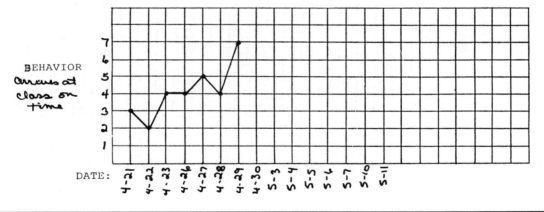

Figure 8-3a. **An example of a completed worksheet.**

feelings. This self-ranking may be important data for charting purposes and documenting a trend, but it is obvious that there is no way to precisely determine if the increment from 1 to 2 is the same as the increment from 9 to 10.

The activities in Figures 8-1 through 8-8 have provided opportunities for the development of the skills of: 1) accurately observing behavior, 2) stating the behavior and condition in terms that are clear, and 3) assessing how the behavior can best be measured. These skills are used daily by the occupational therapist to define behaviors and to chart progress.

In the clinic or classroom, the intermediate task between identifying the target behavior and reporting progress, is to establish a measurable behavioral objective. A well written behavioral objective has six parts: 1) the child, 2) the behavior (a verb), 3) the setting, 4) the person(s) or trainer(s) involved,

5) the stimuli (or instruction), 6) the criteria (method of counting or charting).

In the example below, 1) the child = Michael, 2) the behavior = load and bring, 3) the setting = regular chair at school lunch, 4) the person(s) involved = teacher aide, 5) the stimuli = school lunch presented, and 6) the criterion = 10 bites per meal, for 4 of 5 days. A long term goal for Michael is independent feeding. Progress is documented as he accomplishes short term objectives and new relevant, understandable, **m**easurable, **b**ehavioral, and **a**chievable objectives replace them.

The current measurable behavioral objective for Michael is: "Sitting in a regular chair during school lunch, Michael will independently load the spoon, and bring the filled spoon to his mouth, with the manual guidance of the teacher's aid for

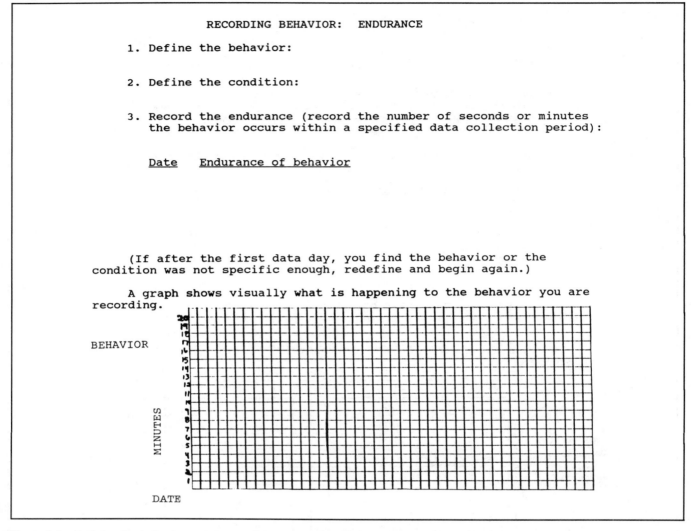

Figure 8-4. Defining the behavior and the condition, and recording and graphing endurance across data days.

ten bites per meal, four of five days." Michael can be observed and the occupational therapist (or another team member) can chart the behavior and state "yes" or "no," the objective has or has not been met. If the behavior is different, either below the expectation (i.e., he's still requiring help in scooping) or above the expectation (he is also independently bringing it to his mouth), that can be reported clearly. Figure 8-9 provides behavioral objective practice guides. Every service provision model requires the occupational therapist to report measurable behavioral objectives, although they may be called something other than objectives. These skills are basic to all professionals who are accountable for the services they provide.

A = ACHIEVABLE. Is your plan achievable for this child within the time period specified by agency or regulatory guidelines? One must step back from a desk full of data and consider not only the child's characteristics, but also the service provision system and the child's environment. Even if very small increments must be established for designated time frames, this enables the team to recognize progress; this is very important for families as well as other professionals, especially when serving children with severe and multiple handicaps.

In summary, the RUMBA test is a method for assessing one's own documentation skills, as well as for checking each objective written. Good documentation is **r**elevant, **u**nderstandable, **m**easurable, **b**ehavioral, and **a**chievable. These skills are important to team members. Occupational therapy documentation is for: 1) the child and 2) the *TEAM*.

Guidelines and Regulations

According to Acquaviva and Malone (1981), the writer must know whose questions the reports, notes, or plans will answer. Although occupational therapists universally write for the child, the team and the family, there are vast differences in documentation requirements across service provision models.

How does the occupational therapist know what questions the agency's documentation must answer? How does one

RECORDING BEHAVIOR: ENDURANCE

1. Define the behavior: *remain seated*

2. Define the condition: *With verbal encouragement, but no physical restraint, Jody will remain at the school lunch table - 20 minutes.*

3. Record the endurance (record the number of seconds or minutes the behavior occurs within a specified data collection period):

Date	Endurance of behavior (*minutes*)
2-5	5
2-8	5
2-9	8
2-10	12
2-11	5
2-12	7
2-15	10
2-16	10
2-17	12

(If after the first data day, you find the behavior or the condition was not specific enough, redefine and begin again.)

A graph shows visually what is happening to the behavior you are recording.

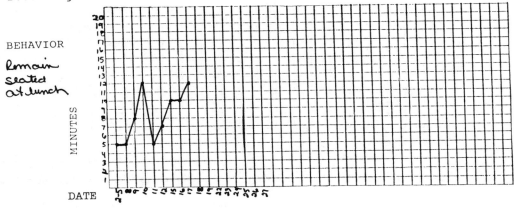

Figure 8-4a. An example of a completed worksheet.

determine the content, timing, and frequency of documentation? In considering the specific content and format, there are three considerations relative to guidelines and regulations: 1) the specific requirements of the accrediting or governing agency, 2) the requirements of reimbursing agencies, and 3) professional guidelines.

Accrediting or Governing Agencies

What is accreditation? It is an independent third party process which sanctions or makes credible an organization, by certifying that the organization meets particular predetermined state or national standards. The process of accreditation has been established to provide consumers, providers, and third party reimbursers a measure of standards-achievement.

Accreditation typically involves the center's participation in a structured and guided self-study, followed by an on-site visit by a team of trained professionals. Examples of accrediting agencies are The Joint Commission for the Accreditation of Hospitals Organization (JCAHO), Commission on Accreditation of Rehabilitation Facilities (CARF), and the Accreditation Council on Services for People with Developmental Disabilities (ACDD). To achieve and maintain accreditation, documentation must comply with specific guidelines.

Not only must therapists attend to accreditation standards, but documentation must also conform to the requirements of federal and state laws, rules and regulations. Examples include the stipulations of Medicaid, and the Division of Services for Crippled Children (DSCC). Often, state governments are called upon to administer (and sometimes co-fund) federal programs, (i.e., a variety of public school programs).

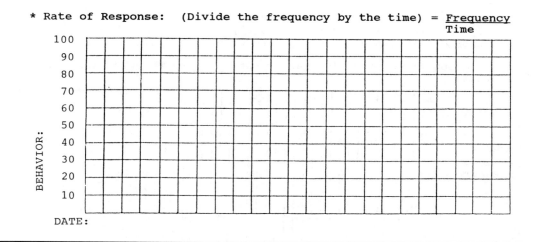

RECORDING BEHAVIOR: RATE OF RESPONSE

1. Define the behavior:

2. Define the condition:

3. Record the rate of response (record the number of times the behavior occurs, as well as the number of seconds, minutes, or hours during which recording occured) :

Date   Frequency of behavior Total   Total time   Rate of Response*

* Rate of Response: (Divide the frequency by the time) = $\dfrac{Frequency}{Time}$

Figure 8-5.   Defining the behavior and the condition, and recording and graphing rate of response across data days.

Reimbursing Agencies

Each facility or agency must also respond to those who pay the bills. In some situations, accrediting or governing agencies and reimbursing agencies overlap (e.g., in school settings). In other settings, the regulating agency and the reimbursing party may be two different agencies, each imposing documentation mandates (i.e., hospital settings attempt to meet JCAHO standards and standards set by third party reimbursing agencies, public and private). Therefore, documentation formats must not only facilitate the communication of factual information mandated by accrediting and governing bodies of the center, but also must attend to any content area which further clarifies data required by the payors. Although occupational therapy personnel are not liable for knowing whether a patient's health plan covers occupational therapy, therapists should know about coverage and help their patients be informed (Scott, 1988, ix). In all cases, those who

pay for occupational therapy services (as well as other rehabilitative and education services) deserve, and in most cases mandate a mechanism to determine what they're getting for their financial investment.

No program or intervention plan, no progress note or report, no discharge plan, consultation note, or home program should be put on paper until the writer has an understanding of the guidelines and regulations of: 1) the accrediting body, 2) the law governing the agency, and 3) the reimbursement system. In other words, when documenting, the writer must know, before starting to write, what the regulators and reimbursers want to know about what is done, and what is planned for the infant, toddler, child, or adolescent.

Professional Guidelines

Although the practice opportunities in pediatrics are diverse within the occupational therapy profession, good occupa-

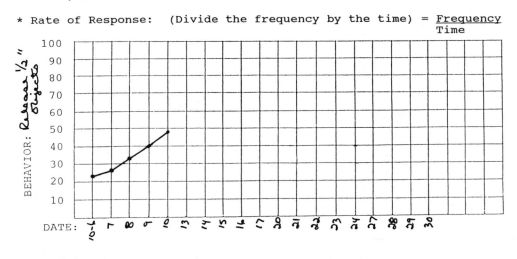

RECORDING BEHAVIOR: RATE OF RESPONSE

1. Define the behavior: *release objects of ½" diameter or less (eg. puzzle piece, bead, pencil, marble)*

2. Define the condition: *Seated in wheelchair with lapboard during fine motor group and 1:1 therapy. Stars used for positive reinforcement.*

3. Record the rate of response (record the number of times the behavior occurs, as well as the number of seconds, minutes, or hours during which recording occured) :

Date	Frequency of behavior	Total	Total time	Rate of Response*
10-6	ʬ II	7	30 min.	.23
10-7	ʬ ʬ ʬ	15	55 min.	.27
10-8	ʬ ʬ ʬ II	17	50 min.	.34
10-9	ʬ I	6	15 min.	.40
10-10	ʬ ʬ II	12	25 min.	.48
10-13				
10-14				
10-15				

* Rate of Response: (Divide the frequency by the time) = $\frac{Frequency}{Time}$

Figure 8-5a. **An example of a completed worksheet.**

tional therapy documentation provides evidence to the reader that in all arenas, occupational therapy's concern is human performance and facilitation of an adaptive response (Kleinman and Bulkley, 1982). The American Occupational Therapy Association (AOTA) has published documents which serve as guides for occupational therapists in the documentation process. A listing of these relevant documents is provided in Figure 8-10.

Besides being familiar with AOTA Official Position Papers, Roles/Functions Papers, Standards, and Guidelines, relative to one's particular practice, occupational therapists are encouraged to be familiar with the *Guidelines for Occupational Therapy Documentation* (AOTA, 1986). This document is presented in its entirety in Appendix B. This resource serves as a guide for content and clarification of the various com-

ponents in a record, such as: parameters for the recording of the client's identification and background information, assessment and reassessment, treatment planning, treatment implementation, and discontinuation of services.

Across service provision models, the names of the types of documentation vary (i.e., treatment plans may be termed *plan of care, program plan, individual education program, individual family service plan*, etc.). The AOTA Guidelines were established as a model, and may clarify the content within each type of documentation, even though the document names may vary. Each therapist must investigate the unique needs of his or her documentation system.

As a child's true story is told (documented), the writer must keep in mind the predetermined questions which need to be answered. With practice, the professional team members come

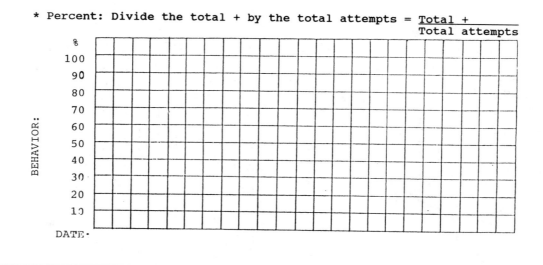

RECORDING BEHAVIOR: TIMES/TRIALS

1. Define the behavior:

2. Define the condition:

3. Record the rate of response (record the number of times the behavior occurs, as well as the number of seconds, minutes, or hours during which recording occured) :

	Record a + for each successful attempt and a – for each	Total		
Date	unsuccessful attempt	attempts	Total +	Percent*

$$* \text{ Percent: Divide the total + by the total attempts} = \frac{Total\ +}{Total\ attempts}$$

Figure 8-6. Defining the behavior and the condition, and recording and graphing times/trials across data days.

to organize their thinking in relation to this framework of questions, not as a limitation to creativity, but as a mechanism for thoroughness. Although following the guidelines doesn't guarantee good documentation, not following the guidelines does guarantee inappropriate documentation. As cognitive beings, with an innate tendency to try to organize their surroundings, occupational therapists can utilize the imposed structure of regulating agencies to make documentation tasks more manageable, rather than perceiving this structure as restricting. In developing a documentation system, or reassessing one which is in place:

Step one: Attend to external regulations and guidelines
—Government regulations
—Accrediting agencies
—Reimbursement systems
—AOTA documentation standards.

Step two: Attend to internal standards
—The setting's interpretation of the guidelines
—Setting-specific procedures
—Local vocabulary and abbreviation guidelines
Step three: Custom-design documentation
—As a team member, devise a data collection and reporting system which provides the required answers (for external and internal communication) in a brief, clear, thorough, and organized format.
Step four: Refocus on the child
—Documentation must facilitate integrated, sequenced, and prioritized intervention.

These four steps are applicable to all occupational therapy settings. In moving from one service provision model to an-

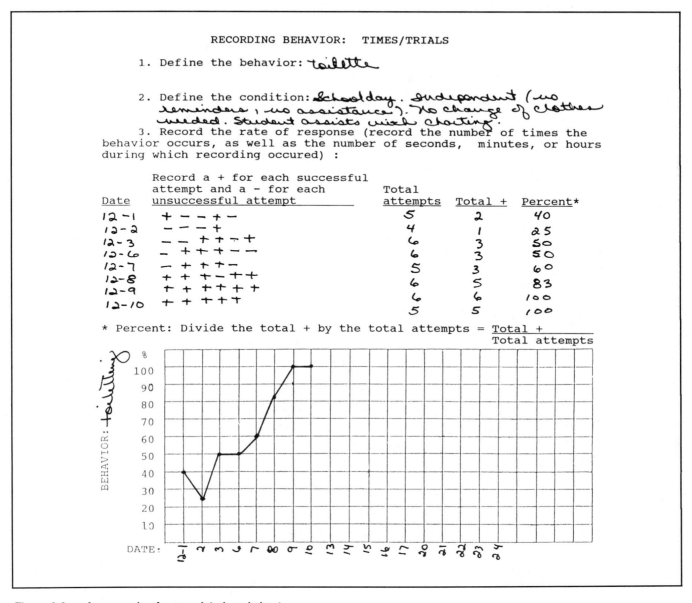

RECORDING BEHAVIOR: TIMES/TRIALS

1. Define the behavior: *toilette*

2. Define the condition: *School day. Independent (no reminders, no assistance). No change of clothes needed. Student assists with charting.*

3. Record the rate of response (record the number of times the behavior occurs, as well as the number of seconds, minutes, or hours during which recording occured):

Date	Record a + for each successful attempt and a - for each unsuccessful attempt	Total attempts	Total +	Percent*
12-1	+ - - + -	5	2	40
12-2	- - - +	4	1	25
12-3	- - - + + - +	6	3	50
12-6	- + + + - -	6	3	50
12-7	- + + + -	5	3	60
12-8	+ + + - + +	6	5	83
12-9	+ + + + + +	6	6	100
12-10	+ + + + +	5	5	100

* Percent: Divide the total + by the total attempts = $\frac{Total +}{Total\ attempts}$

Figure 8-6a.   An example of a completed worksheet.

other (or even from one employer to another within the same model), it is imperative that therapists become familiar with the agencies' documentation needs. Summaries of the documentation considerations for the more common settings are provided here. Specific interpretations for specific agencies within each model, must be investigated, to assure that local standards are met.

DOCUMENTATION IN SCHOOL SETTINGS

Audience

For whom is the school-based occupational therapist writing? Occupational therapists in school settings must document within the framework established by their local educational agency (LEA), as this agency complies with its state education agency (SEA), and federal regulations. The primary regulations guiding school documentation procedures were initiated by Public Law (PL) 94-142, the Education for All Handicapped Children Act, and the regulations generated by the U.S. Department of Education, which specify implementation procedures. These documents may be obtained by writing to: Superintendent of Documents, U.S. Government Printing Office, Washington D.C. 20402. Request the most recent revision of 34 Code of Federal Regulation—Parts 300-399. The most salient portions have been printed in *AOTA's Guidelines for Occupational Therapy Services in School Systems*, 2nd edition (American Occupational Therapy Association, 1989). Thorough reviews and interpretations are documented in the literature (AOTA, 1987; Turnbull & Turnbull, 1982; Turnbull, Strickland, & Brantley, 1982). These regulations will be discussed in Chapter Ten, although key

RECORDING BEHAVIOR: NOMINAL ASSESSMENT

1. Define the behavior:

2. Define the condition:

3. Record the behavior:

RESPONSE OPTIONS:

```
          _____  _____  _____  _____
----------------------------------------------------------------
MONDAY

----------------------------------------------------------------
TUESDAY

----------------------------------------------------------------
WEDNESDAY

----------------------------------------------------------------
THURSDAY

----------------------------------------------------------------
FRIDAY

----------------------------------------------------------------
SATURDAY

----------------------------------------------------------------
SUNDAY

================================================================
```

1. Define the behavior:
2. Define the condition:
3. Record the behavior:

RESPONSE OPTIONS:

```
          _____  _____  _____  _____
----------------------------------------------------------------
8:00-9:00
----------------------------------------------------------------
9:00-10:00
----------------------------------------------------------------
10:00-11:00
----------------------------------------------------------------
11:00-12:00
----------------------------------------------------------------
12:00-1:00
----------------------------------------------------------------
1:00-2:00
----------------------------------------------------------------
2:00-3:00
----------------------------------------------------------------
3:00-4:00
================================================================
```

A data collection system can double as a positive reinforcer. You may devise any calendar-like data sheet, and place a happy face sticker, gold star, or simple + on each data period that the desired behavior occurred.

Establish any time frame (charting once an hour, every five minutes, etc.). Use the nominal recording method as part of an assessment or behavioral program. If after recording initial data, the behavior or the condition was not specific enough, redefine and begin again.

Figure 8-7. Defining the behavior and the condition, and recording nominal responses.

RECORDING BEHAVIOR: NOMINAL ASSESSMENT

1. Define the behavior: Student refrains from hitting, kicking, biting, and throwing objects

2. Define the condition: All three shifts chart on specific four behaviors. Record sheet marked

3. Record the behavior: at 8:00 AM daily. No reminders.

RESPONSE OPTIONS:

	yes	no	In time-out room: no data	
MONDAY		✓		
TUESDAY			✓	✓
WEDNESDAY		✓		
THURSDAY	★			
FRIDAY		✓		
SATURDAY	★			
SUNDAY	★			

1. Define the behavior: Splint on (L) hand (correctly)

2. Define the condition: Arrive at school with splint on daily.

3. Record the behavior:

RESPONSE OPTIONS:

	On-correct	On-wrong	Forgot	Broken
MONDAY	✓			
TUESDAY		✓		
WEDNESDAY		✓		
THURSDAY	★			
FRIDAY	✓			
SATURDAY				
SUNDAY				

Figure 8-7a. An example of a completed worksheet.

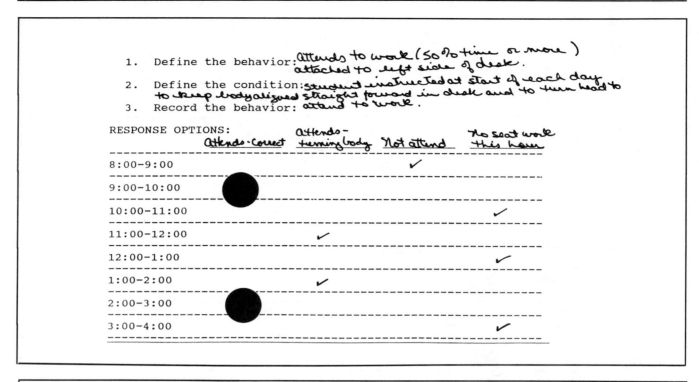

1. Define the behavior: *Attends to work (50% time or more) attached to left side of desk.*
2. Define the condition: *student instructed at start of each day to keep body aligned straight forward in desk and to turn head to*
3. Record the behavior: *attend to work.*

RESPONSE OPTIONS:

	Attends–Correct	Attends– turning body	Not attend	No seat work this hour
8:00–9:00			✔	
9:00–10:00	●			
10:00–11:00				✔
11:00–12:00		✔		
12:00–1:00				✔
1:00–2:00		✔		
2:00–3:00	●			
3:00–4:00				✔

1. Define the behavior: *awake and refrains from (bang head, bite, hit, or scratch) self-abusive behavior*
2. Define the condition: *in day room or classroom. Charted awake must include 50 min. awake time per hour.*
3. Record the behavior:

RESPONSE OPTIONS:

	Awake, non-abusive	Awake, Abusive	asleep	
8:00–9:00			✔	
9:00–10:00		✔		
10:00–11:00	✔			
11:00–12:00	✔			
12:00–1:00			✔	
1:00–2:00		✔		
2:00–3:00	✔			
3:00–4:00	✔			

Figure 8-7a. *Continued.*

points, directly affecting documentation in the school setting, will be discussed here. In school settings, accreditation and funding are tasks shared by the federal government, SEA's, and LEA's.

Brief History

PL 94-142 created a legal right for all children to receive those services that enable them to profit from educational experiences, and prescribed due process procedures for identifying, placing, and teaching handicapped students (Hargrove, 1982). With the advent of specificity in programs, came fiscal and program controls. The federal government interfaces with SEA's and LEA's via funding and regulations. Compliance to the regulations is a major objective of the LEA's, to qualify for a variety of available funds. The law and regulations clearly detail who (by diagnostic definition) is eligible for special education services, and what services are

RECORDING BEHAVIOR: ORDINAL ASSESSMENT

1. Define the behavior:

2. Define the condition (the meaning of the ranking scale or
   terminology are included):

3. Record the ranking: The ranking can be 1) charted and
   transferred to a graph, similar to the exercises in Figures 3
   through 7, 2) it can be charted on a data collection form
   without graphing, or 3) or the ranking can be recorded directly
   on the graph:

Date	Ranking
	1 2 3 4 5 6 7 8 9 10
	1 2 3 4 5 6 7 8 9 10
	1 2 3 4 5 6 7 8 9 10
	1 2 3 4 5 6 7 8 9 10
	1 2 3 4 5 6 7 8 9 10
	1 2 3 4 5 6 7 8 9 10
	1 2 3 4 5 6 7 8 9 10
	1 2 3 4 5 6 7 8 9 10
	1 2 3 4 5 6 7 8 9 10

(If after the first data day, you find the behavior or the
condition was not specific enough, redefine and begin again.)

A graph shows visually what is happening to the behavior you are
recording (although this particular data collection method can be
visual as charted above, without additional graphing).

RECORDING BEHAVIOR: ORDINAL ASSESSMENT

1. Define the behavior: *rate self-esteem*

2. Define the condition (the meaning of the ranking scale or
   terminology are included): *Following A.M. O.T., the
   following scale will be used to self-rate
   esteem. He will turn in the self rating when
   he reports for lunch.*
   1 = Bummer
   3 = Low
   5 = OK
   7 = Good
   10 = Terrific

3. Record the ranking: The ranking can be 1) charted and
   transferred to a graph, similar to the exercises in Figures 3
   through 7, 2) it can be charted on a data collection form
   without graphing, or 3) or the ranking can be recorded directly
   on the graph:

Date	Ranking
8-20	1 2 ③ 4 5 6 7 8 9 10
8-21	1 ② 3 4 5 6 7 8 9 10
8-22	1 2 ③ 4 5 6 7 8 9 10
8-23	1 2 ③ 4 5 6 7 8 9 10
8-24	1 ② 3 4 5 6 7 8 9 10
on pass	1 2 3 4 5 6 7 8 9 10
8-26	1 2 3 ④ 5 6 7 8 9 10
8-27	1 2 3 4 ⑤ 6 7 8 9 10
8-28	1 2 3 4 5 ⑥ 7 8 9 10

(If after the first data day, you find the behavior or the
condition was not specific enough, redefine and begin again.)

A graph shows visually what is happening to the behavior you are
recording (although this particular data collection method can be
visual as charted above, without additional graphing).

Figure 8-8.   Defining the behavior and the condition, and recording and graphing the ranking of behaviors across data days.

BEHAVIORAL OBJECTIVES

Preparation:
    <u>Brief</u> statement of the problem:

    Synthesize the problem into one verb:_____
    (This becomes the target behavior below.)

COMPONENTS OF A MEASURABLE BEHAVIORAL OBJECTIVE:

1. Child _____

2. Behavior (verb)_____

The condition:

3. Setting_____

4. Trainer _____

5. Stimuli _____

The charting:

6. The Criterion (time limit, frequency, number of times/trials, etc.).
    The <u>count</u>.

Re-write the above information into a BEHAVIORAL OBJECTIVE.

Preparation:
    <u>Brief</u> statement of the problem: *Tony rarely gets finger foods to her mouth*

    Synthesize the problem into one verb: *feed*
    (This becomes the target behavior below.)

COMPONENTS OF A MEASURABLE BEHAVIORAL OBJECTIVE:

1. Child *Tony*

2. Behavior (verb) *feed*

The condition:

3. Setting *high chair / home*

4. Trainer *mother*

5. Stimuli *high interest food with supervision*

The charting:

6. The Criterion (time limit, frequency, number of times/trials, etc.).
    The <u>count</u>.
      50% accuracy in 4 of 5 data days (times/trials) by Jan. 1

Re-write the above information into a BEHAVIORAL OBJECTIVE.

    Tony will feed herself high interest finger foods (cheese crackers, animal crackers, etc.) while seated in a high chair at home with her mother supervising, with 50% accuracy in 4 of 5 data days by Jan 1.

Figure 8-9. Defining the components of the behavioral objective, and combining these elements into a statement.

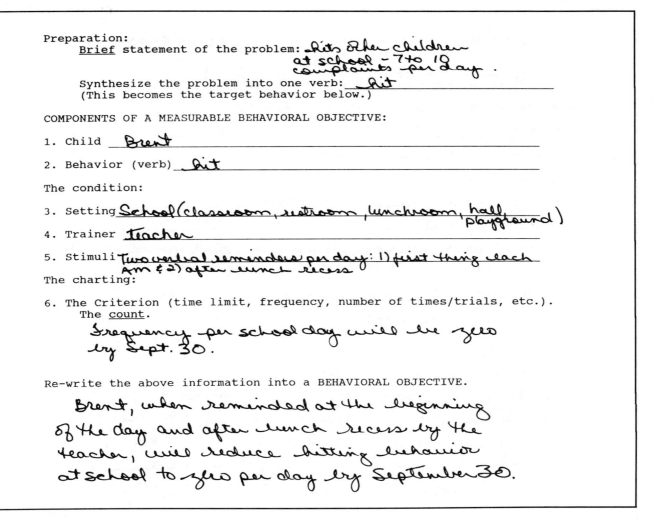

Preparation:
  Brief statement of the problem: _Hits other children at school - 7 to 10 complaints per day._

  Synthesize the problem into one verb: _Hit_
  (This becomes the target behavior below.)

COMPONENTS OF A MEASURABLE BEHAVIORAL OBJECTIVE:

1. Child _Brent_

2. Behavior (verb) _Hit_

The condition:

3. Setting _School (classroom, restroom, lunchroom, hall, playground)_

4. Trainer _Teacher_

5. Stimuli _Two verbal reminders per day: 1) first thing each AM & 2) after lunch recess_
The charting:

6. The Criterion (time limit, frequency, number of times/trials, etc.).
   The count.

   Frequency per school day will be zero by Sept. 30.

Re-write the above information into a BEHAVIORAL OBJECTIVE.

  Brent, when reminded at the beginning of the day and after lunch recess by the teacher, will reduce hitting behavior at school to zero per day by September 30.

Figure 8-9. *Continued.*

to be made available, although the SEA's interpretation and implementation varies. Therefore, it is important for occupational therapists to not only become familiar with the federal law and regulations, but also to obtain a copy of their state and local guidelines regulating special education services.

The movement of occupational therapists into the public school system occurred, not as a chance happening, but as an occurrence which followed major social and philosophical changes in the role of the federal government in education. Providing an appropriate education in America was originally the responsibility of parents and local communities. Exploration of pertinent legislation comes to life when one appreciates the real life dramas leading up to the laws, and the actual changes they facilitate.

Occupational therapists' posture in school settings is a direct result of the Civil Rights Movement of the 1960's. According to Turnbull and Turnbull (1982), Congress incorporated into PL 94-142 points which are direct conclusions of court rulings, involving specific children's rights. This historical perspective is important, as therapists continue to advocate for the rights of the handicapped children who make up their caseloads in school settings.

Prior to PL 94-142, in 1973, there were 950 occupational therapists working in the public schools. By 1978 (post-PL 94-142), 2,500 occupational therapists were in the schools (Gilfoyle, 1981); and by 1986 approximately 5,900 occupational therapists were at work in school settings (American Occupational Therapy Association, 1988). The implementation of the Rules and Regulations for PL 99-457, mandating intervention for children with handicaps, between the ages of 0–3, is similarly affecting intervention models and documentation standards. Individual Family Service Plans are documents which guide service provision for this younger age group.

Mandates

Legal mandates brought an increasing number of occupational therapists into school settings, and documentation of occupational therapy services must demonstrate that the law is being followed. Occupational therapy documentation, as well as service provision itself, had to shift in this setting from a medical model to an educational model. Documentation in the school setting must provide data to clearly dis-

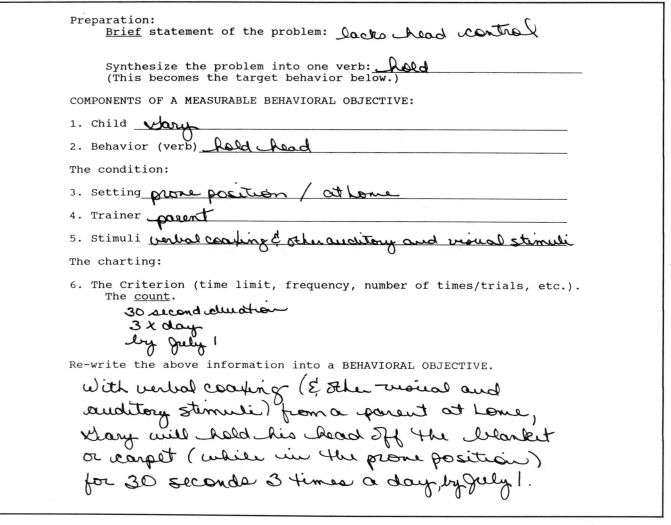

```
Preparation:
    Brief statement of the problem: lacks head control

    Synthesize the problem into one verb: hold
    (This becomes the target behavior below.)

COMPONENTS OF A MEASURABLE BEHAVIORAL OBJECTIVE:

1. Child  Mary
2. Behavior (verb) hold head

The condition:

3. Setting prone position / at home
4. Trainer parent
5. Stimuli verbal coaching & other auditory and visual stimuli

The charting:

6. The Criterion (time limit, frequency, number of times/trials, etc.).
    The count.
        30 second duration
        3 x day
        by July 1

Re-write the above information into a BEHAVIORAL OBJECTIVE.

    With verbal coaching (& other visual and
    auditory stimuli) from a parent at home,
    Mary will hold his head off the blanket
    or carpet (while in the prone position)
    for 30 seconds 3 times a day, by July 1.
```

Figure 8-9. *Continued.*

tinguish occupational therapy's role as a **related service** for the school-aged child. Occupational therapy in an educational setting includes: improving, developing, or restoring functions impaired or lost through illness, injury, or deprivation; improving ability to perform tasks for independent functioning when functions are impaired or lost; and presenting, through early intervention, initial or further impairment or loss of function (Rules and Regulations, 1977). Documentation in the schools must show that occupational therapy services fall within these parameters. As a related service, occupational therapy's role is to maximize the child's ability to benefit from special education.

Every handicapped school aged child must have an Individualized Education Program (IEP) to receive special services in school settings. The IEP, as mandated, has two main parts: 1) the IEP meeting, and 2) the IEP document. The concepts of the IEP meeting and the IEP document were perhaps more foreign to the education community, than to those with a history in the medical model. They are in essence: 1) the team meeting, and 2) the team treatment plan

and progress/discharge note. Occupational therapists are not required by law to be present at the IEP meeting, although it is optimal. The plan is to be a collaborative one. If unable to attend the IEP meeting, occupational therapists must send a report with assessment findings and recommendations relative to services and time commitment (Turnbull & Turnbull, 1982).

a) The IEP meeting serves as a communication vehicle between parents and school personnel, and enables them, as equal participants, to jointly decide what the child's needs are, what services will be provided to meet those needs, and what the anticipated outcomes may be.

b) The IEP process provides an opportunity for resolving any differences between the parents and the agency concerning a handicapped child's special education needs; first, through the IEP meeting, second, if necessary, through the procedural protections that are available to the parents.

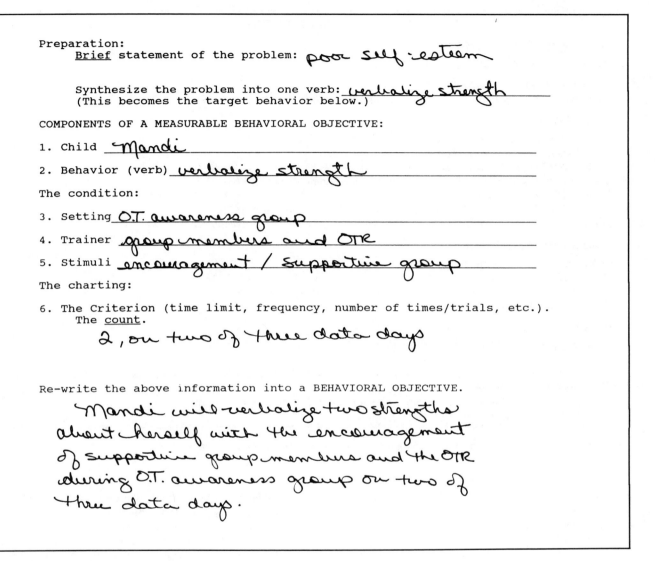

Preparation:
Brief statement of the problem: *poor self-esteem*

Synthesize the problem into one verb: *verbalize strength*
(This becomes the target behavior below.)

COMPONENTS OF A MEASURABLE BEHAVIORAL OBJECTIVE:

1. Child *Mandi*
2. Behavior (verb) *verbalize strength*

The condition:

3. Setting *O.T. awareness group*
4. Trainer *group members and OTR*
5. Stimuli *encouragement / supportive group*

The charting:

6. The Criterion (time limit, frequency, number of times/trials, etc.).
The count.

2, on two of three data days

Re-write the above information into a BEHAVIORAL OBJECTIVE.

Mandi will verbalize two strengths about herself with the encouragement of supportive group members and the OTR during O.T. awareness group on two of three data days.

Figure 8-9. *Continued.*

c) The IEP sets forth in writing a commitment of resources necessary to enable a handicapped child to receive needed special education and related services.
d) The IEP is a management tool that is used to ensure that each handicapped child is provided special education and related services appropriate to the child's special learning needs.
e) The IEP is a compliance/monitoring document, which may be used by authorized monitoring personnel from each governmental level, to determine whether a handicapped child is actually receiving the free appropriate public education agreed to by the parents and the school.
f) The IEP serves as an evaluation device for use in determining the extent of the child's progress toward meeting the projected outcomes ("Assistance to States", p. 5462).

The Rules and Regulations for PL 99-457, in clarifying and defining the Individualized Family Service Plan (IFSP) for infants, toddlers and their families, constitutes a collaborative planning process. The IFSP emphasizes family-centered care. Occupational therapists in early intervention and school settings will face a challenge and an exciting task, as they maintain an informed status, advocate for families, and implement their own states' interpretation of these mandates. AOTA's *Guidelines for Occupational Therapy Services in Early Intervention and Preschool Services* (1989b) provides a copy of the 1986 Amendments to the Education of the Handicapped Act, historical information, and specific implementation guides.

Implementation

In comparing IEP documents from LEA to LEA, many different forms are found, with a trend toward computerization. On first glance, it may appear that there are no similarities. However, if one looks closely, the following elements are noted in all IEP documents, as they are mandated by the

---

AOTA DOCUMENTS

	Source*
ROLES/FUNCTIONS PAPERS	
Roles/Functions of OT in Mental Health, 1985	1, 2
OFFICIAL POSITION PAPERS	
OT Services in Early Intervention and Pre-school Services, 1988	1
STANDARDS	
OT Product Output Reporting System & Uniform Terminology, 1979	1, 2
Standards of Practice for Occupational Therapy, 1979	1, 2
Standards of Practice for OT Services in Schools, 1987	1, 2
Standards of Practice for OT Services for the Developmentally Disabled, 1979	1, 2
Standards of Practice for OT Services in a Home Health Program, 1979	1, 2
Standards of Practice for OT Services in a Mental Health Program, 1979	1, 2
Standards of Practice for OT Services for Clients with Physical Disabilities, 1979	1, 2
GUIDELINES/HIERARCHIES	
Guidelines to OT Documentation, 1986	1, 2
Guidelines for OT Services in Early Intervention and Preschool Services, 1988	3
Guidelines for Occupational Therapy Services in School Systems, 2nd ed, 1989	3
Home Health Guidelines, 1987	3
OTHER	
Payment for Occupational Therapy Services, 1988	3

*1 = *Reference Manual of Official Documents of the American Occupational Therapy Association, Inc.* (Available for AOTA Products).
*2 = *December archival issues of American Journal of Occupational Therapy.*
*3 = Available for purchase from AOTA Products.

Figure 8-10.   AOTA Documents relative to regulations and the documentation process.

law's regulations: 1) Current levels of performance; 2) Annual goals and short term objectives; 3) Special education and the related services involvement, as well as the extent of participation in the regular classroom; 4) Amount of regular classroom placement; 5) Projected dates for initiation and anticipated duration of services; and 6) Evaluation procedures criteria, and schedules for measuring objectives on at least an annual basis (Turnbull & Turnbull, 1982). Appendix C provides diverse examples with elements 1–6 labeled.

Remember that the IEP is actually a process (team meeting) *and* a document (written team treatment and monitoring plan). The IEP document must flow from the process. Although the six mandated elements are relatively self-explanatory, the process is less concrete. The actual identification and implementation of the IEP elements (i.e., annual goals, short term objectives, intervention plans) call for attention not only to the letter of the law, but to the spirit of the law. Optimally, this mechanism will structure the team's collaboration, so that team members provide the particular expertise of their professions. The process can facilitate perception of the child as a whole person. It is not optimal to consider the child as a constellation of unrelated problems (i.e., language problems, educational problems, coordination problems, emotional needs, dietary deficits, cognitive limitations, etc.). The spirit of the law calls for the team's cooperative effort to arrive at annual child-centered goals. Although an annual goal may

relate primarily to a particular discipline, more often it will be impacted by more than one service.

Team members' contributions interface with each other at various times in the IEP process. Figure 8-11 illustrates, via flow chart, the program planning process. The team collaborates from the beginning, as a problem is identified (Step 1) and data is gathered and remediation is attempted within the classroom, in an attempt to circumvent a full team evaluation (Steps 2 and 3).

States typically provide a structured process to maximize opportunities for a child's classroom success, prior to providing a costly and time-consuming full team evaluation. It is important for occupational therapists to know their LEA's and SEA's pre-assessment policies, as they may be asked to provide ideas for simple classroom adaptations, as a means to circumvent educational problems which might otherwise lead to a full team evaluation and more invasive intervention and restrictive environments. Examples of pre-assessment suggestions may be found in Figure 2-14 in the chapter on screening. Some LEA's or SEA's provide specific documentation guidelines for the pre-assessment procedures. In other settings it may be less formal, but it is important for the occupational therapist to produce a good paper trail of classroom adaptations and strategies attempted prior to full team evaluation. Documentation of the successful approaches taken will serve as good resources for future children. However, if

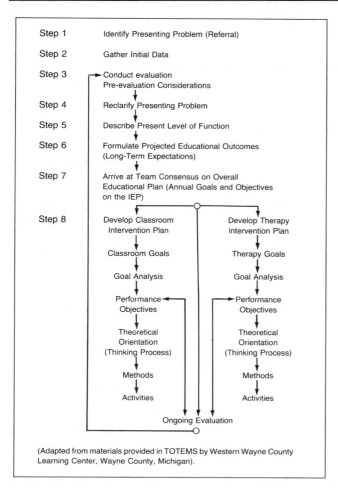

Step 1	Identify Presenting Problem (Referral)
Step 2	Gather Initial Data
Step 3	Conduct evaluation Pre-evaluation Considerations
Step 4	Reclarify Presenting Problem
Step 5	Describe Present Level of Function
Step 6	Formulate Projected Educational Outcomes (Long-Term Expectations)
Step 7	Arrive at Team Consensus on Overall Educational Plan (Annual Goals and Objectives on the IEP)
Step 8	Develop Classroom — Develop Therapy Intervention Plan — Intervention Plan Classroom Goals — Therapy Goals Goal Analysis — Goal Analysis Performance Objectives — Performance Objectives Theoretical Orientation (Thinking Process) — Theoretical Orientation (Thinking Process) Methods — Methods Activities — Activities Ongoing Evaluation

(Adapted from materials provided in TOTEMS by Western Wayne County Learning Center, Wayne County, Michigan).

Figure 8-11.   Steps in the program planning process. *Note: from Development of the Individualized Education Program and Occupational Therapy Intervention Plans (p. 8-3) by W. Dunn, in AOTA's Guidelines for Occupational Therapy Services in School Systems. Reprinted by permission.*

the pre-assessment suggestions do not eliminate the need for a full team assessment, the responses of the child to the adaptations will provide useful data for further planning.

One of PL 94-142's key elements is the proviso that children be placed in the least restrictive environment. Children with handicaps are to be integrated into settings with the non-handicapped population whenever possible. Settings for children with handicaps are to be as similar as possible to those settings provided for the non-handicapped students. Issues which continue to evoke controversy, include the relative importance of the student's academic achievement, social achievement, self concept, acceptance by peers who are non-handicapped, teacher attitudes, and integration into the community. Most LEA's and SEA's determine a continuum or cascade of services, with a ranking of least invasive to most restrictive. Placement of the child in the most "appropriate" setting continues to be a much-debated issue.

When the problem is not resolved via the pre-assessment attempts, team members are called upon to reclarify the pre-

senting problems, to determine what assessments are most appropriate for the child; and following evaluation (formal and informal) to describe the present level of function from their professional perspectives (Steps 4 and 5 in Figure 8-11). Once a child has been provided a full team assessment, and has been diagnosed, an IEP meeting must occur within 30 days. Areas of strength and weakness are reported as the team formulates long term objectives (Step 6). The annual goals (AG) and short term objectives (STO) are part of the IEP document prepared by the team, and must be stated so that there is no doubt in the mind of the reader that they are educationally relevant. Annual goals (AG) are statements which describe reasonable outcomes for a twelve month period. Short term objectives (STO) are logical intermediate steps between the current levels of performance and the annual goals. Note that Step 7 is the point at which the six mandated IEP elements are finalized (current levels of performance, annual goals and short term objectives, special education and the related services involvement and regular classroom placement, projected dates, and evaluation criteria and schedules for measuring objectives on at least an annual basis). However, note in Step 8, that each discipline, in establishing its intervention plan, is also responsible for establishing performance objectives (measurable behavioral objectives) to achieve the goals. Intervention plans are written by each discipline and flow from the STO's.

Whether the LEA's format lists AG's and STO's on separate pages, or sequentially together, it should be apparent that the STO's logically lead to the attainment of the AG's. It should also be apparent that each discipline's intervention plan leads to the attainment of the STO's. (The skills presented in Figures 8-1–8-9 are preparation for the writing of STO's and discipline-specific performance objectives.) Figure 8-12 provides a few examples of short term objectives and annual goals. LEA's may dictate a particular format to which you must adhere. Recently, schools have implemented the use of computerized IEPs. These programs can be very helpful in streamlining the documentation process. They do not relinquish the professional's responsibility to ensure that the writing represents the individualized needs of the child. Therapists frequently need to add objectives, sentences and paragraphs to these programs to complete the links from performance-component needs to functional performance of life tasks.

The IFSP must contain the following elements (Johnson, McGonigel and Kaufmann, 1989): a. present levels of function based on acceptable objective criteria; b. a statement of family strengths and needs; c. criteria, procedures and timelines for expected outcomes; d. a list of needed early intervention services; e. dates of initiation and anticipated duration of services; f. name of the case manager; and g. a transition plan when the child and family are moving to a new service. The family focus is evident in these criteria, and set the stage for further growth in collaborative efforts among agencies, professionals and families.

In summary, the occupational therapist participates in the IEP and IFSP processes as a team member and service provider. The occupational therapist's documentation style must conform to the agency's interpretation of state and federal guidelines.

ANNUAL GOALS (AG) AND SHORT-TERM OBJECTIVES (STO)

AG: To increase self-help skills

STO: Given a regular school lunch, the student will feed herself, requiring assistance only for the opening of packages, and the cutting of meat, in 8 of 10 meals.

STO: Given a 5 minute head start, the student will put on her own coat in time for recess and school dismissal in 9 of 10 attempts.

STO: Given assistance with buckles, but not zippers, the student will manage toiletting in 5 minutes or less in 8 of 10 attempts.

STO: Given no prompts, the student will self-initiate her toileting needs 100% of the time by the end of the first quarter.

AG: To increase fine motor skills.

STO: Given a set of one inch blocks, the student will stack 10 of them in a vertical position in 8 of 10 attempts in 60 seconds.

STO: Given a pencil, the student will imitate 10 specific geometric shapes in 9 of 10 attempts in 60 seconds.

STO: Given regular blunt nose scissors, the student will cut a circle 6 inches in diameter without leaving the line more than ½ inch in 2 minutes by the end of the first semester.

AG: Increase gross motor skills.

STO: Given a wide range of sensorimotor experiences over a nine week period, the student will be able to walk between standard rows of desks independently without bumping a desk on either side in 10 of 10 attempts by the end of the first quarter.

STO: Given no assistance, the student will be able to remove a book from any of the four bottom library shelves in 8 of 10 attempts.

STO: Given no assistance, the student will be able to climb a full flight of stairs (minimum of 10 steps) in 3 minutes, in 10 of 10 attempts.

Figure 8-12. Sample Annual Goals and Short-Term Objectives.

DOCUMENTATION IN HOSPITALS

Audience

Occupational therapists working in hospitals are also guided in their written work by regulations. The Joint Commission of Accreditation of Hospitals Organization (JCAHO) is the major accrediting body, with most state licensing boards requiring acute care facilities to be JCAHO accredited. Third party reimbursing agencies, both public and private, have come to rely upon JCAHO standards. Rehabilitation hospitals and rehabilitation units are accredited by the Commission on Accreditation of Rehabilitation Facilities (CARF).

Brief History

Even before the creation of the Joint Commission of the Accreditation of Hospitals (JCAH) in 1951, many hospitals had joined together for voluntary monitoring to assure quality health care. By 1955 JCAH had instituted a widespread audit method for increasing accountability. During the 1960's and 1970's, the federal government became increasingly involved in hospital regulations, and it was mandated that hospitals be JCAH accredited to participate in Medicare.

In 1972 the Professional Standards Review Organizations (PSRO) were established to set up local peer review groups to monitor health care. By 1974 this audit method had become sophisticated, based primarily on outcome measures. The Peer Review Improvement Act of 1982 called for the establishment of Peer Review Organizations (PRO). This law mandated that, by 1984, each state was to establish a single PRO (Joe, 1985).

Entering the 1980's, even though hospitals had become sophisticated in their record keeping, there was a question about the relationship between good documentation and good medical care. Accountability methods for determining quality and appropriate patient care evolved through the years; presently there is an emphasis on quality assurance (QA) monitors. Centers continually tailor their documentation techniques to facilitate compliance with JCAHO monitoring standards.

The current system encourages concurrent, rather than retrospective report monitoring. The goal of QA monitoring is not to simply report data, but to instigate improvement. The purpose of the data collected for QA is to make a particular thing happen (Bair and Gray, 1985).

As data collection systems improve, therapists are better prepared not only to increase the quality of intervention, but also to demonstrate within diagnostic categories of patients, the efficacy of intervention. Appendix D presents sources which document the difference made by occupational therapy intervention with a variety of diagnoses, as well as some practical resources. Pediatric therapists are encouraged to gather similar information, to establish a data base regarding the impact of occupational therapy's intervention upon the quality of life of children with common pediatric diagnoses.

Reimbursement for occupational therapy services by major insurance carriers also has a rich history, and critical issues continue to evolve with the complexities of health care delivery. Occupational therapists, therefore, have a critical role to play in an ethical sense, to increase the cost-effectiveness of intervention and, in an advocacy sense, to help individuals and their families to get their needs met.

Mandates

The significance of JCAHO standards cannot be overemphasized. Not only do JCAHO standards establish the criteria for hospital accreditation, they also serve as a model for a variety of reimbursement agencies and federal reimbursement programs.

JCAHO publishes an *Accreditation Manual for Hospitals*. Occupational therapists may typically obtain the most current edition of this document in the office of their institution's medical records department or medical library.

Occupational therapy services are defined by JCAHO as "services provided for goal-directed, purposeful activity to aid in the development of adaptive skills and performance capacities by individuals of all ages who have physical disabilities and related psychological impairment(s). Such therapy is designed to maximize independence, prevent further disability, and maintain health" (JCAHO, 1988, p. 197). According to this agency, occupational therapy practice includes, but is not limited to: 1) the assessment and treatment of occupational performance (independent living skills, prevocational/work adjustment, educational skills, play/leisure abilities, and social skills), performance components (neuromuscular, sensori-integrative, cognitive, and psychosocial skills); 2) therapeutic interventions, adaptations, and prevention; and 3) individual evaluations of performance based on observations of individual or group tasks, standardized tests, record review, interviews, and activity histories. Occupational therapy treatment goals are achieved through the use of techniques which include (but are not listed to): 1) task oriented activities (simulation or actual practice of work, self care, leisure and social skills and their components, or the use of creative media, games, computers, and other equipment); 2) prevocational activities; 3) sensorimotor activities; 4) patient/family counseling and education; 5) fabrication or guidance in the use of orthotic devices; 6) adaptation of the environment; 7) body mechanics/joint protection; and 8) positioning (JCAHO, 1988).

Providing services outside the scope of the practice described, or not documenting thoroughly, can jeopardize accreditation. Furthermore, since many reimbursement agencies model their guidelines on JCAHO standards, noncompliance can jeopardize reimbursement.

The Commission for the Accreditation of Rehabilitation Facilities (CARF) was established at a time when rehabilitation, following the acute medical stage, more often occurred in a facility outside the hospital. Although rehabilitation services are currently provided in both models (free standing rehabilitation setting and rehabilitation unit within a hospital setting), the free standing rehabilitation setting is most often accredited by CARF, whereas the rehabilitation unit in the hospital setting will need JCAHO accreditation (because it is part of the hospital). JCAHO provides specific standards for

a rehabilitation unit. Rehabilitation units also attempt to meet federal requirements which allow them to be exempt from the acute care Diagnostic Related Group (DRG) requirements, as a rehabilitation patient's length of stay is usually extended. These procedures also have particular documentation requirements for therapists, relative to content and therapy time per day. Rehabilitation units within hospitals may also elect to apply for CARF accreditation, to improve their status for purposes of public relations and reimbursement.

JCAHO Standards relative to occupational therapy services, and documentation in general rehabilitation, rehabilitation units, psychiatric units, home health, and institutions for clients with mental retardation or psychiatric problems, as well as quality assurance guidelines, are available in the *Accreditation Manual for Hospitals*. CARF standards relative to documentation in these facilities should also be reviewed.

It is impossible to outline the mandates of third party reimbursers, because specific requirements vary from one company to another, and even within the same company from one state to another, or from one particular plan to the next. However, some common points to keep in mind will be included in the next section.

Implementation

Hospital-based occupational therapists must attend to the specific guidelines regarding the scope of occupational therapy practice, record keeping guidelines, and the mandates of quality assurance monitoring. Occupational therapists in hospital settings should align their medical records procedures with the JCAHO standards, and check for compliance point by point.

The most widely accepted documentation systems in hospital settings are based upon a problem-oriented medical record (POMR) system (Berni & Readey, 1978; Kuntavanish, 1987). SOAP notes are one type of problem oriented medical record (Kettenbach, 1990). SOAP notes provide for a tracking of specific problems, as sequential records attend to the subjective data (what the patient said), objective data (what you observe, formal and informal tests), assessment (professional opinion), and plan (next steps), of specific patient problems.

The POMR may be written in forms other than a SOAP note. Two types of POMR (SOAP note and non-SOAP POMR) documentation are in Appendix F. The more quantifiable the data, the more useful they are as quality assurance monitors. The more functional the data, the more clearly they will pass reimbursing criteria.

"Designing a quality assurance monitor requires designation of the activity, its objectives, measurable criteria, data sources, frequency of monitoring, and responsibility for monitoring and reporting" (Bair and Gray, 1985). Through QA monitoring, measurable improvement can be documented, and ideas may be generated for the establishment of additional standards. There are a variety of methods for the establishment of monitors. Because most rehabilitation departments are accustomed to a medical record system which is patient-problem based, many occupational therapy departments utilize problem-based quality assurance. The steps involve an analysis of an aggregate of data to: 1) identify the

---

SAMPLE QUALITY ASSURANCE (QA) MONITORS

The problems identified in this figure are examples and are in no way a thorough or exhaustive list.

1. PROBLEM IDENTIFICATION AND STANDARD SETTING (continuous-monitoring system).
   a. Initial intake evaluation will be performed and documented within two days of receiving referral. Standard: 95%. Frequency: quarterly. Monitors: secretary/concurrent audit.
   b. The problems identified and goals established are consistent with the physician's orders. Standard: 100%. Frequency: quarterly. Monitors: secretary/concurrent audit.
   c. The problems identified and goals established are consistent with the patient's goals. Standard: 90%. Frequency: quarterly. Monitors: O.T. coordinator observation and documentation at weekly team meetings.
   d. Evaluation addressed all elements of diagnosis per established departmental criteria. Standard: 95%. Frequency: quarterly. Monitors: secretary/concurrent audit.
   e. The goals are based upon evaluation results. Standard: 95%. Frequency: quarterly. Monitor: O.T. coordinator audit.
   f. The problems identified are measurable. Standard: 100%. Frequency: quarterly. Monitors: O.T. coordinator observation and documentation at weekly team meetings.

2. PROBLEM MEASUREMENT (continuous monitoring system)
   a. Documentation of progress or lack of progress is recorded in the patient chart every 5 to 7 days. Standard: 95%. Frequency: quarterly. Monitors: Secretary/concurrent audit.
   b. Documentation of patient progress is understandable to other team members. Standard: 95%. Frequency: quarterly. Monitors: O.T. coordinator concurrent audit at weekly team meetings.
   c. Documentation reflects the patient's functional status. Standard: 95%. Frequency: quarterly. Monitors: O.T. coordinator concurrent audit at weekly team meetings.

3. IMPROVEMENT PLANNING (analysis of continuous monitors)
   a. Were standards met? Were they realistic?
   b. Did analysis of monitors uncover another problem that warrants monitoring?
   c. Were those responsible for recording/auditing monitors on-task?
   d. Was frequency of monitoring maintained?

4. IMPLEMENTATION OF AN IMPROVEMENT PLAN (reestablishment of quality assurance monitors or quality indicators)
   a. Specific tasks are established to ensure the meeting of standards not met (i.e., staff inservice, revision of documentation protocol sheets, specific instruction to particular staff in non-compliance, revision of monitor [indicator] to make it more measurable, assign monitor to more appropriate personnel, etc.).
   b. Monitors which have met the standards can be deleted.
   c. New monitors addressing other possible problems are established.
      1) Restate continuing monitors and define new monitors.
      2) Establish acceptable standards.
      3) Define means and personnel responsible for monitoring.
      4) Determine frequency for formal monitoring of each indicator (monitor).

5. MEASUREMENT TO DETERMINE WHETHER STANDARDS HAVE BEEN MET (continuous monitoring system).
   a. Were ongoing and new standards met? Were they realistic?
   b. Did analysis of monitors uncover another problem that warrants monitoring?
   c. Were those responsible for recording/auditing monitors on-task?
   d. Was frequency of monitoring maintained?

Figure 8-13.   Problem-based quality assurance monitors relative to occupational therapy intervention.

problem and establish the standard, 2) measure the problem, 3) plan improvement, 4) implement an improvement plan, and 5) measure to see if the standards have been met (Bair and Gray, 1985, p. 260). Examples of QA monitors which deal with common occupational therapy problems are presented in Figure 8-13. Kuntavanish's (1987) *Occupational Therapy Documentation: A System to Capture Outcome Data for Quality Assurance and Program Promotion*, published by AOTA, provides further concrete examples of medical records and a system for producing quality assurance monitors.

To facilitate reimbursement, the following points should be kept in mind when submitting claims in a medical setting: 1) Include a physician's referral; 2) Attain a referral for a medical problem rather than an educational problem; 3) Report how the child's medical or neurological problem affects learning, adaptive play, and self help skill (include functional activities); and 4) Report services provided as occupational therapy, not neurodevelopmental therapy or sensory integration (Scott, 1988).

DOCUMENTATION IN COMMUNITY SETTINGS

Audience

For whom is the community-based care provider writing? Because accrediting and reimbursement sources vary, (at times even within the same agency), the occupational therapist must carefully explore the agency's regulators.

Reimbursement sources for public health agencies, home health agencies, voluntary agencies, outpatient clinics, private practice, and day care include the Division of Services for Crippled Children (DSCC), private insurance agencies, health maintenance organizations (HMO's), Medicaid, Easter Seals programs, United Way, public schools, and others. According to an informal survey by the Home Health Task Force of AOTA's Commission on Practice, the top three sources are DSCC, private insurance, and HMO's (AOTA, 1987).

Brief History

The provision of rehabilitative services to children on a home health basis, and in other community settings, has grown as a result of a number of social and health care trends. The normalization principle, or the implementation of the deinstitutionalization movement of the early 1970's, has decreased the proportion of children institutionalized, and returned a portion of previously institutionalized children with severe or multiple handicaps to their home communities (Gardner and Chapman, 1985; Flynn and Nitsch, 1980). Because of the cost containment measures instituted in acute care and rehabilitation facilities, patients of all ages are discharged in record time, often taking home with them limited levels of health and independence. The home health and rehabilitative needs of children are, as a result, increasingly dealt with by a variety of types of outpatient and community agencies. Since the mid 1970's and the implementation of PL 94-142's Rules and Regulations, public schools' role has increased relative to the educational and educationally related needs of all children with disabilities, not just children able to attend a classroom.

Mandates and Implementation

Division of Services for Crippled Children (DSCC) guidelines are mandated as part of Title V of the Social Security Act of 1935. Federal funds are available for the infant to 21-year-old who has chronic organic diseases or conditions that may interfere with normal growth and development. Each state submits a program plan to the federal government to become eligible for payments. The programs are state administered. Crippled Children's services are approved after other resources have been exhausted. Occupational therapists employed by hospitals to provide community services, should know the JCAHO Standards relative to Home Care Services (HC).

Medicaid guidelines are also state-specific, within federal guidelines, and therefore cannot be generalized from state to state. Medicaid is the second largest national health care expenditure for a single program, second only to Medicare (Scott, 1988). The Medicaid Program (Title XIX of the Social Security Act: Medical Assistance for the Poor) carries the vast responsibility of home health care for low income families. Therapists employed in medicaid-approved agencies should clearly understand the medicaid guide-lines in their state. Occupational therapy, along with physical therapy and speech-language pathology, are not funded in all states (Rourk, 1984).

Those in private practice must explore their state's regulations relative to record keeping. Additionally, private practitioners should prepare a printed descriptive document of their particular service. According to Hershman (1984), this document should contain the therapist's professional background, license (if applicable), philosophy of practice, referral system, specific services offered, payment policies, location, office hours, and telephone number. This document should be made available to patients, referring physicians, medical managers, vocational counselors, and third party payers. Because private practitioners are not regulated by a traditional accrediting agency, therapists in private practice may need to be proactive in securing approval for third party payment for their clients, by submitting documents necessary for approval of their practice. Guidelines for service provision and for documentation within public and private agencies which provide community-based services and home visits for children, are typically governed by local, state, or regional boards of directors. Occupational therapists must be knowledgeable about their agency's interpretation of service provision and documentation guidelines.

DOCUMENTATION IN RESIDENTIAL SETTINGS

Audience

For whom do those in residential settings write? Documentation in residential settings is strictly regulated by federal and state laws. Those who are least able to care for their own needs are more strictly protected by legal mandates. Federal legislation has, in fact, created an advocacy system for this population.

Brief History

The deinstitutionalization movement which was brought about by the normalization principle of the 1970's, not only decreased the proportion of children in institutions, but also increased the regulations governing those who remained in residential settings. Normalization is "the utilization of means which are as culturally normative as possible, in order to establish or maintain personal behaviors and characteristics which are as culturally normative as possible" (Gardner & Chapman, 1985). This movement has led to an intensive effort to protect the civil rights of those placed in residential facilities. Residential facilities serving children are primarily care facilities for those with severe cognitive or mental health deficits, with particular programs designed for individuals with mental retardation or psychiatric diagnoses. As community support increases for persons to live, learn, work and play within regular environments, institutions will no longer be needed.

Mandates and Implementation

Residential facilities, whether public or private, must comply with federal guidelines, as administered by the state. The three major federal laws protecting children in residential settings are: 1) the Rehabilitation Act of 1973 (PL 93-112), 2) the Developmental Disabilities Assistance and Bill of Rights

Act (PL 94-103) and the Developmental Disabilities Act of 1984 (PL 98-527), and 3) the Education for All Handicapped Children Act (PL 94-142).

The Rehabilitation Act of 1973 serves to protect the civil rights of persons with handicaps. It requires educational programs to make reasonable accommodation to meet the needs of special populations.

The Developmental Disabilities Act of 1970 was revised in 1978 to provide a functional definition of developmental disabilities. Because children in residential settings typically have severe or multiple handicaps which interfere with functional performance, and because occupational therapists are well prepared to document functional performance, the occupational therapist's documentation is crucial in documenting the severity of the problem and it's affect on performance. This documentation may impact the qualification for services. Under this Act, one is developmentally disabled if he or she has mental or physical impairment or a combination of mental and physical impairment, which is manifested before the person attains the age of 22 and is likely to continue indefinitely, resulting in function limitation in three or more of the following areas: self care, receptive and expressive language, learning, mobility, self-direction, capacity for independent living, and economic self-sufficiency (Gardner & Chapman, 1985). The Developmental Disabilities Act of 1984, PL 98-527, prohibits the use of federal funds in residential programs which do not meet certain standards. It provides a structure under which State Plans must be organized, including a plan for record-keeping and auditing.

The mandates of PL 94-142 have been thoroughly discussed. LEA's clearly bear responsibilities in providing special education programs. The mechanisms whereby the LEA's assist with their educational responsibilities toward those in residential care facilities vary from state to state.

Medicaid guidelines play a major role in the documentation procedures in residential care facilities. Those serving intermediate care facilities for individuals with mental retardation "must develop and maintain a record keeping system that includes a separate record for each client and that documents the client's health care, active treatment, social information, and protection of the client's rights" (Conditions of Participation for Long Term Care Facilities, June 3, 1988). This mandate, from Part 483 of the Department of Health and Human Services Health Care Financing Administration; Medicaid Program; Conditions for Intermediate Care Facilities for the Mentally Retarded; Final Rule, set specific standards for client records, services provided with outside sources, and protection of the patient's rights relative to his finances, staff treatment and qualifications, services provided, living environment, privacy, etc.

Those working in residential facilities for individuals with mental retardation are advised to be familiar with the content of the federal mandates, and the facility's guidelines in implementing them relative to therapy programming and documentation. Furthermore, therapists are advised to inquire about the facility's accreditation body. Is it accredited by the Accreditation Council on Services for People with Developmental Disabilities (ACDD), the Division of Services for Crippled Children (DSCC), the Joint Commission for the Accreditation of Hospitals Organization (JCAHO) or other accrediting agencies? Updated documentation guidelines must be as-

certained, as well as the facility's procedures to meet the guidelines.

In order to serve as advocates for children and adolescents, occupational therapists working in residential settings need to be well informed regarding reimbursement. Are documentation standards affected by particular public funding requirements or third-party reimbursement requirements? The documentation format must be that which is in the best interest of the child being served.

Similarly, those who serve public or private residential settings for children and adolescents with mental health diagnoses should be informed of current legislation. Not only must the state implementation of federal rules and regulations be followed, but also the accrediting standards must be met (typically Joint Commission on the Accreditation of Hospitals Organization or the Commission on Accreditation of Rehabilitation Facilities). As always, attention must be given to the diversity of payors and their expectations. Depending on the structure of the facility, the financial responsibility may reside with a county or state agency, special interest group, or private funds.

LEGAL CONSIDERATIONS

All health-related professionals have been sensitized to the need to understand the legal framework in which they function, by the rising number of malpractice litigations against physicians. Likewise, those practicing in the education arena are seeing due process being exercised by families who become knowledgeable about their legal rights. Cohen (1986) described occupational therapists as being among those professionals who have "taken cognizance of the foreboding constellation of societal factors that may make them more vulnerable than ever before to the receipt of a summons and complaint alleging malpractice."

Article Five of the Constitution declares that "no person shall be . . . deprived of life, liberty, or property without due process of law." Due process has been further defined in the Bill of Rights. These rights are guaranteed to all U.S. citizens. As described herein and in more detail in Chapter Ten, a number of statutory rights result from laws which have been enacted specifically to protect children, and in some cases, particularly to protect children with handicaps. Protection guaranteed through this legislative process may change as the laws are changed. Rules and regulations developed to implement legislation are also a part of statutory law. People are entitled to constitutional and statutory rights, unless through a due process procedure in court, the rights are restricted. To ensure conformity with laws and regulations, many accrediting agencies and/or individual facilities have developed policies and procedures.

In addition to the laws discussed under the specific intervention models, pediatric therapists need to be aware that all states currently have laws which specify a mandate to report children who are suspect of abuse. This usually pertains not only to physical and sexual abuse, but also mental suffering and neglect (Heymann, 1986). In most states, the reporter is provided with immunity, and failure to report will incur criminal penalties.

Occupational therapists are advised, and often are required to be protected by malpractice insurance. The basis of a

1. Timeliness: Keep records following the established time guidelines. ANYTHING you think may be relevant should be documented as close to the time it happened as possible.
2. Sign and date all entries.
3. Write legibly and completely, using only approved abbreviations.
4. Make all entries permanent (black pen is preferred).
5. Make alterations carefully. Draw a thin line through errors, allowing original content to be legible. Date and initial the change. In some cases you may need to have a correction witnessed.
6. Avoid gaps, both in content and in format. Write on every line of the record.
7. Be specific and objective. Avoid derogatory remarks about patients and judgmental comments about other professionals or institutions.
8. Avoid unsupported assertions and opinions. Base your documentation upon well founded measurable behavioral objectives.
9. Know what level of professional signature you need on what types of documents (i.e., have student's and COTA's notes co-signed, etc.).
10. Double check your work.

Figure 8-14. Writing for litigation: Guidelines for all documentation, to provide protection if documents are called into court.

lawsuit can arise from a wide variety of perceived impingements on the patient or client's rights, including but not limited to complaints about least restrictive environment, failure to report abuse, confidentiality and privacy, right to refuse service, and lack of informed consent. If served with a summons alleging professional misconduct, therapists are advised to notify their malpractice insurance carrier immediately, and not to discuss or make any documentations relative to the case with anyone, except under the advice of an attorney (Cohen, 1986).

All documentation should be written with this in mind: one's organized thoughts which are transferred into written words may, when least expected be called into court and provide evidence to: 1) protect the rights of patients or clients, or to 2) protect oneself against litigation. Figure 8-14 provides guidelines to keep in mind when writing for litigation.

SUMMARY

Often documentation is perceived as a chore and drudgery that consumes time better spent in productive child-centered activities. This perception regards documentation as an activity separate from "therapy." As activity-oriented professionals, rich in skills of task analysis, occupational therapists are well prepared to organize the documentation process so that it becomes the pulse of intervention. As creative documentation systems attend to the mandates of governmental regulations, accrediting agencies, and the payors, while providing structure for efficacious treatment and team communication, clinical reasoning is facilitated. A regard for the advocacy role played by the regulations which impact documentation, as they protect the rights of children with handicaps (and provide financial coverage of special programs), can lead to a more positive attitude toward documentation and a renewed attempt to meet the imposed guidelines.

Documentation can serve as an opportunity for expression of pride in the profession, as well as confidence in one's therapeutic abilities. Outside referral sources, policy makers, and consumers respond to data which shows in print the efficacy of occupational therapy. Not only are the needs of

the child, the team/family, the payer, and the governmental and accrediting agency best met via good documentation, but documentation also provides an opportunity to promote the profession of occupational therapy.

EXPAND YOUR NEWLY ACQUIRED KNOWLEDGE

1. For each of the following behavior recording systems design a data collection form, collect data for at least one time period, and design a graph for recording data across time: a. duration and frequency, b. duration, c. frequency, d. rate of response, e. times/trials (percent), f. ordinal, and g. nominal.
2. Choose one case from the application chapters (Chapter 4 and 7). Write two measurable behavioral objectives.

References

Acquaviva, F. A., & Malone, R. A. (1981). *The power of positive persuasion.* Laurel, MD: RAMSCO Publishing Company.

Acquaviva, F., & Malone, R. A. (1981). Writing for publication. *The power of positive persuasion* (p. 10). Laurel, MD: RAMSCO Publishing Company.

American Occupational Therapy Association (1986). Guidelines for occupational therapy documentation. *American Journal of Occupational Therapy, 40,* 830–832.

American Occupational Therapy Association (1987). *Guidelines for occupational therapy services in home health.* Rockville, MD: Author.

American Occupational Therapy Association (1987). *Guidelines for occupational therapy services in the school systems.* Rockville, MD: Author.

American Occupational Therapy Association (1988). *Member Data Survey Printout.* Rockville, MD: Author.

American Occupational Therapy Association (1989a). *Uniform Terminology for Occupational Therapy* (2nd ed.). *American Journal of Occupational Therapy, 43,* 808–815.

American Occupational Therapy Association (1989b). *Guidelines for occupational therapy services in early intervention and preschool services.* Rockville, MD: Author.

American Occupational Therapy Association (1989c). *Guidelines for occupational therapy services in school systems* (2nd ed.). Rockville, MD: Author.

Bair, J., & Gray, M. (1985). *The Occupational Therapy Manager.* Rockville, MD: The American Occupational Therapy Association, Inc.

Baum, C. M. (1983). Management of finances, communications, personnel, with resources and documentation. In H. L. Hopkins and H. D. Smith (Eds), *Willard and Spackman's Occupational Therapy* (6th ed.), pp. 815–826. Philadelphia: J. B. Lippincott Company.

Bernie, R., & Readey, H. (1978). *Problem-oriented medical record implementation* (2nd ed.). St. Louis: The C. V. Mosby Company.

Cohen, R. J. (1986). The professional liability of behavioral scientists: An overview. In L. Everstine and D. S. Everstine (Eds.), *Psychotherapy and the Law*, pp. 251–267. New York: Grune & Stratton, Inc.

Conditions of Participation for Long Term Care Facilities, Part 483, Subpart D, Conditions of Participation for Intermediate Care Facilities for the Mentally Retarded (June 3, 1988). *Federal Register, 53*, p. 107.

Department of Education, Office of Special Education and Rehabilitation. (1987). The state vocational rehabilitation services program. (*Federal Register, 52*, (222, 44366–44374, 34 Code of Federal Regulations, Part 361). Washington, D.C.: U.S. Government Printing Office.

Flynn, R. J., & Nitsch, K. E. (1980). *Normalization, social integration, and community services*, Baltimore: University Park Press.

Gardner, J. F., & Chapman, M. S. (1985). *Staff development in mental retardation services: A practical handbook.* Baltimore: Paul H. Brookes Publishing Co.

Gilfoyle, E. M. (1981). *Training: Occupational therapy educational management in schools.* Rockville, MD: The American Occupational Therapy Association, Inc.

Glasnapp, D. R., & Poggio, J. P. (1985). *Essentials of statistical analysis for the behavioral sciences.* Columbus: Charles E. Merrill Publishing Company.

Hargrove, E. C. (1982). Strategies for the implementation of federal education policies: Compliance and incentives. *Peabody Journal of Education, 1*, 20–33.

Hershman, A. G. (1984). Reimbursement in private practice. *American Journal of Occupational Therapy, 38*, 299–306.

Heymann, G. M. (1986). Mandated child abuse reporting and the confidentiality privilege. In L. Everstine and D. S. Everstine (Eds.), *Psychotherapy and the Law*, pp. 146–156. New York: Grune & Stratton, Inc.

Assistance to states for education of handicapped children; Interpretation of the individualized education program (January 19, 1981, Vol 46, No 12). *Federal Register*, p. 5462.

Joe, B. E. (1985). Quality assurance. In J. Bair and M. Gray (Eds.), *The Occupational Therapy Manager*, pp. 251–266. Rockville, MD: The American Occupational Therapy Association, Inc.

Johnson, B. H., McGonigel, M. J., & Kaufmann, R. K. (eds) (1989). Guidelines and Recommended Practices for the Individualized Family Service Plan. Cosponsored by: National Early Childhood Technical Assistance System, Chapel Hill, and Association for the Care of Children's Health, Washington, DC.

Joint Commission on Accreditation of Healthcare Organizations (1988). *Accreditation manual for hospitals, 1989.* Chicago: Author.

Kettenbach, G. (1990). *Writing S.O.A.P. Notes.* Philadelphhia: F. A. Davis Company.

Kleinman, B. L., & Bielkley, B. L. (1982). Some implications of a science of adaptive responses. *American Journal of Occupational Therapy, 36*, 15–19.

Kuntavanish, A. A. (1987). *Occupational therapy documentation: A system to capture outcome data for quality assurance and program promotion.* Rockville, MD: The American Occupational Therapy Association.

Rourke, J. D. (1984). Funding health services for children. *American Journal of Occupational Therapy, 38*, 313–319.

Rules and Regulations (1977). Assistance to States of Education of Handicapped Children. *Federal Register, 42*, (250, 65082–65085). Washington, D.C.: U.S. Department of Health, Education, and Welfare.

Scott, S. J. (ed.) (1988). *Payment for occupational therapy services.* Rockville, MD: American Occupational Therapy Association, Inc.

Tiffany, E. G. (1983). Psychiatry and mental health. In H. L. Hopkins and H. D. Smith (Eds), *Willard and Spackman's Occupational Therapy* (6th ed.), pp. 267–334. Philadelphia: J. B. Lippincott Company.

Turnbull, A. P., Strickland, B., & Brantley, B. (1982). *Developing and implementing education programs* (2nd ed.). Columbus: Charles E. Merrill.

Turnbull, R., & Turnbull, A. (1982). *Free appropriate public education: Law and implementation* (3rd. ed.). Denver: Love Publishing Co.

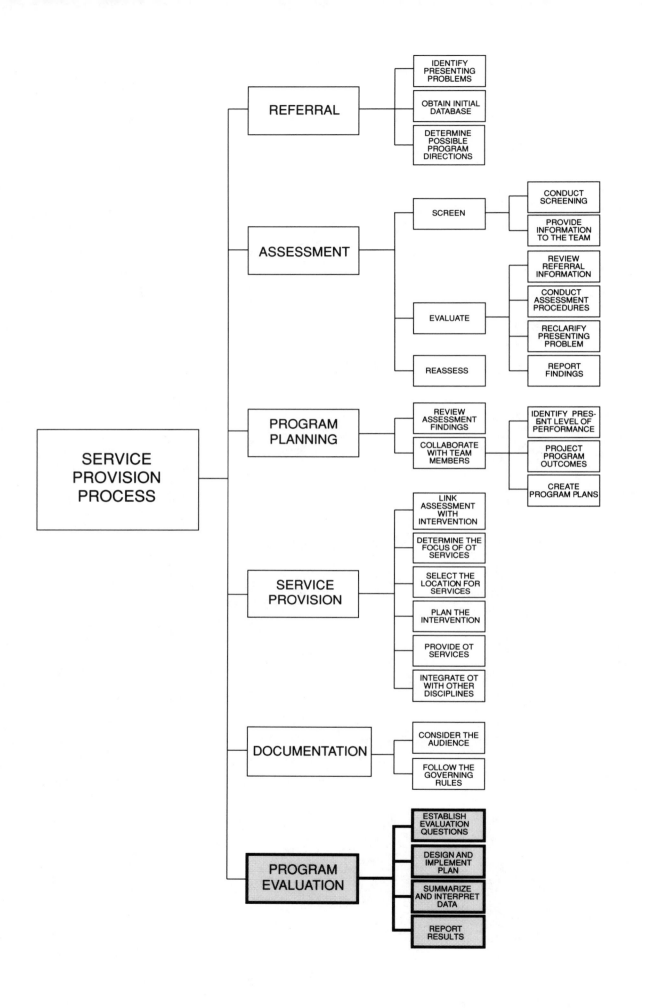

CHAPTER 9

Evaluating Pediatric Occupational Therapy Programs

Philippa H. Campbell, PhD, OTR

"Progress cannot be determined in the abstract. One must ask: Progress towards what? Measured by what? Once a relationship to a target or goal is established, the following qualifiers must be considered: How much change? What kind of change? Therefore, to answer the question, 'What is child progress?' it is first necessary to answer these three questions:

- *What content (e.g., benchmarks of development or standards of performance) is to be measured?*
- *What quantity of change toward acquisition of this content constitutes progress?*
- *What quality of change towards acquisition of this content constitutes progress?"*

Bricker & Gumerlock, 1985

All pediatric occupational therapists are responsible for evaluating children's performance and for planning, implementing, and documenting interventions designed to optimize children's functional skills in home, school, community and work environments (see Section I). Documentation procedures allow therapists to record information about the therapeutic activities used to influence children's performance of target therapy objectives. Information for accrediting and financing agencies is provided through documentation, resulting in a longitudinal information base about each child on a therapist's caseload. Program evaluation procedures, in contrast, are used to provide information about the occupational therapy services as a whole (Shaw, 1985). These procedures either are designed separately from, or are built directly upon documentation methods. Occupational therapy personnel may be involved in collecting data used for program evaluation activities or these data may be collected, summarized and interpreted by supervisory staff, or by other persons who are outside the occupational therapy service system.

Program evaluation studies are conducted for many reasons, and provide information about occupational therapy services that may not be available through other sources (Linder, 1983). The types of information that result from evaluation studies focus on issues such as: a) program impact on different organizations, agencies or individuals including the community-at-large, staff, families or children (Bricker, Sheehan, & Littman, 1981); b) effects of therapy on children's performance in home, school, and community environments (Campbell, 1988); or c) agency-related issues such as effects of inservice training activities on staff performance or staff satisfaction with agency (Linder, 1983). A comprehensive program evaluation consists of one or more individual studies, and occurs when administrators, staff and consumers design an evaluation plan that represents each of the key components of the service system (e.g., Sheehan & Gallagher, 1983; Suarez & Vandivier, 1978). The number of agencies requiring program evaluation activities in addition to documentation of

service provision is growing, but program evaluation is not required as of yet by many agencies such as school systems. Conducting these studies provides valuable information for occupational therapy and other agency personnel, which can be used to improve service provision and provide high quality services for children and families.

The purpose of this chapter is to enable occupational therapists to design and implement procedures to evaluate programs provided for children. Specifically, the chapter outlines procedures to: a) determine and state evaluation questions; b) design and implement an evaluation plan; c) summarize and interpret data; and d) report data and summarize results. Each of these activities is an essential and interrelated component of meaningful program evaluation.

ESTABLISHING EVALUATION QUESTIONS

Program evaluation provides data used to answer specific questions and/or address specifically identified service provision issues. For example, a supervisor or administrator may want to know about staff development activities, or a therapist may be interested in whether or not children perform better under a consultation, or direct service plus consultation service provision model. In the first instance, the supervisor or administrator is using evaluation to determine information about the program function of staff development. In the second instance, a therapist is using evaluation to provide information about the effects of the service provision model on children's performance. Each of these instances results in an examination of one component or function of a total program of occupational therapy.

Components, Goals, and Objectives of Pediatric Programs

Comprehensive program evaluation results when each component of a program has been defined and evaluated. Pediatric service programs as a whole, as well as occupational therapy programs, have various components which relate to the purposes of the program. A component is defined as an individual function of a program, including functions such as staff development, parent activities, service provision, team functioning, supervision, or administration. Each component is further defined by goals and objectives. Program evaluation plans and procedures are derived directly from statements of the program's purpose and from statements of goals and objectives. A first step in beginning to plan for evaluation is to establish or review the written statements of the program's purpose and goals and objectives (Shaw, 1985).

A pediatric occupational therapy program may be organized as one therapist, a private practice of one or more individuals, or a department of personnel, for example, in a school district, early intervention program, or hospital. Goals and objectives for the program as a whole are established in written form by an individual therapist, the members of the department or private practice, or the supervisor or administrator. Program goals define the purpose of the program. The purpose of occupational therapy services, for example, may be to provide high quality services for all identified or referred children. Objectives outline areas of emphasis within a particular goal and may be time-limited. Establishing a school-district-wide screening program to ensure that all eligible children are identified, is an example of an objective that will help the organizational unit attain the overall program purpose and goal of high quality service provision. An objective of identifying ten eligible children per year through the screening program, is an example of a time-limited objective.

Table 9-1 outlines the goals and objectives established for an occupational therapy department in a school-district which serves children from three through 21 years of age. This department has four component functions that define the program's purpose: a) assessment and identification; b) service provision; c) staff development; and d) administration. Table 9-2 outlines the goals and objectives for an early intervention program that includes occupational therapy services, and has six program component functions: a) public awareness and identification; b) family involvement; c) service provision for infants, toddlers, and their families; d) staff development; e) program evaluation; and f) administration. Statements of the program's purpose by component functions underlie design of program evaluation studies. A comprehensive evaluation of the program addresses all defined component functions through program evaluation. Evaluation of an individual component function, separate from all other functions of the program, is also possible when overall program purposes are defined by their individual components.

A process for defining program purposes, establishing component functions and writing goals and objectives is outlined on Figure 9-1a. Goals and objectives that are clearly written, contain only one idea per statement, and include measurable outcomes, are translated easily into program evaluation questions and studies. For example, (figure 9-1b) determining the extent to which ten new referrals per year have been generated, as a result of undertaking a specific public awareness program about pediatric occupational therapy services, is easier to judge than whether a public awareness program has been effective. Objectives that state the desired outcome (e.g., ten new referrals per year), are more

easily incorporated into program evaluation studies than are those where measurable outcomes are not defined. The measurable outcome in a goal or objective statement, establishes a dependent measure by which the activity outlined in the objective will be judged. Dependent or outcome measures are established separately when not included in the goal or objective statement. For example, in order to evaluate the extent to which a program goal of "establishing an effective public awareness effort" was achieved, staff creates measures by which to judge effectiveness. Such measures typically include: a) the percent increase in the number of referrals; b) the percent increase in the number of sources for referrals; c) the number of inquiries made about occupational therapy services; or d) the percent increase in the numbers of children and families receiving services. These dependent measures are determined as part of the process used to establish program components, goals, and objectives, or as the initial step in establishing program evaluation questions.

Evaluation Questions

Goals and objectives that define a program become the basis for formulating questions that can be addressed through program evaluation studies. Questions that derive from the goals and objectives previously illustrated on Tables 9-1 and 9-2 are outlined on Tables 9-3 and 9-4. Those statements that were written to include defined outcomes are easily reworded into evaluation questions. For example, the objective of "establishing a public awareness program that will yield ten new referrals per year," is easily reworded into an evaluation question of: "To what extent does the public awareness program yield ten new referrals per year?". Evaluation questions that specify the desired outcome(s) are written for goals or objectives that do not include the dependent (outcome) measure in their wording.

Use of program goals and objectives as a total basis for program evaluation, limits the possible information gained through evaluation activities. An administrator may be able to document that all staff attended at least three inservice training sessions provided during a school year, but may desire additional information about staff development. The extent to which staff were satisfied with the sessions attended, or the impact of those sessions on staff's ability to provide assessment and intervention services, or to interact with children's families may also be of interest. Evaluative information that is most often needed or desired can be classified into four areas: a) program impact; b) program efficacy; c) program satisfaction; and d) program operation. Evaluative information gained through measuring outcomes of program goals and objectives yields data concerning program operation, whereas separately formulated evaluation questions are needed to address each of the other three areas. Table 9-5 outlines evaluation questions related to impact, efficacy, and satisfaction.

DESIGNING AND IMPLEMENTING A PROGRAM EVALUATION PLAN

Program evaluation is based on studies that address one or more questions, and yield either formative or summative

TABLE 9-1. Goals and Objectives for a School System Occupational Therapy Program for One School Year

Component	Goal	Objectives
Assessment and Identification	Screen all special and regular education students for eligibility	Contact all schools prior to school year to arrange screening program to be conducted for: (a) all special education students; (b) all regular education students. Implement screening protocol for all entering special education students (200 district wide). Implement screening questionnaires with all district regular education teachers (400 district wide) to determine O.T. needs of entering students (900 district wide). Review screening data and develop a schedule for all eligible entering students to receive necessary assessments (estimate 90 consultations; 20 full assessments).
	Complete consultation or child-based assessments for all referred or screened students.	Conduct appropriate assessments for all children identified through screening by November 15.
Service Provision	Provide direct, consultation, monitoring, or combinations of service models for all eligible students.	Schedule all retained students for appropriate provision and initiate services by September 15 (estimate 90 previously enrolled students). Schedule all newly eligible students for appropriate service provision and initiate services by November 30.
	Complete all documentation for all students.	Write an intervention or consultation plan for every student prior to initiation of services. Establish a plan for documenting services provided. Write documentation information for each student, as specified in the plan.
Staff Development	Implement a comprehensive program of inservice training.	Conduct a needs assessment to determine staff interests and areas of strength/weakness. Design a staff development program of inservice training, co-therapy, ourside consultation, or other activities designed to increase knowledge and skill levels of staff. Schedule activities throughout the school year, documenting staff attendance.
	Enable staff to attend outside workshops and conferences.	Develop a policy for attendance at outside workshops or conferences including released time and payment information and procedures for requesting attendance. Communicate policy to staff. Document the number of requests made and number of events attended.
Administration	Implement plan of operation.	Write a plan of operation by September 15 that includes activities, person, and projected time-lines for each of the program objectives. Review the plan monthly in staff meetings. Document monthly accomplishment of activities, any needed changes, or any added activities.
	Coordinate with agency administration.	Meet monthly with agency supervisor/administrator. Document discussions at these meetings.

data (Sheehan & Keogh, 1981). Formative data are collected throughout a program, and are used to ensure consistency in addressing program objectives or to make decisions to improve the functioning of program operation. Summative data provide information about program impact and outcome. These data may be collected either prospectively or retrospectively. Prospective evaluation occurs when data are collected in conjunction with the program component function being evaluated. When program evaluation is included as a component function of a program's overall purpose, prospective evaluation studies are more frequently selected. Retrospective evaluation studies are undertaken after the activity being evaluated has occurred. These studies are used,

for the most part, when program evaluation has not been viewed as a planned function of a program, but when information about the program's impact, efficacy, satisfaction, or operation is desired. Collecting information from parents about their interaction with their infants each time the parent-infant dyad attends an intervention session, is an example of a prospective study. Data are collected in conjunction with the activity being evaluated. Interviewing parents to determine their perceptions of frequency of interactions with their infants after parent-infant dyads have been enrolled in intervention sessions for one year, is an example of a retrospective study. These data are being collected after sessions have occurred, rather than concurrent with service provision. Both of these

TABLE 9-2. Goals and Objectives for an Early Intervention Program		
Component	**Goal**	**Objective**
Public Awareness and Identification	Identify infants and toddlers with disabilities in Wyoming County.	Develop a brochure describing services available. Distribute brochures to all pediatricians and family practice physicians within Wyoming County by visiting the office of each physician, explaining the program to the physician and office staff, and asking that brochures be distributed to appropriate families. Mail brochures to all agencies providing services for infants and toddlers.
	Identify those infants and toddlers who are eligible for services.	Screen referrals/contacts to determine whether eligibility criteria met. Conduct developmental and other assessments to confirm eligibility.
Family Involvement	Provide families with needed services.	Determine family needs through discussion or questionnaire/interview. Establish/locate a range of family services including parent support, family training, respite care, information networks, and make services available to families. Individualize plans to address family needs for services on the IFSP; review regularly and document services received.
Service Provision for Infants, Toddlers and Families	Provide infants, toddlers, and their families with early intervention services.	Conduct multidisciplinary assessment procedures, identify family needs and strengths to provide families information about their children, to provide data for determining how children/families may achieve desired outcomes, and to write statement about present levels of function. Develop an IFSP that is based on outcomes desired by the family for themselves and their child. Determine the services and actions to be undertaken to address desired outcomes. Provide services/actions as outlined on the IFSP and in accord with detailed intervention plans. Document service provision. Review IFSP service provision on at least a six month basis; conducting additional assessments as necessary.
Staff Development	Increase staff skills in working appropriately and effectively with families.	Provide training in family-centered service provision.
	Improve staff skills as team members, increasing their abilities to include family members as team members and to work effectively with each other.	Provide ongoing training in team interaction skills including group process, collaborative consultation, and other relevant areas.
Program Evaluation	Determine the extent to which early intervention services improve the functioning of infants and toddlers.	Develop a plan for evaluating the impact of team services on infants. Implement the plan.
	Determine the extent to which early intervention services improve the capacity of families to optimize the growth and development of their infants and toddlers.	Develop a plan for evaluating the impact of services on family members. Implement the plan.
Administration	Ensure timely processing of children through steps of program eligibility, assessment, assignment to service model, and provision of services.	Establish a data teaching system so that each eligible child is receiving services within 45 days following determination of eligibility.
	Provide supervisory activities that are individualized around the strengths and concerns of each staff member.	Develop an individualized plan of supervision for each staff member that includes goals and objectives of the supervisory process; implement the plan so that each staff person receives appropriate supervision.

studies address an evaluation question of: "To what extent does participation in parent-infant intervention sessions impact on the frequency of parents' interactions with their infants?". In these examples, direct observation data are collected when the question is answered through a prospective study, where perception data are used when the question is addressed retrospectively.

The program evaluation plan derives directly from the questions that will be addressed. The first step in planning is to determine the type of design which will provide the data necessary to answer each program evaluation question. The second step is to outline the activities necessary to implement each study design.

Program Evaluation Study Designs

Undertaking individual or comprehensive program evaluation studies is similar to designing and implementing a series of research studies. Program evaluation studies may involve simple to complex research, depending upon the design selected to address each question. Descriptive, single subject, or group designs are used in program evaluation studies.

Descriptive Designs

Studies that summarize outcome data, without use of statistical or comparative procedures, are referred to as descriptive. These designs may be implemented either prospectively or retrospectively. Summarizations of the numbers of children who received services through direct, monitoring, consultation, or combinations of service provision models, before and after occupational therapy staff received training in collaborative consultation, is an example of an evaluation study using a descriptive design. Summarization of the changes in pre- and post-test scores, on a test of information presented before and after a one day training session, is another example of a descriptive design. Distributing a questionnaire to school district teachers to elicit their degree of satisfaction with occupational therapy services, and summarizing the results by type of service provision model (e.g., direct, monitoring, consultation), is a third example of a descriptive study. Descriptive data may be used to address any number of evaluation questions related to program impact, satisfaction, or operation, but are less useful when evaluating program efficacy questions.

Descriptive designs report outcomes directly or allow for simple numerical comparisons of data from different groups, or under different conditions. Descriptive designs do not require control or comparison groups, therefore, only simple statistical procedures may be used to analyze data. Statistical procedures are used to summarize numerical data by obtaining the average (or mean) score, the standard deviation of the scores in the group, or other measures of central tendency. Mean scores may also be subject to parametric and non-parametric statistical procedures, when more than one set of data are available for comparative purposes. Procedures, such as the t-test or chi-square analyses, determine the extent to which any differences are significant statistically. For example, the pre- or post-test scores of parents of children with cerebral palsy, before and after attending a training session on positioning, were calculated in terms of differences in scores before and after training. The average score of the group of parents was higher following training. The

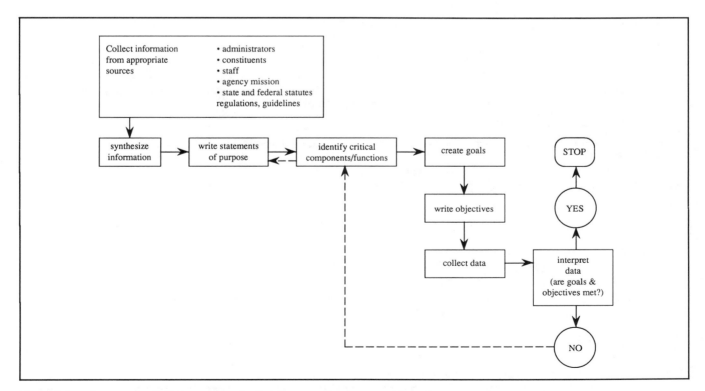

Figure 9-1a. Process for Defining and Evaluating Program Purposes and Functions.

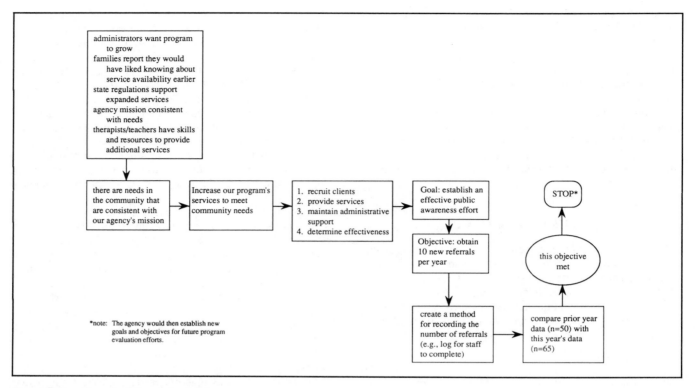

Figure 9-1b. Sample Process for an Agency.

TABLE 9-3   Examples of Selected Program Evaluation Questions for a School-based Occupational Therapy Department

Assessment, Identification, Service Provision:

How many special education students were screened for eligibility to occupational therapy services? What percent of the total special education enrollment as of October 1 were screened?

Of those students screened, what number (and percent) were eligible for assessment?

What percent of students eligible for assessment received assessments by November 15?

What percent of students needing occupational therapy services were scheduled for service provision by November 30? by January 30?

What percent of students needing occupational therapy services were not scheduled during the school year?

Staff Development:

To what extent did staff members gain knowledge through staff development activities?

To what extent did staff members acquire new skills and/or broaden existing skills.

Did staff members attend new workshops and training sessions during the school year when compared with attendance of previous years?

Were staff members satisfied with the staff development program?

Administration:

To what extent were timelines adhered to in implementing program objectives?

How often did meetings occur with the agency supervisor/administrator?

TABLE 9-4 Examples of Selected Program Evaluation Questions for an Early Intervention Program that Includes Occupational Therapy

Public Awareness/Identification:

How many brochures were distributed to which physicians and agencies?

How many referrals were received from each physician/agency?

How did the number of referrals received compare with the previous year's referral rates?

How many screenings were administered in comparison with the number of the previous years?

What percent of children screened met eligibility criteria?

Family Involvement:

What were the numbers and types of services available to families? Which services were added during this year?

What percent of families participated in each available service?

How satisfied were families with: (a) the types of services available; and (b) the service(s) in which they participated.

Service Provision:

Did infants/toddlers benefit from services provided?

How satisfied were families with the services provided for their children?

Staff Development:

Did staff increase knowledge about elements of family-centered service provision?

To what extent did staff apply new knowledge when interacting with families?

Program Evaluation:

How many program evaluation activities (studies) were implemented?

To what extent did data from studies impact on the service provision process for infants? families? program staff?

Administration:

What percent of eligible children were receiving services within 45 days following eligibility?

What were the patterns of supervision for each staff member? To what extent did these patterns reflect individualization for strengths and concerns?

---

mean scores for before and after training were compared statistically, using a *t*-test for the difference between related means. The *t*-test score indicated that the group mean following training was not *significantly* higher than the mean score before training.

Single Subject Designs

These designs are used most often in program evaluation studies to investigate the efficacy of service provision for individual children or family members (Campbell, 1988). Single subject designs are easily superimposed on documentation activities carried out as part of individualized planning for students through the IEP, IFSP or similar plans, providing a mechanism for easily combining clinical practice and research (Ottenbacher & York, 1984).

Single subject designs require that data are collected prospectively—concurrently—with the intervention (treatment) being provided. Both the intervention being provided, and the desired outcome, are defined before single subject designs are implemented. The intervention is defined as the independent variable, the activity that is being provided for the child or family. The desired outcome is defined as the dependent variable, the behavior that will be measured. For

example, a mother identified a need to have her child eat more quickly during mealtimes. The occupational therapist consulted with the mother by observing the feeding process during several lunchtimes, and concluded that the child was taking a long time to eat due to poor lip and jaw closure. The therapist subsequently taught the mother to use techniques to activate jaw and lip closure during mealtimes, as a means of decreasing the length of time necessary to feed the child. The independent variable, in this example, consists of the techniques used to activate lip and jaw closure. The dependent variable is the length of time for the child to eat the meal. The therapist designed a data sheet, and asked the mother to record the length of time necessary for the child to eat, and the amount of food that the child consumed. These prospective data were used to measure the effectiveness of the intervention program of techniques to activate lip and jaw closure.

Various types of single subject designs may be used to investigate effects of intervention (Alberto & Troutman, 1982; Campbell, 1988; Ottenbacher & York, 1984; Worley & Harris, 1982). Those that are most useful in clinical situations are outlined on Table 9-6 and include: a) reversal; b) multielement; c) changing criterion; d) multiple baseline; e) alternating treatment; and f) decreasing treatment. Single subject de-

TABLE 9-5 Sample Evaluation Questions

Area	Questions	Sample Data Sources
Impact	What is the impact of services provided for children on their parents?	Questionnaires mailed to families on a monthly basis. Telephone interview with a random sample of families.
	What is the impact of program evaluation on staff development efforts for all department staff?	Record satisfaction with staff development pre and post questionnaire to staff to determine differences in satisfaction.
	What is the impact of occupational therapy services on children as perceived by teachers?	Interview with all teachers to determine perceptions about the purpose of occupational therapy and the impact of services on child progress.
Efficacy	What is the number of children who demonstrated change in a target behavior following occupational therapy intervention?	Analysis of progress on behavior target for each student in the program; Rate each target behavior in terms of P, NP, S
	To what extent did children with CP learn to feed themselves independently?	Review all records to identify children with CP and those on self-feeding program. Interview teachers, therapist, parent to identify competency level in self-feeding. Observe each child during lunch and document competencies in self-feeding. Summarize data across children.
Satisfaction	Are families of children who receive occupational therapy services satisfied with services provided?	Satisfaction rating scale completed by parent of each child.
	Are occupational therapy department staff satisfied with personnel benefits and policies?	Rank order analysis of most to least preferred benefits.

signs vary the conditions under which intervention is provided to the same subject. Each condition is labeled with a different letter (e.g., A, B). Typically, the A condition represents the condition where no specific intervention is provided and is labeled as the baseline condition. Other letters and their order

indicate the ways in which the intervention is provided. An ABBA reversal design, for example, indicates that an equal number of baseline and intervention sessions were provided, and that baseline preceded and followed the intervention sessions. An ABC multielement design indicates that one con-

TABLE 9-6 Single-Subject Designs

Design	Component	Distinguishing Feature(s)	Reference
Reversal	ABA; ABBA; ABAB	Treatment is reversed, which should result in a return to baseline performance.	Tawney & Gast, 1986
Multielement	ABCD . . .	Different types of treatment procedures are used as required, or the number of treatment procedures is systematically decreased over time.	Murphey, Doughty, & Nunes, 1979 Ullman & Sulzewr-Azeroff, 1975
Changing criterion	ABCD . . .	The criterion for performance changes over time.	Hartmann & Hall, 1976
Multiple baseline	A B C	Data are simultaneously taken on several types of behavior, but only one behavior is the target of treatment at any time.	Hall, Cristler, Cranston, & Tucker, 1970
Alternating treatment	AB; ABC	Several treatment procedures are used to address the same behavior; treatments may be alternating or randomly provided (e.g., AACBACBBC).	Kazdin & Kopel, 1975

Campbell, P. (1988). Using a single-subject research design to evaluate the effectiveness of treatment. American Journal of Occupational Therapy, 42(11): 732–738. Used with permission.

dition without intervention was provided, followed by two different types of intervention.

Single subject designs allow comparisons of a child's performance on the dependent measure under different conditions. Interpretation of the effect of intervention is made on the basis of differences in performance, under conditions of intervention and no intervention. A child whose rate of reaching, for example, is 1 per minute under baseline, and 5 per minute under intervention conditions, reaches more often with than without intervention. In this circumstance, the probability is that intervention is the variable influencing the child's rate of reaching. Judgements of the effect of intervention, on a child's performance in single subject designs, are made on the basis of visual inspection of graphed data or numerical analyses of data (e.g., Hersen & Barlow, 1976; Tawney & Gast, 1984). Graphed lines that are clearly separate, and that do not overlap, are interpreted more clearly than are those that illustrate performance that is similar in one or more intervention conditions. Figure 9-2 illustrates two graphs of reaching performance. The top graph (figure 9-2a) illustrates a situation in which intervention is the variable influencing rate of reaching. The effect of intervention on rate of reaching is not interpreted easily from the graph illustrated on the bottom (figure 9-2b).

Single subject designs may also be used to compare performance of individual subjects within a group. Multiple baseline designs are commonly used for this purpose (Hall, Cristler, Cranston, & Tucker, 1970; Kazdin & Koppel, 1975). The same intervention is used with more than one subject, but the initiation of intervention is delayed for each subject. Each subject functions as his own control subject, as well as the control subject for other children included in the group. Figure 9-3 illustrates the results of a multiple baseline design, across

subjects that tested an intervention of training students with severe disabilities, to operate switch interface devices (e.g., Campbell & Mulhauser, 1989). Other single subject designs also may be used across different children, but are summarized and reported by individual subjects. Those most typically combined include reversal and multielement designs (e.g., Campbell & Stewart, 1986).

Single subject designs that allow comparisons among groups of children are an essential component of program evaluation (Campbell, 1988). These designs allow therapists (as well as other professionals) to measure overall progress in children who are served through programs, while grouping results to evaluate overall program effectiveness. Single subject measures, summarized across participating children, not only document, but also evaluate the effectiveness of a program. These objective measures may be reported for all students as a group, or by various characteristics, such as: a) diagnosis; b) severity of children's disabilities; c) age of children; d) intervention procedures or techniques used; or e) model of service provision.

Group Designs

These designs are most applicable to program evaluation questions that involve provision of some sort of intervention for children, their families, or program staff, and are analyzed statistically to determine differences before, during, or after intervention (e.g., Slavin, 1984). As with single subject designs, group designs are constructed in terms of independent (intervention being provided) and dependent (outcome) variables. Comparisons in performance among experimental (receives intervention), and control (does not receive intervention) groups are the essential feature in most group designs

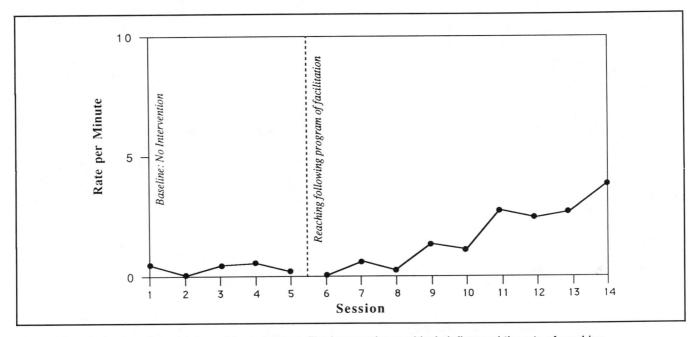

Figure 9-2a. A graph on the rate of reaching behaviors. The intervention positively influenced the rate of reaching.

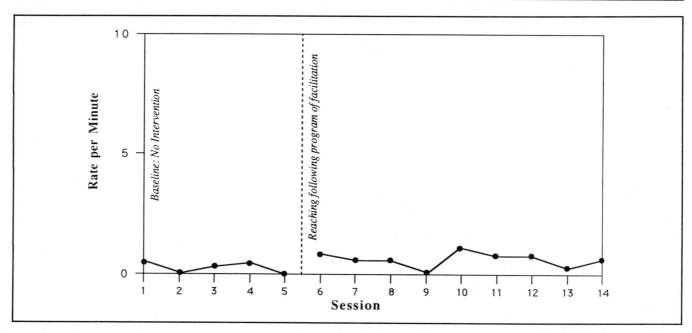

Figure 9-2b. A graph on the rate of reaching behaviors. The intervention does not have a clear affect on reaching.

used in program evaluation studies. A judgement that the intervention has been effective cannot be made with validity in the absence of some sort of control group with whom to compare the performance of the experimental group.

Group designs are the least often used designs in program evaluation activities, due to the complexities involved, and the resources required to implement these designs accurately. Obtaining necessary dependent measures on a true control group may be difficult for several reasons. First, fully withholding any intervention from children, families, or staff may not be possible within schools, early intervention programs, or other types of service provision agencies. A standard practice control group, a similar group that is receiving an intervention, but is not receiving the intervention being evaluated, may be used as a control group. The dependent measures are obtained on both the experimental and standard practice control group. The intervention being evaluated is provided to the experimental group, while the standard practice control group receives the services that are typically available.

Standard practice control groups may be available within the same program, or may be obtained through other schools or community programs. For example, an occupational therapist was interested in evaluating the extent to which consultation services adequately addressed needs of students enrolled in the school districts to which she was assigned. She randomly picked one school district, and provided services to all children in that district through consultation, and randomly selected a second district where standard practice was provided. Two dependent measures were used to evaluate service provision: a) attainment of IEP goals and objectives; and b) repeated measures that assessed teachers perceptions of the usefulness of occupational therapy services for students. The therapist designed a questionnaire to assess teacher perception, and asked all teachers in both districts to complete the questionnaire at the beginning, middle, and end of the school year. The IEP's of all experimental and standard practice control groups students were examined at the beginning and end of the school year, and records were maintained of the number of IEP objectives attained by each student. All data were compiled at the end of the school year and summarized for analysis. These data provided the information that allowed the therapist to conclude that consultation was superior to standard practice. Experimental students, those that had received consultation, attained a greater number of IEP goals than those who had received standard practice occupational therapy services only. In addition, teachers of experimental subjects perceived occupational therapy services of greater importance than did teachers of children receiving standard practice therapy.

A second reason why group experimental designs are difficult to use in program evaluation, are the number of resources required to implement designs accurately. In addition to difficulties encountered in locating control group subjects, the appropriate number of children, families, or staff required to implement a design, may not be available easily within a program. A minimum of ten experimental and ten control group subjects are required to implement most group designs. Evaluating services through group designs, for example, for children of particular characteristics, such as Down syndrome, may not be feasible due to the small number of children in a particular diagnostic category who are enrolled in a program. Another problem concerns the resources necessary to collect dependent measures on both experimental and control group subjects. Designing and obtaining dependent measures may require time above that typically used in the service provision process, necessitating that staff time be allocated specifically for program evaluation. A final prob-

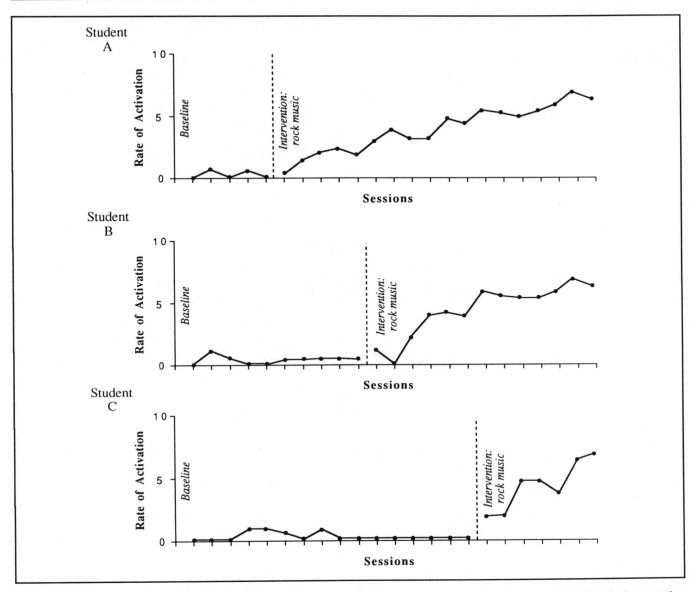

Figure 9-3. Graphs of a multiple baseline design across subjects. The graph depicts rate of activation of a switch. With the intervention of rock music, the rate of performance increases.

lem concerns levels of expertise. Using group designs for program evaluation purposes requires basic knowledge of research design and statistical analysis, skills that may not be within the repertoires of clinically-trained occupational therapists, but that may be obtained through use of other personnel within an agency, or by hiring outside consultants.

The majority of program evaluation questions are addressed through descriptive studies (Bricker & Littman, 1982). These designs lack a control group of any type, making the resultant data more difficult to interpret clearly than data resulting from single subject or group designs. Group designs are an important component of program evaluation despite the limitations to their easy use. Certain evaluation questions are best addressed through use of group designs. Program evaluation activities that rely on use of single subject and group designs yield information that fulfills two purposes: a)

program evaluation; and b) contribution to the overall knowledge base in occupational therapy.

Evaluation Activities

Identifying the component functions of a program, formulating evaluation questions, and selecting the design that will be used to address those questions, are the beginning steps in designing a program evaluation plan. Subsequent steps outline the process that will be used to obtain the data desired to address each question. Table 9-7 outlines a complete plan for comprehensive evaluation of a program of occupational therapy services provided in one school district. The plan is divided into the following seven sections: a) program component function; b) evaluation questions; c) design; d) evaluation activities; e) data to be collected; f) person(s) respon-

TABLE 9-7 Program Evaluation Plan for a School-Based Occupational Therapy Program

Program Component Function	Evaluation Questions	Design	Data to be Collected	Evaluation Activities	Person(s) Responsible	Timeline
Assessment and ID	What % of special education students were screened for eligibility for OT services?	Descriptive—Total number of special education students. Number screened for OT	Records reviews—Number of special education students; number who were screened for OT	Design OT screening form.	Mary & Susan	April/May 89
				Train special education staff in use of OT screening form.	Bldg. OT staff	August 89
				Review all special education files to determine presence/absence of OT screening form.	Bldg. Secretary	Throughout school year
	Of students who met screening criteria, what number & % also met assessment criteria?	Descriptive—Total number of students meeting screening criteria. Number meeting assessment criteria	Record review—is decision correct according to criteria? Number meeting screening; number meeting assessment; total number of students	Determine cutoff score—screening.	OT staff	May 89
				Determine criteria for full assessment.	OT staff	May 89
				Design method for recording information.	OT supervisor	Summer 89
				Review files to collect data.	OT supervisor	Fall 89
	What % of students who needed an OT assessment received one by Nov. 15?	Descriptive—Meet timeline	Record review—Date of OT assessment. List those incomplete by Nov. 15	Create list of those who meet OT assessment.	OT staff	Summer-Fall 89
				Record date OT assessment performed.	OT staff	Fall 89
Service Provision	What % of students who require OT services were scheduled for services by Dec. 1? by Jan. 1?	Descriptive—meet criteria for scheduling	OT Services student lists—therapist schedules—dates of onset of service—dates of eligibility decisions	Prepare a master list of students receiving OT services.	OT supervisor	Dec. 1, 89
				Obtain therapist schedules.	Spec. Ed. Dir.	Dec. 89
				Record dates of service provision.	Spec. Ed. Dir.	Dec. 89
				Compile master list of service provision dates.	OT staff	Ongoing—submit to date each month. Monthly
				Determine total number of students eligible by each month; determine number who have been scheduled by target date.	Secretary	
				Calculate percent receiving service by targeted dates.	OT Supervisor	Jan. 90
	What is the impact of various OT services on student performance as judged by teachers?	Descriptive—overall ratings overall awareness	Teacher questionnaire interview re: student progress identify their level of awareness of OT contribution	Create ratings/awareness scales.	Jim & Arlene (OTs)	Fall 89
				Create interview questions.	Sandra (OT)	Fall 89
				Create demographic form for students receiving OT services.	Sam (OT)	Summer 89

TABLE 9-7 *Continued*						
Program Component Function	**Evaluation Questions**	**Design**	**Data to be Collected**	**Evaluation Activities**	**Person(s) Responsible**	**Timeline**
				Complete and submit demographic forms.	OT staff	Monthly
				Complete scales/interviews.	Teachers/admin. assistant	April/May 90
				Compile information	Admin. asst.	June 90
				Report information.	OT supervisor	June 90
		Group comparison sort data by: 1. educ. diagnosis 2. buildilng 3. type of placement 4. type of services		Reorganize data by targeted subgroups.	Admin. Asst.	Summer 90
				Analyze data.	Information analyst	Summer 90
				Report findings.	OT supervisor	August 90
	How many students demonstrated a change in target behaviors following OT intervention?	Descriptive comparison	Record number of mastery of IEP goals and objectives/intervention plan goals and objectives	Provide copy of IEP for each student receiving OT services.	OT Staff	Fall 89
				Identify goal attainment on IEP.	Teacher/case manager	May 90
				Calculate overall %.	OT supervisor	June 90
	What % of students with postural control needs improve in their ability to complete seatwork tasks?	Single subject AB design Across subjects (multiple baseline)	Review records to locate students with postural control concerns; conduct skilled observation in seatwork period to collect data on on-task behaviors.	Identify students who fall into focus of study.	OT Staff Teacher/case manager	August 89
				Collect baseline data on each student.	OT supervisor OT supervisor	Sept. 89
				Note when intervention occurs.	OT (not the person providing service)	Ongoing
				Collect some data during intervention.	Data collector Data collector	Ongoing
				Compare across subjects for changes.	OT supervisor	June 90
	Are teachers satisfied with OT services provided?	Descriptive—level of satisfaction	Likert scale on satisfaction with services—teachers report	Write satisfaction questionnaire.	Marie & Georgia	Fall 90
				Identify teachers who have a student receiving OT services.	Special services office	Fall 90
				Distribute questionnaire to appropriate teachers.	Special services office	May 90
Staff Development	To what extent did staff gain knowledge through staff development activities?	Descriptive—knowledge gained	Pre/post test data on knowledge gained	Create a pre/post test for staff developmental programs.	Speaker	Ongoing
				Administer pre/post tests.	Inservice manager	Ongoing

sible for data collection; and g) timeline. Implementation of a plan such as this one, results in data concerning all aspects of the program including impact, operation, efficacy, and satisfaction.

Evaluation activities describe the steps necessary to implement the designs specified and to collect the desired data.

Activities may include: a) designing an instrument for use in program evaluation, for example, a questionnaire or a series of interview questions to collect data on staff satisfaction; b) obtaining and selecting subjects when group or single subject designs are used; or c) determining the timing for collecting various types of data. Planning and writing the proposed

						TABLE 9-7 Continued

Program Component Function	Evaluation Questions	Design	Data to be Collected	Evaluation Activities	Person(s) Responsible	Timeline
				Tally & report results.	Admin. Asst.	Ongoing
	Did staff attend at least as many continuing education experiences this year compared to last year?	Descriptive—number of continuing education experiences	Records reviews 88–89—number of continuing education experiences.	Obtain list of last year's continuing education efforts.	Admin. Asst.	June 90
				Create & maintain current list.	Admin. Asst.	June 90
			Collect list of continuing education experiences 89–90.	Complete comparisons.	Admin. Asst.	June 90
	To what extent did staff apply above new skills?	Single subject AB design across subjects.	Therapist weekly records of service provision schedules.	Obtain weekly record of service provision provided.	Admin. Asst.	Ongoing
		Descriptive—patterns of performance	IEP's of students.	Obtain IEP of each student.	Admin. Asst.	Ongoing
				Graph on charts by number of units in direct, monitor, and consult.	Admin. Asst.	Ongoing
				Provide inservice on consultation.	Invited expert	Dec. 89
				Continue to record data from weekly records.	Admin. Asst.	Ongoing
				Mark when IEP is renegotiated.	Admin. Asst.	Ongoing
				Compare before/after inservice.	OT supervisor	Summer 90
				Compare across therapists.	OT supervisor	Summer 90
				Compare original IEP pattern to new IEP patterns.	OT supervisor	Summer 90
				Report findings.	OT supervisor	Summer 90
	Were staff satisfied with staff development activities?	Descriptive—overall ratings	Satisfaction ratings	Create Likert scale for staff development activities.	Admin. Asst.	Ongoing
				Distribute scale after each staff development activity.	Admin. Asst.	Ongoing
				Tally and report results.	Admin. Asst.	Ongoing
	What is the impact of program evaluation activities on staff development efforts?	Descriptive—overall ratings	Obtain satisfaction ratings from staff on program evaluation activities; obtain ratings on usefulness of activities.	Create a Likert scale to determine satisfaction/usefulness.	Admin. Asst.	Fall 89
				Distribute scales.	Admin. Asst.	May 90
				Tally and report results.	Admin. Asst.	Summer 90
Administration	What % of staff personal goals were met during the year?	Descriptive—goal attainment	List of personal goals. Number of goals obtained.	Identify personal goals.	OT staff/OT supervisor	Aug. 89
				Keep data on personal goals.	OT staff	Ongoing
				Report goal completion.	OT staff	May 90
				Calculate % of goals met.	OT supervisor	June 90

TABLE 9-7 Continued

Program Component Function	Evaluation Questions	Design	Data to be Collected	Evaluation Activities	Person(s) Responsible	Timeline
	Are staff satisfied with personnel benefits and policies?	Descriptive—level of satisfaction	Likert scale rating of benefits and critical policies	Create Likert scale for benefits and policies.	Benefits Officer	Fall 89
				Distribute scale.	Benefits Officer	Fall 89
				Tally and report results.	Benefits Officer	Spring 90
	What % of eligible students were receiving services within one month of the eligibility determination?	Descriptive—meet criteria	Lists of students receiving OT services. Lists of team decisions/dates. Lists of OT service initiation dates.	Prepare a master list of students receiving OT services.	Spec. Ed. Director	Dec. 89
				Obtain list of eligibility determination dates.	Spec. Ed. Director	Dec. 89
				Obtain list of starting dates.	Spec. Ed. Director	Jan. 90
				Calculate the length of time to initiate services.	Admin. Asst.	March 90
				Report results.	Spec. Ed. Director	April 90

activities that need to occur is an important step. Pieces of the program evaluation may become lost when implementation plans are not developed. For example, a repeated measures design was selected in order to assess the degree of parent stress evidenced at different points in time, with parents of children who were enrolled in a program, and those who were not yet enrolled. A committee was formed to identify and review existing measures of parent stress and to recommend several to be used in the proposed program evaluation study. The program evaluation consultant was designated as the individual to make the final decision concerning the measure to be used. Completion of these two steps was required prior to the initiation of the program evaluation study itself, therefore, timing was of critical importance. Implementation of the study depended upon the successful implementation of planned activities.

Implementation of the Program Evaluation Plan

The main purpose of the program evaluation plan is to produce reliable data that can be interpreted systematically to answer specific evaluation questions. The types of data to be collected, at what time periods, and by what type of person, are the essence of implementation of the program evaluation plan.

Data To Be Collected

The types of data to be collected relate directly to the program evaluation question being addressed. Several types of data typically are collected in a comprehensive program evaluation. Data may be collected through interview, questionnaire, completion of tests, or direct observation. Live observations are made at the same time the behavior being observed is occurring, or behavior may be recorded through videotape or audiotape for later observation. Direct or coded notations of the behavior being observed are made continuously or at fixed time periods. The type of data collected must match the question being addressed. For example, a question such as "to what extent do oral stimulation procedures improve lip closure," is best matched with an observation of lip closure during eating, vocal production or speech, or during both situations. Similarly, test performance or perception questionnaire data is appropriate to address a question of "to what extent do staff improve their knowledge of family systems theory, following a one-day inservice training session?". If the question were "to what extent do staff apply their knowledge of family systems theory in writing an IFSP for an infant and family," direct observation of staff performance during the ISFP process is necessary to produce the type of data necessary to address the question.

Reliability

Determining reliability is an essential issue in all data collection, and is particularly important in program evaluation studies that use single subject, or group designs based on observation of performance. Data collected by two or more people at the same time, and with similar results, are considered reliable. Reliability data are collected on 20% to 33% of all data points in each condition (phase) of a single subject design, and on a randomly selected 20% to 33% of all subjects in each condition (phase) of a group design that uses observational outcome measures. The effects of an intervention designed to increase postural tone with infants with low tone in the trunk musculature were measured, for example, using repeated administrations of a scale designed to rate postural tone, and a system for measuring the degree of alignment in sitting. Measures were completed before intervention began (baseline condition), during each of ten intervention sessions, and for six weeks following the termination of the intervention.

Ten infants were included in the study. Four infants were randomly selected in each condition (pre-intervention baseline; intervention; post-intervention baseline), and two therapists completed the ratings of these infants.

A number of different methods may be used to calculate reliability of the data. The measure most commonly used in single subject design is called percentage of agreement. The number of agreements are divided by the number of agreements, plus the number of disagreements, and multiplied by 100. Most researchers desire a percentage of agreement that ranges from 85% to above 90% agreement, dependent on the type of data. Other measures, such as correlation coefficients, may be used to calculate reliability with numerical data when the number of subjects are large. For the most part, program evaluation studies in pediatric programs do not meet the criteria necessary to administer statistical tests for reliability, other than percent of agreement.

Reasonable levels of reliability may be difficult to obtain without training of the individuals conducting the observations. Two approaches are typically used. Two (or more) observers (therapists) observe behavior, and compare their ratings until the point that reasonable reliability is achieved. This approach allows the observers to discuss the areas of disagreement, and to develop refined definitions of any observational categories being used. In the second approach, a videotaped sample of behavior is rated, and used as a basis for discussion and clarification of definitional categories. The videotape is repeated until all observers have reliability agreements of above 85% to 90%.

Scheduling reliability observations may be difficult in pediatric service provision programs. The second observer does not have to be the same discipline, or have the same level of expertise, when training has been provided and the two individuals are reliable observers of behavior. A Certified Occupational Therapy Assistant (COTA), an aide, the teacher, a parent or any other available individual, may function as a second observer when reliability data are being collected. Reliability measurements are essential in program evaluation research. Observational data may fluctuate due to differences in child behavior, differences in observations, or for other reasons. Reliability measures indicate that behavior is changing as a function of the intervention being provided, not as a function of differences in observations.

Persons Responsible for Data Collection

Two types of individuals typically are responsible for data collection. Individuals who are employed within the program being evaluated are assigned responsibility for various aspects of data collection (e.g., Campbell & Stewart, 1986). Therapists, for example, may be responsible for collecting data on child performance, that will be used in studies designed to evaluate the efficacy of service provision. An administrator or supervisor may collect data on staff performance. These individuals who are employed by the program are defined as inside evaluators. Individuals who collect data within a program, but who are not employed or associated with the program, are defined as outside or third party evaluators. There is always an implication that inside evaluators may be biased, due to their involvement with a program, and therefore, inadvertently may bias the evaluation results in favor of the program.

Outside evaluators, on the other hand, are not biased as to the outcome of program evaluation, but may have difficulty obtaining data, particularly if the outside evaluation is conducted on a short-term basis. Outside evaluators typically are individuals who either specialize in third-party evaluations, or are known to be experts in the program area being evaluated. Consumer-based program evaluation, however, may be conducted by a group of consumers, and/or individuals from the community at large. A school-district or agency may appoint a representative evaluation committee, and give the committee responsibility for designing, conducting, and reporting program evaluation studies. In other instances, state and national funding sources may conduct an on-site program review to evaluate the extent to which the program is on target with proposed activities, or to conduct an impartial program review and evaluation (Shaw, 1985).

Both community-based evaluation committees and on-site program evaluations by funding sources, are different from monitoring committees or teams. State monitoring or accreditation teams have responsibility for ensuring that a program meets either national, state, or local standards and requirements, or those outlined by the accreditation agency. For example, most states review school districts periodically to determine compliance with the federal *Education for the Handicapped Act*, and the standards and requirements adopted by a state to ensure compliance with the federal statute. Accreditation agencies, such as the Council for the Accreditation of Rehabilitation Facilities (CARF), or the Joint Commission for the Accreditation of Hospitals (JCAH), review agency programs to determine compliance with minimal standards. These types of program review are beneficial for participants, but do not provide an evaluation of all aspects of a program.

Well-orchestrated comprehensive program evaluations are based on data collected by both types of individuals. In addition, programs may hire consultants in program evaluation who assist in establishing the program evaluation plan, and in reviewing the results, but who are not responsible for the evaluation process itself. Outside evaluators are particularly helpful in evaluating program function components that involve staff or families and other program consumers. Both staff and consumers have vested interests in the program, and an inherent potential for being penalized, if favorable program evaluation information is not presented. Therefore, members of these groups may not be fully accurate in reporting data to program insiders, particularly if the insiders are believed to have the power to inflict penalties.

Timeline

Establishing a timeline for data collection, and adhering to the proposed timeline as closely as is feasible is important. Certain types of data are useful only if collected at the right points in time. A measure designed to determine differences in test scores before and after a parent training course, for example, is of little value if data are not collected at the right points in time. Similarly, performance data for a child who is receiving intervention are of no value if sufficient data have not been collected first under a condition of no intervention. Planning a timeline is only the first step in ensuring that data are collected at the right points in time. The plan has to be implemented, as designed, for data to be interpretable. One strategy for ensuring that the plan is implemented, is to designate one or more persons as responsible for reviewing data collection for the total plan, or for specific studies within the plan. Another strategy is to schedule regular meetings where all involved persons review the data collection that has been undertaken to date. Problems that may be occurring (e.g., children's absences, changes in staff development activities, rescheduling of an on-site visit by an outside evaluator), are discussed in these meetings, and the original plan for data collection is modified to accommodate solutions for recurring problems. Once the timeline for data has been established in the program evaluation implementation plan, ongoing review is necessary with whatever strategy appears best within the program being evaluated.

SUMMARIZING AND INTERPRETING DATA

Raw data are organized and summarized following data collection, in order to complete any statistical procedures being used for analysis, or to represent the data in ways others will understand. The initial step in this process is to transfer raw data onto a data summary sheet that will be used as the basis for graphing single subject results, calculating tendency measures (e.g., mean or average scores, standard deviation), or performing statistical tests. This process is illustrated in Figures 9-4, 9-5, and 9-6, which provide examples for descriptive, group, and single subject designs. A descriptive study was designed to measure the impact of a program to train teachers and other school personnel in use of tech-

---

Technology Training Project Follow-up Phone Study
Teacher Summary

Number of students: _____105_____

Number of teachers: _____100_____

% Responding _____95%_____

1. Was specific piece of equipment recommended?
   ___71___ Yes ___18___ No ___11___ Don't Know
2. Was equipment obtained?
   ___47___ Yes ___51___ No ___2___ Don't Know
3. Is child using equipment currently?
   ___35___ Yes ___2___ No ___10___ Don't Know
4. Is child using equipment successfully?
   ___29___ Yes ___6___ No ___0___ Don't Know

Figure 9-4. Form used to summarize data from Technology Training Project follow-up phone study.

Data Summary Sheet

	Mothers with Training				Mothers without Training		
Subject No.	Pre-test Score	Post-test Score	Difference		Pre-test Score	Post-test Score	Difference
1	22	41	+19		20	21	+1
2	21	47	+26		21	23	+2
3	15	40	+25		22	19	−3
4	21	42	+21		19	18	+3
5	22	43	+21		18	20	+2
6	20	40	+20		17	20	+3
7	14	46	+32		26	25	−1
8	17	45	+28		17	24	+7
9	19	48	+29		14	18	+4
10	20	41	+21		25	28	+3
11	21	42	+21		22	24	+2
12	22	45	+23		21	26	+5
13	19	49	+30		15	20	+5
14	18	46	+28		21	23	+2
15	17	41	+24		14	16	+2
16	26	50	+24		20	22	+2
17	23	51	+26		17	20	+3
18	21	53	+22		19	21	+2
19	14	39	+25		21	24	+3
20	17	43	+26		22	22	0

Figure 9-5. Summary of data collected on two groups of mothers who have a child with a disability.

<u>Independent Ambulation</u>

NAME: _____   DATE: _____

TRAINER: _____

<u>A</u>   Trainer places child in standing position on floor. Trainer instructs the child to walk a given distance to a wall or bench or mark on the floor.

<u>B</u>   Child walks independently the given distance with the following quality items correct.

<u>C</u>   SR+ or other appropriate consequence/reinforcement

Session 14- Raw Data

Date: 11/4/87	+ - correct				0 - incorrect			NR - no response		
Trials	1	2	3	4	5	6	7	8	9	10
Distance	1	0	2	0	2	1	0	2	0	0
Base no wider than shoulders	+	+	+	+	+	+	+	+	+	+
Neutral pelvis a/p	+	+	+	+	+	+	+	+	+	+
No forward trunk flexion	+	+	+	+	+	+	+	+	+	+
Hip neutral rotation	0	0	+	0	+	0	0	+	0	0
Hip knee extension stance leg	0	+	+	0	+	0	0	+	+	0
Foot flat stance leg	0	0	+	0	+	0	0	+	0	0
Equal diagonal weight shifts	0	0	+	0	+	0	0	+	0	0
TOTAL RESPONSE	0	0	+	0	+	0	0	+	0	0

Figure 9-6a. Sample of grid format used to collect raw data in Independent Ambulation study.

nology. Recommendations of the technology training team, whether or not the student obtained the recommended equipment, and the extent to which the student was successful in using the equipment, were recorded on the raw data sheet and summarized as illustrated in Figure 9-4. The pre-test and post-test scores of two groups of mothers of children with disabilities were recorded using the forms illustrated in Figure 9-5. One group of mothers received a ten session training program, designed to enhance their abilities to teach their young children self-care skills. The second group of mothers did not receive training. Figure 9-6a illustrates the raw data sheet used to record the number of times a toddler with cerebral palsy reached during the classroom day (Nov. 4; data point 14), and figure 9-6b illustrates the sheet used to summarize the data across baseline and intervention sessions.

Summarizing data often is a lengthy and time consuming process which requires accuracy. Errors occur easily in trans-ferring data from one sheet onto another, as well as in the mathematical calculations that may be done. Therefore, some sort of checking system is necessary in order to prevent errors, and discover and correct those that have been made inadvertently. A checking system is accomplished easily, by having an individual who has not participated in the study check the work of the person with responsibility for summarizing data.

Some program evaluation study designs require statistical analyses in order to interpret data as accurately as possible. Data generated from single subject or group designs across a group of children, families, or staff, may be analyzed statistically if the numbers of subjects included in the group are sufficiently large (e.g., Bruning & Kintz, 1977). Two general types of statistics may be used. Parametric tests, such as t-tests or analyses of variance (ANOVA's), are the most commonly used tests to determine differences among groups, where the subject group(s) include at least ten members, and

Data Summary Sheet

Discipline: Motor/Classroom/Speech

Goal: Independent Ambulation _____ Child's Name: _____

Date	Data Point	# Trials	Number Correct #	Number Correct %	Number Incorrect #	Number Incorrect %	#	%	#	%	#	%	Comments
6/29	1	10	–	–	10/10	100							Baseline
7/1	2	10	–	–	10/10	100							
7/20	3	10	–	–	10/10	100							
7/22	4	10	–	–	10/10	100							Intervention:
7/29	5	10	–	–	10/10	100							2 ft. ceiling
9/14	6	10	–	–	10/10	100							walk in hallway
9/28	7	10	–	–	10/10	100							
10/5	8	10	–	–	10/10	100							
10/7	9	10	–	–	10/10	100							walk to bench
10/14	10	10	–	–	10/10	100							2 feet away
10/19	11	10	–	–	10/10	100							
10/21	12	10	1/10	10	9/10	90							
10/26	13	10	0	0	10/10	100							
11/4	**14**	**10**	**3/10**	**30**	**7/10**	**70**							
11/9	15	10	2/10	20	8/10	80							
11/16	16	10	3/10	30	7/10	70							
11/18	17	10	4/10	40	6/10	60							
11/23	18	10	8/10	80	2/10	20							
11/25	19	10	9/10	90	1/10	10							
12/7	20	10	0	0	10/10	100							raise ceiling
12/9	21	10	1/10	10	9/10	90							to 5 feet
12/14	22	10	0	0	10/10	100							walk to fence
12/16	23	10	3/10	30	7/10	70							
12/20	24	10	2/10	20	8/10	80							

Figure 9-6b. Grid designed to analyze data collected in the Independent Ambulation study. (See Figure 9-5a.)

where the data generated are numerical. Non-parametric tests, such as chi-square, are used when at least ten members are included in each subject group, and where the data are ranked. Data, such as the number of times (frequency) that a child reached during snack time, are numerical, whereas scores obtained from a rating scale where parents rated the extent of satisfaction with various aspects of a program, are ranked. Data from the first example are analyzed using parametric statistics. Non-parametric tests are used to analyze those in the second example. The use of statistical procedures is determined during the planning phase of program evaluation, to ensure that the data will be generated in ways that meet the criteria for use of various tests. Consultants may be helpful in determining the types of analyses that are appropriate, and in performing the necessary calculations, once data have been collected and summarized.

The majority of studies undertaken to evaluate various aspects of a program do not require statistical analyses. Data are reported descriptively, in the text of a report, or in summarized tables, or through graphs or charts. Table 9-8 and 9-9 show the final summarizations of data, for data previously illustrated in Figures 9-4 and 9-5. The summarization of single subject design data (see Figure 9-6) is illustrated as a graph in Figure 9-7. These final representations of data are included in written reports of program evaluation studies, or are used to illustrate data presented verbally.

REPORTING PROGRAM EVALUATION RESULTS

Reporting of program evaluation results is related to the purpose for conducting program evaluation. Audiences interested in the results range from program personnel, and their supervisors and administrators, to national audiences, and include program consumers, including families of participating children, related community agencies, and the community-at-large, state and local policy makers, accreditation bodies, funding sources, university faculty, as well as personnel from similar programs (Shaw, 1985). Dessemination of program evaluation results is quite important, since these results communicate to others about the quality of the program being provided for children and their families. Communicating results of program evaluation efficacy studies is important for two reasons. The first reason is to explore and document the effectiveness of service provision being provided in a particular program. The second reason is to report

---

TABLE 9-8

DATA SUMMARY
TECHNOLOGY TRAINING PROJECT

	YES	NO	DON'T KNOW	NO RESPONSE
specific equipment recommended n=100	**71**	**18**	**11**	**0**
equipment obtained n=100	**47***	**51**	**2**	**0**
child using equipment correctly *n=47	**35****	**2**	**10**	**0**
child using equipment successfully **n=35	**29**	**6**	**0**	**0**

TABLE 9-9 Data Summary

	Mothers with Training				Mothers without Training			
	No. of Subjects	Pre-test Score	Post-test Score	Difference	No. of Subjects	Pre-test Score	Post-test Score	Difference
Totals	20	389	882	491	20	391	438	47
x̄:		19.45	44.1	24.55		19.55	21.9	2.35
Standard deviation:		3.268	3.553	3.605		3.268	2.854	2.159
$t_{(.05)}$: 23.626 > 2.093								

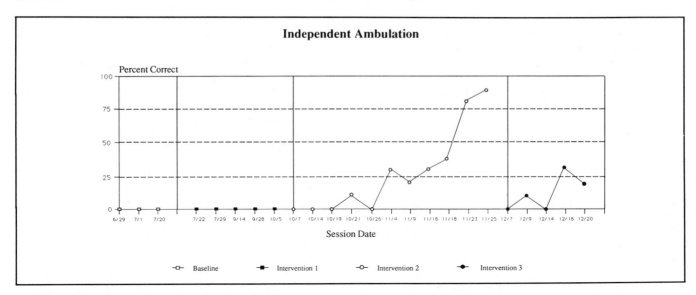

Figure 9-7.   Example of use of graph format to summarize single subject design data. (See Figures 9-6a and b for raw data.)

to interested professionals the interventions that were used in service provision, that were effective with children, as a whole, or particular groups of children (e.g., Campbell, 1988).

The types of reporting required are generally determined by the audience to which results will be presented. Audiences are classified as either internal (inside the agency administering the program), or external (outside the agency administering the program). Compiling and communicating results for the community-at-large, for example, through an article in a local newspaper, is quite different from preparing a report of program evaluation for a funding source.

Communicating With Internal Audiences

Internal audiences include: a) immediate program staff; b) program supervisors and administrators; c) consumers; and d) the Boards of the program or the agency. The purpose of conducting the evaluation guides decision making in terms of what information to present using what mechanisms.

Program staff are likely to be most interested in using data for decision making. Formative or ongoing studies that yield information that may be used to improve program functioning are of most interest. Knowing that parents would view the program as more effective if parent training were provided, for example, provides staff and administration with the data to support establishing such a program. Similarly, determining through review of ongoing data that the intervention being provided for a child or group of children is not having the desired effect, allows program staff to change the intervention being provided. Data may be presented to staff and administration verbally or through short written reports. Verbal presentations that are timely, and are included as a regular part of staff meetings or other group meetings, are often most effective. The data are used in these situations to provide program staff with immediate feedback about current status of the program. This feedback in turn provides a basis for group discussion, and for decisions concerning program organization and services.

Internal administrative and supervisory staff are typically more interested in summative outcome data that describe the effectiveness or impact of the program, than on formative data that is used as a basis for ongoing decision making. Outcome studies provide critical information about the characteristics and demographics of the children receiving services, the impact of services on those children and their families, the cost of services, the quality of the staff and other related issues (Linder, 1983; Shaw, 1985).

Consumers in pediatric programs include a variety of audiences dependent on who is purchasing and using services. Parents, for example, are indirect consumers for their young children with disabilities, but older children may function directly as consumers of services. Other community agencies are consumers when a pediatric program sells services to agencies. For example, occupational therapy services may be provided by a school district, but that district may also contract with an outside agency to provide a specific service, such as evaluation or technology services. In this instance, the consumer for the outside agency is the school district, in addition to families and children who may receive the services through the outside agency. Consumers may be interested in a number of aspects of program operation and impact, but particularly value information about the extent to which the program operates efficiently, and impacts positively on a program, or on children and families. Information may be communicated verbally, through meetings with consumer groups or discussion with individual consumers, but information may reach all consumers only when communicated through a written report or working paper.

Board members are a very important audience to which evaluation results are communicated. These individuals are responsible for making policy and financial decisions that impact on the provision of services for children. Board members are most interested in demographic studies that report services and their changes or improvements, or that describe needed improvements. Being able to demonstrate, for example, that the number of children served by occupational therapy services has increased across a time span, may be important information for program policy personnel such as Board members. Studies that report consumer satisfaction and illustrate the extent to which occupational therapy services further the mission of the agency or organization as a whole, also are meaningful for Board members. Results of program evaluation studies are likely to be reported to audiences of this type through written or verbal reports. Requesting to be included on the Board meeting agenda is acceptable in some agencies, whereas in other agencies, presentations are invited by the Board chairperson or arranged by the program's director or superintendent.

Communicating With External Audiences

Audiences that are external to a program or agency include the community in which a program's services are offered, other professionals, including university faculty, accreditation bodies, funding sources, and state and national policy makers. Information from program evaluation studies can be of interest to any of these groups if presented in ways that address their interests and needs. For example, residents of a community may be interested in knowing that the tax dollars that support an agency, such as the public schools, are being spent in ways that benefit children in general, or specific groups of children. An article in a local newspaper that describes the program, and its benefits for those individuals receiving services, is one way of communicating selected program evaluation information. Many private agencies have newsletters, annual reports or internal house magazines that are distributed to a wide range of individuals in a community. These publications are another good location for stories or short articles about the ways in which services are provided and their impact on individuals being served.

Other professionals are interested in successful models of service provision, the effects of particular intervention techniques or strategies on children, staff development programs and their effects, or other unique and successful features of programs. The extent to which a particular occupational therapy department (or other service provision unit) provides quality services is of less interest than are descriptions of specific features of a program that can be replicated in other similar situations. Communicating the methods used and the outcomes obtained from selected program evaluation studies can be achieved in a variety of ways. Information may be shared verbally through presentations or discussions at local meetings of professionals (e.g., a local or state occupational therapy association; a local early intervention collaborative group; or a local study group composed of various discipline school-based therapists). In this instance, professionals within a particular locality become knowledgeable about a particular program study, (e.g., a study that examined the differences in children's performance under service provision models of consultation, or direct individual therapy). Similar presentations may be developed for state and national conferences, where the audience affected represents larger geographical areas.

A second way of informing other professionals is through written documentation that may be submitted for publication. Newsletters are received by a wide range of professionals dependent on the type of newsletter. Some are received by all occupational therapists or professionals in a state or in the country, whereas others may be sent only to those who identify particular specialty interests, or are members of particular groups outside, (for example, the American Occupational Therapy Association, AOTA). A journal is a second type of publication. Journals are distributed nationally to those professionals who either belong to the sponsoring organization, or who subscribe separately to the journal. Other journals are distributed on a subscription basis only, and do not have a sponsoring professional organization. For the most part, journals publish articles that focus on a particular issue or topic. Program evaluation studies that present descriptive, single subject, or group data, may be appropriate for submission to journals. A single, well-done program evaluation study on a particular topic is likely to be more appropriate for journal submission, than an evaluation study of the overall program. Journals vary considerably in terms of the amount and type of data collection and analysis that is considered appropriate by the journal's editor(s) or review board. The type of article that is appropriate for a particular journal may be determined by reviewing past issues to determine the types of articles that have been published or by discussing the type of article being prepared with the journal's editor. All journal articles are prepared according to predetermined guidelines, which are published in each issue (or periodically) under a heading such as "Guidelines for Authors." Following these guidelines will ensure that the description of the program evaluation study is written in the format and manner used by the journal to which the article will be submitted.

Funding sources and accreditation bodies are important audiences to which program evaluation study outcomes are communicated. Funding sources are most interested in the studies that examine the cost-effectiveness of services being paid for by the source, or the outcomes of services being provided to particular individuals (e.g., individuals being funded by the source). Information may be added to documentation information being submitted to the funding source, may be prepared as a separate report, or shared verbally with appropriate personnel within the funding agency. Information gained through program evaluation studies often relates directly to the kinds of information required by accreditation bodies and links to the types of documentation required. Being able not only to provide documentation of services, but also to report evaluation data about the impact of those services on individuals or groups of individuals, is gaining importance with accreditation bodies. Review of the standards and requirements of accreditation bodies assists in determining the types of program evaluation studies that will be of greatest interest and relevance.

State and national policy makers are an external audience who are instrumental in determining state and national policies that underlie service provision for children. Most national organizations, including AOTA, employ individuals whose responsibility is to monitor federal and state policies, and to influence policy makers by providing information at critical points in the development of policy. One route for influencing federal policy development, is to communicate program evaluation data to the individuals employed in governmental relations. These individuals, in turn, use program evaluation data when communicating with governmental relations personnel of other national organizations and with federal policy makers. Activities undertaken to inform state policy makers typically occur through members of a professional organization within a state, and often are less formal than those used at a federal level. Becoming knowledgeable about the activities of a state professional organization, is a first step in knowing how to communicate program evaluation information. State congressional representatives from the district in which a program is located may have some interest in evaluation studies that involve their local constituents, but these studies are more likely to be of interest to those representatives whose responsibility includes education or health issues. Policy makers, whether at a federal or state level, are the constant recipients of information from all sorts of special interest groups, constituents, and other individuals. Effective communication with these individuals is more easily accomplished through coordinated and collaborative approaches, rather than by isolated contacts.

EXPAND YOUR NEWLY ACQUIRED KNOWLEDGE

1. Create a program evaluation plan for a pediatric arthritis program. Include strategies for adapting the program, and demonstrating effective feedback mechanisms from the data collected.

References

Alberto, E., & Troutman, S. (1982). *Applied behavior analysis for teachers.* Columbus: Charles E. Merrill.

Bricker, D., & Gumerlock, S. (1985). A three-level strategy. In J. Danaher (Ed.) *Assessment of child progress* (p. 7). North Carolina: University of North Carolina at Chapel Hill.

Bricker, D. D., & Littman, D. (1982). Intervention and evaluation: The inseparable mix. *Topics in early childhood special education, 1*(4), 23–33.

Bricker, D., Sheehan, R., & Littman, D. (1981). *Early intervention: A plan for evaluating program impact.* Monmouth, Oregan: WESTAR Series Paper #10.

Bruning, J. L., & Kintz, B. L. (1977). *Computational handbook of statistics* (2nd Ed.). Glenview, IL: Scott Foresman Publisher.

Campbell, P. H. (1988). Using single subject research design to evaluate the effectiveness of treatment. *American Journal of Occupational Therapy, 42*(11), 732–738.

Campbell, P. H., & Mulhauser, M. B. (1989). Use of electronic switch interface devices in discrimination training with severely multihiandicapped students. Manuscript submitted for publication.

Campbell, P. H., & Stewart, B. (1986). Measuring changes in movement skills with infants and young children with handicaps. *Journal of the Association for Persons with Severe Handicaps, 11*(3), 153–161.

Hall, R. V., Cristler, C., Cranston, S. S., & Tucker, B. (1970). Teachers and parents as researchers using multiple baselines. *Journal of Applied Behavior Analysis, 3*(4), 247–255.

Hersen, M., & Barlow, D. H. (1976). *Single case experimental designs: Strategies for studying behavior change.* New York: Pergammon Press.

Kazdin, A. E., & Kopel, S. A. (1975). On resolving ambiguities of the multiple baseline design: Problems and recommendations. *Behavior Therapy, 6*, 601–608.

Linder, T. (1983). *Early childhood special education: Program development and administration.* Baltimore: Paul Brookes.

Ottenbacher, K., & York, J. (1984). Strategies for evaluating clinical change: Implications for practice and research. *The American Journal of Occupational Therapy, 38*(10), 647–659.

Shaw, K. J. (1985). Program evaluation. In J. Bair & M. Gray (Eds.), *The occupational therapy manager* (pp. 235–249). Rockville, MD: The American Occupational Therapy Association, Inc.

Sheehan, R., & Gallagher, R. J. (1983). Conducting evaluations of infant intervention programs. In S. G. Garwood & R. R. Fewell (Eds.), *Educating handicapped infants: Issues in development and intervention* (pp. 495–519). Rockville, MD: Aspen Systems Corporation.

Sheehan, R., & Keough, B. (1981). Design and analysis in the evaluation of early childhood special education programs. *Topics in Early Childhood Special Education, 1*(4), 81–88.

Slavin, R. E. (1984). *Research methods in education: A practical guide.* Englewood Cliffs, NJ: Prentice-Hall, Inc.

Suarez, T. M., & Vandivier, P. (Eds.) (1978). *Planning for evaluation. A resource book for programs for preschool handicapped children: Documentation.* Chapel Hill, NC: Technical Assistance Development System.

Tawney, J. W., & Gast, D. L. (1984). Single subject research in special education. Columbus, OH: Charles E. Merrill Publishing Co.

Worley, M., & Harris, S. R. (1982). Interpreting results of single-subject research designs. *Physical Therapy, 62*(4), 445–452.

APPENDIX

Selected Sources of Information on Study Design and Statistics

Campbell, P. H. (1988). Using single subject research design to evaluate the effectiveness of treatment. *American Journal of Occupational Therapy, 42*(11), 732–738.

Slavin, R. E. (1984). *Research methods in education: A practical guide.* Englewood Cliffs, NJ: Prentice-Hall, Inc.

Tawney, J. W. & Gast, D. L. (1984). *Single subject research in special education.* Columbus, OH: Charles E. Merrill Publishing Co.

Support for the
Service Provision Process

CHAPTER 10

Impact of Federal Policy on Pediatric Health and Education Programs

Barbara E. Hanft, MA, OTR/L, FAOTA

"Today's programs for exceptional children and youth are to a large extent a direct result of organized advocacy efforts, legislative campaigns, and litigation of the 1970's. But present conditions actually had their roots in the beginning of special programs for the handicapped at the turn of the century. And a number of events of the 1960's and early 1970's greatly accelerated progress on behalf of the handicapped, setting the stage for formulation of public policy that we now accept as essential. For the most part, these events have been couched in civil rights movements, with an emphasis on removing race, sex, and age barriers. Civil rights policy making provided and foundation and climate for bringing about needed changes on behalf of the handicapped."
Meyen, 1982

INTRODUCTION

Federal policy is reflected in legislation passed by Congress, regulations promulgated by federal agencies, and decisions handed down by the federal courts. It is also reflected in the daily decisions and actions of federal administrators and politicians. Federal policy evolves in a developmental process that reflects and responds to public opinion and research, as well as professional, personal, and political experience.

Current federal support for health and education services for children evolved out of three general trends in public policy: health care for the disadvantaged in the early 1900's, rehabilitation and vocational education of the wounded soldiers after World Wars I and II, and civil rights for individuals with disabilities. The lack of any federal programs for children until the early 1900's reflected popular opinion, which viewed children as possessions of their parents, devoid of rights or individuality until they matured. Treated as miniature adults, children had no unique health care needs.

Slowly, it was recognized that, if infants were going to survive childhood, then parents and professionals needed to know more about child rearing, health care, and treating specific disabilities. Dr. Thomas Rotch, the first chair of pediatrics at Harvard Medical School, stated in 1888:

> "To intelligently understand the fully developed man in health and disease, it seems self-evident that the anatomy and physiology not only of the final state of growth should be studied, but also that the various stages of development, from embryo to infant, and the infant to child, and child to adult, should successively be dealt with. This in the past, however, has been but little done. On the contrary, the very opposite method has been adopted; the most careful attention being paid to adult anatomy and physiology, and then deductions made backward from adult to child—a retrograde means of acquiring knowledge, which has proved eminently unsuccessful." (Public Health Service, 1976, p. 9).

The concepts articulated by Dr. Rotch at the end of the 19th century provided the foundation for a new specialty, pediatrics, for many health care professions including occupational and physical therapy, nursing, medicine, social work, and psychology. The stages of child development establish a common foundation for providers of pediatric health care, education, and habilitation services.

When development is viewed as a continuum between the typical and atypical, a continuum of service needs, from generalized to specific, also emerges. For example, a child with a developmental disability, such as Down Syndrome, may experience the "typical" childhood illnesses of colds, flu, or chickenpox, as well as the "atypical" symptoms associated with Down Syndrome. Thus, this one child will need health and education services generally available to all children, as well as services for children with special needs.

Such a continuum of general and specific health and education services for children has developed only in the last 70 years. Public policy trends during this time can be tracked by studying federal legislation effecting special education, developmental disabilities, and maternal and child health services. It is important for occupational therapy practitioners specializing in pediatrics to recognize that federal policy has a dual impact on services to children: it both shapes and is shaped by trends in health and education practice. Legislation, regulations, and administrative policies reflect current practice, as well as shape future services. The continuum of child and policy development, each with its own successive stages and markers, establishes a guideline for the provision of pediatric occupational therapy services.

HISTORICAL PERSPECTIVE OF FEDERAL POLICIES ON PEDIATRIC CARE (1800–1949)

Programs for the Disabled

One of the forerunners of federal policy for children's services was the development of programs for the disabled. During the 1800's, state and local policies of benevolent shelter for individuals with mental disabilities translated into home and community care (Finch, 1985). The earliest federal role in education for the disabled occurred during this period, with the creation of special schools for the mentally ill, blind or deaf between 1820 and 1870. This paralleled a similar movement at the state level, when state schools for the handicapped were established as early as 1823 (LaVor, 1976).

Early in 1900, a new set of policies evolved, called the "eugenics movement". People with disabilities, particularly developmental disabilities, were viewed as "defectives" and "deviates", likely to be dangerous, promiscuous, and unable to improve their condition. During this period, institutionalization became the treatment of choice. Although originally designed to cure and train the resident with disabilities, institutions became far too crowded, with little habilitation potential. Large facilities quickly deteriorated, providing custodial care, social control, and isolation from family and community life (Rothman, 1971).

The Evolution of Public Health Programs for Children

The present United States Public Health Service evolved from the Marine Hospital Service authorized by Congress in 1798. This was the first federal program concerned with the care of persons with disabilities (i.e., sick or disabled seamen). Early in 1900, the service's name was changed to the Public Health and Marine Hospital Service, when it became responsible for the control of communicable diseases in all the states (Mountin, 1949). In 1912, the name was simplified to its present designation. Over the years, the Public Health Service has assumed major responsibilities for the health care of children.

The federal government first focused on issues affecting the health of children when it established the Children's Bureau in 1912. Created largely in response to social reformers' concerns about the problems of child labor, the Bureau's mandate was limited to information gathering and investigation. Such issues as maternal mortality, unmarried mothers, child labor, aid to mothers with dependent children, and the control of juvenile delinquency were among its studies. The Bureau's first investigation of infant mortality was also the first of its kind in any nation, and identified family income, housing, and sanitation as crucial factors in determining whether infants and mothers lived or died (Davis & Schoen, 1978).

Julia Lathrop, the first chief of the Children's Bureau, presented a plan for the "Public Protection of Maternity and Infancy" in her annual report to Congress in 1917. She detailed the need for the following nationwide services: public health nurses for instruction and service to mothers, university curriculums covering hygiene, centers for the examination of well children, and city and rural-based services for mothers and children (Eliot, 1972). Eventually, the Children's Bureau helped influence Congress in 1921 to enact the Maternity and Infancy Act, also known as the Sheppard-Towner Act.

The enactment of the Sheppard-Towner Act marked the first time the federal government provided grants-in-aid to the states for human services (previously, federal aid to states was given for agriculture and road construction). Specifically, these federal grants provided direct maternal and child health services. State activities included the promotion of birth registration, fostering cooperation between public health authorities and health providers, and establishing infant welfare and maternity centers, as well as educational classes for mothers, midwives, and mothers' helpers (Bailey, 1983).

Unfortunately, political support for the program was extremely limited, as it was perceived to interfere with family life. During original debate in the Senate, the bill had been branded as coming from the "radical, socialistic and bolshevistic philosophy of Germany and Russia" (Public Health Service, 1976, p. 30). It was also ridiculed as being a departure from common sense since:

> "The mother of today has enough sense to know in general what her baby needs. When she is in doubt she resorts to the assistance of her husband, the counsel of some good old mother, and the advice of the family doctor." (Public Health Service, 1976, p. 30).

In 1929, Congress failed to reauthorize the Act. In its eight years of existence, the Sheppard-Towner Act helped bring about expanded public health care for mothers and children. The American Academy of Pediatrics was also established in 1930, as a direct result of the professional dissent surrounding the Act. Physicians who had been members of the opposing American Medical Association broke away, and formed their own association to develop relationships with other organizations interested in the health and medical care of children.

The Great Depression and Social Security

The Great Depression, following the stock market crash in 1929, presented the federal government with nationwide problems that required a unified response. By the spring of 1933, unemployment had reached an estimated fifteen million people, many of whom protested through demonstration and hunger marches (Public Health Services, 1976). One of the federal programs developed in response was the Public Works Administration, authorized in the National Industrial Recovery Act of 1933. Funds were available to construct public buildings, including institutes for the mentally retarded and state psychiatric hospitals (Braddock, 1987).

By 1935, the United States had a higher maternal death rate than nearly all other industrialized countries, and childbirth represented the second leading cause of death among women age 20 to 45. In addition, about one child in every 100 was physically handicapped, with only a very small percentage receiving timely treatment (Senate Committee Report, 1935).

The Social Security Act was signed into law on August 14, 1935. Title V of this Act established two state grant programs, one for maternal and child health (MCH) services, and the other for crippled children's services (CCS).[1] Neither program was designed to provide services to children with mental handicaps, however. The state MCH programs generally focused on preventive health care services, such as prenatal clinics, maternity-nursing services, and immunization and school health programs.

---

[1] The Children's Bureau is now part of the U.S. Department of Health and Human Services, as are the CCS and MCH programs. Federal legislation in 1986 changed the designation of Crippled Children's Services to Children with Special Health Needs.

The CCS programs initially treated children who needed orthopedic services or plastic surgery. The minutes of the 1936 Crippled Children's Service National Advisory Committee contained the recommendation that "children with incurable blindness, deafness, or mental defect . . . and those requiring permanent custodial care, should be beyond the scope of the Program" (Braddock, 1987). Services were expanded in the 1940's to treat children with rheumatic heart conditions, and were again expanded in the 1950's to cover children with congenital heart disease (Davis and Schoen, 1978).

In 1965, Social Security was again amended to establish Title XIX, a federal-state medical assistance program (Medicaid). States are given broad flexibility in providing services; however, they all must provide early periodic screening, diagnosis, and treatment (EPSDT) services for individuals under age 21. Eligibility for Medicaid services is based on financial need. Each state submits a Medicaid plan to the federal government defining the extent, scope and cost of services. In addition to EPSDT, the state must provide nine other core medical services, and then can choose from 20 other optional services. Occupational therapy and other "related services" fall within the state option, and may or may not be included in any given state's plan. The federal government pays the state 50% to 80% of the cost of Medicaid services, adjusted annually, based on the average annual per capita income in the state.

Vocational Education and Rehabilitation Program

Although the federal government's first role in education was to establish special schools for the disabled in the 1800's, no further federal activity occurred until World War I and II spurred the government into providing vocational education and rehabilitation programs (Boggs, 1971). The Smith-Hughes Act of 1917 authorized grants to states for vocational education activities. This program was the first major program in public education, as well as the nation's first state formula grant program in the broad areas of health, education, and welfare. Unfortunately, services to persons with disabilities were not authorized.

The following two laws were the forerunners of the landmark Rehabilitation Act of 1973, which established important treatment programs and civil rights for individuals of all ages with disabilities (see the Act for further discussion). The Civilian Vocational Rehabilitation Act of 1920 authorized rehabilitation services to civilians with physical disabilities. Vocational rehabilitation services to individuals with mental handicaps were not available until 1943, when the Barden-LaFollete Act was passed (Braddock, 1987).

KEY PEDIATRIC HEALTH AND EDUCATION LEGISLATION (1950 — PRESENT)

From 1950 through the 1970's, there was a significant expansion of federal education and health programs for individuals with disabilities, especially children. This shift in federal policy was based on five major factors (Menzler, 1986). The first was the need for rehabilitation created by returning World War II veterans. Public understanding of disability issues increased and federal programs for people with disabilities expanded. Social Security was revised and Medicare, Medicaid, and Supplemental Security Insurance (SSI) programs were enacted.

The second factor was the development of new treatment techniques and technology, which made prevention and habilitation possible. This, in turn, created the need for new services and programs. Advances in the treatment of disabling conditions reduced the public's misperception about the cause of disability, particularly mental retardation and mental illness.

The Civil Rights movement for minorities in the 1960's was the third factor. This, together with the principle of normalization, set the stage for legislation guaranteeing the rights of individuals with handicaps. Normalization views an individual with a disability as a person, not a "disabled" person, entitled to the same education, habilitation, and employment opportunities as able bodied people.

The fourth factor was the development of parental rights and advocacy for the disabled, which helped individuals with disabilities establish the right to control their own lives. Founded in 1950, The National Association for Retarded Children (later changed to the Association for Retarded Citizens) presently has 160,000 members, the majority of whom are parents or family members of individuals with disabilities (Marchand, 1987). Simultaneously, a consumer movement throughout the country created the climate to analyze and judge services of all kinds, including those for individuals with handicaps.

The fifth factor was the expanding economy in the 1960's. Federal funds were allocated for health, education and social welfare programs for many Americans, not just those with disabilities. The administration of President Lyndon Johnson was labeled the "Great Society" because of its policies increasing services to the disadvantaged. This funding also fueled an expansion of services for people with disabilities. Table 10-1 contains a summary of the federal legislation which has impacted pediatric services from 1960–1988.

Reconciliation and Austerity

During the 1980's, economic changes and political questioning of the value of some services, as well as the roles of federal and state government in providing programs to the disabled and economically disadvantaged, have contributed to an attitude of reform and change. The Omnibus Budget Reconciliation Act of 1981, P.L. 97–35, authorized extensive budget cuts in domestic and social programs while increasing defense spending. Large, multipurpose block grants to the states replaced separate, categorical programs, allowing states to make their own funding choices.

Nevertheless, several essential laws guaranteeing services to children with disabilities have been expanded during the past five years. These laws, and their recent modifications, are discussed in detail below.

EDUCATION OF THE HANDICAPPED ACT (EHA)

The Education of the Handicapped Act (EHA) provides funds to states and local educational agencies to assist them

TABLE 10-1. Federal Legislation Impacting Pediatric Health and Education Programs (1960–1988)

Date Enacted	Public Law Number	Name Legislation	Impact on Education and Health Care for Children
1963	PL 88-164	Mental Retardation Facilities and Community Mental Health Centers Construction Act	Provided financial aid for building community based facilities for people with developmental disabilities and mental illness and authorized research centers and university affiliated facilities (UAF's)
1963	PL 88-156	The Maternal and Child Health and Mental Retardation Planning Amendments (to social security)	Established the Maternal and Child Health Program to improve prenatal care to high risk women from low income families.
1963	PL 88-210	Vocation Education Act of 1963	Recognized that individuals with special needs required assistance to achieve success in regular vocational programs.
1964		Economic Opportunity Act of 1963	Established Project Head Start offering health, education, nutritional and social services to economically deprived preschool children. In 1972, PL 92-424 set aside a minimum of 10% of Head Start enrollment for children with handicaps.
1965	PL 89-97	Social Security Amendments	Established Medicare/Medicaid, providing public funding for the poor, aged and disabled. This was one of the legislative reforms recommended by the Presidents's Panel on Mental Retardation (Kennedy, 1961).
1970	PL 91-230	ESEA Amendments of 1970 creates the Education of the Handicapped Act (EHA)	Consolidate several separate special education statutes into a single Title VI, referred to as the "Education of the Handicapped Act." Increased funds for schools to buy equipment and build facilities.
1970	PL 91-517	The Developmental Disabilities Services and Facilities Construction Amendments	Expands PL 88-164 into a comprehensive statute that also require every state to establish a governor's council on developmental disabilities. First time the term "developmental disabilities" was used, replacing "mental retardation." People with cerebral palsy and epilepsy are now eligible for services under this new definition.
1972	PL 92-223	Social Security Amendments	Authorized "Intermediate Care Facilities" to be reimbursed under Medicaid if states ensured that residents received "active treatment." The ICF/MR program became the single largest federal expenditure for operating state institutions.
1972	PL 92-603	Social Security Amendments	Established Supplemental Security Income to standardize assistance programs to people in need, including those with developmental disabilities.
1973	PL 93-112	Rehabilitation Act, Section 504	The first legislation to focus on rehabilitation services for people with severe disabilities. Section 504 established civil rights protection for all people with disabilities by prohibiting all recipients of federal funds from discrimination against the handicapped.
1978	PL 95-602	Rehabilitation Comprehensive Services and Developmental Disability Act	Defined "Developmental Disabilities" in functional terms and emphasized the severity and chronicity of these functional impairments. Identified priority areas for state Developmental Disabilities Councils to address.
1980	PL 96-265 Section 1619 a and b	Social Security Amendments	Established a three year demonstration project to allow individuals with developmental disabilities to keep Social Security benefits while working.
1981	PL 97-35 Section 2176	Omnibus Reconciliation Act, "Home Based Waiver"	Allowed states to finance (through Medicaid) a wide variety of community based services for the developmental disabled rather than in institutional settings, if states demonstrated such services would be less expensive than institutional care.
1982	PL 97-248	Social Security Amendments, ("Katie Beckett" Amendments)	Permitted states to use Medicaid for certain children with disabilities, 18 years of age or younger, to remain living at home rather than be institutionalized.

Federal Legislation Impacting Pediatric Health and Education Programs (1960–1988). *Continued.*

Date Enacted	Public Law Number	Name Legislation	Impact on Education and Health Care for Children
1984	PL 98-248	Carl Perkins Vocational Technical Education Act	Mandated development of quality vocational education programs with 10% set aside to train individuals with disabilities.
1984	PL 98-527	Developmental Disabilities Act Amendments	Amended the purpose of the Developmental Disability Act to ensure that individuals receive necessary services and to establish a coordination and monitoring system. Definitions were added for "independence," "integration," "supported employment" and "employment-related activities."
1987	PL 100-146	Developmental Disabilities Assistance & Bill of Rights Amendments of 1987	Revised priority service areas and added "family support service". Funds were pinpointed for training by University Affiliated programs to address the needs of persons with developmental disabilities in the area of early intervention.
1987	PL 100-203	Omnibus Budget Reconciliation Act of 1987	Amended Medicaid to allow states to enroll pregnant women and children (0–1 yr.) with incomes up to 185% of federal poverty line.
1988	PL 100-407	Technology Related Assistance for Individuals	Provided funds to assist states in developing technology-related assistance programs for individuals of all ages with disabilities. Studies of financing issues as well as setting up a national information and program referral network were also initiated.
1988	PL 100-360	Medicare Catastrophic Coverage Act	Clarified that Medicaid funds can pay for the cost of "related services" in a school aged child's IEP or IFSP, if the services would have been paid for if PL 94-142 was not in effect.

TABLE 10-2. Education of the Handicapped Act

Subpart	Description
A	General Provisions and definition
B	Funding formula, procedural safeguards, evaluation plan
C	Centers and services to meet special needs of the handicapped
D	Training special education, related services and early intervention personnel
E	Research and demonstration projects
F	Instructional media, captioned films
G	Technology
H	Early intervention

in educating children with disabilities.[2] The EHA has eight subparts, A through H. (see Table 10-2)

Part B, commonly known as Public Law 94-142, was passed in 1975, and provides the framework for special education. The remaining subparts define terms and authorize grant programs aimed at supporting Part B services with research, demonstration, training, technical assistance, dissemination, and model projects. Key provisions guaranteed by the law include:

- Free, appropriate public education for all children with disabilities;
- Special education and related services, including occupational therapy, to meet the unique educational needs of students with disabilities;
- Written Individualized Education Programs (IEP) for all students receiving specialized services;
- Due process rights for parents related to identification, evaluation and placement procedures for their children;
- Placement in the least restrictive environment (i.e., children with disabilities are educated with their peers, to the maximum extent appropriate).

Why the EHA Was Enacted

Until the early 1970's, public schools across the country did not provide equal educational opportunities for children with disabilities. Supporting the need for enacting P.L. 94-142 in 1975, Congress found that one-half of the eight million children with disabilities in the United States were not receiving appropriate educational services, and that one million of these children were excluded from attending school at all [20 U.S.C.b 1401 (b)]. School practices ranged from creating

[2] The EHA uses the term "handicapped children" to identify students who are mentally retarded, hard of hearing, deaf, speech impaired, visually handicapped, seriously emotionally disturbed, orthopedically impaired, other health impaired, deaf-blind, multi-handicapped, or as having specific learning disabilities, who because of those impairments need special education and related services. The 1990 amendments to the EHA proposed in Congress would change the label of "handicapped children" to "children with disabilities," recognizing all students as children first, who also have a specific disability.

waiting lists; to admitting only selected students with the same disability, to refusing admittance to all children with disabilities. Different admission policies for the handicapped were also created, with some excluding children with retardation, because they created behavioral or disciplinary problems. State funding for special education personnel was also restricted (Turnbull, 1986).

Several key court decisions in the early 1970's helped lay the judicial foundation for enacting special education legislation. These decisions were based on a landmark case on school desegregation, Brown v. Board of Education (1954). In this case, the U.S. Supreme Court held that racial segregation in public education violated the Constitution's fourteenth amendment, ensuring equal protection to all people within each state, despite sex or race. Relying on the Brown decision, similar arguments have since been made for children with disabilities (i.e., that a child with disabilities has the same rights to education as any other child).

Two subsequent court cases, Pennsylvania Association for Retarded Children (PARC) v. Commonwealth of Pennsylvania, and Mills v. D.C. Board of Education, have actually made the Brown decision meaningful in terms of educating children with disabilities. In both PARC and Mills, courts held that education was essential to enable a child to function in society, and that all children can benefit from education. Moreover, schools were required to provide a public education that would be appropriate to the student's capabilities, by providing programs and facilities "suited to their needs".

Formation of the EHA: Legislative Preludes

Congress first turned its attention to the problems of educating children with disabilities in 1966, when it added Title VI to the Elementary and Secondary Education Act of 1965 (P.L. 89-750). Title VI established a grant program to help states educate children with disabilities, and created a Bureau of Education for the Handicapped (BEH) within the Office of Education in the United States Department of Health, Education, and Welfare (BEH is now called the Office of Special Education Programs in the Department of Education and is located in the U.S. Department of Education).

In 1970, Congress replaced Title VI with P.L. 91-230, The Education of the Handicapped Act (EHA). The Bureau and the state grant program were retained. Funding was authorized for regional resource centers for deaf and/or blind children, experimental early education programs, and personnel training. However, there still was no *guarantee* that children with handicaps were entitled to a public education.

Congress enacted P.L. 93-380 in 1974, in response to judicial decisions handed down in PARC and Mills, giving children with disabilities access to public education. Now federal aid to states for special education was substantially increased. Due process protection, as well as requirements that children be taught in the least restrictive environment with able bodied peers, was put in place. The essential piece missing was a national deadline requiring state departments of education to provide education to children with disabilities.

This timetable was finally provided in 1975 with the enactment of P.L. 94-142, the Education for All Handicapped Children Act. Congress set 1980 as the deadline for providing a free, appropriate education, if each state wanted to continue to receive federal funds. A 12% cap was placed on the number of students a state could classify as "handicapped," in order to receive federal funds.

Each student also is entitled to receive an annual, written individualized education program (IEP). This is the legal document that defines the student's service plan. Public schools are required to provide related services, such as occupational therapy, only if included on the student's IEP, and then only if needed to help the student benefit from special education.

Major Principles of the EHA

Turnbull (1986) summarized the major principles of EHA as follows.

Zero Reject

No child with a disability can be excluded from a public education. This policy ensures that children with disabilities are entitled to the same educational services and programs as other children. It also goes one step further, by ensuring that all children with disabilities have equal opportunities to develop their own capabilities. Thus, schools must provide programs and facilities for each student to meet his or her needs. Individual strengths and needs must be assessed student by student, not by diagnosis or handicapping condition.

Nondiscriminatory Evaluation

Congress recognized that discrimination, through the misuse of testing and inappropriate classification, presents a major obstacle to receiving a free and appropriate education (U.S. Senate Report, 1975). The EHA therefore requires the public schools to assure that testing and placement of children with disabilities will not be racially or culturally biased.

Multidisciplinary evaluations are required and must be administered in the child's native language or, in the case of a child with a hearing loss, in their mode of communication, unless it is clearly not feasible to do so. The 12% cap on the number of children who may be identified as handicapped prevents states from over classification in order to receive federal funds. Procedural safeguards entitle parents to notice of the school's actions, a fair hearing, and the right to appeal. Access to professional records is also granted.

Testing procedures require that all personnel, including occupational therapists, use assessments that will give the student a fair and unbiased chance to perform to the best of his or her ability. Assessing the visual perceptual skills of a child who has limited manipulation by using a paper and pencil test, rather than a motor-free test, will not elicit fair performance.

Individualized and Appropriate Education

The EHA provides for appropriate education by requiring that education be individualized. This is achieved through the IEP, as developed by the student's teacher and parents, the student, a representative of the public school, and other individuals chosen by the parents or school. The IEP must include statements addressing the following:

- Present levels of education performance;
- Annual goals and short-term instructional objectives;

- Specific educational services to be provided, as well as how much the student can participate in regular education;
- Projected dates for services;
- Criteria, evaluation procedures and timelines for determining whether or not the IEP objectives are met [20 U.S.C. 1402 (19)].

Appropriate education is also protected by the requirement of placement in the least restrictive program. This means having the opportunity to interact and learn with able bodied children, to the extent possible. An "appropriate" education under EHA is one that results from a process of non-discriminatory evaluation, IEP development, and placement in the least restrictive program.

In 1982, the U.S. Supreme Court further clarified "appropriate" education to mean giving students with disabilities the same opportunities as other students (Board of Education v. Rowley). This, however, does not mean the best education, or one designed to help the child reach his or her maximum potential. Occupational therapy services in the school system, therefore, are not intended to help a student develop his or her full potential, but should assist the student in benefitting from special education.

Another landmark U.S. Supreme Court decision, addressing appropriate education with regards to related services, was made in 1984 (Irving Independent School District v. Tatro). This decision distinguished between related and medical services. A medical procedure, such as catheterization, that can be provided by parents and educational personnel *with minimal training*, would be considered a related service under EHA.

Least Restrictive Environment

This provision ensures that children with disabilities have the right to placement in an integrated or "regular" educational environment, if appropriate for the individual student. This does not depend on whether the school can conveniently place the student in a regular classroom, or whether the teachers or other students find the placement acceptable. Students with disabilities also have a chance to participate in extracurricular activities such as sports, recreation, clubs, field trips, lunch, recess, and transportation on the school bus.

The principle of the "least restrictive" placement rests on whether the education is appropriate for the individual student. This varies from student to student, depending on the severity of the disability and individual learning and coping styles. For example, not all students with the diagnosis of cerebral palsy are mentally retarded or have severe physical limitations.

Procedural Due Process

These provisions give families and advocates the right to protest how the state or local educational agencies educate the student. Two previously discussed court cases, PARC and Mills, set the precedent for establishing the following parental rights under the EHA:

- Access to all relevant school records;
- Independent educational evaluation by a qualified examiner not employed by the school;
- Written notice in the parent's native language for any change or initiation in the identification, evaluation, or placement of the student;
- Assignment of a parent surrogate, if the child's parents are unavailable;
- Opportunity for an administrative hearing before an impartial officer, with appeal to the state education agency or state or federal courts, if necessary [20 U.S.C. 1415 (b) (1)].

In 1986, Congress passed P.L. 99-372, The Handicapped Children's Protection Act, which clarified a parent's right to reimbursement (from the public schools) for attorney's fees in civil court cases where parents are the prevailing party. Parents can also be reimbursed for attorney's fees expended at administrative hearings, if the school system is found in violation of EHA provisions.

EHA Amendments of 1986 (P.L. 99-457)

In October, 1986, Congress enacted P.L. 99-457, the Education of the Handicapped Act Amendments of 1986. This law expanded P.L. 94-142 to provide special education and related services to preschool children with disabilities, age three to five years. Occupational therapy, as a related service, must be available by school year 1990–1991 to children who need this service, in order to benefit from special education.

P.L. 99-457 also established an early intervention state grant program, Part H of EHA, for young children (0–3 years) and their families. Under Part H, occupational therapy is considered a *primary* early intervention service, and can be provided solely on the child's need, regardless of what other medical or educational services are provided or needed.

The intent of Congress in passing P.L. 99-457, was to acknowledge the urgent need for services, for all preschool age children with handicaps, to minimize future education and institutionalization costs to society. Rather than making Part H mandatory, Congress provided increased monetary incentives to the states for providing early intervention services.

Preschool Service (3–5 years)

Federal grants, known as "preschool incentive grants," have been available since 1975 to assist state and local educational agencies in providing services to preschoolers. These grant monies were dramatically increased under P.L. 99-457, to encourage states to serve the estimated 70,000 preschool children with disabilities (3–5 years), in need of special education and related service (U.S. Congress, 1986). By school year 1990–1991, states applying for federal educational funds will have to assure that they are providing a free, appropriate public education to every eligible child with a disability, ages 3 to 21 years.

Preschool children, ages three to five years, who have a handicapping condition *and* are in need of special education, are also eligible to receive occupational therapy services. Schools are allowed flexibility in varying the length of the school day from part to full time. They can also provide services in a center, school or home. All preschool programs will be administered through state and local educational agencies. However, other public and private non-profit programs, agencies, and providers may be contracted to offer a range of services. Failure to provide special education and related services to preschoolers with disabilities by school year 1990–1991 (1991–1992 if certain federal funding levels are not appropriated), will result in the loss of the state's preschool grant and P.L. 94-142 funds for three to five year old students.

Early Intervention Services (Part H)

A critical difference between Part H early intervention, and Part B preschool programs funded under the EHA, is that interagency responsibility for programs is required. Serving infants and toddlers with disabilities necessitates the involvement of many different agencies, as well as the school system. State departments of education, health, developmental disabilities, and mental health must collaborate to provide comprehensive programs to infants and their families.

Early intervention services under Part H must be designed to meet the developmental needs of the infant or toddler, in one or more of the following areas: physical, cognitive, language and speech, psychosocial, or self-help. Children are eligible for services if they are experiencing developmental delay in at least one of these five areas, or if they have a diagnosed physical or mental condition which has a high probability of resulting in developmental delay. States have the option of providing services to children "at-risk" of becoming substantially delayed. Each state is given the authority to define "developmental delay."

Occupational therapy is included as one of ten *primary* developmental services in the definition of "early intervention services," as follows:

i. Family training, counseling and home visits,
ii. Special instruction,
iii. Speech pathology and audiology,
iv. Occupational therapy,
v. Physical therapy,
vi. Psychological services,
vii. Case management services,
viii. Medical services only for diagnostic or evaluation purposes,
ix. Early identification, screening, and assessment services, and
x. Health services necessary to enable the infant or toddler to benefit from the other early intervention services [20 U.S.C. 1472 (2) (E)].

Thus, occupational therapy can be provided independent of the infant's or family's need for other medical, health, and education services. In another departure from P.L. 94-142, Part H lists "special instruction," not special education, as an early intervention service critical for this age group.

P.L. 99-457 also emphasizes the role of the family in the intervention process (Shelton, T., Jeppson, E., & Johnson, B., 1987; AOTA, 1989b). Early intervention services will be documented on an Individualized Family Service Plan (IFSP), developed by a multidisciplinary team including the parent or guardian. Each child will receive an annual evaluation and the family will be provided with a review of the IFSP at six month intervals.

Similar to the IEP, the IFSP will contain a statement of the infant's present level of development, and the family's strengths and needs *related to enhancing the child's development*. The services, procedures, criteria, and timelines necessary to meet the unique needs of the infant, as well as his or her family, must also be included (Johnson, B., McGonigel, M., & Kaufman, R., 1989).

Federal funds under Part H are to be used for planning, developing, and implementing statewide systems for providing early intervention services. All services must be provided at no cost, unless state or federal law allows fees; such fees must be on a sliding scale. Funds may also be used for the general expansion and improvement of services. However, for direct program services, federal funds are the "payer of last resort" [20 U.S.C. 1431 (a)]. This means that EHA funds may not be used when there are other public, private, federal, state or local monies available. For this reason, it becomes critically important to achieve efficient and effective interagency participation in each state.

To be eligible for federal funds, each state must:

- Adopt a definition of "developmentally delayed;"
- Develop a timetable to provide services within five years;
- Provide for timely evaluations and needs assessments;
- Use individualized family service plans, including case management;
- Establish a comprehensive child find and referral system;
- Conduct a public awareness program;
- Compile a central directory of services and resources;
- Develop a comprehensive system of personnel development;
- Establish a lead agency to administer, supervise, and monitor the program;
- Establish a contracting process or make other arrangements with service providers;
- Develop a payment system;
- Develop personnel standards;
- Develop a data collection process.

There is no specific date by which services must be provided nationwide, since Part H programs are discretionary. Each state must set up its own identification, evaluation, and intervention programs according to a five year timetable. However, all states and territories applied for federal funds in 1987, and will be required to provide "hands-on" early intervention services in 1991, in order to continue receiving federal dollars.

Impact of EHA on Occupational Therapy Services

The EHA has had a major impact both on the number of occupational therapy personnel providing services in the school system, as well as how services are provided. The early intervention program laid out in Part H will create still further challenges for occupational therapy practitioners (Hanft, 1988). By 1985, approximately 10,000 certified occupational therapists and assistants provided services to children in school settings (AOTA, 1986). The majority (70%) of these personnel were salaried employees; the remainder had contractual arrangements through hospital or private practice to serve children in one or more schools (AOTA, 1985a).

School systems are now the second largest employer of occupational therapists and occupational therapy assistants (AOTA, 1986). Keeping pace with this increase in employment has been an expanded professional interest in pediatrics. In 1974, 25% of the profession reported they worked primarily with children, birth to 18 years of age. In 1985, that percentage jumped to 33%, with an additional 20% of occupational therapists reporting a mixed caseload of children, adults, and elderly (AOTA, 1986).

Despite the significant increase in the number of occupational therapy personnel working in the school system, a severe shortage of personnel remains to fill positions (AOTA, 1985b). Critical shortages have also been reported in other pediatric settings, such as early intervention programs (Meisels, Harbin & Modiglian, 1988; Yoder & Coleman, 1990).

This manpower crisis, in addition to related services restrictions in the EHA, have shaped *how* occupational therapy services are provided in the school system. Several provisions set the boundaries for how preschool and school-aged children receive occupational therapy services, as follows:

1. Occupational therapy is a related service and is available only to children with disabilities who need special education to learn in school.
2. Occupational therapy, when provided as a related service, must be directed to helping a child benefit from special education.
3. Occupational therapy can be provided to help a child with a disability receive an appropriate education, not develop his or her potential to the maximum extent possible.
4. Occupational therapy can be provided through different service models, including consultation, monitoring and direct service (AOTA, 1989b; Dunn, 1988). What related services are needed, and how they are provided, is determined by an educational team, including the child's parents or guardians. An occupational therapist or occupational therapy assistant may be included on the educational team.

This fourth point illustrates how practice and policy influence one another. The provision of occupational therapy services is affected by the manpower shortage. In school year 1986–1987, there were 4,421,601 children with handicaps, from birth to age 21, receiving special education services in the school system (U.S. Department of Education, Tenth Annual Report to Congress, 1988). With approximately 10,000 occupational therapists and certified assistants to provide services, it is clearly a monumental task to provide direct "hands-on" intervention to all the special education students needing them.

Hence, a public debate has erupted over whether occupational therapy services should be direct, provided by occupational therapy personnel, or indirect, provided through consultation and/or supervision of other educational staff or families (Dunn, 1988). Decisions by hearing officers at due process hearings have been made on a case-by-case basis, but indicate clearly that services provided by educational staff and monitored by the occupational therapist, can also meet the intent of the EHA (Education of the Handicapped Law Report, 1986) as long as it matches the student's needs.

As such decisions become policy and are institutionalized, occupational therapists will be expected to know how to function effectively as consultants in the school system (Royeen, 1988). This requires knowing, not only how to assess an individual student's educational strengths and needs, but also the teacher's experience and availability, so that appropriate therapeutic strategies can be integrated into classroom activities to achieve the IEP goals and objectives (Coutinho & Hunter, 1988).

REHABILITATION ACT OF 1973: SECTION 504

Rehabilitation legislation can trace its origins back to 1920, when the National Civilian Vocational Rehabilitation Act established a system of state vocational rehabilitation agencies to help individuals with disabilities relearn work skills. Major revisions to the program were adopted in 1954, and again in 1973, when P.L. 93-112, the Rehabilitation Act of 1973 was enacted.

Title V of P.L. 93-112 contains essential safeguards to the civil rights of children, since all individuals with disabilities, irrespective of age, are protected. Section 504 of Title V prohibits discrimination solely on the basis of a person's disability in all federally assisted programs and activities as follows:

"No otherwise qualified handicapped individual in the United States . . . shall, solely by reason of his handicap, be excluded from the participation, be denied the benefits of, or be subjected to discrimination under any program or activity receiving Federal financial assistance, or under any program or activity conducted by any Executive agency or by the United States Postal Service.

Under Section 504, a "handicapped individual" includes a child who has a physical or mental impairment that substantially limits one or more major life activities, has a record of such impairment, or is regarded as having such an impairment. Major life functions refers to normal growth and developmental tasks, such as caring for oneself, performing manual tasks, walking, seeing, hearing, speaking, breathing, learning, and working. With respect to education, a "qualified handicapped individual" is someone who is guaranteed a free, appropriate public education under the EHA (Turnbull, 1986).

Relationship of EHA and Section 504

The EHA is a federal grant program to the states, while Section 504 is civil rights legislation that affects all recipients of federal funds. These two federal laws cover all children with disabilities, no matter where they reside, assuring them the right to receive a free, appropriate education, and protection against discrimination by any public agency providing special education and related services. Even if a state or local agency does not receive EHA funds, they must comply with Section 504, if they receive any funds from the Department of Education or other federal agency.

Section 504 guarantees the major provisions of the EHA: a zero-reject policy against excluding any child from a school program, a free and appropriate education, non-discriminatory testing, placement in the least restrictive environment, and due process. However, there are several notable distinctions between the two laws.

The definition of who is "handicapped" is far broader in Section 504, not only if a categorical label such as hearing-impaired is applicable, but if the child *functions* as though "handicapped." Under the EHA, a child with a disability must fit into a categorical label, *and* be in need of special education. Second, Section 504 prohibits discrimination against individuals of all ages, while the EHA addresses only children and youth, birth to 21 years.

DEVELOPMENTAL DISABILITIES ASSISTANCE AND BILL OF RIGHTS ACT

The Developmental Disabilities Assistance and Bill of Rights Act, P.L. 94-103, had its beginning over 20 years ago as a federally funded program supporting the construction of facilities for people with mental retardation. Today, it is a consumer directed system for providing and promoting services to individuals with a broad range of severe disabling conditions. The term "developmental disability" was first used in legislation enacted in 1970, replacing the definition of mental retardation, as follows:

" . . . a severe, chronic disability of a person which (a) is attributable to a mental or physical impairment or combination of mental or physical impairments; (b) is manifested before the person attains age twenty-two; (c) is likely to continue indefinitely; (d) results in substantial functional limitations in three or more of the following areas of major life activity: (1) self-care, (2) receptive and expressive language, (3) learning, (4) mobility, (5) self direction, (6) capacity for independent living, and (7) economic sufficiency; and (e) reflects the person's need for a combination and sequence of special interdisciplinary, or generic care, treatment, or other services which are of lifelong or extended duration and are individually planned and coordinated" [72 U.S.C.].

There are four major programs of P.L. 94-103: basic state grants for planning, protection and advocacy, university affiliated facilities, and special projects.

Basic Grants for Planning and Services

To receive funds under this section, a state or territory must establish a Developmental Disabilities Planning Council, composed of representatives of the state agencies serving persons with developmental disabilities, as well as providers and consumers. This Council is responsible for developing and submitting a state plan to specify needs and choose priority service areas defined in the law. It is also responsible for services, model programs, activities to enhance the ability of institutions and agencies to provide services, and the coordination, training, and outreach of providers.

Grants to Protection and Advocacy (P&A) Systems

The basic mission of the state protection and advocacy system is to pursue legal and administrative remedies, insuring that persons with developmental disabilities receive appropriate care and treatment. The P&A systems were first incorporated in the 1975 amendments to the developmental disabilities legislation, after a television documentary exposed the neglect, abuse, and lack of programming at a state institution for people with mental retardation in New York (Ellis, 1987). In order to provide for individuals with developmental disabilities, each state protection and advocacy system must be independent of all provider groups and services, including the state developmental disabilities council.

Grants to University Affiliated Facilities (UAF)

Part D of this Act authorizes grants to public or nonprofit facilities associated with a college or university, to provide interdisciplinary training to prepare personnel, including occupational therapists, to work with the developmentally disabled. Funding for UAF's is also provided by the U.S. Department of Health and Human Services, Division of Maternal and Child Health. Since the reduction of institutionalization was a particular goal of the 1984 amendments, funds may also be used to demonstrate model services, and deliver technical assistance to providers, in order to increase the independence, productivity, and integration of individuals with developmental disabilities in the community. In addition to interdisciplinary training, the UAF's strive to create exemplary service programs and conduct ongoing research related to developmental disabilities.

Special Projects

Funds are authorized to support demonstration and technical assistance projects which "hold promise of expanding or otherwise improving services to persons with developmental disabilities" [42 U.S.C. 6081]. Such projects include training policy makers, developing data collection systems, or coordinating interagency initiatives.

Legislative History

The Developmental Disabilities Assistance and Bill of Rights Act had its initial beginnings in the Hill-Burton Construction Act, enacted in 1946. This Act authorized funds to states to construct hospitals in communities with the greatest need, especially rural areas. Between 1958 and 1964, the Hill-Burton Construction Act was the primary source of federal assistance for building state institutions, activity centers, and workshops for people with mental retardation throughout the country (Braddock, 1987). In 1963, the Mental Retardation Facilities Construction Act, P.L. 88-164, was enacted. This legislation was based on recommendations of a panel of experts, called together by President John Kennedy in 1962, to address the needs of individuals with mental retardation across the country. P.L. 88-164 authorized funds for building community facilities, such as research centers and university affiliated training facilities.

In 1970, the Developmental Disabilities Services and Construction Act, P.L. 91-517, expanded previous legislation, and emphasized the importance of statewide planning for the mentally retarded. Developmental Disability Councils were established, comprised of state and local agencies, nongovernmental organizations, and community service providers and consumers. One-third of the membership of each Council had to be made up of individuals with disabilities, or their parents or guardians. Although other federal programs required public review and participation on advisory boards by consumers of services, the number of consumer members on the Councils made this program distinctive (Menzler, 1986). Federal funds were authorized to support the planning, monitoring, and administrative function of the Council in each state, as well as the development of a state plan. Pilot projects in one of 16 service areas such as daycare, education, or diagnosis could also be funded.

Also in 1970, the term "developmental disability" was used for the first time to replace mental retardation. Although recognition was given to the fact that a developmental disability begins during childhood before the age of 22, the disability extends throughout the individual's adulthood and old age, requiring extensive interdisciplinary services. The scope of the developmental disabilities program was also broadened to include the needs of individuals with cerebral palsy, epilepsy, and other related neurological conditions.

The program was again expanded in 1975 to include individuals with dyslexia, in association with other conditions, and autism. The amendments, P.L. 94-103, placed an emphasis on community-based services, by requiring each state developmental disability plan to develop and incorporate a deinstitutionalization plan. A Bill of Rights emphasized that people with developmental disabilities were entitled to services that would maximize their potential, and be provided in the least restrictive setting of the person's personal liberty. In 1975, at the same time that the IEP was incorporated in P.L. 94-142, an Individualized Habilitation Plan (IHP) was included in P.L. 94-103 for those served by this legislation.

The Rehabilitation, Comprehensive Services and Developmental Disabilities Amendments of 1978, P.L. 94-602, significantly changed the definition of developmental disability. Now an emphasis was placed on the severity of functional impairments, rather than diagnosis. This new definition eliminated specific medical diagnoses as eligibility criteria, and substituted language which required functional limitations in three of seven major life areas: self-care, language, learning, mobility, self-direction, independent living, and self-sufficiency. Children with chronic problems in any three of these functional areas would, therefore, be eligible for state services for the developmentally disabled.

As a result of the definition change, consumer members of the Councils were redefined, and increased to 50% of the membership. One-third of the consumer members had to be individuals with developmental disabilities, and another third were to be immediate relatives or guardians of individuals with a mentally impairing disability. Also, service priorities were reduced to: case management, child development, alternate community living arrangements and services, and nonvocational, social development services.

In 1984, P.L. 98-527 reinforced the goal of deinstitutionalization, by promoting services which encourage independence, productivity, and integration into the community. Individualized habilitation plans were also required to address this issue. A new emphasis was placed on promoting opportunities for people with developmental disabilities to become productive community members, by defining and adding "employment related activities" to the priority service areas. A definition of "supported employment" was also added. These amendments reflected the current public debate concerning access to services for individuals with the most severe disabilities, and their ability to become meaningfully employed.

In 1987, P.L. 30-10 reauthorized the programs of the developmental disabilities program for three years. These amendments require each Council to review the effectiveness of its respective state agencies in serving the developmentally disabled. A plan must be recommended by 1990, designating responsible agencies for providing services to traditionally underserved groups (i.e., individuals with developmental disabilities who have a combination of physical and mental impairments or who have only severe physical impairments). An additional primary service area, "Family Support Systems," was added. The UAF's also received additional funds to support interdisciplinary training projects to prepare allied health professionals, including occupational therapists, to provide early intervention services.

SUMMARY

Federal policy both shapes, and is shaped, by pediatric health care and education services, including occupational therapy. Federal legislation, regulations, and judicial decisions influence treatment programs for children with special needs. Federal policy not only defines eligibility criteria, but often is a major factor in determining the provider, service provision model, setting, and frequency of services.

Rapidly changing federal policies present a complex maze to the families of children with special needs. It is the responsibility of occupational therapy personnel, and other health and education providers, to inform themselves and consumers of these federal policies. It is only through increased awareness and efforts to inform consumers, that the full range of services mandated by federal policy will indeed be made available to children. A summary of federal legislation impacting pediatric health and education programs (1960–1988) is contained in Table 10-1.

EXPAND YOUR NEWLY ACQUIRED KNOWLEDGE

1. Describe the interrelated components of our culture in the 1960's (political priorities and service priorities). Explain how one component affects the other, and how they both in turn affect the next decade's priorities.

2. Trace the political and service priorities for the 1960's, 1970's and 1980's. Consider the direction and patterns of change, to create a hypothesis about where both political and service priorities will be by the turn of the century.

References

American Occupational Therapy Association (1986). *Member data survey*. Rockville, MD: Author.

American Occupational Therapy Association (1989b). *Guidelines for occupational therapy services in early intervention and pre-school services*. Rockville, MD: Author.

American Occupational Therapy Association (1989a). *Guidelines for occupational therapy services in school systems*, Second Edition. Rockville, MD: Author.

American Occupational Therapy Association, Commission on Practice (1985a). *School systems task force survey*. Rockville, MD: Author.

American Occupational Therapy Association (1985b). *Occupational therapy manpower: A plan for progress*. Rockville, MD: Author.

Bailey, S. (1983). *The Maternal and Child Health Services Block Grant, Title V of the Social Security Act* (Report No. 83093EPW). Washington, D.C.: Congressional Research Service.

Board of Education v. Rowley. (1982). 458 U.S. 176, 102 S. Ct. 3034, 73 L. Ed, 2d 690.

Boggs, E. (1971). Federal legislation affecting the mentally retarded. In Wortis, *Mental Retardation, III*. New York: Grune and Stratton.

Braddock, D. (1987). *Federal policy toward mental retardation and developmental disabilities*. Baltimore: Paul H. Brookes Publishing Co., Inc.

Brown v. D.C. Board of Education (1954). 347 U.S. 483.

Coutinho, M., & Hunter, D. (1988). Special education and occupational therapy: Making the relationship work. *American Journal of Occupational Therapy, 42*(11), 706–712.

Davis, K., & Schoen, C. (1978). *Health and the war on poverty: A ten-year appraisal*. Washington, D.C.: The Brookings Institute.

Dunn, W. (1988). Models of occupational therapy service provisions, in the school system. *American Journal of Occupational Therapy, 42*(11), 718–723.

Eliot, M. (1972). Six decades of action for children. *Children Today, 1*(2). Washington, D.C.: Department of Health, Education and Welfare.

Ellis, E. (1987) *NAPAS and the Protection and Advocacy Systems: 1977–1987*. Paper presented at the annual meeting of the National Association of Protection and Advocacy Systems, Washington, D.C.

Finch, Ellen (1985). Deinstitutionalization: Mental Health and Mental Retardation Services. *Psychosocial Rehabilitation Journal*. VIII(3), 36–47.

Hanft, B. (1988). The changing environment of early intervention services: Implications for practice. *American Journal of Occupational Therapy, 42*(11), 724–731.

Irving Independent School District v. Tatro (1984). ___U.S.___, 104 S. Ct. 3371, 82 L. Ed. 2d 664.

Johnson, B., McGonigel, M. & Kaufman, R. (1989). *Guidelines and recommended practices for the individualized family service plan*. Washington, DC: Association for the Care of Children's Health.

LaVor (1976). Federal legislation for exceptional persons: A history. In Weintraub, et al. (Ed.) *Public Policy and the Education of Exceptional Children*. Reston, VA: Council for Exceptional Children.

Marchand, P. (1987). Director of Government Affairs, Association for Retarded Citizens. Personal communication.

Meisels, S., Harbin, G., Modiglian, K. (1988). Formulating optimal state early childhood intervention policies. *Exceptional Children, 55*(2), 159–165.

Menzler, C. (1986). *The advocacy for change training manual*. Washington, D.C.: National Association of Developmental Disability Councils.

Meyen, E. L. (1982). *Exceptional children in today's schools: An alternative resource book* (p. 35, 587). Colorado: Love Publishing Co.

Mills v. D.C. Board of Education. (D.D.C. 1972). 348 F. Supp. 866.

Mountin, J. W. (1949). The history and functions of the United States Public Health Service. In J. S. Simmons (Ed.), *Public health in the world today*. Cambridge, MA: Harvard University Press.

Pennsylvania Association for Retarded Children (PARC) v. Commonwealth of Pennsylvania, 334 F. Supp. 1257, 343 F. Supp. 279 (E.D. Pa 1971, 1972).

Public Health Service (1976). *Child Health in America*. ((HSA) 76-5015). Washington, D.C.: Department of Health, Education and Welfare.

Public Law 89-750 (1965). Elementary and Secondary Education Act of 1965. Washington, D.C.: U.S. Government Printing Office.

Public Law 91-230 (1970). The Education of the Handicapped Act. Washington, D.C.: U.S. Government Printing Office.

Public Law 93-112. (1973). The Rehabilitation Act of 1973. Washington, D.C.: U.S. Government Printing Office.

Public Law 94-103. (1975). The Developmental Disabilities Assistance and Bill of Rights Act of 1975. Washington, D.C.: U.S. Government Printing Office.

Public Law 94-142. (1975, November 29). The Education for All Handicapped Children Act. Washington, D.C.: U.S. Government Printing Office.

Public Law 94-602. (1978). The Rehabilitation, Comprehensive Services and Developmental Disabilities Amendments of 1978. Washington, D.C.: U.S. Government Printing Office.

Public Law 98-527. (1984). Developmental Disabilities Act Amendments of 1984. Washington, D.C.: U.S. Government Printing Office.

Public Law 99-372 (1986). The Handicapped Children's Protection Act. Washington, D.C.: U.S. Government Printing Office.

Public Law 99-457. (1986). The Education of the Handicapped Act Amendments of 1986. Washington, D.C.: U.S. Government Printing Office.

Rothman, D. J. (1971). *The discovery of the asylum: Social order and disorder in the new republic*. Boston: Little, Brown & Co.

Royeen, C. (1988). Occupational therapy in the schools. *American Journal of Occupational Therapy, 42*(11), 697–698.

Shelton, T., Jeppson, E., & Johnson, B. (1987) *Family-centered care for children with special health needs*. Washington, DC: Association for the Care of Children's Health.

Turnbull, R. (1986). *Free appropriate public education: The law and children with disabilities*. Denver: Love Publishing Company.

U.S. Congress (1986). *Report accompanying the education of the handicapped act amendment of 1986*, (House Report No. 99-860), (p. 17 ff). Washington, D.C.: U.S. Government Printing Office.

U.S. Congress, Senate Committee on Finance. (1935). Report accompanying H.R. 7260 (House Report No. 628), (p. 20). Washington, D.C.: U.S. Government Printing Office.

U.S. Department of Education (1988). *Tenth Annual report to Congress on the Implementation of the Education of the Handicapped Act*. Washington, D.C.

U.S. Senate. (1975). Report accompanying P.L. 94-142 (No. 94-168) p. 26–29). Washington, DC: U.S. Government Printing Office.

Yoder, D., & Coleman, P. (1990). Allied health personnel: Meeting the demands of Part H, Public Law 99-457. Chapel Hill, N.C.: University of North Carolina at Chapel Hill.

CHAPTER 11

Marketing

Elizabeth A. Cada, MS, OTR/L
Elizabeth J. Maruyama, MPH, OTR/L

"Throughout the planning cycle the role of marketing is to validate the mission of the organization in relation to the people and organizations to be served. Basic to that role is the organization's understanding and balancing its own wants and needs with those of the target market." Olson & Urban, 1985

Marketing is most commonly thought of as selling and advertising, when, in fact, that is only one aspect of the marketing process. Marketing is meeting people's needs in the most efficient, and therefore profitable manner (Jacobs, 1987). In the past, health care providers were most concerned with providing the services that they thought the consumer wanted or needed. The real purpose of marketing is to discover and understand what the consumer truly wants and needs, by investigating and surveying. Marketing focuses on the consumer as the touchstone for data gathering, strategic planning, product design, and profitability (Jacobs, 1987).

So why is marketing necessary? Why is it important to meet actual needs, rather than provide services you think are important? A product that is not actually needed will not be purchased. With more pronounced competition for health care dollars, the potential for under-utilized resources, better educated consumers, and more proactive legislation to support issues and services, it is essential that the occupational therapist not waste time and resources on developing products that will not be utilized.

The concept of marketing is relatively new to the health care field. Many health care professionals are reluctant to identify their expertise as a product. They overlook the associated costs of their time and expertise. Therapy services must be clearly articulated and defined as products to establish their value to the consumer. To market successfully, the occupational therapist must be able to integrate sound business practices with clinical expertise (Hopkins & Smith, 1978).

MARKETING: AN INTERVENTION PLAN FOR THE PRODUCT

Occupational therapists are most familiar with clinical practice; in this frame of reference the client services are based on evaluation and a sound intervention plan. Smith and Tiffany (1978) describe evaluation as a process of collecting and organizing the relevant information about a client, so that the therapist can plan and implement a meaningful and effective program.

The marketing plan is comparable to an "intervention plan" for the product. The marketing plan, like an intervention plan, establishes a variety of goals, objectives, and strategies to attain these goals. Clear-cut marketing plans are designed for each of the target markets (see Figure 11-1).

In marketing, evaluation occurs while collecting and organizing information about what the consumer needs and wants. The data are then analyzed to determine whether a product can be provided that meets the consumer's need. If the desired product can be provided, then a marketing plan is developed to promote that product to a specific consumer group. These specific groups are called target markets (Jacobs, 1987). Target markets have particular expectations of the product. A first time buyer has different expectations and needs than the experienced buyer. The first time consumer may have minimal expectations in terms of convenient location or price, and may be simply interested in finding a qualified service provider at any cost. Persons who have already purchased occupational therapy services may be more critical and selective since they are familiar with one occupational therapy product. Sometimes the price or location of services figure more prominently in the decision to purchase the product. Keep in mind that the consumer's expectations of a product and the consumer's needs change over time. That is why marketing is a dynamic process.

MARKETING CONCEPTS

When reviewing literature related to marketing health care, references to the "four P's" come to the reader's attention. The four P's are: product, price, place, and promotion (Olson & Urban, 1985). Olson refers to a fifth "P," position, as a significant factor in a marketing plan (ibid.). The product is the occupational therapy service that is available, and must be defined at the consumer's level. Price is determined by considering the actual cost of the product, what the competition is charging, the desired amount of profit, and what the consumer is willing to pay. The price of the product must be commensurate with its perceived value. Place involves how the product is made accessible to the consumer. The product should be distributed in the most efficient manner possible. Promotion is the communication of information to the consumer audience. This communication should include the product's merits, place, and price. Promotion involves advertising, sales promotion, publicity, and personal selling. Position, as Olson & Urban (1985) describes it, is the relative

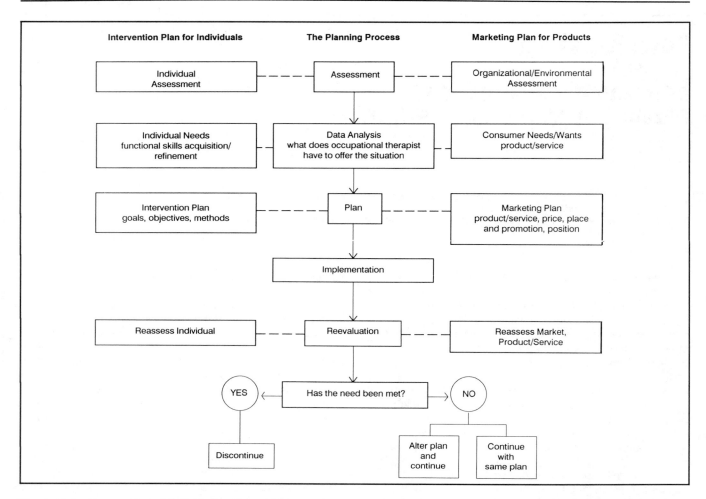

Figure 11-1. Comparison of individual and intervention planning process and the marketing planning process.

place that a product holds in the marketplace. A unique product may be more desirable, and thus have a better position in the marketplace.

Product

The occupational therapists' products are the specific services the therapist has to offer. The product is clearly defined, so that consumers can match the definition of the product with their need for it. The therapist also considers what additional products the consumer may desire after using one product. For example, will providing consultation services to a local day care center, eventually provide referrals for evaluation and intervention? Preferably, the therapist offers a group of products associated by a common theme (Olson & Urban, 1985); this is called a product line. In pediatric occupational therapy, a product line could include consultation, evaluation, intervention, fabrication of adaptive devices, and family education. However, these product names do not tell the consumer how the products can meet their needs. Intervention is a nebulous term for the consumer, unless it is connected to a desired outcome. Parents seek occupational therapy intervention, for their child who has cerebral palsy, to improve functional abilities such as dressing, eating and

playing. This makes the product tangible, something that the consumer recognizes when they purchase it. Consumers also need to recognize that the product will bridge the gap between what they want, and what they have.

The product definition is very important. A product labelled occupational therapy consultation, can mean different things in different settings: the definition of consultation must clearly state what these services will entail. One setting may indicate that consultation is inservice education, while another setting may define consultation as assistance with new program development.

Price

After deciding on a product, price is determined. Pricing can be a complex process because there are many factors to consider. The product's price is based on the costs associated with it. Remember *all costs* must be considered (see Chapter twelve)—not just the direct costs that are most easily identified with the product, such as the therapist's salary, equipment and training expenses. Indirect costs are those shared among the products, such as rent, utilities, secretarial services, insurance, promotion, etc. Figure 11-2 summarizes primary direct and indirect costs. Ideal product line manage-

Direct Costs	Indirect Costs
salary	rent/space
training	secretarial/administrative
equipment	utilities
promotion	insurance

General Principles for Costing a Product

1. Trace as many costs as possible to each specific product. These are considered direct costs.
2. The remaining costs that can not be directly traced to a specific product should be allocated as fairly as possible to each product.
3. You must know your true costs both direct and indirect, don't guess. If you are guessing you will not get a true picture of what a specific product costs. This misinformation may cause you to discontinue a product because it appears to be too expensive to provide.

Figure 11-2. A summary of direct and indirect costs associated with a product's price and how to use them to price a product.

ment suggests converting as many indirect costs to direct costs as possible, to create a true picture of the expenses associated with providing the product. By examining how much of the therapist's time, how much equipment, space, etc., is used to provide each product, one determines how much of the indirect costs can be attributed to each product. Figure 11-3 provides a flow chart for pricing a product.

Effective pricing revenues also include a profit margin. Frequently, providers offer some services for less than, or at cost, to entice consumers to buy additional products or services. For example, for a nominal fee, the occupational therapist could train a pediatrician's staff to administer developmental screening assessments, as part of the well baby checkup. The staff may then identify children who could benefit from occupational therapy services.

One must also consider what the competition charges for similar products. Every day the consumer is becoming better educated in comparison shopping. An excellent product that is overpriced for its market will never be provided. Currently, there is an effort to encourage the consumer to choose Health Maintenance Organizations (HMO's) and Preferred Provider Organizations (PPO's) over traditional insurance. These newer programs may limit the amount of payment available for products. Even traditional insurance coverage frequently specifies the type and amount of eligible services.

Place

Place is another important aspect in selling the product, and is related to family priorities. If time is a priority for the consumer, and therapy services are available from either a homebound program or clinic site ten miles away, the consumer would most likely choose the homebound program. On the other hand, a consumer, with few contacts with other parents of children with handicaps, may choose to come to a clinic setting, which provides an informal meeting place for parents. A convenient location will make a product more desirable. Convenience means easy access to a central location, ample parking, ramps, and elevators. The environment in which the product is distributed can also have a positive or negative effect on the consumer. A child who has had

numerous hospitalizations, or invasive medical procedures, may be anxious in an intervention setting that reminds the family of a hospital environment. This parent may specifically seek an environment that is homelike. Easy access and the comfort of the consumer are important when choosing a place to provide a product.

Promotion

Promotion is more easily recognized as a part of marketing. Promotion communicates to the consumer all the desirable qualities of your product. Promotional efforts focus on specific target markets. Examples of target markets in pediatrics would be parents, schools, physicians, and professional associates. Promotion involves advertising, sales promotion, publicity, and personal selling. Of these techniques, personal selling is the most effective, and probably the most widely used by occupational therapists. An occupational therapist participating in pediatric rounds, might suggest an occupational therapy evaluation for a child who is developmentally delayed. In a school setting, an occupational therapist might suggest a referral for a child who has poor fine motor skills. Active participation in professional associations is another form of personal selling. A department might offer to host a meeting of the local chapter of the state Occupational Therapy Association, or one representative might speak at a parent association meeting. These interactions provide an opportunity to tell others about the product, and alert them to its availability. Community organizations should not be overlooked. Joining and participating in the local Chamber of Commerce, political and fraternal organizations, Parent/ Teachers Associations (PTAs), etc., provide high visibility in the community. Taking part in a community health fair is an example of interacting with the community. Advertising about the product in the newspaper, or getting the newspaper to write a human interest story about the services, can also be advantageous. Designing a brochure about the services, or writing letters of introduction to specific target markets, can inform consumers and other potential referral sources, of the availability and desirability of your product. Giving away promotional items, such as balloons and stickers, will improve name recognition. These items might prompt a consumer to ask questions about the products. Most importantly, promotional campaigns need to be repeated periodically, at appropriate intervals, to ensure continued interest in products. Promotion takes time. Developing promotional materials and making personal contacts, may take time away from revenue producing activities. Considering that promotion is critical to the selling of the product, it is imperative to budget time and resources to promote the product.

Position

Position in the market place will be the telling factor in the success of the product. The unique qualities of the product will enhance its position (Olson & Urban, 1985). Is your location more convenient? If the target market is families, in which both the parents are employed full time, do you offer evening and weekend hours? Do you offer day care for the siblings of your clients? If the target market needs other re-

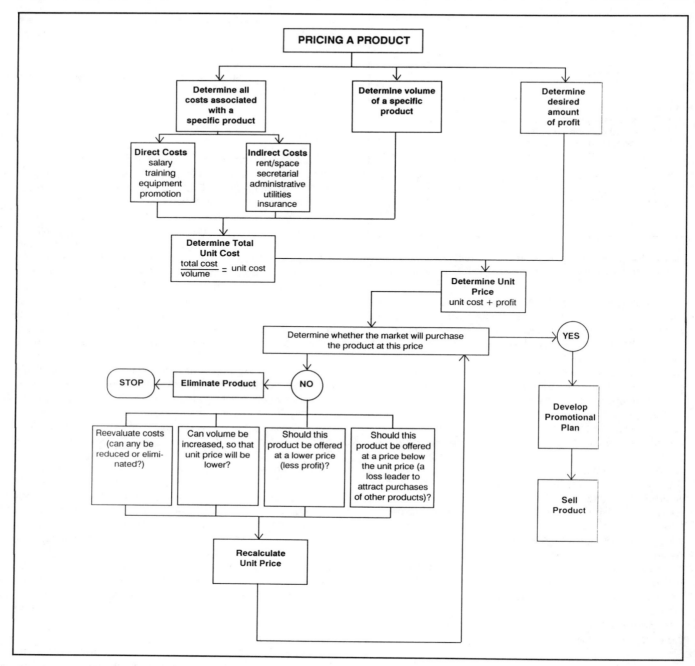

Figure 11-3.   Pricing a product.

lated therapy services, do you offer these? Is scheduling these additional services easy? Will purchasing services from your agency be less expensive, than going to an outside agency for the additional services? Do you have a greater expertise, or are your products more specialized than the competition? All of these qualities may make your product more desirable to the consumer, and thus enhance its position in the marketplace.

ESTABLISHING A MARKETING PLAN

When establishing a marketing plan, one evaluates the environment and organization to discover what the consumer needs, and what products can be provided. This is sometimes called marketing research.

Environmental Assessment

Environmental assessment entails gathering all information about the environment to reveal possible consumers of products. This includes information about the consumer, such as: Is the population predominatly employed?; Do they have children living at home?; What are the parents' education levels?; Do they generally have medical insurance, or do they rely on state or local funding for health care? Other environmental issues include information about the professional community.

Is there a large professional community, and are they familiar with occupational therapy? Are there other agencies, schools, or hospitals also providing occupational therapy services? What are those services or products? If occupational therapy is being advertised, is the manpower available to provide those services? Is there a market glut of occupational therapists in the area? This component of marketing research is investigating unmet consumer needs, not determining product preferences.

There are many ways to collect this information. Living in the target community, provides some idea of the employment patterns and educational level of the residents. One could also gain information by relying on census data, reading the local newspaper, talking with realtors, surveying the local medical facilities, and visiting public and private educational facilities. In addition, one could interview community officials, and contact the local chapter of a professional organization, such as the Occupational Therapy Association, to obtain even more data. Figure 11-4 provides a sample environmental assessment worksheet.

Organizational Assessment

Organizational assessment is completed simultaneously, but independent of the environmental assessment. Analyzing one's organization begins with an examination of the agency mission: What is the organization's purpose? What are the products already being provided? Do these products reflect the mission? What are the skills of the providers, and are they being fully utilized? Does the structure of the organization give you the authority to initiate new products? What products would you like to offer? Will further training be needed to provide these products? Have the location, equipment, and supplies been secured to distribute these products? Answering these questions will help determine if resources are available to respond to the consumer's needs. Figure 11-5 summarizes the data needs for organizational assessment.

Analyzing the Data

Environmental assessment enables an organization to discover information about the community, potential consumers, and competition. This information enables professionals to decide if products meet consumer needs, and if not, to develop new products or redesign current products to meet consumer needs. Matching the consumer's need with a product establishes target markets. An organization then prioritizes the products and markets, to determine which ones to pursue. It is important to "blend" these markets to best utilize resources. Figure 11-6 provides a mechanism for analyzing market data.

Figure 11-7 provides an example of a completed Data Analysis Worksheet for a small private practice group. The group wanted to add additional products to the existing product line. The current products included evaluation, intervention, and consultation. Although the products were being purchased at the targeted rate, the owners wanted to provide additional products. Rather than guessing what the consumer might want, the owners decided to evaluate who the potential consumer was, and what the environment had to offer. By comparing these data with the information about the organization, existing products, and personnel, the owners systematically analyzed what products could be offered to meet consumer needs. (See Figure 11-7 for details.)

Plan and Implementation

The "intervention plan" for the product is designed for a specific target market. State the goals, objectives, and methods to define the product, to price it, to determine how to distribute it, and how to promote it.

For example, through market assessment, an experienced pediatric therapist determines that a local school district has a need for an occupational therapist to provide direct services for ten students. How can this therapist match the product (pediatric occupational therapy intervention), with the school's need (occupational therapy services for ten school children)? The first step of assessing the environment is complete, having matched the product to the consumer's need; now there is a need to define the product so that the consumer (the school) will understand what the therapist has to offer. The therapist might define the product to include expertise in providing occupational therapy, as an educationally related service in another school. The therapist might also determine the price for the product. The price should exceed the direct and indirect costs, be competitive, and reflect what the market will bear. In this particular example, personal selling appears to be the most effective means of marketing the product. The therapist might make an appointment with the school administrator, describe the product, and communicate the price and place. If the consumer (the school) buys the product (the occupational therapist's services), the marketing has been a success.

Reassessment

When a therapist serves an individual's needs, an intervention plan is followed. The therapist reassesses the individual's condition regularly, to determine progress toward achieving the stated goals and objectives. Reassessing the product involves the same process. Markets change, and in order to continue to be responsive to consumer needs, products may have to be modified. Keep a clear view of the environment to be aware of changes. Consumer needs change over time, and products that no longer meet a need will not be purchased. Sometimes, products have to be eliminated, or new products created. By keeping abreast of changes in the environment and organization, new opportunities and means to serve the consumer will be recognized. Over time every product can be replaced with a substitute, so don't "fall in love" with the product. Occupational therapy services and products are greatly influenced by who pays for them. Goods and services that are not reimbursable, may not be as desired by the consumer, and thus not profitable to the provider. Without revenue, the provider jeopardizes other products. Marketing is a dynamic process, and if done successfully, will ensure the longevity of the product.

ENVIRONMENTAL ASSESSMENT WORKSHEET

I. Survey the Targeted Consumer Population Through Vital Statistics
   Population statistics:
   Overall population:

   birth rate: _____
   death rate: _____
   neonatal death rate:

   persons birth—5 yrs: _____

   6–12 yrs: _____   median age: _____
   13–19 yrs: _____
   20–40 yrs: _____
   41–60 yrs: _____
   61–80 yrs: _____
   81 yrs+: _____

   Social structure
   Two parent families: _____   Other: _____
   One parent families: _____   Describe: _____
   Single persons: _____
   Employment patterns—percentage of unemployed
   % unemployment: _____   Types of employment:
   Factory: _____   Education: _____
   Industry: _____   Arts: _____
   Farming: _____
   Business: _____   Other: _____

   % on government assistance: _____
   Median income: _____
   Median educational levels: _____
   Medical needs:
   Disease rates: _____
   Trauma rates: _____
   Common health concerns: _____
   Incidence of handicapping conditions: _____
   Psychosocial needs:
   Hospitalization rate: _____
   Utilization patterns: _____

II. Survey the Physical Environment
    Rural _____   Urban _____
    Major industries in the area (list):

    _____   _____

    Medical facilities in area (list):
    public: _____
    services offered: _____   private: _____
    Educational system: services offered: _____
    public: _____
    services offered: _____   private: _____
    Social Services Agencies in the area—services offered: services offered: _____
    1. _____   1. _____
    2. _____   2. _____
    3. _____   3. _____
    4. _____   4. _____
    5. _____   5. _____
    Professional Population

Profession:	Name of Individual or group	Possible referral (indicate reason)	Possible competitor (indicate reason)
M.D.			
R.N.			
O.T.			
P.T.			
Speech Therapy			
Psychologist			
Social Worker			
Other			

    Transportation System
    type   convenience   accessibility
    _____   _____   _____

Figure 11-4. Environmental assessment worksheet.

ORGANIZATIONAL ASSESSMENT WORKSHEET

I. Survey the Organization
    Is the Facility: for profit: _____ not for profit: _____
    Organization mission or purpose: _____
    Organization's strategic plan: _____
    _____

    Strengths of the Organization: _____
    _____
    _____
    _____
    _____

    Weaknesses of the Organization: _____
    _____
    _____
    _____
    _____

II. Survey the Organization's Structure
    Who has the authority to initiate products and/or eliminate them?

    _____   _____   _____
    _____   _____   _____
    _____   _____   _____
    Title   Person   For which products
    Who has input into the decision process/planning process?

    _____   _____   _____
    _____   _____   _____
    _____   _____   _____
    Title   Person(s)   For which decisions
    Who is responsible for marketing the organization?

    _____   _____
    _____   _____
    Title   Person(s)

III. Survey the Organization's Personnel
     Who is responsible for provision of product?

    _____   _____   _____
    Title   Person(s)   For which products

    Expertise necessary for each product

    Are there skills that are not currently being utilized? (list)

    _____   _____   _____
    _____   _____   _____

    Do staff lack skills necessary to provide new products? (list)

    _____   _____   _____
    _____   _____   _____

IV. Survey the Organization's Current Products

List the products	Do they match organizational mission?	Frequency of product purchases	Does this meet agency's expectations?
_____	_____	_____	_____
_____	_____	_____	_____
_____	_____	_____	_____
_____	_____	_____	_____
_____	_____	_____	_____
_____	_____	_____	_____
_____	_____	_____	_____

    Are these products purchased at the levels expected by the organization?
    Are some specific products purchased from frequently than others?

Figure 11-5. Organizational assessment worksheet.

Data Analysis Worksheet

I. Identify Environmental Features
   A. Develop general consumer profile
   B. Develop general environmental profile
   C. Hypothesize consumer needs based on consumer and environmental profiles (compare consumer to environment)
   D. Determine unmet vs. met needs

II. Identify Organizational Features
   A. Develop general organization profile
   B. Develop profile of organization personnel
   C. Develop profile of organization's current products
   D. List potential new products

III. Compare Environmental Features to Organizational Features
   A. Determine if organization fits in the environment
   B. Determine if organization's current products meet *all* consumer needs

IV. Plan of Action
   A. Determine what specific products could meet any unmet needs
   B. Determine if the organization could provide those specific new products
   C. Prioritize new products
   D. Implement marketing of new products
   E. Reassess utilization of established and new products

Figure 11-6. Data analysis worksheet.

SUMMARY

Marketing is necessary in today's changing health care and educational environment. As competition increases for decreasing health care dollars, and the consumer becomes better educated and selective, it is critical that occupational therapists provide products that effectively meet the consumer's needs. Successful marketing includes analyzing the environment and your organization, clearly defining your product, pricing it competitively, distributing it conveniently, and actively promoting it. Following these guidelines can assure occupational therapists a place in the continually changing health care & education arena.

EXPAND YOUR NEWLY ACQUIRED KNOWLEDGE

1. Identify a group or area that may be underserved by occupational therapy services in the community. Create a marketing plan.
2. Discuss how you would analyze a program that is not getting an adequate amount of referrals, but which seems to meet a community need. How might you alter the marketing plan to improve the referral base?

CASE STUDY—EXAMPLE OF DATA ANALYSIS

I. ENVIRONMENTAL FEATURES
   A. *Consumer Profile*
      • Large growing community
      • Numerous families, young population (60% under 50 years old)
      • Middle class group, low unemployment
      • Median income for a family of four ($40,000)
      • Median educational level (13 + years)
      • Increased incidence of handicapping conditions (childfind state dept. education)

   B. *Environmental Profile*
      • Suburban area, within a high-tech industry corridor
      • One general hospital in town-no pediatric OT services
      • Three general hospitals within 15 miles of the town
         Two of these hospitals have a NICU and provide OT services on a limited basis
      • One rehabilitation hospital within 10 miles of town that has several general pediatric beds
      • Progressive school districts:
         30 elementary schools
         3 secondary schools
         Limited OT, PT and ST services are available to special education students
      • Private educational facility
         birth to 3, developrnentally delayed children
         recreational programs, alternative living facility
      • Public health department
         Prenatal screenings
         well baby clinic, immunizations
         home health nursing care
      • Adequate number of day care facilities
      • Professional Population:
         50 pediatricians (10 mile radius)
         2 orthopedists (pediatric specialty)
         2 neurologists (pediatric specialty)

Figure 11-7. Data analysis worksheet.

20 speech pathologists (pediatric specialty)
5 school psychologists
30 physical therapists (pediatric specialty)
22 occupational therapists (pediatric specialty)
- Transportation:
  primarily by private car
  public bus transportation is available on a limited basis
  arrangements can be made for wheelchair accessible public transportation

C. *Hypothesized Needs*:
specialized health care services
outpatient clinic facilities with evening and Saturday hours
day care facilities
health education re: child development and raising the "model" child

D. *Met Needs*:
general health care needs
general special education needs
additional OT intervention

Unmet Needs:
coordination of health care services
OT evaluation
OT intervention
consultation to medical facilities
consultation to educational facilities
patient and family education

II. ORGANIZATIONAL FEATURES:
A. *Organization Profile*:
- Small for-profit agency located in suburban area
- Owned and managed by two partners who are OTs
- The mission is to provide quality OT services to children and their families
- Strategic plan includes:
  increasing the volume of intervention services provided
  establishing a consultation contract with the local public school system
- Decision making is done by the partners with staff input
- All members of the organization participate in marketing
- Strengths of the Organization:
  highly experienced and progressive staff
  minimal staff turnover
  well respected in community
  conveniently located, well equipped clinic
  well established network of referral sources
- Weaknesses of the Organization:
  limited parking and intervention space at the clinic site
  small number of staff
  limited number of support staff
  service personnel time is taken up with nonrevenue producing activities

B. *Profile of Organization Personnel*
- Managing partners:
  each have masters degrees
  each have 14+ years of experience in pediatric occupational therapy
  highly skilled in intervention
  strengths in consultation in non-traditional settings
  strength in program development
  inservice education and presentation skills underutilized
- staff
  five contract OTs
  each with 10+ years of experience
  skilled primarily in evaluation and intervention
  less experience with consultation in non-traditional settings
  diagnostic skills are under utilized due to time spent in intervention
  education and presentation skills underutilized

C. *Product Profile*
- direct intervention
- evaluation
- consultation to private and public schools
- providing services to developmentally disabled children
- consultation to public health care agencies for program development

Figure 11-7. *Continued.*

III. *Compare Environmental and Organizational Features*:
A. a profitable organization matches the economically stable and progressive environment.

B. current products only meet the needs of a very specific consumer, children with disabilities and their families.

IV. *Plan of Action*
A. New Products
developmental diagnostic services for community health agencies
developmental diagnostic services for pediatricians
continuing education programs for professionals
parent education programs for the community
specialty clinics for community concerns:
—handwriting
—improved sports coordination
—homework organization skills
—sports readiness clinic
—play skill development
group intervention programs
case management

B. The organization has qualified personnel to provide new products, but may need additional personnel, finances, resources and space to expand into new products.

C. Prioritize:
consider:
those products most likely to succeed
who is the apparent target market
taking a comfortable degree of risk
these are the products that will be chosen:
—parent education programs for the community
—group intervention programs
—developmental diagnostic services for pediatricians

D. Marketing new products
budget and promotional plans will be developed for the products selected

E. Review and reevaluate
determine utilization patterns at 3, 6 and 12 month intervals

Figure 11-7. *Continued.*

References

Hopkins, H. L., & Smith, H. D. (1978). *Willard and Spackman's Occupational Therapy* (p. 151) (5th ed.). Philadelphia: J. B. Lippincott Co.

Jacobs, K. (1987). Marketing occupational therapy. *American Journal of Occupational Therapy*, 41(5), 315–320.

Olson, T., & Urban, C. (1985). Marketing. In J. Bair and M. Gray (Eds.), *The Occupational Therapy Manager*, Rockville, MD: The American Occupational Therapy Association.

Smith, H., & Tiffany, E. (1978). Assessment and evaluation—An overview. In H. Hopkins & H. Smith (Eds.), *Willard and Spackman's Occupational Therapy*, (5th ed.). Philadelphia: J. B. Lippincott Co.

CHAPTER 12

Financing the Pediatric Program

Elizabeth A. Cada, MS, OTR/L
Elizabeth J. Maruyama, MPH, OTR/L
Philippa H. Campbell, PhD, OTR

"The budgeting process not only contributes significantly to management functions, but it also can exert a positive influence on behavior . . . . The plans represented by the budget reflect expected performance and provide direction for the organization. Because the organization's internal and external environments constantly change, planning and budgeting are continuing, dynamic processes." Laase, 1985

The current health care and educational environments are affected by the tenuous availability of financial resources. Consequently, competition for limited financial resources has increased. Occupational therapy is faced with challenges of providing quality services in cost effective ways. Being versed in clinical practice is not enough. Today, occupational therapists in different types of pediatric settings and programs are required to establish coherent plans for current and future service provision, develop budgets, understand reimbursement patterns, interface with financial personnel, and interact with a variety of agencies and service providers.

Traditionally, pediatric therapists have been more concerned with providing high quality services, and less interested in participating in, and being accountable for financial resources necessary to support the services. Fiscal responsibility goes hand in hand with service responsibility even for clinical and nonmanagerial therapists. Developing a mind set for quality of care, cost, and reimbursement considerations is important. Essentially, without financial resources, there is no service. Put simply: (a) dollars represent financial resources; (b) resources are used to provide services and to maintain an organization, practice, or therapists; (c) better services result when information about where and how to use resources effectively is known; (d) services represent products; (e) knowledge of products that are being marketed, the consumer for those products, and the cost that the consumer is willing to pay is important; and (f) planning and decision making for program services is enhanced by accurate knowledge about resource utilization (Vitner, 1984).

Most occupational therapists have little to no formal training in financial decision making and acquire these skills through experience, or continuing education opportunities. Competence in developing fiscal plans and making responsible financial decisions is important for all practicing pediatric therapists. These skills are essential for therapists employed as agency program mangers, or department directors, or for those who contract services or practice privately. Competent financial decisions are made on the basis of a variety of sources of information. Accounting personnel are employed directly in larger organizations, and retained by private practice or contract pediatric therapists to report and account for the use of funds. Accounting information, such as a profit and loss statement, is one source of financial information used to make decisions about resource allocation and management. Information about what resources are needed is obtained through fiscal planning and budgeting. Knowledge of funding sources, as well as any trends in public policy that may influence financing, enables therapists to determine the best use of available resources to achieve program aims and objectives.

Pediatric occupational therapy programs are established within private or public agencies or organizations, as companies that contract or directly sell therapy services, or by one or more self-employed therapists. Therapists have responsibility for financial decisions within each of these service structures, a responsibility that may include working collaboratively with accountants, financial consultants, or the management and financial divisions of an organization. Collaborative working relationships result in a team approach to program financing that allows therapists to use knowledge of quality services, resource availability, and public policy trends to interpret and make decisions on the basis of financial information provided by others. Together, teams address six interrelated functions essential to financing any pediatric program of occupational therapy, including: (a) defining current programs and services, as well as those that may be provided in the future; (b) planning budgets; (c) making ongoing decisions; (d) locating sources of revenue; (e) collecting funds; and (f) financial accounting. Each of these functions are addressed in a subsequent part of this chapter.

DEFINITION OF PROGRAMS AND SERVICES

Financing begins with development of a plan to specify goals for a pediatric therapy program as a whole, or for the specific services that will be made available through fee-for-service, contracting, grant funding, or other financing mechanisms. The plan outlines activities and costs necessary to address a specific problem or service need in a particular manner. The purpose of planning at this level is to generate an information base for use in determining costs in development and/or operation phases. A plan of operation outlines the goals and objectives for the program or service, the activities that will be undertaken in development and/or operation phases, the resources needed to complete planned activities, and a projected timeline for accomplishment of each activity. Operational plans for new programs or services differentiate costs for development and operation phases. Many development activities are necessary on a one time basis only, and may entail expenditures of time and effort that are not characteristic of, or required once programs are operational. Developing and distributing brochures as one means of informing potential consumers of the service, for example, is an activity that may be included in the development, but not the operational phase.

Operational plans are required by most external funding sources in applications for funds that will support an entire service program. For example, federal agencies may recommend particular planning formats in applications for discretionary grant funds, whereas state agencies may require other formats. In essence, the plan of operation for a grant-funded program outlines for the funding agency the activities for which funds will be used. Judgments concerning cost-effectiveness and other desired outcomes are made on the basis of the proposed operational plan. Operational plans used within pediatric therapy departments, contracting, or other types of fee-for-service financing systems provide a basis for budgeting and ongoing financial decision making. Discretionary grant funds are more likely to be used for activities that develop a service program, which will be maintained, once implemented, through other sources of funds (e.g., fee-for-service).

An example of a plan of operation, developed by a therapist in private practice, to guide development and operation of a home-based service to address family needs for their young children with delayed development is included in Table 12-1. Plans of operation are a critical first step in defining services. The activities that will be undertaken to initiate or maintain a service, or a total program of services, are the central factor in accurate estimation of needed resources, projection of costs, and financial decision making.

Plans of operation are, in fact, plans. Many factors may influence implementation of the plan. Some components of a plan are more critical than others. For example, the plan outlined in Table 12-1, required hiring of a therapist with particular types of training. Other activities, such as making home visits or developing a referral base, cannot be implemented until this position is filled. The plan specifies a six month period for recruitment and hiring, and describes activities that will be undertaken by this individual following hiring. In the event that a qualified individual is not hired within the projected six month period, other activities that are dependent on this hiring step cannot be carried out as described in the plan. Complete and detailed systems for projecting the impact of activities and timelines are available to increase the flexibility of the planning process. Various operational planning systems (e.g., PERT) allow projection of adjustments.

FISCAL PLANNING AND BUDGETING

Budgeting is a dynamic process that is used as a planning tool, and to provide capacity to anticipate and adapt to change. The budget planning process begins after services have been defined and provides financial direction. This process involves translating the service provision plans for a given period of time into financial terms. Most often, budgets are prepared a year at a time, and reviewed monthly to compare the actual with the budgeted revenue and expenses. This review provides opportunities to make adjustments in program operation without waiting until the year end. Monthly revenue may vary and directly depends on the sources of revenue. For example, school contracts may cover only nine of the 12 month budget period. Revenue may also fluctuate if a primary referral source does not provide the expected number of clients each month or if competition increases in a targeted geographical area. Likewise, projected expenses may change from month to month.

In practical terms, why prepare a budget? A budget describes the services, identifies the prices charged for the services, specifies the number of units of service, and lists expenses necessary to provide the services. The revenue estimate is derived by multiplying the number of units of service with the price charged. All this planning is necessary so that a determination can be made about whether a projected service will produce enough revenue to cover expenses and provide a profit. Is profit necessary? Replacing equipment, expanding services, meeting salary increases, or responding to any unexpected needs will be difficult if revenue equals expenses with no money left over. Therefore, a profit makes good sense, even when services are provided within a large agency or organization (Cada, 1984).

Determining Expenses

Expenses are usually categorized as either variable or fixed. Variable expenses are those that change based on the volume of service provided. Salary is the largest variable expense, followed by supplies, continuing education, travel, and marketing. Fringe benefits also may be a large variable cost depending on the package available to employees. Salary expenses, for example, vary when a greater number of therapists are required in order to provide more services. Variable expenses seem very obvious when thinking about providing services, but fixed costs must also be remembered. Fixed expenses are those that are not affected by the number of patients seen or treatments provided, and include rent, utilities, equipment, and insurance. Accounting, secretarial, and maintenance services are also fixed expenses in most cases. These costs must be covered by revenues generated within a program or agency, even though many therapists believe that fixed costs are someone else's responsibility. Rent on an office space to treat 100 patients will remain constant even though the patient load may fluctuate. Rent is a fixed expense, because the space is still being paid for whether or not it is being used. Obviously, it is important to match your space with your patient load. Revenues from services provided are expected to cover the fixed and variable expenses in most organizations. Organizations do not tolerate an inability to meet expenses (Cada, 1984).

Revenue

Revenue is money that is exchanged for goods or services. The amount of revenue is dependent on pricing of services,

TABLE 12-1. Plan of Operation.

Problem/need: Families of young children with developmental delays require a home-based service option. There is a desire to expand services to meet this need in the community.

Goal	Objectives	Activities	Timeline (month)
Hire a qualified therapist	Create an appropriate job description	Obtain pediatric job descriptions from other agencies	1
		Identify specialty skills needed; incorporate these into the job description	1
	Advertise the position	Write the advertisement	2
		Select location for advertisement	2
		Submit advertisement, payment and desired schedule for the ad	2
	Screen applicants	Review applicant materials with respect to job description requirements	3
		Notify those who do not meet the minimum criteria	3
		Rank order the remaining applicants in regard to general qualifications	3
	Interview applicants	Schedule selected applicants	4
		Conduct interviews	4
		Contact references for further information	4
	Hire a therapist	Make an offer to the therapist of choice	5
		Negotiate salary, benefits, working conditions, and expectations	5
		Determine appropriate starting date with regard for present employer	6
Develop a referral base	Identify present community sources	Create an informational flyer specifying the need to be addressed and stressing the advantages of the services for families	3
		Contact local pediatricians to explain services and solicit referrals	4–5
		Contact community developmental evaluation center to explain services and solicit referrals	4–5
		Contact parent support group to explain services	5
		Give flyer to families in present caseload.	6
Obtain materials and equipment to support the home-based services	Identify core materials and equipment for the initial services	Obtain catalogues from pediatric supply companies	5
		Obtain office materials and equipment to support services	5
		Review initial referrals to identify core needs	5–7
		List priority items required for initial services (newly hired therapist)	6
	Purchase core materials and equipment using start up funds	Order materials and equipment on a monthly plan	6–12
Provide quality home-based services	Receive referrals	Maintain contact with referral sources	Ongoing
	Schedule home visits	Contact parents to determine their family schedule	Ongoing
		Organize visit schedule to accommodate an efficient travel plan	Ongoing
	Visit families to provide services	Obtain initial data-history, concerns, environmental characteristics	Ongoing (Mo 7 on)
		Create a plan with the family	Ongoing (Mo 7 on)
		Collaborate with other professionals who are involved with the child and family	Ongoing (Mo 7 on)
		Provide regularly scheduled services	Ongoing (Mo 7 on)
	Document services efficiently	Create a method to organize initial data information summary/report	7
		Create a program plan format	8
		Create a progress rate/plan adjustment format	10
Evaluate program effectiveness	Identify quality indicators for home programs	Determine family member's view of quality services	10
		Record professional views of quality services	11
		Identify indicators of need to move out of home programming and into new program	12
	Create methods for systematic data collection	Design raw data collection formats	9
		Design data summary methods	11
		Create visual displays for data	12

as well as on other sources of departmental income. There are several ways to price services. The simplest way is to research prevalent prices for similar services within a defined service area. The next step is to determine whether your service is superior or inferior to the competition. If your services are comparable, you can charge the same price, slightly lower to enter the market, or decide to even charge a higher price to distinguish yourself from the competition. Information about what the market will bear is considered when making pricing decisions. Another way to price services involves determining expenses (both fixed and variable), and dividing by the number of units of service to be provided. This equals a minimum price without any profit. Next, examine the competition's price for similar services. Then decide your price for services based on minimum price information and your market (Cada, 1984).

BUDGETING AND DECISION-MAKING

The process of budget planning and decision-making is illustrated by the two examples in Tables 12-2 and 12-3. Making assumptions, calculating the results, and determining if the outcomes are acceptable are the three major steps in this process. Assumptions are changed when the outcomes are not acceptable, and information is recalculated until the outcome is fiscally and programmatically acceptable.

The following assumptions have been made in these examples: (a) you have determined through a market analysis that you are going to sell two services from your Occupational Therapy department; (b) services will be called Treatment A and Treatment B; and (c) Treatment A will cost $50 per unit and Treatment B will cost $100. The budget illustrated on Table 12-2 reflects that Treatment A will generate a projected revenue of $50,000, based on provision of 1,000 units of treatment. Variable costs associated with Treatment A are $40,000 and the fixed costs are $5,000, resulting in total costs for Treatment A of $45,000. A profit of $5,000 is projected by subtracting the total cost of $45,000 from the projected revenue of $50,000.

TABLE 12-2. Proposed Budget.

Items	Treatment		Both Products
	A	B	
Price	$ 50	$ 100	
Quantity	1,000	500	
Total Revenue	$50,000	$50,000	$100,000
Costs			
Variable Costs			
Salaries	30,000	25,000	
Supplies	5,000	5,000	
Marketing	5,000	10,000	
	$40,000	$40,000	
Fixed Costs			
Space Rental	2,000	4,000	
Equipment	1,000	3,000	
Utilities	1,000	3,000	
Support Costs	1,000	3,000	
	$ 5,000	$13,000	
Total Costs	$45,000	$53,000	$ 98,000
Profit (Loss)	$ 5,000	($3,000)	$ 2,000

TABLE 12-3. Adjusted Budget.

Items	Treatment		Both Products
	A	B	
Price	$ 50	$ 100	
Quantity	1,000	600	
Total Revenue	$50,000	$60,000	$110,000
Costs			
Variable Costs			
Salaries	30,000	25,000	
Supplies	5,000	5,000	
Marketing	5,000	15,000	
	$40,000	$45,000	
Fixed Costs			
Space Rental	1,000	4,000	
Equipment	1,000	3,000	
Utilities	1,000	3,000	
Support Costs	1,000	3,000	
	$ 4,000	$13,000	
Total Costs	$44,000	$58,000	$102,000
Profit (Loss)	$ 6,000	$ 2,000	$ 8,000

Treatment B is priced at $100 per unit with projections of 500 service units to be provided, generating an income of $50,000. Variable costs of $40,000 and fixed costs of $13,000 result in total costs of $53,000. A projected loss of $3,000 results when the total costs are subtracted from total projected revenues. Finally, if the $5,000 profit from Treatment A is added to the $3,000 loss from Treatment B, the net profit from both services is $2,000. The net profit of $2,000 for providing Treatment A and B is not going to be an adequate cushion to meet any unexpected needs. In addition, budgeting losses for services is not a good practice. Providing both treatments is important to the department, and a profit from both services is desirable.

New assumptions were made and the budget was recalculated as illustrated in Table 12-3. A determination was made that rental space could be reduced after discussing the amount of space required to provide Treatment A. This adjustment decreased space rental costs from $2,000 to $1,000. Total revenue remained the same at $50,000, but total costs decreased to $44,000. The resulting projected profit from Treatment A increased to $6,000. Treatment B appeared to be where the greatest changes needed to occur. A determination was made that the quantity of treatments projected could be increased from 500 to 600 by increasing the marketing effort. The total revenue increased to a projected $60,000, which projected a $2,000 profit with expenses remaining at $58,000. Adding the profit from both treatments together resulted in a combined projected total profit for both programs of $8,000, resulting in a reasonable cushion to cover any unexpected needs.

A budget maps out revenues and expenses for planned services within a projected time period. Some expenses, however, will be incurred before revenue is generated. Space, for example, is rented before the first child receives services. How does one pay these initial fixed and variable expenses? These are examples of start-up costs. Available cash is needed to cover start-up costs and the first several months of expenses. There are a variety of potential sources for these funds. A small business loan may provide money to organize and operate the business while waiting for revenue to be realized. Local banks or the Small Business Administration are sources of funds for eligible recipients. Profits from existing programs may be used to finance new services in larger organizations. Lastly, private funds or a combination of funding sources may be used to invest in a new service program.

COLLECTING FUNDS

Billing is an extremely important aspect of financing occupational therapy services because the payment schedule and, specifically, cash flow is affected. Consequently, billing procedures should be organized, consistent, and clear, and include proper documentation, appropriate reimbursement information, and timely collection.

Documentation begins with the initiation of a contract between the service provider and the consumer. The individual consumer enters into a verbal contract with the provider to purchase services on a scheduled basis and pay in a timely manner. There is usually no written agreement between the consumer and the provider, but a therapist documents treatment times and uses this information to generate a bill. A written contract or letter of agreement outlines the specific services that are being purchased when providing therapy services on a larger scale, such as consulting or contracting with a health care or educational agency. This contract also details the price of services and the billing and payment policy. This written agreement is then signed by each party and kept on file for the length of the contract. The service provider documents days or hours of service, treatment hours, individual treatments, or special services provided to generate a bill to the contracting agency.

Keeping track of service hours is accomplished using a variety of methods, including a calendar system, time sheet records, or computer entries (Figures 12-1, 12-2, and 12-3 provide examples of documentation strategies). Use of a primary system and a backup system ensures accuracy and provides a failsafe procedure.

The bill itself may take several different forms, depending on the party being billed. An individual patient bill or "statement" usually includes the patient's name and address, the provider's name and address, and a complete listing of the charges specifying type of treatment and dates of service. Billing an insurance company directly requires the service

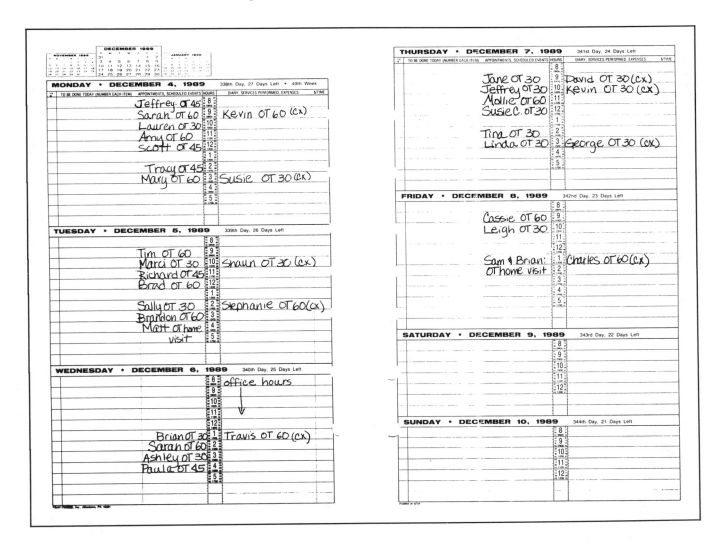

Figure 12-1. Calendar system of recording charges.

TIME SHEET

TO: Smithfield Public School (contracting agency)

FROM: Pediatric Rehabilitation Services (servicing agency)

Service	Date	Time (hours)	Amount Due
OT Treatment			
J. Doe	3/6/88	1	$ 55.00
B. Brown	3/6/88	1	55.00
S. White	3/6/88	1	55.00
E. James	3/6/88	1	55.00
OT Consultation			
Staff	3/6/88	2	100.00
Parent meeting	3/8/88	3	150.00
Program development	3/10/88	3	150.00
staff	3/13/88	2	100.00
OT Treatment, J. Doe	3/13/88	1	55.00
OT Treatment, B. Brown	3/13/88	1	55.00

Total

Treatment		6	
Consultation		10	$500.00
TOTAL DUE:			$830.00

Figure 12-2. This form is used to record occupational therapy service hours in order to bill another agency. The therapist would keep track of working hours and note how time was used. Items listed on the time sheet might include: specific patients that were treated, time spent in treatment, time spent consulting with or in-servicing staff and parents, time spent on program development, and the datesfor each of these services.

LIST OF OCCUPATIONAL THERAPY PROCEDURES

Search	Procedure Description	Amount	Pro Code	Statement
OT-Ed1	OT Education	$ 45.00		OT Education
OT-Ed2	OT Education	22.50		OT Education
OT/PT60	OT/PT60	55.00		OT/PT 1 hour
OT30	OT30	35.00		OT 30 minutes
OT45	OT45	45.00		OT 45 minutes
OT60	OT60	55.00		OT 60 minutes
OTConsult	OT60Consult	50.00		OT Consultation
OTEval	OTEval	85.00		OT Evaluation
OTGroup	OTGroup	27.50		OT Group Treatment
OTHome	OTHome	60.00		OT 60 minutes—Home
OTSCSIT	OTSCSIT	200.00		OTSCSIT Eval
OTSIPT	OTSIPT	300.00		OTSIPT Eval

Figure 12-3. This is a sample list of occupational therapy charges that would be maintained in the computer billing data base. The therapist would choose from this list when recording her daily charges into the computer. To record charges, the therapist would call up the patient's name from the data base and enter the date and type of treatment that was provided. By the end of the month, all the charges will be accumulated in the computer and a bill is generated according to the charges that were entered throughout the month. Checking computer entries against a manual calendar assures more accurate record keeping (Refer to Figure 12-4 for illustration of patient bill).

Pediatric Rehabilitation Services
4701 Auvergne Av. Suite 2
Lisle, Illinois 60532

1-31-88
STATEMENT DATE

JOHN JONES

DATE	DESCRIPTION	CHARGES	PAYMENTS & CREDITS
1-5-88	OT- 60 minute treatment	$55.00	
1-12-88	OT- 60 minute treatment	$55.00	
1-19-88	OT- 60 minute treatment	$55.00	
1-26-88	OT- 60 minute treatment	$55.00	
1-28-88	Insurance Payment		$176.00
1-30-88	Patient Payment		$ 44.00

THIS COPY IS MAINTAINED FOR PATIENT FILE

	PREVIOUS BALANCE	TOTAL PAYMENTS & CREDITS	CURRENT CHARGES	PAY THIS AMOUNT
Jane and Jack Jones
1111 Smith Blvd.
Anywhere, Il. 60000	$220.00	$220.00	$220.00	$220.00

33

ACCOUNT NO.

Pediatric Rehabilitation Services
4701 Auvergne Av. Suite 2
Lisle, Illinois 60532

Pediatric Rehabilitation Services
4701 Auvergne Av. Suite 2
Lisle, Illinois 60532

1-31-88
STATEMENT DATE

THIS COPY MAILED TO PATIENT

JOHN JONES

DATE	DESCRIPTION	CHARGES	PAYMENTS & CREDITS
1-5-88	OT- 60 minute treatment	$55.00	
1-12-88	OT- 60 minute treatment	$55.00	
1-19-88	OT- 60 minute treatment	$55.00	
1-26-88	OT- 60 minute treatment	$55.00	
1-28-88	Insurance Payment		$176.00
1-30-88	Patient Payment		$ 44.00

	PREVIOUS BALANCE	TOTAL PAYMENTS & CREDITS	CURRENT CHARGES	PAY THIS AMOUNT
Jane and Jack Jones
1111 Smith Blvd.
Anywhere, Il. 60000	$220.00	$220.00	$220.00	$220.00

33

ACCOUNT NO.

Pediatric Rehabilitation Services
4701 Auvergne Av. Suite 2
Lisle, Illinois 60532

Figure 12-4. Pediatric services statements.

provider to include more extensive information on the bill. The patient's name and address, all insurance identification information, the patient's diagnosis, the referring physician, the provider's address and tax identification number or Social Security number, and a list of the charges identifying the type of treatment and the dates of service are all necessary data for the insurance company to process the claim (Figures 12-4 and 12-5). Some insurance companies require service providers to use Current Procedural Terminology (CPT) codes to describe treatment (see Figure 12-6), or to use specific diagnostic categories from DSM manuals. It is important for the occupational therapist to be familiar with these codes, and know how and when to apply them. In addition, the provider should ask the patient to sign over benefits to the provider if the insurance company is to pay the service provider directly. Billing another agency may simply require a list of

HEALTH INSURANCE CLAIM FORM

READ INSTRUCTIONS BEFORE COMPLETING OR SIGNING THIS FORM

☐ MEDICAID ☐ MEDICARE ☐ CHAMPUS ☒ OTHER

FORM APPROVED
OMB NO. 0938-0008

PATIENT & INSURED (SUBSCRIBER) INFORMATION

1. PATIENT'S NAME (First name, middle initial, last name)	2. PATIENT'S DATE OF BIRTH	3. INSURED'S NAME (First name, middle initial, last name)
JAMES M. Jones	3 15 1981	JACK Q. Jones

4. PATIENT'S ADDRESS (Street, city, state, ZIP code)
1111 Smith Blvd.
Anywhere, Illinois 60000
TELEPHONE NO. 312 999-0010

5. PATIENT'S SEX MALE ☐ FEMALE ☐

6. INSURED'S I.D., MEDICARE AND/OR MEDICAID NO. (Include any letters)

7. PATIENT'S RELATIONSHIP TO INSURED SELF ☐ SPOUSE ☐ CHILD ☒ OTHER ☐

8. INSURED'S GROUP NO. (Or Group Name)
51160 AM

9. OTHER HEALTH INSURANCE COVERAGE - Enter Name of Policyholder and Plan Name and Address and Policy or Medical Assistance Number
NONE

10. WAS CONDITION RELATED TO:
A. PATIENT'S EMPLOYMENT YES ☒ NO ☐
B. ACCIDENT AUTO ☒ OTHER ☐

11. INSURED'S ADDRESS (Street, city, state, ZIP code)
1111 Smith Blvd.
Anywhere, Il. 60000

12. PATIENT'S OR AUTHORIZED PERSON'S SIGNATURE (Read back before signing)
I Authorize the Release of any Medical Information Necessary to Process this Claim and Request Payment of MEDICARE Benefits Either to Myself or to the Party Who Accepts Assignment Below.
SIGNED Signature on file   DATE 1-31-88

13. I AUTHORIZE PAYMENT OF MEDICAL BENEFITS TO UNDERSIGNED PHYSICIAN OR SUPPLIER FOR SERVICE DESCRIBED BELOW
signature on file
SIGNED (Insured or Authorized Person)

PHYSICIAN OR SUPPLIER INFORMATION

14. DATE OF: ILLNESS (FIRST SYMPTOM) OR INJURY (ACCIDENT) OR PREGNANCY (LMP)
birth

15. DATE FIRST CONSULTED YOU FOR THIS CONDITION
2-28-82

16. HAS PATIENT EVER HAD SAME OR SIMILAR SYMPTOMS? YES ☐ NO ☐

16a. IF AN EMERGENCY CHECK HERE ☐

17. DATE PATIENT ABLE TO RETURN TO WORK

18. DATES OF TOTAL DISABILITY FROM   THROUGH
DATES OF PARTIAL DISABILITY FROM   THROUGH

19. NAME OF REFERRING PHYSICIAN OR OTHER SOURCE (e.g., public health agency)
Dr. Jane Doe

20. FOR SERVICES RELATED TO HOSPITALIZATION GIVE HOSPITALIZATION DATES
ADMITTED   DISCHARGED

21. NAME & ADDRESS OF FACILITY WHERE SERVICES RENDERED (If other than home or office)
Pediatric Rehab Services 4701 Auvergne Lisle, Il.

22. WAS LABORATORY WORK PERFORMED OUTSIDE YOUR OFFICE? YES ☐ NO ☒ CHARGES:

23. NATURE OF ILLNESS OR INJURY. RELATE DIAGNOSIS TO PROCEDURE IN COLUMN D BY REFERENCE NUMBERS 1, 2, 3, ETC. OR DX CODE
1. cerebral palsy
2.
3.
4.

EPSDT YES ☐ NO ☐
FAMILY PLANNING YES ☐ NO ☐
PRIOR AUTHORIZATION NO.

24 A DATE OF SERVICE	B PLACE OF SERVICE	C FULLY DESCRIBE PROCEDURES, MEDICAL SERVICES OR SUPPLIES FURNISHED FOR EACH DATE GIVEN PROCEDURE CODE (IDENTIFY)	(EXPLAIN UNUSUAL SERVICES OR CIRCUMSTANCES)	D DIAGNOSIS CODE	E CHARGES	F DAYS OR UNITS	G T.O.S.	H LEAVE BLANK
01-05-88		97110,97145	OT 60 minute treatment		55. 00			
01-12-88		97110,97145	OT 60 minute treatment		55. 00			
01-19-88		97110,97145	OT 60 minute treatment		55. 00			
01-26-88		97110,97145	OT 60 minute treatment		55. 00			

25. SIGNATURE OF PHYSICIAN OR SUPPLIER
(I certify that the statements on the reverse apply to this bill and are made a part hereof.)
Elizabeth J. Maruyama
SIGNED Elizabeth J. Maruyama, OTR/L DATE 1/31/88

26. ACCEPT ASSIGNMENT (GOVERNMENT CLAIMS ONLY) (SEE BACK) YES ☐ NO ☐

27. TOTAL CHARGE 220. 00

28. AMOUNT PAID

29. BALANCE DUE 220. 00

30. YOUR SOCIAL SECURITY NO.

31. PHYSICIAN'S OR SUPPLIER'S NAME, ADDRESS, ZIP CODE & TELEPHONE NO.
Pediatric Rehab Services
4701 Auvergne Av. Suite 2
Lisle, Illinois 60532
312 964-4707

32. YOUR PATIENT'S ACCOUNT NO.
33

33. YOUR EMPLOYER I.D. NO.
00-00111

I.D. NO.

*PLACE OF SERVICE AND TYPE OF SERVICE (T.O.S.) CODES ON THE BACK

REMARKS
AETNA LIFE AND Casualty
1111 Brown Street
SMITHFIELD, IL. 60111

APPROVED BY AMA COUNCIL ON MEDICAL SERVICE 5/80
APPROVED BY THE HEALTH CARE FINANCING ADMINISTRATION & CHAMPUS
Form **AMA-OP-409**
Form **HCFA-1500 (4-80)**
Form CHAMPUS-501

Figure 12-5. Health insurance claim form.

the dates of service, a description of what was provided, and the specific services and charges.

The actual billing process may be lengthy and time consuming, or very brief depending on the number and type of bills to be produced. The billing cycle, or how often a patient is billed may be influenced by the number of patients, frequency of service, and the established policy of the service agency. A 30 day billing cycle means that the patient is billed every 30 days (or once per month) for the current month's charges and any previous outstanding balance. An insurance company may take anywhere from 30–90 days to process a claim and issue payment, so in some instances it may be beneficial to bill insurance companies every 15 days to establish a better cash flow. Part of the billing process may be eliminated when patients pay at the time of receipt of service. The patients would then be responsible for submitting bills to their insurance company for reimbursement.

Payment for services is often deferred 30–90 days. There-

CURRENT PROCEDURAL TERMINOLOGY (CPT)

CPT Codes used in billing for medical procedures.

Procedures listed under "Physical Medicine" in the CPT Code Book refer to procedures performed by a therapist or physician. The following are a few of the codes used with pediatric occupational therapy services.

97110 = Physical medicine treatment to one area, initial 30 minutes, each visit; therapeutic exercises.
97145 = Physical medicine treatment to one area, each additional 15 minutes.
97112 = Neuromuscular reeducation
97114 = Functional activities

These codes would be listed on the insurance statement and would correspond to the treatment description on the bill (refer back to Figure 12-5).

Figure 12-6. Current procedural terminology and CPT codes used in billing for medical procedures.

---

fore, providing agencies or hospitals often have an accounts receivable equal to at least one month's total billing. Stated simply, the accounts receivable is all the money owed to the provider that has been billed out. These funds represent income that has not yet been collected. The efficiency and accuracy of the billing process can make a tremendous impact on reducing the accounts receivable, which in turn improves the cash flow. The payment process may be streamlined by providing the patient or insurance company with the correct and necessary information on the initial bill. Using incorrect procedural codes, or omitting a diagnosis may delay payment, negatively influence cash flow, and increase accounts receivable.

SOURCES OF FUNDING FOR OPERATING EXPENSES

Establishing contracts with other service agencies may provide steady revenue. Providing services to another agency on a weekly or monthly basis, with 30 day terms, generates predictable revenue each month. Contracts provide a more stable income than regular patient treatment, which is dependent on attendance and financing sources. Contracting for a specific number of service hours, versus a specific number of treatments, results in payment that is not tied directly to patient attendance.

Third Party Reimbursement

Another source of payment for services is third party reimbursement. This category includes private medical insurance, Health Maintenance Organizations (HMOs), and Preferred Provider Organizations (PPOs). Each insurance company has specific plans that may or may not cover occupational therapy treatment. The service provider assists the consumer in researching plan benefits to determine if occupational therapy is a covered service. Each insurance company may have individual requirements for reimbursement, but generally the service must be provided under certain conditions. Most plans require that a physician provide a diagnosis and referral for treatment. In addition, certain plans only pay for inpatient treatment, or outpatient treatment performed at certain locations such as a hospital or physician's office, rather than in the patient's home or at a private therapy clinic. An indi-

vidual may have a copayment of 10–20% of the bill after a deductible has been met under third party payment. Still other insurance plans do not cover occupational therapy unless an illness or injury has occurred. A family with insurance may be self-paying for occupational therapy if the child's diagnosis does not meet required criteria.

A PPO is a group of providers who agree to provide health care to subscribers for a discounted negotiated fee (Davy, 1984). This reimbursement plan requires a service provider to approach the PPO sponsor to have Occupational Therapy recognized as a preferred provider. Occupational therapists then compete with their colleagues for preferred provider status. An HMO is a prepaid health plan that is a comprehensive, coordinated medical service. Consumers who join an HMO may be limited in their choice to those providers that are members of the HMO. Insurance companies may perform periodic case reviews to determine if a patient is making progress, or simply being maintained through treatment, or may limit the number of treatments that a patient may receive regardless of the diagnosis. A child with cerebral palsy might use up his allotted treatment sessions in the first six months of the year, and have to go without paid services until the following January. Situations where treatment sessions are allotted make provision of consistent treatment extremely difficult. Occupational therapy could have been provided twice a month in a longer treatment session, rather than every week, if the service provider had known that a specific allotted number of sessions would be covered, and could have made better use of the limited allocations for treatment.

Federal and State Programs

Occupational therapy services may be supported through state and federal educational or health care funds. A federal program with which most pediatric therapists are familiar is P.L. 94–142, the Education of the Handicapped Act (EHA), passed by Congress in 1975. Occupational therapy is included in this Act under a designation of "related services." Funds are available to states to use in ways designated by individual state policies, including provision of occupational therapy as an educationally related service within a school system. Each state varies somewhat in the way in which federal funds are distributed to individual districts. Some states pass funds through on an individual child basis, whereas others distribute funds on the basis of units (Rourk, 1984). P.L. 99–457, the Education Amendments of 1986, identifies families and their infants who are developmentally delayed, or at risk for delayed development, as the focus in early intervention. Occupational therapy is listed as one of many early intervention services that may be provided for families and infants. States are required, under this new legislation, to develop and implement state-wide systems of comprehensive and multidisciplinary early intervention services (Hanft, 1988). Currently, funds may be used for planning and developing, or for the provision of services. Ultimately, funds will be available to provide services that have not already been available under other programs. This legislation has been referred to as "glue money," rather than as a source of ongoing funds for support of services. The intent of federal involvement in state services for infants and toddlers and their families is to provide the mechanism needed to coordinate existing funds used for services (i.e., Medicaid), and to supplement available federal funds with those from other programs, as well as from direct financial support at the state level (Gallagher, Trohanis, & Clifford, 1989).

The Social Security Act of 1935 created Title V to provide special grants to improve the health care of preschool and school-aged children, and especially those from low income families. This law provides for a wide range of services including screening, diagnosis, preventative services, dental care, remedial care, and treatment. Federal grants may also be made to medical schools, teaching hospitals, crippled children's agencies, and state health agencies to pay for 75% of comprehensive health services. Title XIX is an amendment to the Social Security Act which assists states in providing medical care to needy persons of all ages. The individual state determines eligibility through income level. States plan and operate their own programs. Occupational therapy services may be reimbursed under certain conditions, such as being provided in a hospital on an inpatient or outpatient basis. Occupational therapy also may be reimbursed when provided in a nursing home or through an approved home health agency.

Other funding sources may be available in particular states dependent on the policies and practices of the state. Some of these programs are supported fully through state funds, although others match state and federal funds, or use federal support alone. For example, states such as Wisconsin or Michigan have state family support legislation that allows families to obtain funds to pay for a variety of services to support the care of children who are medically complex, or who have severe or profound disabilities. The Medicaid waiver program may cover occupational therapy services for children who are technologically dependent, or for individuals who are mentally retarded and are being moved to the community from residential care institutions. Being knowledgeable about the sources of funds that are available to cover occupational therapy services for infants and children, with a variety of disabilities, in the state in which a therapist is practicing is essential, even when pediatric therapists are employed by school systems or in organizations and agencies. Of even greater importance is accurate information about eligibility criteria for receiving funding. Programs available in many states are so confusing for consumers that other individuals, such as case managers, frequently are necessary to enable

individuals to become familiar with sources of funding, complete required application procedures, and actually secure payment for needed services.

Federal and State Discretionary Programs

Many departments and agencies within both the federal and state government operate discretionary grant programs that support development, training, and research activities. These funds are awarded on a limited and competitive basis in accord with annual published priorities established by the agency, frequently with the assistance of consumer groups or professional organizations. These funds are most useful for program development activities, and do not support ongoing service provision as a general rule. The Department of Education, Office of Special Education Programs (OSEP), which administers P.L. 94–142, for example, operates a number of discretionary programs in training (Division of Personnel Preparation) and research (Division of Innovation and Development). In addition, specific demonstration programs for individuals with severe handicaps, in early intervention and preschool, and for children and youth who are deaf or blind are administered through the Division of Educational Services. Each of these divisions within OSEP is responsible for administering a specific Part of P.L. 94–142 in accord with the statute and its regulations.

Announcements soliciting applications by specific deadlines for priorities under each of these categories are published regularly in the *Federal Register*. These announcements frequently are picked up and published by secondary sources (such as *OT Week*) in order to give broad public notice of the availability of funds. Applicants then complete a proposal that outlines the ways in which the priority will be responded to, and the costs entailed in providing the program. Application procedures and guidelines for preparing applications are published in the *Federal Register* with the notice announcing the deadline for application. All applications are reviewed by peer review panels and recommendations for funding are made. These recommendations are rank-ordered and matched with available funds. The top scoring proposals are awarded funds.

Other federal agencies, such as the National Institute of Disability and Rehabilitation Research (NIDRR), the Small Business Administration Innovative Grant Award program, various divisions of the Department of Health and Human Services, such as the Division of Maternal and Child Health (MCH), or the Administration of Developmental Disabilities (ADD), also are sources of funds for discretionary grant programs. Notices for these funds are also published in the *Federal Register*, with the review and award processes generally following a sequence similar to that used by the Department of Education. Funds administered through P.L. 94–142 are restricted to programs involving children with disabilities from birth through 21 years of age, whereas those available through other agencies and programs (such as NIDRR) may support programs for individuals of all ages. Knowing what funding is available through discretionary programs is most easily accomplished by reading newsletters, or by belonging to a service where individuals are employed to read the *Federal Register* and other publications, and pass on relevant information. Being associated with a university may enable local practitioners to use the services of the university's grant office.

MODERATORS

A variety of issues impact on the current and future design of an occupational therapy practice. Awareness of current state and federal legislation, health care trends, and economic factors is necessary to establish or maintain a visible practice. Many different types of legislation affect the provision of, and payment for occupational therapy services. Pediatric practice is primarily influenced by legislation in the educational or health care areas. (see Chapter 10). Legislation in both of these areas, even when federal in origin, is often implemented in unique ways at a state or local level.

Legislation enacted at a state level may determine whether or not your facility or practice will be eligible for reimbursement for occupational therapy services. An example is the state service for children with special health care needs (formerly called Crippled Children's Services). Each state determines the diagnoses eligible, and the types and amount of services that are reimbursable. Awareness of these mandates allows positioning of services to take full advantage of eligibility requirements and payment practices.

Trends in health care are good indicators of future markets. With a movement toward prevention, occupational therapy programs may need to gear their services toward children at risk, as well as baby and family issues. Less health care dollars are available, so self-payment becomes a greater possibility. It becomes important to provide services that the consumer wants and is willing to purchase. Developments in technology are improving the survival rate of severely ill babies and prolonging the lives of chronically ill children. As a result, there are greater numbers of children in need of specialized health care services. Special education legislation provides occupational therapy services for children with educationally relevant needs. There are some children who have needs that could be addressed by occupational therapy, but who are not eligible for occupational therapy within the school system. Occupational therapists need to be sensitive to the variety of systems and how they interact, so that there are no missed opportunities to provide services that are desired and supported by some financial structure.

As we all know, the economy plays a major role in our lives. Medical costs continue to rise as more consumers utilize health care services. There have been a variety of programs developed to control health care costs, both in the public and private sectors. Business and industry have increasingly moved toward self-insurance programs as a means for controlling these costs. These programs, along with HMOs and PPOs, provide opportunities for occupational therapists to negotiate services for subscribers. At the same time, each occupational therapist must be aware of the current economic status of those businesses and industries in their immediate service area. For example, imagine that 90% of patients are covered by insurance benefits provided by a local steel mill. If this plant suddenly closes, laying off the work force, patients will lose medical coverage, putting the occupational therapy program reimbursement at risk. This points out the importance of being attuned to economic indicators, and relying on a variety of sources of revenue.

SUMMARY

Knowledge and skill in financial planning is a necessary tool in the occupational therapist's repertoire for future pediatric service provision. Recognition of the impact of financial resources on the effective provision of pediatric occupational therapy is a first step. Through planning and projecting needs and trends, pediatric services will remain viable in the market place.

EXPAND YOUR NEWLY ACQUIRED KNOWLEDGE

1. Create a plan of operation for providing consultation services to a respite core system within your community. Be sure to include time to determine family perspectives & needs.

References

Cada, K. G. (1984). CPA Personal Communication. Annson Corporation, IBM Corporation, *Doctor's Office Manager*, software, Boca Raton, FL.

Davy, J. D. (1984). PPOs. *American Journal of Occupational Therapy, 38*(5):313–319.

Gallagher, J., Trohanis, P. L., & Clifford, R. M. (1989). *Policy implementation in P.L. 99-457: Planning for young children with severe needs.* Baltimore: Paul H. Brookes.

Hanft, B. (1988). The changing environment of early intervention services: Implications for practice. *American Journal of Occupational Therapy, 42*(12):724–731.

Laase, S. M. (1985). Financial management. In J. Bair & M. Gray (Ed.). *The occupational therapy manager* (p. 114–115). Rockville: The American Occupational Therapy Association, Inc.

Rourk, J. D. (1984). Funding health services for children. *American Journal of Occupational Therapy, 38*(5):313–319.

Vinter, R. D. (1984). *Budgeting for not-for-profit organizations.* New York: Free Press.

CHAPTER 13

The Special Education Administrator's Perspective

Charlotte Brasic Royeen, PhD, OTR, FAOTA
Martha Coutinho, PhD*

"People tend to resent the connotation of mandates. This is particularly true when mandates relate to professional roles. . . . They have required professionals to change practices that were popular and were considered sound by many. At the same time, the mandates have offered only limited guidance on how to accomplish the change. The inference was that educational practices of the past were not appropriate for the handicapped and that changes were warranted." Meyen, 1982

In an article by Ottenbacher (1982), an excellent analysis of the disciplinary differences between occupational therapy and special education is put forth. Ottenbacher suggests that both disciplines are in the process of developing a unique body of knowledge, but that special education is more concerned with end products of performance, whereas occupational therapy has more often been associated with a medical model concerned with identification and remediation of the underlying dysfunction hindering performance. For example, one may say that occupational therapy is more concerned with the process of how the student engages in educationally related activity, whereas the special education administrator is more concerned with the quality of the product regarding the educational activity. Ottenbacher concludes that:

> All professionals involved in providing service under the mandates of P.L. 94-142 must develop an understanding of their historical and philosophical differences and similarities and a realization that all conceptual and treatment models are limited in their capacity to deal effectively with the many and varied problems existing within the developmentally disabled population (Ottenbacher, 1982, p. 84).

Herein lies one of the primary problems regarding related services in special education, and most specifically occupational therapy services in a special education setting: there is a marked and detrimental lack of understanding between the two disciplines.

This lack of understanding can be related, in part, to a lack of effective communication between the two disciplines. In describing common problems concerning educational program effectiveness, Patton (1981) identified "communication problems" as a pervasive phenomenon. Similarly, there appears to be a communication problem between the fields of special education and occupational therapy. The reasons for the communication problem between the two disciplines may be similar to the reasons for communication problems suggested by Patton. First, there is the previously identified difference in operational strategies which underlie the two disciplines (i.e., special education being more "product" oriented and occupational therapy more "process" oriented). Second, the language used by the two disciplines is different. Much of the language employed in occupational therapy is medically oriented, or grounded in anthropological or natural science; whereas special education language is more grounded in educational and psychological science. A third reason accounting for the communication problem between the two disciplines has to do with a lack of common experience. To illustrate, the education and training experiences of special educators and occupational therapists are different. Special educators are trained in universities and school systems. However, occupational therapists are usually trained in universities and hospitals, as well as community centers, rehabilitation centers, etc. Many occupational therapists are hired for school system positions when, in fact, little of their didactic or practical training involved the school system. Lacking a common educational experience, it is not surprising that a foundation for understanding between the two disciplines is lacking.

Given the communication problem between special education and occupational therapy, it is probably an accurate assessment to suggest that many special education administrators may not understand the provision of occupational therapy services in the public schools as specified by P.L. 94-142. Furthermore, many school-based occupational therapists may not clearly understand occupational therapy in their public schools, as specified by the requirements of P.L.-142, since an occupational therapist may or may not have received adequate orientation to school systems, special education, and P.L. 94-142 as part of their professional training.

Considering this, the occupational therapy practitioner in the public school system has the following responsibilities:

• To understand how occupational therapy in the school serves the intent of P.L. 94-142;

---

* This work was done in this author's private capacity; no official endorsement by the Department of Education should be inferred.

• To develop effective strategies for communication with special education administrators regarding how occupational therapy in the schools serves the intent of P.L.-142.

Consequently, this chapter on the special educator's perspective regarding occupational therapy in the school system has been designed to provide the basic conceptual framework, or background, necessary for an occupational therapist to fulfill these two responsibilities. Specifically, this chapter will educate occupational therapists in the schools regarding the viewpoints of the special education administrator; will further identify the type of information the occupational therapist working in the public schools needs to convey to the special education administrator; and will delineate communication patterns the occupational therapist may wish to establish with the special education administrators within the school system.

However, because these stated purposes are rather broad, they may be best accomplished by analysis of six major issues of concern to special education administrators and occupational therapists. These are as follows:

1. The special education perspective;
2. Roles and functions of occupational therapy as an educationally related service;
3. Models of service provision for occupational therapy in the public schools;
4. Effective communication on the part of the occupational therapist in the schools;
5. Cost considerations regarding occupational therapy, and;
6. Parent's rights and due process.

Each of these will be elaborated upon in subsequent sections of this chapter.[1]

THE SPECIAL EDUCATION PERSPECTIVE: THE MANDATE TO PROVIDE A FREE AND APPROPRIATE PUBLIC EDUCATION

Administrators of special education programs perceive the provision of occupational therapy to students with handicaps from a particular set of beliefs and knowledge. Specific federal and state requirements dictate some of their attitudes and beliefs. In part, they are influenced by commonly held philosophies regarding education, judicial precedents, local or regional cultural practices, etc. Of course, individual experiences and professional training also influence views. In sum, administrators are guided and influenced in many ways as they seek to oversee the provision of instructional and other educational services to children and youth.

In 1975, Public Law 94-142, "The Education of the Handicapped Act" (EHA) was passed. This Federal law mandated the provision of a free, appropriate public education to all children who are handicapped, regardless of the severity of the handicapping condition. The EHA was passed in response to a long term effort by parents, educators, and others to better serve children with special needs. Congress, in exercising its authority to enact law passed the EHA; and then President Ford signed the Act, and it became law. To carry out the law, implementing regulations were developed by the then Department of Health, Education and Welfare, an executive agency. In 1980, this function was vested in the newly created Department of Education. All agency regulations must be based on authority found in the legislation. Given a particular context, we may speak of the EHA itself and/or its implementing regulations, which are codified in the *Code of Federal Regulations* (CFR) at 34 CFR Part 300. Most often, and in this chapter as well, however, reference is made to the implementing regulations; for example, the definitions of handicapped conditions are provided at 34 CFR 300.5.

The EHA embodies the aforementioned broad mandate to provide a free and appropriate public education (FAPE) to all children who are handicapped. Under the EHA, there are many provisions regulating and guiding the provision of services and programs. State regulations and implementation must be consistent with the *Federal Regulations*. However, because either certain interpretations and variations are legally permissible, or the regulations are silent on a particular policy issue, state regulations actually vary to some extent from one another. For example, currently the age range for mandated provision of services is from 5 through 17. Many states have developed and implemented regulations that mandate services to children and/or youth beyond the age of 17.

The EHA consists of many subparts; through Part B, it provides monies to states and local education agencies (and ultimately, schools). In this sense, the EHA is a federal grant program. To participate and receive funds under the EHA, a state must agree to conform with its provisions and requirements. Certain subparts of the EHA contain provisions for states, other institutions, and/or individuals to apply for other, discretionary monies. These monies are appropriated for the purpose of encouraging, for example, provision of services to preschool-aged children, or to support research or demonstrations projects in a variety of areas.

In sum, when the funds for providing occupational therapy are to be provided by a public agency, then occupational therapy is associated with special education in a specific, legally defined manner. Responsibility for the provision of related services such as occupational therapy, requires that special education administrators make occupational therapy available, when required to meet the unique needs of children identified as handicapped. In reality, the practice of occupational therapy in schools varies. The beliefs and knowledge held by individual special education administrators regarding the role of occupational therapy in the schools, affect the extent to which services are provided in an appropriate, cost effective manner.

Several provisions of the EHA may be identified which affect directly the role of occupational therapists who work in public schools. From the special education administrator perspective, occupational therapists most often work in settings in which students with handicaps are integrated, at least partially, with students who are not handicapped. Therefore, reference here generally will be to situations encountered in public schools. The requirements under the EHA apply, however, in any setting a public education agency either provides

---

[1] This article was prepared by the authors in their private capacity. No official support or endorsement by the U.S. Department of Education was intended or should be inferred.

or arranges for services. Many children with handicaps, for example, receive publicly funded services in special schools, hospitals, or private facilities.

One provision contained in the EHA that has linked special education and occupational therapy in a particular way, are the definitions of terms and services. Students who are handicapped as defined by the EHA are children, "who because of [specifically defined] impairments need special education and related services," (34 CFR 300.5). Special education, in turn, represents "Specially designed instruction . . . to meet the unique needs of a handicapped child," (34 CFR 300.14). Thus, in a very specific way, related services are linked in the regulations to special education. They are defined as "developmental, corrective, and other supportive services as are required to assist a handicapped child to benefit from special education," (34 CFR 300.13). Occupational therapy is provided only when necessary to assist a handicapped child to benefit from the specially designed instruction.

The consequence of this particular definition, and relationship among terms, is that occupational therapists whose services are funded by special education monies in public agencies, may serve only children who are handicapped and in need of special education. In a comment to the regulations where special education is defined, the federal intent regarding special education and the provision of related services was stated directly, ". . . a related service must be necessary for a child to benefit from special education. Therefore, if a child does not need special education, there can be no "related services," and the child (because not "handicapped") is not covered under the Act" (comment to 34 CFR 300.14).

In addition to stating the conditions required before the provision of occupational therapy is allowable under the EHA, occupational therapy is itself defined in the implementing regulations of the EHA, at 34 CFR 300.13 (b) (5) as:

   i. Improving, developing or restoring functions impaired or lost through illness, injury, or deprivation;
   ii. Improving ability to perform tasks for independent functioning when functions are impaired or lost; and
   iii. Preventing, through early intervention, initial or further impairment or loss of function."

Because of this specially defined relationship between occupational therapy and special education, occupational therapists serve as a part of a team providing special education and related services to a child. Hence, they are affected by the requirement that the services provided are appropriate and designed to meet the unique needs of a child who is handicapped.

PROCEDURES GOVERNING THE REQUIREMENT TO DEVELOP AN INDIVIDUALIZED EDUCATIONAL PLAN (IEP)

To insure children who are handicapped receive a free and appropriate public education (i.e., specially designed instruction to meet unique needs), the EHA requires an individualized educational plan (IEP) be developed for each child (34 CFR 300.340). The IEP requirement itself is represented by:

1) an IEP document which is a written statement describing the kinds of special education and related services the child is to receive, and 2) IEP meeting(s) at which parents and school personnel meet to develop, review and revise a handicapped child's IEP. The significance of this requirement is that: first, decisions about the program a child is to receive must be made on an individual basis; and, second, parents are given the opportunity to participate in decisions about their child.

In addition to the IEP requirement itself, the EHA provides for the manner in which eligibility, programming and placement decisions are determined. A set of protections governing evaluation procedures, parental participation, and confidentiality of information (records, etc.) accompanies those procedures. These provisions impact on an occupational therapist in significant ways. Specifically, one role of occupational therapists is the assessment and evaluation of students to determine the need for, and type of, intervention necessary. Under the EHA, the occupational therapist functions as a member of a multidisciplinary team which includes, but is not limited to, the child's teacher, parents, and other specialists to conduct preplacement evaluation, as a first step to determine eligibility for services (i.e., identification as handicapped). A meeting is held to review the evaluation team's findings. Often, the occupational therapist will be asked to participate in the meeting to describe the particular evaluation procedures used, and the results obtained.

If the multidisciplinary team, one member of which is the child's parent, determines the child to be handicapped, an IEP is developed at the same, or a subsequent meeting. The occupational therapist is responsible in this instance for insuring team members have all recommendations the occupational therapist has formulated, and these are in a form that is comprehensible to other team members, including parents. All team members' recommendations are translated into an IEP for the child. Because state regulations vary, states may require additional information, but federal regulations require (34 CFR 300.342 and 300.346 (c)) that the IEP state the related services to be provided. To conform with federal requirements at 34 CFR 300.346, an IEP must include, in addition to other information, a statement of annual goals and short term instructional objectives, and provide objective criteria and evaluation procedures for determining, at least annually, if goals are being met. From the point of view of a special education administrator, one role of an occupational therapist would be to make certain that the sections of the IEP, as related to the provision of occupational therapy, accurately reflect the type of occupational therapy to be provided. On a more general level, the occupational therapist must assure that the occupational therapy to be provided truly does serve to: 1) assist the child to benefit from special education services and 2) is designed to meet the unique needs of the child.

Once an IEP is developed, and parental consent for initial placement is obtained, services are initiated. Occupational therapy, as recommended in the IEP, would also commence. The role of the occupational therapist would be to work with the staff to coordinate the provision of all services, given a child's particular special education program and placement (e.g., regular class, self-contained class, special day school, etc.). In addition to informal periodic review of the child's program, a child's IEP must be reviewed by a team, at least annually (34 CFR 300.343 (d)), and a comprehensive re-evaluation (i.e., one that conforms to the requirements under 34 CFR 300.532) must be carried out every three years, or "more frequently if conditions warrant or the child's parent or teacher requests an evaluation" (34 CFR 300.534). As before, the occupational therapist would serve as a part of a team to describe: 1) the results of the occupational therapy evaluation, 2) the occupational therapy services recommended, and 3) the outcomes expected from the actual intervention. As before, the therapist is likely to also participate in decisions regarding the child's entire program of regular and special education and related services.

THE LEAST RESTRICTIVE ENVIRONMENT MANDATE

In addition to the requirement to provide free, appropriate education (FAPE), uniquely suited to meet the individual needs of a child with handicaps, the EHA embodied a second, equally important mandate. Referred to as the Least Restrictive Environment (LRE) provision, the EHA requires that services be provided within the least restrictive environment. LRE is explicit, and impacts directly upon the way in which occupational therapists make programmatic recommendations for children with handicaps, and select among service provision models. In keeping with society's historical preference, apparent in our Constitution as well as civil and criminal law, any curtailment or infringement upon an individual's personal freedom is permissible only in certain conditions, and then only to the minimum extent necessary to meet a carefully defined purpose.

Historically, individuals with disabilities, or who were "different" in some way from other children, were denied an education (Cruickshank & Johnson, 1975). Individuals with disabilities were excluded, typically, because public schools had no program available, and the handicapping condition(s) were perceived to be too severe, or the amount of disruption to others too great, to accommodate the students with handicaps in the existing school program (Turnbull, 1986).

Many students who were retarded, sensory impaired, or in other ways difficult to serve, were also excluded, effectively, from the opportunity to receive a free and appropriate education, by virtue of the placement of these individuals in special classes. Often, this required placement in different settings than those where regular education took place. In addition to precluding handicapped students from an opportunity to interact with non-handicapped peers, many of the special classes or schools were inferior with respect to curricular, teacher and other resources. In sum, the educational services provided to many individuals with disabilities, who had been placed in segregated schools and/or classes, rarely approached the quality or comprehensiveness of those available to children not labelled handicapped. Moreover, most often the child with handicaps, who received services in segregated settings, could not interact, learn, or socialize with non-handicapped peers; in effect denying both handicapped and non-handicapped the critical opportunity to interact when growing up, in ways that would be required as adults. In sum, publicly funded placement in segregated facilities, schools, or classes was to still deny many handicapped individuals the opportunity to receive a free and appropriate education.

Parents of children with disabilities, acting alone or as a member of associations dedicated to the education and/or welfare of individuals with disabilities (e.g., The Association for Retarded Citizens), sought judicial remedies, initially, to redress this imbalance, and to compel schools to provide free and appropriate educational services to students with handicaps. Several of these cases, many of which became landmarks in the drive to establish rights for handicapped individuals, were litigated successfully (e.g., Pennsylvania Association for Retarded Children (PARC) v. Commonwealth of Pennsylvania, 1972; Mills v. D.C. Board of Education, 1972, 1980).[2] Collectively, the decisions rendered in these cases provided a stimulus for the enactment of federal legislation that would mandate a free and appropriate public education for students with handicaps, in all, rather than in some states and localities, and would require the provision of services in the least restrictive environment.

With the passage of P.L. 94-142, the federal intent was made clear at 34 CFR 300.550 (a):

"1) That to the maximum extent appropriate, handicapped children, including children in public or private institutions or other care facilities, are educated with children who are not handicapped, and

2) That special classes, separate schooling or other removal of handicapped children from the regular educational environment occurs only when the nature or severity of the handicap is such that education in regular classes with the use of supplementary aids and services cannot be achieved satisfactorily."

Lack of an existing appropriate placement or program was not a sufficient cause to remove a child from a mainstream or general education environment:

"Each public agency shall insure that a continuum of alternative placements is available to meet the needs of handicapped children for special education and related services" (34 CFR 300.551 (a)).

Although P.L. 94-142 was passed over ten years ago, many barriers and obstacles confront educators and specialists seeking to educate children with handicaps in the least restrictive environment (Rostetter, Kowalski, and Hunter, 1984). Some of these stem from the attitudes of parents, educators, or the general public. Some of the factors are administrative (e.g., a sparsely populated district, with a low resource base, finds the only existing program for a severely impaired, medically fragile child is located 100 miles away). Many of the obstacles are fiscal, in that some funding patterns encourage segregation. For example, total cost for services at a residential facility may be less than that required to develop a comprehensive program at the neighborhood high school. Finally, school staff, especially regular educators, may lack the skills and knowledge to either teach full-time, or effectively share responsibility for the education of particular students with handicaps.

All of these factors will affect the kinds of services an occupational therapist is asked, or prefers to provide. Clearly, P.L. 94-142 requires the occupational therapist to consider

---

[2] Turnball (1986) provides a comprehensive, broad view of judicial and legislative initiatives which have affects on the education of handicapped individuals.

the requirement of least restrictive environment at many points in the overall planning and placement process. First, at the point at which the child first experiences difficulty, a decision must be made whether or not to investigate further. Despite the suspicion of a specific disorder, the occupational therapist must ask: Has educational progress been affected significantly?

An occupational therapist's evaluation of the child must be consistent with the purpose of determining whether or not the child is making satisfactory progress in the regular classroom, and not just represent an assessment of the presence and nature of a specific disorder (e.g., gravitational insecurity, irrespective of whether the existence of this disorder adversely affects the child's capacity to learn) (see Chapter 3 on Assessment). As importantly, the evaluation addresses not only recommendations regarding any supplemental aids or services, but must also encourage and enable placement in the least restrictive environment (e.g., the regular class in the neighborhood school). A strictly child-centered evaluation may overlook important system characteristics—characteristics which will critically affect the type of occupational therapy intervention to recommend, and the role the occupational therapist is to assume (e.g., direct or indirect service provision). In sum, in recommending a particular level and kind of service, the occupational therapist must determine if the information collected justifies the provision of a service, performed by a specialist, not a regular educator, in a setting that does not include contact with non-handicapped peers. Does a "pull out" intervention, implemented by the occupational therapist twice a week, reflect FAPE? Is the handicap so severe that placement out of the regular classroom is appropriate, and reflects the least restrictive environment for that particular child? (see also Chapter 6).

Other points in the process at which the occupational therapists must take into account least restrictive considerations, include program planning and review. At the point an IEP is developed, are the services uniquely suited to meet the child's needs in a least restrictive manner? When program reviews are made, has consideration been given to how goals and objectives might be met by indirect, rather than direct services, and/or some direct services provided in the regular classroom in cooperation with the classroom teacher? When developing intervention plans, from a multidisciplinary perspective, in a residential or hospital facility, can it be argued that the occupational therapy services recommended, in fact, do assist the child to benefit from the special education services offered?

Occupational therapists must be cautioned that they need to develop skills that will enable them to work effectively with regular and special education staff. In trying to make coordinated and appropriate recommendations that fully meet the spirit of the least restrictive environment mandate, occupational therapists may encounter incredible resistance. Regular teachers may not wish to work directly with a particular child who is handicapped; funding may not encourage the therapist to work in an indirect manner with other service providers, etc.

It is important to note here, that to function effectively, the occupational therapist will need to know more than how to implement an intervention with a child needing occupational therapy. Occupational therapists must possess skills and knowledge that enable them to work with other specialists, classroom teachers, and administrators, so that they can teach their own "expertise" to others when appropriate, and they can provide occupational therapy services in an integrated and truly related manner.

RECENT AMENDMENTS TO THE EHA

In 1986, the EHA, P.L. 94-142, was amended by P.L. 99-457, "The Education of the Handicapped Amendments." Certain provisions of the EHA were expanded or modified (e.g., additional data reporting requirements were added). The mandate to provide a free and appropriate education, within the least restrictive environment, was unaffected. All of the provisions regarding parental participation, confidentiality, due process, evaluation procedures, etc., were retained. However, section 619 of EHA extended the mandated age for provision of services to three through five year olds, effective 1991–1992 school year. Part H of EHA is an amendment to the EHA, and may be best represented as incentives to states to create a statewide system of early intervention services to infants and toddlers with handicaps and their families. Occupational therapists, employed by programs funded under the provisions of Part H are affected by the specific provisions of this amendment, with respect to the kinds of services and nature of participation that is required. Although participation in programs provided for under Part H is discretionary, all states chose to participate in the first three years of the program. At this time, states are allowed and encouraged to conduct specific activities, and if they choose to participate, they must conform to certain requirements. On the other hand, they are not mandated to provide these specific services to infants and toddlers.

States receiving funding under Part H must develop and enhance the capacity to provide a multidisciplinary, coordinated, and inter-agency program of early intervention services for handicapped infants and toddlers and their families. A "handicapped infant and toddler" is defined in a specific way under Part H. The definition departs from how children are defined as handicapped under P.L. 99-142. Section 672 of Part H defines a handicapped child as those infants and toddlers needing services because they:

"a) are experiencing developmental delays, as measured by appropriate diagnostic instruments and procedures in one or more of the following areas: Cognitive development, physical development, language and speech development, psychosocial development, or self-help skills, or

b) Have a diagnosed physical or mental condition which has a high probability of resulting in developmental delay.

Such term may also include, at a state's discretion, individuals from birth to age 2, inclusive, who are at risk of having substantial developmental delays if early intervention services are not provided."

Early intervention services are defined as "developmental services," and occupational therapy is included as one type of service. The services provided must be designed to meet developmental needs in the areas of physical, cognitive, self-help, language and speech, or psychosocial development. This definition departs significantly from how occupational therapy is defined under the EHA. As stated previously, occupational therapy is a related service, only, under EHA, and is provided only when necessary to assist a child determined to be handicapped in benefiting from special education. Occupational therapists working in programs funded under Part H should be alert to this distinction in the definition of allowable services. If working with handicapped infants or toddlers in a discretionary program, funded and regulated by Part H, occupational therapists are providing a direct form of developmental services, given that it is designed to meet needs in the aforementioned developmental areas.

Occupational therapists, who work in programs for infants and toddlers funded under P.L. 99-457, should familiarize themselves with the particular procedures in the state in which they work; for example, the designated lead state agency is not necessarily an educational one. Therapists need also to become knowledgeable with applicable federal and state requirements under 99-457, pertaining to parental procedural safeguards, the nature and minimum components of the "individualized family service plan," and "case management services," as well as those related to the federal and state standards regarding the definition of a "qualified" service provider.

ROLES AND FUNCTIONS OF OCCUPATIONAL THERAPY IN THE SCHOOLS

It is imperative that those occupational therapists working in the school system become adept at explaining how occupational therapy services meet the intent of P.L. 94-142, in a way that special education administrators can understand. Most descriptions of occupational therapy in the schools employ language consistent with the medical model. To illustrate, most of the goals are stated in biophysical terms; their relationship to education, and educational readiness or progress is not evident. They are not stated in educational terms that administrators, teachers, and parents can easily understand. There is a need, therefore, to delineate the roles and functions of occupational therapy within the context of an educational model.

As stated, P.L. 94-142 provides that a child with a handicapping condition receives occupational therapy services, if those services are necessary for the child to benefit from special education services. What is not always clear to special education administrators, is what occupational therapy can do to facilitate a child's performance in special education. To illustrate, during a national meeting of school system administrators (personal communication, December 15, 1985, Barbara Hanft, American Occupational Therapy Association), two questions were repeatedly posed by school system administrators. These questions were:

- What services of school based occupational therapists are related to the education of handicapped children?
- How do such services relate to the education or educational readiness of handicapped children?

To elaborate, analysis of proper positioning of a child during seated activities may be a school-based service of occupational therapy, as related to the education of children with handicapping conditions. An example of how such a service may relate to the educational readiness of children follows: "Proper positioning can allow for stability of the child's body at the desk. Better body stability can allow a child with a handicap to read more easily, and attend to the teacher, since less attention needs to be directed to maintenance of body position, when properly seated with positioning devices." Further specification of what and how occupational therapy services are educationally related, is a critical need to be addressed by school-based occupational therapists.

Examples are presented in Figure 13-1 as illustrations of ways to explain occupational therapy in the schools. These examples have been adapted from Gilfoyle and Hays (1979), who used data from the 1978 AOTA membership survey to identify roles and functions of the school-based occupational therapist. These examples are not meant to be a comprehensive overview of roles and functions of occupational therapy in the schools. Rather, it is simply to serve as clarification of ways to make occupational therapy concepts more understandable for special educators. And, these examples are for general functions and are not related to specific IEP goals. Figure 13-1 presents examples using traditional occupational therapy terminology, as well as the same example presented in more common language.

The functions of occupational therapy as a school-based service, is but one of the related services specified in P.L. 94-142. The intent of P.L. 94-142 was that related services should be available to any handicapped child needing them to benefit from special education. And, as previously stated, occupational therapy is considered but one of various related services. Differentiation and explanation of the similarity and differences between occupational therapy, and other services designated as related services, is also important.

The overall conceptualization of occupational therapy as an education related discipline is philosophically and theoretically different from other disciplines. One unique characterization of occupational therapy in the schools, is that it employs a developmental approach geared to sensory as well as motor development, in the context of overall central nervous system maturation. An occupational therapy goal may be to build up the underlying central nervous system foundation for automatic function of skills and educational readiness.

For example, a special education teacher may use a behaviorally based approach to enhance mouth closure and reduce drooling in a student with severe disability. Thus, the student may be "rewarded" every time he closes his mouth in response to the teacher snapping her fingers. Somewhat differently, the occupational therapist might feel this requires too much "cognitive energy" on the part of the student, and siphons off energy which could otherwise be directed to learning. Therefore, the occupational therapist may employ neuromuscular facilitation techniques, based upon touch and deep pressure to the muscle of the jaw, in order to facilitate automatic mouth closure in the student.

Generally speaking, the school based occupational therapist is trained to consider the following:

- The internal environment of the child; the underlying neurological foundation of educational readiness.
- The interaction between the child (internal environment) and the environmental demands (external environment).

Traditional	Revised
Improve gross and fine motor skills.	Improve motor skills necessary for interaction with the environment ranging from mobility to manipulation of objects.
Improve sensorimotor integration function.	Improve child's ability to receive, process, and use sensory information allowing for more normal environmental interaction.
Prevent developmental disability, dysfunction, and deformity.	Promote development of motor skills, reduce effects of motor dysfunction and prevent deformity which limits function.
Improve ability in activities of daily living.	Improve self care skills (feeding, dressing, grooming, and toileting) through use of adapted equipment and strategies to compensate for disability.
Increase joint range of motion.	Increase movement available at all joints to allow for better positioning during activities and rest as well as to allow for more functional use of arms, legs, and head.
Increase school adjustment.	Increase child's ability to function within classroom and made adaptations necessary within the classroom to allow the child to function most efficiently and effectively.

Figure 13-1. Examples of General Functions of School Based Occupational Therapists in Tradition and Revised Language. *Royeen, C. B., & Marsh, D., 1988. Promoting occupational therapy in the schools. American Journal of Occupational Therapy, 42(11), 714. Traditional examples adapted from Gilfoyle and Hays (1979). Occupational therapy roles and functions in the education of the school-based handicapped student. American Journal of Occupational Therapy, 33(9), 565–576. Acknowledgment is given to Joan Dostal, OTR, for help in generating this figure.*

Another critical difference between special education and occupational therapy in the schools is that, generally speaking, a special educator would look to teach to strengths, and compensate for deficit skills by drill and practice; whereas the occupational therapist would intervene, to remediate or ameliorate the underlying dysfunction or weakness. The occupational therapist is more often concerned with the underlying sensorimotor or neurological foundation of the child's educational readiness. And, the occupational therapist intervenes by building up the underlying foundation by environmental manipulations or facilitation/inhibition of components of the child's internal environment, to allow for better child/ environment interactions and consequent learning.

Given the distinction presented between special education and occupational therapy, other related disciplines need to be identified. A summary of the similarities and differences between occupational therapy, and other related service disciplines is presented in Figure 13-2. Given this discussion of occupational therapy as a related service, the chapter will now address models of service provision.

MODELS OF SERVICE PROVISION FOR OCCUPATIONAL THERAPY IN THE SCHOOLS

The actual service provision model of occupational therapy within the school system can take many forms, but can usually be characterized as one of three main categories. These are: a) direct service, b) consultation, and c) monitoring. Each of these is briefly explained and references provided in Figure 13-3.

Traditionally, occupational therapy curricula have trained occupational therapy personnel in the direct service model. In the past seven years, there has been an increasing trend to train personnel competent to function in the consultation and monitoring role, as well as in the role of direct service. This has occurred in response to the need to provide a greater breadth of services in the school system. In fact, the variety of models of service provision for occupational therapy in the schools, may be essential to the continued provision of occupational therapy services in the school setting (Dunn, 1987).

There is an increasing pressure to assume consultation and monitoring roles, with a corresponding decrease in direct treatment. Considering this, the issue is not which model is best. It is not a value judgement that direct treatment is inherently better than monitoring, which is inherently better than consultation. Nor is it a value judgment that the opposite is true, i.e., that monitoring is "better" than consultation, which is better than direct treatment, because it is the most inexpensive form of occupational therapy services. Rather, the issue is one of student needs, and meeting student needs in an: a) individualized, and b) appropriate manner. Children with certain types of problems or needs require direct intervention. Other children, with different types of needs or problems, require consultation. And still others, with yet different problems, require monitoring.

Therefore, the issue is identification of student dysfunction or need, and matching it to the appropriate form of service provision. It is not a matter of investigating which model works best overall. This is an important, yet complex concept, which occupational therapists need to understand themselves, and then communicate to special education administrators.

It should also be noted that the method of service provision will also change over time, as student needs or dysfunction will change over time.

EFFECTIVE COMMUNICATION

In a previous section of this chapter, the need to communicate to special education administrators was identified.

Discipline	Role and Function in the School System	Relationship to Occupational Therapy
Adaptive Physical Education	Concerned with sports activities and fitness of handicapped children.	Common concern with physical activity and fitness of handicapped children. Adaptive physical education uses more generalized strategies and group activities. Occupational therapists can prescribe individual treatment program geared to ameliorate specific dysfunction.
Perceptual Visual Motor Trainers and Optometrists	Concerned with visual perception and function.	Perceptual motor trainers and optometrists are concerned with visual motor integration primarily related to gross motor activity. Occupational therapists are concerned with visual motor integration as related to gross and fine motor as well as sensory processing.
Physical Education	Concerned with sports activities and fitness.	Common concern with students' engagement in physical activity and fitness. Occupational therapists are concerned with students' other limitations which may interfere with physical education.
Physical Therapy	Assess, remediate and habilitate physical and motor dysfunction.	Common concern with motor function. Occupational therapists are concerned with motor function in relationship to engagement in occupation or activity.
Psychologist	Concerned with psychological and intellectual processing of the child.	Occupational therapists are concerned with sensory motor processing as a substrate of intelligence, and sensory motor processing as a substrate of the child's social/emotional/psychological state.
Speech Pathologist	Assess, remediate and habilitate speech/language and communication disorders.	Common concern with oral motor function. Occupational therapy intervention focused more on oral development as related to eating, reduction of drooling or in motor skill to utilize adaptive communication device.
Vocational Educator	Preparation for and training in vocational skills leading to employability.	Both concerned with engagement in vocational activities. Occupational therapists are more involved in sensory, motor, and technological adaptation necessary to allow the individual to function most effectively.

Figure 13-2. Overview of Similarities and Differences Between Occupational Therapy and Other Related Services. *Royeen, C. B., & Marsh, D., 1988. Promoting occupational therapy in the schools. American Journal of Occupational Therapy, 42(11), 715. In part, adapted from S. Cermack and L. Cermack, Neuroanatomical and neurophysiological aspects of apraxia in adults and children. Institute presentation at the American Occupational Therapy Association Annual Conference, 1979. Detroit. Also comments by Joan Dostal, OTR, are gratefully acknowledged.*

In addition, there are other considerations of which to be aware, when planning a strategy for communication with special education administrators. These considerations have more to do with the process of communication; that is, how one communicates, rather than the content of what is communicated.

Sharing of information (Neighor and Schulberg, 1982) is a hallmark of effectively provided occupational therapy services in the schools. Sharing of information with the special education administrator needs to be thought out deliberately, and planned, based upon the time and medium for communication. These factors shall be discussed in turn.

Occupational therapists in the schools are well aware of student variation in preferred learning modalities. Similarly, special education administrators may have preferred modalities for communication. Some may like formal verbal presentations, while others may prefer handwritten notes. Still others may choose informal give-and-take sessions. The occupational therapist needs to assess and respond in the preferred mode of communication of the special education administrator. Attempts to communicate what the school-based occupational therapy program is accomplishing, also need to be tailored to the preferences of the particular administrator.

The time of communication may similarly be tailored to the

Category of Service	Definition	Examples
Treatment/Direct Service	Evaluation and treatment of a handicapped child. Treatment delivered on a one-to-one basis or in small group setting.	Children displaying gravitational insecurity or tactile defensiveness. Children at high-risk for aspiration of food: once stabilized, child can go to monitoring.
Monitoring/Indirect Service	Evaluation of a handicapped child with the intervention strategy planned by the occupational therapist but executed by another such as the classroom teacher, aide, etc. under the supervision of the occupational therapist.	Often used with self care skill training such as dressing or eating, toileting, or use of adaptive equipment such as a wheel chair, communication device, splint, etc.
Consultation/Indirect Service	Sharing of professional knowledge on an "as needed" basis from case problems.	Explanation of certain behavioral idiosyncracies associated with particular disabilities, or estimation of performance potential in activities of daily living.

Figure 13-3.   Models of Service Provision in School Based Occupational Therapy. Acknowledgement is given Joan Dostal, OTR, for help in generating this figure.

special education administrator's preference. Certain administrators may prefer a time early in the morning, whereas others may prefer after school hours. The school-based occupational therapist should initiate and maintain communication with the special education administrator. Moreover, the occupational therapist needs to constantly monitor and evaluate the effectiveness of a chosen communication strategy, and modify the strategy as necessary.

COST CONSIDERATIONS REGARDING OCCUPATIONAL THERAPY IN THE SCHOOLS

To date, occupational therapy services within public schools have been accepted, if not always well understood. However, the long standing need for clarification of how the services occupational therapists provide in the public school setting are educationally related, is intensified by the financial pressures bearing on special education. The cost of special education has risen dramatically, and Congress has mandated a national study of the cost of special education, with costs for related services—including occupational therapy, to be documented (U.S. Dept. of Ed., 1988). In Minnesota, the state legislature has mandated a fiscal analysis of occupational therapist services in the public schools (Barbara Hanft, Government and Legal Affairs Division, American Occupational Therapy Association, May 20, 1986). These separate events foreshadow the increasing scrutiny of the costs associated with the provision of all special education services, and for occupational therapy specifically.

Considering costs, many school systems may believe it is more efficient to bus children to occupational therapy services in a central location, rather than have the therapist travel and provide space and equipment in each school. And, many therapists prefer this, since it is more similar to a clinical model. However, unless adequate time is set up to allow the

therapist to be in the classroom, and interacting with teachers, therapy will not be as effective, and therefore, is not cost efficient. Also, in such cases, the effectiveness of the occupational therapy service cannot be judged, as the occupational therapist does not know about carry-over or generalization to the classroom, and the teacher will not be able to attribute gains to what is occurring in occupational therapy.[3]

From one viewpoint, cost is not an issue regarding occupational therapy in the schools, since occupational therapy is required by law as a related service, if, indeed, occupational therapy services are recommended by the team and become part of the IEP. However, from a practical viewpoint, the cost of occupational therapy services is everyone's concern. It may not be surprising that there is an increased pressure on school-based occupational therapy programs, if they are not well understood by the special education administrators.

PARENTAL RIGHTS AND DUE PROCESS PROCEDURE UNDER P.L. 94-142

Parental opportunity to participate in decisions regarding the development, revision, and review of their child's special education program, is a central feature of the EHA (see Subpart E-"Procedural Safeguards"). The right is embodied by the law in various ways, most significantly with respect to the opportunity for parental participation, and the right to pursue due process remedies when a parent disagrees with the decisions recommended by, or the program being provided by the educational agency.

With respect to participation, essentially parents must provide informed written consent for the initial evaluation, if it is suspected the child is handicapped, and the initial placement

---

[3] This section was substantially contributed to by Joan Dostal, OTR.

of the child in a special education program, if it has been determined that the child is handicapped, and therefore eligible to receive special education and related services (34 CFR 300.504(2) (b)). Parents must be afforded an opportunity to participate, by the provision of prior notice by the educational agency, before decisions regarding identification, evaluation, placement, and review or revisions in a program can be made. Additionally, parents have the right to request and obtain an independent educational evaluation at public expense, if the parent disagrees with the evaluation obtained by the educational agency. And finally, parents must be given the opportunity to inspect and review all education records that relate to the identification, evaluation, and educational placement of their child.

In sum, the prior notice requirement applies whenever the public agency (e.g., the local school district or school) seeks, or refuses to initiate or change, the identification, evaluation, educational placement, or provision of a free and appropriate public education to a child (34 CFR 300.504(a)). Occupational therapists need to be aware of these requirements, when working in facilities with children whose programs are supported and bound by P.L. 94-142. For example, before beginning a pre-placement occupational therapy evaluation, the therapist must provide informed notice and obtain consent from the child's parent. Schools and facilities use somewhat varying forms and procedures to reflect, not just federal, but also state and local practices. Therefore, occupational therapists must work with system personnel to identify the correct forms, and to conform with accepted procedures. When a particular occupational therapy intervention is recommended, as a part of the entire special education program and services to be provided, occupational therapists should be certain parents, if not participating directly in the meetings, have at least been given an opportunity to do so. Actual services, when provided for the first time, must not be initiated unless parents have provided their consent. Failure to conform with these safeguards, is sufficient cause for parents to initiate due process procedures.

The due process provisions of P.L. 94-142 enable parents to initiate procedures, when they disagree with all or some of the special education decision affecting their child. These disagreements may range from the initial decision that a child is or is not handicapped (and, therefore, is or is not eligible to receive services), to the actual services provided, the school district's refusal to amend educational records at a parent's request, or the extent to which services are provided in the least restrictive environment. The centerpiece of these rights is the right of a parent (or, importantly, the public agency when it disagrees) to an impartial due process hearing, as required under 34 CFR 300.506-509. If aggrieved by this decision, parents may appeal to the state educational agency and obtain an administrative appeal.[4] If the parents disagree with the decision reached through the administrative appeal, they retain the right to bring a civil action (34 CFR 300.510-511). Finally, in 1986, the EHA was amended by P.L. 99-372, the "Handicapped Children's Protection Act," which al-

lows parents to recover attorney fees and other costs, when they win in a due process hearing or a court case proceeding.

Parental rights are reinforced further by their additional right to file a complaint with the state educational agency, if they believe the local school district has violated, or is about to violate, a federal statue or regulation that applies to a program (34 CFR 76.780-782). This right, which is available as a part of the Education Department General Administrative Regulations, and not the EHA, requires the state educational agency to investigate and resolve the complaint. If not satisfied, the parent has the right to request the U.S. Secretary of Education to review the matter. Parents may also file a complaint under Section 504 of the Rehabilitation Act of 1973, known as civil rights legislation. "Section 504" prohibits discrimination on the basis of handicap in the operation of federally funded programs. Many provisions of Section 504 are similar to those found under the EHA. Specific provisions, conditions, and limitations under each of these laws affect the particular way in which parents can disagree and seek to change school decisions. Clearly, however, parents retain comprehensive rights to participate and challenge public agency (e.g., school) decisions affecting the education of their child.

To function effectively, occupational therapists should be informed and knowledgeable regarding parental participation requirements, and the due process provisions in the conduct of their duties. Special education administrators are charged to insure that the staff and service providers work with parents to jointly make decisions about what a child needs, and how to accommodate those needs, given the mandates and requirements under the EHA. Inevitably, there will still be some disagreements between parents and educators when a full partnership is not achieved. In those cases, an occupational therapist, when involved, may be asked to participate in some fashion, most likely through: 1) the provision of records pertaining to the occupational services provided to the child, 2) the provision of testimony regarding an occupational therapy evaluation or intervention services, or 3) the conduct of an independent evaluation. Understanding the requirements under the EHA, and the conscientious fulfillment of duties, insures the occupational therapist is working in permissible and appropriate ways to meet the unique needs of the individual children served.

EXPAND YOUR NEWLY ACQUIRED KNOWLEDGE

1. Identify three issues that face the special education administrator when dealing with the related services. Design two strategies for dealing with each issue in a positive, effective manner.
2. Explain how service provision decisions are supposed to be made within the educational system.

References

Cruickshank, W. M., & Johnson, G. O. (1975). *Education of exceptional children and youth*, (3rd ed.). Englewood Cliffs, NJ: Prentice-Hall.
Dunn, W. (1987). Development of the individualized education program and occupational therapy intervention plans. In *Guidelines for Occupational Therapy Services in School Systems*. Rockville, MD: American Occupational Therapy Association.

---

[4] In some states, the state educational agency conducts the due process hearing. In those cases, no administrative appeal is conducted by the state. Parents retain the right, however, to bring civil action.

Education for all handicapped children act of 1975 (Public Law 94-142), 20 U.S.C. 1401.

Education of the handicapped act amendments of 1986. (Public Law 99-457), 20 U.S.C., 1400.

Gilfoyle, E., & Hays, C. (1979). Occupational therapy roles and functions for school-based handicapped children. *American Journal of Occupational Therapy, 33*(9), 565–576.

Meyen, E. L. (1982). *Exceptional children in today's schools: An alternative resource book* (p. 35, 587). Colorado: Love Publishing Co.

Neighor, W. D., & Schulberg, H. C. (1982). Evaluating the outcome of human services programs: A reassessment. *Evaluation Review, 6*(6), 731–752.

Ottenbacher, K. (1982). Occupational therapy and special education: Some concerns related to Public Law 94-142. *American Journal of Occupational Therapy, 36*(2), 81–84.

Patton, M. Q. (1981). *Creative evaluation*. Beverly Hills: Sage Publishing Co.

Rostetter, D., Kowalski, R. S., & Hunter, D. (1984). Implementing the integration principle of P.L. 94-142. In N. Certo, N. Haring, & R. York (Eds.), *Public school integration of severely handicapped students*. Baltimore: Paul H. Brookes.

34 Code of Federal Regulations (CFR)—Parts 300-399. Washington, D.C.: U.S. Government Printing Office.

Turnbull, H. R. (1986). *Free appropriate public education: The law and children with disabilities*. Denver: Love.

U.S. Department of Education. (1988). *Tenth annual report to Congress on the implementation of the education of the handicapped act*. Washington, D.C.: Office of Special Education Programs.

CHAPTER 14

The Family Perspective

Jane Case-Smith, EdD, OTR

"Family-centered care must reflect a balanced view of the child and family. That is, in assessing and attempting to address the child's problems, the child's and the family's strengths and resources must be considered as well. Secondly, the individuality of the child and his or her family and their different methods of coping must be respected and supported." Shelton, Jeppson & Johnson, 1987

WORKING WITH FAMILIES

Occupational therapists have long recognized the value of involving families, particularly parents, in intervention with the child. In recent years, the role of the family in the intervention process seems to be expanding, and with the accumulating evidence of the importance of the family to any child's development, it has been proposed that the family be viewed as the center of the service provision process rather than as peripheral team members (Turnbull & Summers, 1987). This perspective requires that therapists balance their goals for the child's achievement with concern for and protection of that child's membership in a family unit (Carney, 1987).

What Is a Family?

The family plays a key role in our society and assumes primary responsibility for the transmission of the culture from one generation to the next. Parents assume the responsibility for transmitting to their offspring the competencies required by the social, economic and political forces of society and community (Fewell, 1986, p. 4).

A universal role of families is to nurture the young child. The family provides for the child's physical needs and fosters the development of an integrated person capable of living in and contributing to society (David, 1979; Lidz, 1963). Parents foster the child's competence and skills to prepare that child for the adult tasks he or she will later assume. Parents teach children those skills essential for coping with society. These skills cross the domains for social, emotional, cognitive, and physical development that enable a person to function in the community (Fewell, 1986, p. 6.). The parent-child relationship is one of the most basic relationships in the human community. It is in this relationship between parent and child that both learn about themselves and the other; there is the opportunity for human experience, joy, and love not duplicated in the human community. The family as a social system has unique characteristics and needs. Individual family members are so interrelated that any experience affecting one member will affect all members (Carter & McGoldrick, 1980).

Families With a Child With a Disability

The strong influence that family members have on each other is particularly important to understanding families with children who have disabilities. The interactions of the parent and the child, the responses of the child to the parent and the parent to the child, are strongly influenced by the child's impairment. This relationship is supported and influenced by all members of the family.

In families who have a member with a disability, everyday events and activities may cause tension and stress in family members. A child who struggles to chew and swallow and is incapable of efficient feeding, may be a constant disruptive force at mealtime. Many children who have severe physical or behavioral problems also have limited social skills. Consequently these children have constant conflicts and disruptive relationships with other children and siblings. They may be a source of great sadness to parents concerned that their child is socially excluded and does not engage in positive relationships with others.

Although the child with a disability may take a physical, social and psychological toll on the family, the child may also provide extraordinary reward and joy. The special needs and vulnerabilities of a child with a handicapping condition can be a major rallying point. Family members can grow closer by sharing the duties of child care and learn more about each other in their intense common struggle. Parents also learn about their own capacities and adaptability. Having a successful meal during which a six-year-old manages to keep food off the floor without spilling milk, can be an extraordinarily satisfying experience (Paul & Porter, 1981, p. 9). Commonplace activities for a typical child such as a party or outing, may be a very special and joyous event for the child with a disability and the family.

The effect of the child with a disability on the family relates to a number of variables. The characteristics of the child with a handicap affect the family's reactions and responses. A child with a terminal illness may cause constant grief and loss. A child with severe or multiple disabilities may have a more intense family impact. Caretaking demands are particularly draining with children who have behavioral problems.

Family Characteristics

The characteristics of families shape their response to the child with a disability. The family's cultural background, socioeconomic status, size and other characteristics can be potential resources to enable the family to cope with their child's disability. Large families have more people available to help with chores and special adaptations. Other siblings may be able to absorb parents' expectations for achievement. Parents may be more philosophically accepting of the child if they also have "normal" children (Turnbull & Turnbull, 1986, p. 29).

The relationship of the parents seems essential to the ability of the family to cope with a child with disabilities. In a recent survey of mothers of children with Down Syndrome, mothers indicated that their spouses were their most important support persons (Fewell, Belmonte, & Ahlersmeyer, 1983). Spouses share in the emotions, the physical care, the nurturance and the concerns about the future. Frederick (1979) reported that mental satisfaction was the single best predictor of a family's positive coping behavior, when rearing a child with a disability.

Cultural and ethnic background and religion greatly influence a family's daily lives. These values and perspectives play an important role in shaping a family's reaction to a child with a disability. They also influence the family's responses to the occupational therapist. Differing child rearing practices are often difficult for service providers to understand or interpret. Typical parents from Central and South America constantly carry their children, which may conflict with the therapist's goals for mobility and exploration of the environment. The goal for independence is not shared or even valued by families of other cultures. In many Mexican, South American, and Chinese families, reliance and dependency on each other is valued as part of the bonding and caring between members. Family well being and caretaking may be valued over individual achievement (Lynch, 1987).

A family's socioeconomic status (SES) has many implications for adaptation to a child with a disability. Although families with higher incomes and education may have more resources available to cope with their child, higher SES does not automatically guarantee better coping. Higher SES families are often more achievement oriented, and may consider a physical or mental disability as a severe disappointment to their aspirations for a child. Parents of a higher SES may have a great sense of control, and may be unusually stressed by the birth of a child with a handicap, which contradicts their belief that they are in control of their lives (Turnbull & Turnbull, 1986, p. 34).

Families that feel in control of their lives are more likely to participate in intervention and activities designed to improve the function of their child. In contrast, poverty families who do not believe in the possibility of controlling their environment, may be more accepting of a child with a disability. The families that feel they have minimal control over their environment may not think that change in the child is possible or important, and consequently may not be motivated to participate in intervention.

Personal characteristics of individual family members affect the way that the family functions as a whole. These personal characteristics can be strengths or drawbacks for the family as a whole. For example, a parent in poor physical health is less able to cope with stressful situations. Parents may have mental problems that can lead to instances of neglect or abuse. Individual family members may vary in the strategies they adopt to deal with stress. Coping styles usually rely on spiritual, social, or professional supports. Coping strategies influence family functioning, satisfaction, feelings of efficacy, and the child's outcome (Zeitlin, Rosenblatt, and Williamson, 1986).

Family Interactions

The family is tremendously influenced by the child, and his or her unique needs and problems. A child with a disability can have both a positive and/or a negative effect on the husband and wife interactions. Many studies have indicated that having a child with a disability is a negative influence on the parent's marriage. Featherstone (1980) vividly described this effect:

> A child's handicap attacks the fabric of a marriage in four ways. It excites powerful emotions in both parents. It acts as a dispiriting symbol of shared failure. It reshapes the organization of the family. It creates fertile ground for conflict (p. 91).

A child with a disability can also be a positive influence on marriage. Some husbands and wives feel closer and stronger as a result of the experience. Gath (1977) reported that almost half of the 30 couples which she sampled, reported that they felt closer, and felt that their marriage had been strengthened by their shared experience. Kazak and Marvin (1984) compared 56 couples with spina bifida children, and 53 couples with normal children, and found that couples with children with spina bifida actually experienced somewhat higher levels of marital satisfaction.

Therefore, assumptions about the interaction between parents can not necessarily be made from the knowledge that the family has a child with a disability. Similarly, the interactions between a parent and a child are always unique. The birth of an infant with impairments often has an immediate effect on the early bonding interaction. The family's dreams and expectations are threatened by the initial diagnosis, and intense feelings of guilt, anger, or disappointment may result. These feelings may disrupt the parent-child interactions as described by parents (Allen & Allen, 1979; Featherstone, 1980). Usually, with time, equilibrium returns and the parent and child begin to form a lasting and mutually satisfying relationship.

The unique nature of the child and the type of disability, contribute to the interactions of parent and child. A difficult child may delay or disrupt the attachment process. Infants with impaired sensorimotor systems are probably less efficient in communicating their needs, feelings, and states. This communication process can be frustrating for parents and may result in inappropriate responses to the child.

Another result is that often the parent tends to exhibit greater control and directiveness in the interaction. This observed "style" of parent-child interaction may result from the parent's eagerness to overcome the child's disability by sheer intensity of effort. Directiveness seems to be associated with the child's developmental level (e.g., capability to respond) rather than the parents' style of interaction. While the effect of parental directiveness and control on the child have been debated, sensitive and positive responses by the parent seem to benefit and enhance development (Crawley and Spiker, 1983; Kasari, 1987).

The interactions between parent and child constitute the foundation of their relationship. This relationship between parent and child is both powerful and enduring. It has a profound effect on the child's ability to function in the community and in society.

Family Roles

The roles of all family members may change in the course of raising a child with special needs. New roles are added to the traditional ones. Caretaking may be more involved and may take more hours in the day. Extended family may become involved in caretaking and provide a source of relief and respite to the parents.

When the child is severely disabled or medically vulnerable, the roles of all family members may change in interaction with the child. The father's expected role may shift. As Gallagher, Cross and Scharfman (1981) note, "the traditional father roles of physical playmate and model for the male child are largely diminished or not present at all" (p. 13). Michaelis (1980) explains that for some fathers, the lack of interaction with the child may be the result of a perceived inability to meet the child's needs (p. 92). In some families, the caretaking responsibilities of the father are greatly increased. Siblings of the child with a handicap must make special adjustments, although the impact on siblings has not been well understood or recognized by therapists (Vadasy, Fewell, Meyer, & Greenberg, 1984). The research on siblings suggests they may have some special concerns as a result of their brothers' or sisters' disability. They may have emotional problems or negative reactions. Siblings often have increased responsibilities to help with physical and caretaking needs of their brother or sister. Grossman (1972) found that siblings in a two child family experience special pressure. Parental attitudes, and reactions to the brother or sister with retardation, had the strongest influence on the normal sibling's acceptance.

Family Time

The time demanded to provide help, support and care for a child with severe impairments, can amount to an intensive, exhausting, never-ending 24 hour care routine (Lyon & Preis, 1983). Parents may feel that they must give all their time to their child with a handicap and may fail to take time for themselves. When first searching for services, the parents often feel great relief and gratitude when they locate a program for their child. However, this "help" also demands part of their time.

The additional demands imposed on parents by the intervention program are intended to foster long term benefits in child skills and parent-child relationships. However, the short term impact of activities recommended by the program can be draining. Featherstone (1980) illustrates the demands on her time and energy as a parent of a child with disabilities.

> I remember the day when the occupational therapist at Jody's school called with some suggestions from a visiting nurse. Jody's course of Dilantin had caused the gums to grow over the teeth. The nurse had innocently recommended that his teeth be brushed four times a day, for five minutes, with an electric toothbrush. The school suggested that they could do this once on school days, and that I should try to do it the other three to four times a day. . . . The new demand appalled me. . . . Jody . . . is blind, cerebral-

palsied, and retarded. We do his physical therapy daily and work with him on sounds and communication. We feed him each meal on our laps, bottle him, change him, bathe him, dry him, put him in a body cast to sleep, launder his bed linens daily, and go through a variety of routines designed to minimize his miseries and enhance his joys and his development. Now you tell me that I should spend fifteen minutes every day on something that Jody will hate, an activity that will not help him walk or even defecate, but one that is directed at the health of his gums. This activity is not for a finite time, but forever. It is not guaranteed to help, but "it can't hurt." And it won't make the overgrowth go away, but may retard it. Where is that fifteen minutes going to come from? What am I supposed to give up? Taking the kids to the park? Reading the bedtime story to my eldest? Washing the dishes? Because there is not time in my life that hasn't been spoken for, and for every fifteen minute activity that is added, one has to be taken away (pp. 77–78).

Family Finances

The presence of a child with a disability can create special economic needs. The family has greater expenses and may have decreased productive capacity (Turnbull, Summers, & Brotherson, 1984). In one study, 29% of the families reported that their child's physical disability had created a financial hardship. The child's special needs can include costly medical bills, expensive equipment, or structural adaptations for the home. Families seldom anticipate these expenses and may be overwhelmed by the costs. Financial resources may also be decreased by factors such as time off work, or a less well paid job (Lonsdale, 1978, p. 117).

Summary

Although families with children with disabilities have inevitable stress, the impact of that stress and their ability to function as a family are related to many complex and interwoven variables. A child with a disability affects each member of a family, the interrelationships of members and the way that a family functions in the community.

Family function is dependent on the ability to cope or adapt to crises, and to everyday life, and is related to values, resources, cultural background and support systems. The ways that families interact and relate determine how the family adapts to crises in everyday events. Strong relationships, positive interaction, and adaptability ultimately enable a family to cope with a child with a disability. Researchers (Hill and Hansen, 1982; McCubbin, Joy, Cauble, Comeau, Patterson, and Needle, 1980) document that families with close emotional bonds that are able to adapt to change are more resistant to crisis and able to recover more quickly from crises. Supportive relationships within families seem more important to their ability to cope than any singular characteristics of families. In addition, bolstering can occur from support systems outside the family. Parent support groups may foster effective coping. Positive interactions with other families provide support and role models.

Pediatric occupational therapists need to understand the families they serve as systems that interact with the child with a disability, with each other, and with the community. By addressing the needs of the family, the therapist ultimately effects the functional outcome for the child. Support to the family can facilitate bonding, coping and adaptability. The second part of this chapter discusses methods for supporting and assisting families as an integral part of occupational therapy with the child.

PRINCIPLES IN WORKING WITH FAMILIES

Assessment

Families are unique and complex systems that defy assumptions or routine structured approaches. A comprehensive family assessment is accomplished by the occupational therapist with other team members. The assessment provides the foundation for establishing appropriate goals and planning effective treatment. Comprehensive family assessment may be separated into three dimensions: *child variables*, *family needs and strengths*, and *interactions between family and child*.

Child Variables

First, child variables are assessed (see also Chapter 3). These variables determine many aspects of the family's function, including the amounts of daily care given and services needed. The child's degree and type of disability, as well as his or her personality and temperament, affect the family's interactions and daily routines. Assessment includes the child's behavior, temperament, and readability (Huntington, 1988).

Specific temperament traits can affect the attitudes and behaviors of parents. Whether a child is difficult, easy, or shy has a impact on his or her relationship with family members. Salient characteristics that may affect relationships within the family are limited sensory awareness, severe physical deformity, or lack of "cuddliness" due to hyper- or hypotonicity (Blacher, 1984). Fundamental social skills, such as smiling, eye contact or vocalizations may not occur, thus inhibiting or delaying the reciprocity that characterizes interactions between mothers and nonhandicapped children. Parents may find their child's cues and responses more difficult to read. The child may exhibit fewer responses and more subtle responses. Behavioral characteristics have implications for family function. Beckman (1983) found that children who were socially unresponsive, displayed repetitive behaviors, and had more caregiving needs created more parental stress and family problems. The number of additional caregiving demands was highly related to the mother's level of stress.

Child characteristics that influence family function can be assessed in a number of ways. Scales to measure the child's temperament usually rely on interview with the primary caretaker and therefore are based on the parent's perception of the child (Thomas, Chess, & Birch, 1968; Carey & McDevitt, 1978; Fullard, McDevitt, Carey, 1984; McDevitt & Carey, 1978). Typical categories used in measuring temperament are activity level, rhythmicity, adaptability, approach, distractibility, and persistence. The parent's perception of the child's temperament is one of the most powerful determinants of parent-child interaction. The child's behavior may be assessed through interview and observation. Three scales based on observation and interaction are the *Early Coping Inventory* (Zeitlin, Williamson & Szczepanski, 1989), the *Coping Inventory*, (Zeitlin, 1985), and the the *Carolina Record of Individual Behavior* (Simeonsson, Huntington, Short and Ware, 1982). These scales measure adaptive behaviors such as: responsiveness, reactivity, goal directiveness, response to frustration, attention span, communication, and sensorimotor skill.

Family Needs and Strengths

The second dimension of family assessment is the family's strengths and needs, which can be assessed using a written survey or an interview. This assessment offers an opportunity for the parents to express their concerns, and to give the therapist important information about home and family life. Family strengths as defined by Dunst, Trivette, & Deal (1988) include a sense of commitment toward promoting family growth and wellness, an appreciation of family members, and an effort to spend time and do things together. Cohesive families share a sense of purpose and a set of rules, values, and beliefs. A family's strengths may include their relationships with each other, friends and extended family. When strong and positive relationships bind a family, the ability to cope effectively with stress and crisis is enhanced. Other family strengths are effective coping strategies and the ability to be positive, flexible, and adaptable. These variables make family life satisfying and fulfilling. Dunst, et al. (1988) state that all families have strengths that constitute valuable resources for meeting needs (p. 27).

To effectively work with families, occupational therapists and other professionals must understand each family's concerns and needs. The family's needs may include the need for additional resources, information, special services, or special considerations. The therapist can not always provide or locate solutions to all of the needs identified, but knowledge of family needs and strengths assists in determining the direction of therapy, and the priority of treatment goals. It may be beneficial for families to prioritize needs or to identify which needs seem to be creating problems for the family. In addition to needs for information, support resources, or services, families may need support systems outside of the nuclear and extended family. They may desire an explanation about the disability to extended family or friends. They may need community services or access to additional financial resources.

A number of scales have been developed to help identify family needs. The *Family Need Survey* (Bailey and Simeonsson, 1988) is organized into six categories listed below:

A. Needs for Information
B. Needs for Support
C. Explaining to Others
D. Community Services
E. Financial Needs
F. Family Functioning.

Dunst and his colleagues have developed several scales that assess specific family needs (Dunst, et al., 1988). The scales measure family functions, resources, and support systems. Categories of these scales are financial support, vocation, child care, transportation, and communication.

Family Interactions

Finally, the interactions between family and child are evaluated. By understanding the nature of the family's transactions with the child, much is learned about the child's daily environment and the relationships within that environment. These transactions have a profound effect on the child's ability to cope, level of motivation, self esteem, and confidence in accepting a challenge or a new situation. Family transactions illustrate the match or "fit" between the unique characteristics of the child and the family as they interact in the environment. A good fit, or strong match between child and family implies positive interactions between child and family. This goodness-of-fit promotes successful interactions between the child and the daily environment. A demanding child may fit into a large family with multiple caretakers to fulfill the child's needs. A child with a low frustration tolerance who is defeated easily and displays a loss of temper, will match well with parents who structure and simplify activities and appropriately discipline loss of temper. Passive or placating parents may not have goodness-of-fit with this child. The implications of this concept is that outcome and family function are predicted not by family characteristics or child characteristics, but by the interactions that occur between family and child.

Many different approaches have been taken in assessing the interactions between the family and child. For reasons that will be discussed later in this chapter, most assessments of interaction are between infants and parents (see Table 14-1). The instruments vary according to their purpose, the characteristics begin assessed, and the behaviors of interest. Bromwich (1981) developed a scale of parental involvement with the infant. This scale assesses six levels of behaviors from maternal enjoyment of the infant to the mother independently providing developmentally appropriate activities. Other assessments of parent-infant interactions, such as the one developed by Mahoney and Powell (1984), evaluate turn-taking and interaction match or the compatibility of parent's and infant's style. The Mahoney and Powell scale assesses the parent's expressiveness, warmth, sensitivity, effectiveness, and directiveness; and the child's activity level, attention span, enjoyment, and expressiveness.

Observational assessments have been developed which rate interaction while the parent is playing with the child. The Parent-/Caregiver involvement Scale (Farran, Kasari, Comfort, & Jay, 1986) evaluates physical involvement, verbal involvement, responsiveness of caregiver to child, play interaction, teaching behavior, control over child's activities, and negative and positive statements. This scale focuses on the parents, and their ability to provide play and teaching experiences to the child in a growth fostering manner (see Table 14-1). While the occupational therapist may not be the team member to administer these scales, often she or he must interpret and understand the results of these assessments.

The subjective opinion of the occupational therapist, regarding the warmth and sensitivity of the family's transactions, and the degree to which these transactions foster and support the child's growth and success, is invaluable.

Family Intervention Principles and Strategies

Family and professional collaboration and partnership is essential throughout the intervention/education process. Collaboration means that occupational therapists, other service providers, and families work toward common goals and join efforts to achieve mutually agreed upon outcomes. In pro-

viding therapy and recommending home activities, it is essential to fit into the family as it defines itself, and respect individual member roles. (Turnbull & Turnbull, 1986, p. 82).

Activities of the occupational therapist should strengthen family interactions and support their ability to cope with and adapt to the consequences of their child's disability. It has been demonstrated that parent-child interactions are not always improved through therapy. Kogan, Tyler, and Turner (1974) compared mother-child interactions of children with cerebral palsy, while mother and child played together and while they were engaged in therapy. While performing therapy, the mother and child showed greater amounts of negative behaviors such as control, hostility and negative voice and content.

Intervention programs may place additional demands on parents that take time away from family life, and conflict with their roles as nurturing caregivers. The role conflict is illustrated by one mother's experience with therapy.

> Mom takes the program home with twenty goals, and drags the diaper bag, special equipment, stroller, screaming baby and her broken heart home (from therapy). There she looks over the list of technical jargon and tries to remember important instructions. Then she wonders if she will ever catch up on the housework and laundry (Gidewall, 1987).

Another mother expressed the role conflict that is often experienced with a child with a handicapping condition.

> I have spent a great deal of the last 22 months trying to think and behave as a therapist and feeling disappointed in myself if I don't. . . . I continually said if I'd only worked fewer hours and spent more time doing therapy (Lyon, 1986).

The parent role of nurturing and caretaking comes first, and should not be diminished by the treatment regimes of therapy programs. Creative and responsive therapy programs can improve everyday caretaking routines and responsibilities. Therapeutic activity suggestions that incorporate different family members or family members together, can facilitate positive interactions and family cohesion.

Therapy may inadvertently make a parent feel incompetent. The therapist's high level of skill may exacerbate a feeling of incompetence and loss of self esteem, particularly when the parent is unable to produce the same responses in the child.

Other mothers report positive feelings resulting from therapy:

> I found myself feeling proud of my child. Her (therapist) was so thrilled to hear of everything she did at home, and was almost as delighted to learn when she first sat up as we were! We called and told her even before we told the grandparents. We felt she had a right to be one of the first to know.

> These sessions were a place where my child was not judged on what he could not do, but rather on what he could and would eventually be able to do. It was clear that we were all working together to make him the very best person he could possibly be. (Moeller, 1986, p. 153).

This mother explains the importance of the parents' first interactions with professionals. Parents may hear the first

TABLE 14-1. Examples of Parent-Child Interaction Scales*

Name	Authors/Date	Purpose	Content
1. Maternal Behavior Rating Scale	Mahoney, Finger, & Powell/1985	Assesses the quality of maternal interactive behaviors during play.	Parent's expressiveness, warmth, sensitivity to the child's state, achievement orientation, social stimulation effectiveness, directiveness; child's activity level, attention span enjoyment expressiveness.
2. Nursing Child Assessment Feeding Scale (NCAST)	Bernard/1978	Assesses parent and child behaviors during feeding to identify potential problems in the interactions of the dyad.	Parent's sensitivity to cues, response to distress, cognitive and social growth fostering; child's clarity of cues, responsiveness.
3. Nursing Child Assessment Teaching Scale (NCAST)	Barnard/1978	Assesses parent and child interactive behaviors in a teaching episode to identify problems.	Parent's sensitivity to cues, response to distress, cognitive and social growth fostering; child's clarity of cues, responsiveness.
4. Parent Behavior Progression	Bromwich/1981	Assesses infant-related maternal behaviors to develop short-term goals aimed at changing maternal attitudes and behavior for the purpose of enhancing maternal-infant interaction.	Parent's pleasure in watching the infant, physical proximity, awareness of signs of distress, comfort, provides stable caregiver, provides variety of stimulation.
5. Parent and Caregiver Involvement Scale	Farran, Kasari, Comfort, & Jay/1986	Assesses parent's involvement in play interaction with the child for purposes of planning intervention strategies.	Parent's amount, quality, appropriateness of involvement in the following areas: physical and verbal, responsiveness, control and directiveness, teaching and play. Positive and negative interactions, affective climate, and learning environment.
6. Teaching Skill Inventory	Rosenberg, Robinson, & Beckman/1984	Assesses the parent's teaching skills with child to plan intervention and to evaluate its effects.	Parent's clarity of verbal instruction, task structure and modification, effectiveness of prompts; child's interest.

*Adapted from Comfort, M. (1988) in D. Bailey & R. Simeonsson, Family Assessment in Early Intervention. Columbus, OH: Merrill Publishing Company.

hopeful words about their child from the teacher or therapist; this positive attitude in a professional can bolster the parent's attachment to his or her child.

While parents of children with disabilities need professional and technical services, they frequently report that the most important aspect of their encounter with a professional is that person's sensitivity to them and the needs of their child (Paul & Beckman-Bell, 1981, p. 125). The sensitivity of the professional is a reinforcement of family dignity. While preservation of family dignity seems to be a natural element of therapy, it can easily be overlooked or abandoned when schedules are tight or when resources are low. This theme is emphasized as parents are incorporated in the assessment, planning, and program evaluation process. Ongoing, efforts are required to encourage parent participation, and at the same time avoid creating dependency and passivity (Simeonsson et al., 1986). The family should decide the extent and the type of involvement they desire in the intervention/education program. The parent's involvement often changes as the child matures and transitions from programs that emphasize developmental skills to ones that emphasize academic and vocational skills. In-

volvement and level of participation also changes as the family's interests, needs, and circumstances change. Parents may choose to be more involved when their child begins the school year, and less involved after they become familiar with the therapists and teachers. Parent involvement should be viewed broadly as a range of alternatives. Peterson (1987) lists the elements that allow for optimal parent involvement:

1. Flexibility, to allow changing levels and types of participation over time.
2. Individualization, to match the style and amount of involvement to meet parent and child needs.
3. Alternative options, to offer choices and the right of choice in order to achieve constructive and meaningful outcomes. Simple consideration of parents' time and resources may allow the parents more enjoyment of their child.

If the parents feel in control of their lives, their confidence about parenting becomes stronger. The impact of having a child with a disability, and their everyday stress of caring for that child while attending a variety of clinics and programs, may greatly reduce the parents' feeling of control. This loss of control can be disabling and disruptive to the relationship with the child. By recognizing and reinforcing parents' strengths, the occupational therapist can assist the parents in gaining or maintaining a sense of control about their situations. Efforts to teach parents intervention techniques can, without intention, have the effect of increasing their passivity and feeling of inadequacy; thus undermining their problem solving skills (Affleck, McGrade, McQueenery, & Allen, 1985). Given the importance of the mother-child relationship, the therapist emphasizes the parent's sense of competence in activities that facilitate the child's successful skill achievement. By promoting parental competence and problem solving skills, the relationship and quality of interactions can improve. It is the "recipient's own belief in him/herself as a causal agent that determines whether the gains will last or disappear" (Dunst, et al., 1988, p. 96).

A strong parent-child relationship is built on a goodness-of-fit between the parent and the child. Goodness-of-fit is particularly important in the parent-infant relationship. The therapists's understanding of sensory systems and motor behaviors can assist the parent in better understanding the infant, and in achieving a better fit. The therapist can also facilitate and promote developmental skills of the child, which may assist in strengthening his or her fit or match with the family. Improving developmental skills, such as control of eye contact or attention span, may improve the infant's ability to interact. Improving the infant's sensorimotor skills may, in and of itself, promote attachment by improving the infant's competence and responsiveness. Fraiberg (1970) also proposes that interventionists should strive to serve as models of competent parenthood; showing pleasure in the infant's achievements and qualities, and sharing his progress and problems with the parents.

The consonance of family interaction is associated with good outcomes of the child and the family (Simeonson, Bailey, Huntington, & Comfort, 1986). To facilitate consonance or goodness-of-fit, the therapist may assist by promoting change in the child, change in the family, or change in the interaction between the child and the family. Therapists' understanding of sensory systems and the basis of behaviors can be extremely helpful to families in understanding the child, and in relating positively to the child. Therapists most frequently address child behaviors and performance, working toward increased competency and function in the child. Generally, increases in skill levels contribute to improved family interactions. Information and techniques to assist in daily management are invaluable to family functioning. Therapists may also promote the family's adaptation to the disability, by addressing the family's needs for information to assist the parents in understanding their child or therapy, or in locating support groups, support systems and community resources.

Studies have demonstrated that the most powerful benefits of support are realized if aid and assistance come primarily from informal sources (Dunst et al., 1988, page 32–33). The best resources are often those closest to the family unit. Therapy is likely to be most effective if it promotes the family's use of natural support networks and neither replaces nor supplants them with professional networks (Dunst et al., 1988, page 96). Helping families develop this network to carry out the child's intervention plan is of greater long term value to families than limiting problem solving to the primary caregiver. An example would be to encourage the parents to make opportunities for their child to play with other neighborhood children. This contact with nondelayed peers may facilitate social play skills, language, and mobility. Optimal development likely occurs when structured, goal directed therapy activities are balanced with family recreation and social activities. One reinforces the other.

ISSUES IN WORKING WITH FAMILIES ACROSS THE CHILD'S LIFE SPAN

Not only do families have unique assets and needs, but these change throughout the sequential phases of the family life cycle. Families change as their life situations evolve, and as their children mature. Priorities may shift, and critical needs may differ during this life cycle. These stages, which characterize all families, may pose special problems to families with children with disabilities. Critical events which occur in all families during the child's lifespan may have a devastating effect on families with a child with a handicapping condition. Critical events may be the first encounter with a diagnosis or changing therapists and intervention programs. When normal developmental milestones are not met, the parents may experience renewed sorrow and apprehension. The following section describes some of the common experiences that families of children with a disability have during the life cycle, and some of the issues that arise from those experiences. Suggestions as to how occupational therapists may assist families in adjusting to these stages and critical events are given.

Early Childhood/Infancy

Infancy is generally characterized by warmth and happiness. The most important task during this time is the formation of the baby's relationship to the parents. This attachment formation depends on the quality of interaction between the baby and parents, the amount of contact, and the individual behaviors of the infant and parents. When a child is diagnosed with a disability, the crisis affects all family members. The immediate reactions of sadness, grief and disappointment are normal. As time passes, parents begin to understand and accept the disability; however, the sorrow tends to linger and periods of anxiety, confusion, and anger recur, often during the critical events. Some authors have attempted to define stages that parents experience, in coming to acceptance of a disability in their child (Farber, 1975). Recently, other authors have commented that the events of grief that occur prior to acceptance are not simple and parents have a wide variety of reactions (Trout, 1983). Learning the diagnosis is probably only one of a series of jolts that the family experiences as they learn more about the child's disability. For young children with serious disabilities or medical problems, this period can be a chain of crises as the child has surgeries or illnesses.

Family Focused Intervention During Infancy

In family focused early intervention programs, *Individualized Family Service Plans* (IFSP) are developed to guide the intervention process. Through this process families choose the level and nature of involvement in early intervention. The occupational therapist, along with other team members, supports the family's participation in the IFSP process so that the completed plan reflects the family's goals and priorities. To prepare for this process, families are given information about service options and available community resources. As families assimilate this information, the intervention team gathers assessment data on the child and the family. Once families and professionals are prepared to fully participate in the IFSP process, they meet to review assessment results, discuss options and priorities, develop outcomes and negotiate strategies. The family's agenda and priorities become the focus of the intervention plan.

Deal et al., (1989) described a number of principles that support and strengthen family to participate in the development of the IFSP.

1. The development of the IFSP is done within the context of collaboration and partnerships between the family and the team members.
2. Any and all information included in the IFSP is done so with explicit permission and authorization of the family.
3. The development and revision of the IFSP should be responsive to the broad based needs of families, although no early intervention practitioner or program should be expected to offer support to meet all family.
4. Both the development and implementation of the IFSP should emphasize promotion of the competence of the family and interdependence with members of the family's community. (p. 36–37).

These principles suggest therapists and other team members are responsible for enabling the family to participate in and benefit from early intervention services. To fulfill this goal, families are linked with other support systems that they can mobilize to procure needed resources. To enable linkage with other service options, occupational therapist should become aware of the continuum of services provided in the community and should know the lines of communication for accessing those services.

Families in this early stage should be allowed to express their grief or anger about their child's disability. Time is needed for parents to work through these feelings, and listening may be what a parent needs most at this stage. Some parents desire extensive information about the disability. These parents probably benefit most from small amounts of information given repeatedly in different forms. As a professional, the occupational therapist may unknowingly inhibit the parents' expression of their sorrow and grief. It is important to recognize when parents need access to other sources, such as other parents, for expressing their feelings. Parents desire honest answers, and professionals who communicate openly, honestly, and realistically about the disability. The occupational therapist can offer the parents hope about the skills and development of their child, without exaggerating the progress achieved or predicting unrealistic outcomes. The trust that families place in their child's therapist should be carefully guarded and respected. In therapy, parents learn about their child and his or her skills, and learn everyday management. These aspects of therapy enable positive interactions of the family with the child.

Family Interactions

Most early interventionists recognize that the interaction of parent and infant constitutes the priority of this stage of the family life cycle. Several authors (Affleck et al., 1985; Simeonsson et al., 1986; Bromwich & Parmelee, 1979) have proposed a model of early intervention which encourages the parents' sensitivity to the child and mutual responsive interactions between parent and infant. A strong parent-infant relationship and attachment has been documented in the beneficial effects on the outcome of the child, and an inadequate parent-infant relationship has been demonstrated to interfere with the child's development. The parent-infant relationship when the infant is disabled, may be at risk for several reasons. The parental emotional crises may reduce sensitivity to the infant's signals, and the infant himself may be less responsive, or difficult to read and interpret. The difficult temperament characteristics typical of infants with disabilities could make everyday care routines unsuccessful and stressful (Connor, Williamson, & Siepp, 1978).

It seems essential that occupational therapists recognize the importance of these early relationships. Occupational therapists have skills in interpreting the infant's behaviors, and in understanding some of the reasons for their behaviors. Helping parents become more effective interpreters of their infant's behavior can enhance the parent-infant relationship.

A careful balance is required in providing treatment to the infant and the family. Therapists recognize the importance of early developmental gains, and may inadvertently push parents to the point of burnout. The viewpoint that "the more the better" is not always in the family's (or the child's) best interest. Home programs should consider what is practical and realistic given the other demands on the parents' time. Disproportionate emphasis on the needs of the child with a disability can disrupt family balance and cause neglect of other family member needs. The therapist-parent interactions in the early stage of intervention set a precedent for future professional-parent relationships. At this time, parents are embarking on a lifetime of responsibility for care of a child who may never become independent. Relative and friend support, family recreation, and relaxation, are as important as the child's therapy, and should be balanced with the activities of the early intervention program. For parents who do not access services, or participate erratically in services, consideration of their need for support or emotional buttressing may come first, before direct occupational therapy intervention will be beneficial.

Case Management

Given the multiplicity of needs of families, in early intervention programs, a variety of resources may be helpful and a number of agencies may be involved. To assist the family in accessing and coordinating services a case manager is selected from the professions most relevant to the infant's and family's needs. (Public Law 99-947, Part H, Section 677 [d]. When the occupational therapists are the primary service providers, they may serve as case managers. The case manager is the single point of contact in helping parents gain services and may engage in any or all of the activities listed in Table 14-2.

Although by law, the family has one case manager, not all service coordination responsibilities rest on one person. The

---

TABLE 14-2. Case Manager Activities

1. Coordinating the performance of evaluations and assessments;

2. Facilitating and participating in the development, review, and evaluation of individualized family service plans;

3. Assisting families in identifying available service providers;

4. Coordinating and monitoring the delivery of available services;

5. Informing families of the availability of advocacy services;

6. Coordinating with medical and health providers;

7. Facilitating the development of a transition plan to preschool services, if appropriate (Federal Register, 54, p 26311).

---

role of the case manager is evolving as early intervention systems develop to provide coordinated and comprehensive care to families. When the occupational therapist is the case manager, she/he may delegate certain activities to other professionals who hold more expertise in that area. For example, the social worker can often provide the family with financial case management. Service coordination or case management activities require the skills listed in Table 14-3.

Occupational Therapists as case managers become invested in many aspects of the family's life. A holistic view of the family is important. By considering all of the systems that affect family life, such as extended family and community groups, the therapist can link the family to valuable resources for raising their child.

Transition to Preschool

Transitions are the periods of time between stages, when the family is adjusting its interactional style and roles to meet

---

TABLE 14-3. Case Manager Skills

1. Communicating with and relating to families with diverse lifestyles.

2. Coordinating and scheduling with many different agencies.

3. Preparing parents to enter into collaboration with professions and professionals to enter into collaboration with parents.

4. Recognizing and nurturing family strengths.

5. Mediating between service providers and resolving conflicts.

6. Promoting the family's communication of their needs to others.

7. Facilitating family involvement in all aspects of intervention.

8. Negotiating the intensity and amount of services.

9. Working with families to develop a transition plan.

10. Helping families through transitions, exploring future alternatives, and identifying options.

11. Linking families with other families.

12. Advocating for best practice and comprehensive service.

13. Teaching families to be advocates. (Zipper, Nash, Rounds, Weil and Bennett, 1990).

---

the needs of the new developmental stage of their child. Because these shifts may result in confusion and conflict, the transition period is almost always a time of stress and anxiety (Neugarten, 1976; Olson, McCubbin, Barnes, Larsen, Muxen & Wilson, 1983). The transition from an early intervention program to preschool is often a critical event, as many aspects of this transition are difficult for the family. The parents must leave a group of professionals that they trust and have befriended. At the same time, the change in programs may result in a loss of developmental skills. In preschool, the parents probably have much less involvement in the child's therapy program. They are separated from the child during the school day or half day, and may feel anxiety about this separation. When the intensity of the parents' involvement is decreased, they may feel a loss of influence in their child's development. At the time of entrance into preschool, the parents may become increasingly anxious regarding the child's accomplishments, or lack thereof. The child may be given a diagnosis for the first time, and the parents may feel more in the public's eye as their child enters the school system.

Preschool/School Age and School Based Intervention

When the child enters a preschool program an *Individualized Education Plan* (IEP) is developed. In contrast to the IFSP, the child, rather than the family is the focus of this plan. The family is invited to be equal participants with school personnel, in developing, reviewing and revising the child's IEP. Many of the principles described for the IFSP process apply to the IEP process. Specifically, the educational team should give parents sufficient information about the IEP process, the program, and available services to prepare them to actively participate in the IEP conference. Communication with parents that avoids professional jargon and is sensitive to the family's culture is critical to eliciting parent involvement. The presence of a "parent advocate" in the IEP conference may facilitate the parent's participation.

Recent studies have examined parental participation in IEP conferences. The research has demonstrated that parents participate at different levels; however, they tend to be passive participants. Generally parents reported satisfaction with both their child's special education program and their relatively low degree of involvement in IEP development (Turnbull & Turnbull, 1986). Parents who first participate in the IFSP process may be better prepared to participate in the IEP process.

Developmental skills seem to be of a priority of parents as the child enters school. Lack of progress, in particular, can cause additional stress. Kogan and Tyler (1973) studied the reactions of parents to their preschool children during therapy and play sessions led by the parent. They concluded that the slow development of the youngster who is physically disabled, has an effect on the social interaction between a mother and her child. This relationship is sometimes more negative when the mother spends long periods of time with the child. They recommend that therapists emphasize the quality, rather than the quantity, of time that parents spend with their child. By spending less time, the child may become more responsive in the interactions, and the mother will have more time for other needs, which can reduce her stress levels.

Model programs recognize that all parents should participate in the therapeutic and educational process to a greater or less degree. Methods for eliciting parent participation are to reinforce parent question asking and to express interest in their input. Questions such as "What are some things that are important to you at home?" and "When are you able to enjoy recreation with your family?" may elicit participation and sharing by the parents.

Parental participation in therapeutic programming for young children with severe neuromuscular disorders, has the potential for reduced parental enjoyment in interactions. In a study by Kogan, Tyler, and Turner (1974), mothers demonstrated a negative affect when engaged in physical therapy procedures. They also showed a decline in warmth and acceptance during free play. These authors advocated less emphasis on the responsibilities of parents in carrying out home programs.

In other school programs, the parent has less contact with the therapist. This may prevent communication between the therapist and parent. Therapists and parents may lack understanding of respective and mutual perceptions. Controversy exists as to the optimal ways to involve parents in school programs. Welsh and Odum (1982) recommend that parents plan, implement and monitor programs, both at home and in school. They concluded that inclusion of parents in school programs was essential. Yet the extent of parent responsibility for teaching and providing other interventions has been questioned. Other researchers have found that parents' non-involvement is not necessarily detrimental to the child, or to his or her therapeutic program. Disappointing parent attendance and participation in some school and therapy programs, may indicate parents' need to be uninvolved. Expectations may be especially high by the occupational or physical therapist, who desires not only for the parent to engage in specific activities with the child, but to perform those activities using specialized techniques. This may cause the parent to excessively focus on the disability and the abnormal movements. Parents need to be constantly reinforced in their child's abilities rather than disabilities. Diamond (1981) provides the prospective of a child with disabilities growing up in a world of therapy:

Something happens in a parent when relating to his disabled child: he forgets they are a kid first. I used to think about that a lot when I was a kid. I would be off in a euphoric state, drawing or coloring or cutting out paper dolls, and as often as not the activity would be turned into an occupational therapy session. "You're not holding the scissors right," or "Sit up straight so your curvature doesn't get worse." That era was ended when I finally let loose a long and exhaustive tirade. "I'm just a kid! You can't therapize me all the time! I get enough therapy in school every day! I don't think about my handicap all the time like you do!" (p. 30).

Therapeutic activities suggested for home should be flexible and adaptable to the day's activities. Therapists should encourage parents to fit therapeutic regimes into play and positive social interactions. By helping parents fit the therapeutic activities into natural, social situations, negative interactions are less likely to occur.

Guidelines for therapists and teachers are summarized by Snell and Beckman-Brinkley (1984). Parents can best follow a home program if they are taught the rationale for activities.

This seems particularly important when the activities occur at school, and are not seen by the parents. Time is spent discussing the reasons why activities are beneficial. If parents understand activities, they are more likely to integrate them into their daily routine, and more likely to generalize them to other situations. Limited time with parents presents a challenge, and a necessity to emphasize the parents' problem solving skills, and to encourage their independence in seeking solutions, or creating adaptations for their child.

Although notes and letters are important for "keeping in touch," face-to-face communication, formally (in a conference), or informally (in the classroom or clinic), is more important. Efforts should be made to meet regularly with parents, and to deal with crises or important decisions in a face-to-face encounter. Decisions about ordering a wheelchair may be routine for a therapist, but are difficult, or at times devastating, for a parent.

A survey of parents expectations for professionals providing services to their children with a handicap (Redman-Bentley, 1982), revealed that the first priority for parents is to have a say in decisions about the child's care. The other expectations that parents have and feel to be important, are explanation of test results, provision of instruction, and information about progress, purpose and role. The parents in her sample desired an active role in the child's intervention, and felt that information was essential. Communication with the parent appears to be an essential link in the therapist-child and family relationship. Mutual respect and honesty is a hallmark of constructive parent-professional relationships.

Professionals need to recognize that at times parents want support more than instruction and information. By listening to parents, and remaining "in tune" with their needs, therapists can gauge their interactions to be more supportive, or more instructional, according to the changing needs of family and child. Parents require greater and lesser amounts of contact, from time to time, and individual parents have differing needs for active involvement in therapy. Carney, Snell & Gressard (1986) found that parents involvement in the IEP process decreased as a function of age. Lynch and Stein (1982) also concluded that parents of older students were less involved than parents of younger students. The parents whose child had a physical handicap, were less involved than parents of students with retardation. The parents' ongoing participation in the therapy program may actually be detrimental when the time and energy that intervention requires takes away from other family needs. The amount of parent involvement is guided by the parents' interest, availability and resources.

Transition Into Adolescence and Young Adulthood

Adolescence is a time of rapid physical and psychological changes. Sexual maturity occurs at this time, and is accompanied with the development of self identity, development of a positive body image, emotional independence from parents, and interest in the opposite sex. Adolescence is normally a challenging time for both the individual and the family. Teenagers may challenge the authority of the parents. Stresses and strains during the transition to adolescence, and then to adulthood, are inevitable.

In the child with a disability, the body may mature, while the mental, emotional, and social state of the child may be delayed. The child may be unable to adjust to physical changes, and may have a pervasive sense of conflict due to these changes. At the same time, a child with a disability may have fewer friends or peers with whom to share feelings, and may be less able to express feelings. The responsibility of finding a peer group and developing social interactions, may fall upon the family.

Often the parents are confronted with the adolescent's rebellion due to lack of peer support. The adolescent may experience great isolation, a growing stigma about his or her handicap, and problems with sexuality. At the same time the parents must absorb the child's conflict and stress, they can become exhausted by physical care needs. Parental anxiety about the future may increase at this transition time, as they watch the child become increasingly isolated, and worry about the future. One mother cites an example of this growing stigma:

> The community accepts our children much more easily when they are small and cute. The problems we face with Lindsay today are partially the result of his growing up and not being "cute" anymore. People are apt to be fearful around him. Doctors and dentists are fearful. It's very hard to give a shot to a six-foot, two-hundred pound man who doesn't want one. Babyish mannerisms are no longer acceptable. Lind has had real problems with his social relationships. (Anderson, 1983, p. 90).

Parents of children without disabilities experience relief from responsibility at this time; however, parents of children with disabilities, particularly those with severe disabilities, may feel that demands increase. Parents of adolescents are older, and may have diminished resources. Adolescents with physical care needs may actually become unmanageable at this time. Parents may realize for the first time, that they will always be caregivers to a son or daughter who is quickly becoming an adult. Residential placement may be considered for the first time at this stage.

If the adolescent is less impaired, decisions must be made regarding the transition from school to a sheltered workshop, supported work setting, or day activity program. Planning for the future should begin early, and should involve multiple professionals of the team. Occupational therapists are involved in vocational readiness activities, or may assist in establishing a suitable environment for vocational placement. Decisions regarding work and community placements are difficult for families who were comfortable with the educational program that carefully graded the standards of performance of their child. Vocational placement creates a new threat of possible failure, and lack of alternatives within the community should failure occur.

Normalization is a trend in educational services across all age groups, but particularly for young adults with disabilities. The idea that these young adults have access to the most normal environment possible is appealing to some professionals and parents. However, a study by Suelzle and Keenan (1981) demonstrated that parents have concerns about their child's isolation and vulnerability. Some prefer sheltered workshops to more independent supported employment situations. The course of action most appealing to professionals may not be attractive to parents. The parents' role in decision making at this point in time should be held as a priority. Their

life experience with their child, now adult, places them as the experts in their child's and family's needs. While the family's decision making is paramount, the options for community placement may be few. Families report much stress as they search for appropriate services to meet their young child's needs (Brotherson, 1985). Research has indicated that parents in later stages of the life cycle, experience greater parent burn-out, less support, less community acceptance, few services and more isolation.

Turnbull (1985) shares some of his concerns about family barriers:

> Jay will pass too soon from public school to adult services. He will move from a school system that must serve everyone to a non-system of multiple programs with usually inconsistent goals, functions, eligibility criteria, funding and governing authorities, and accountability—programs that need not serve him but must merely practice nondiscrimination. He will go from a relatively protective system to one that may impose responsibilities on him that he cannot meet. And he will graduate from a system in which I can legally and functionally command services and accountability to a system that is far less amenable to my importunings. (p. 119).

The role of the parent as an advocate is clearly indicated at this stage, but the parents' time and energy may be exhausted.

Occupational therapists may be involved in this transition, by supporting the work process, developing the skills required for independent living, or assisting in adapting an accessible work environment. One strategy to be incorporated at this time to help reduce stigma for both the individual with a disability and family members, is to provide age-appropriate activities and materials. The adolescent is encouraged to wear socially acceptable clothing, and to participate in social events or sports activities. Independent experiences, such as shopping or visiting museums, are important for building confidence and in learning to cope. Intervention with the adolescent with a physical disability changes, and may be incorporated into other physical activities, such as swimming or horseback riding. Yet the occupational therapist tends to remain a trusted and respected consultant, on whom the family relies for practical advice and support.

SUMMARY

Issues in working with families change throughout the developmental stages of the child and the family life cycle. The needs of the family with a young child with a disability are very different from the needs of a family with an older child or young adult. Transitions, even when handled well, are times of stress and anxiety for families. Several needs seem to prevail through every phase of the family life cycle. Families need support to maintain their cohesiveness and their ability to adapt to, and cope with, their child with a disabling condition. The occupational therapist's sensitivity and understanding can reinforce the family's adaptation and coping. The occupational therapist and other team members form a collaborative partnership with families. This partnership includes complete confidentiality and recognizes the family's rightful role in deciding what is important for the family unit.

To be effective in working with families, therapists must want to hear what parents have to say and must be truly interested in understanding the family's concerns and needs (Stoneman, 1985). The professional who listens and genuinely tries to understand families, promotes their sense of dignity and control. Therapy programs that promote the child's development also promote the family's competence and their ability to access and utilize resources. When needs are met by enabling acquisition of knowledge and skills in the family, positive changes lin the family and their interactions with the community are discernible. The effectiveness of occupational therapist is increased when activities "fit" into the family's routines and daily life, respond to the family's priorities, and draw on the family's strengths. By listening to parents and adapting programs to fit family needs, the occupational therapy will provide the most meaningful and beneficial intervention to the child.

EXPAND YOUR NEWLY ACQUIRED KNOWLEDGE

1. Describe three critical features of successful family interactions.
2. Design three strategies that you could use to involve siblings in the therapeutic process.

References

Affleck, G., McGrade, B. J., McQueenery, M., & Allen, D. (1985). The promise of relationship-based early intervention. *Journal of Special Education, 16,* 413–430.

Allen, D., & Allen, V. (1979). *Ethical issues in mental retardation: Tragic choice/living hope.* Nashville: Abingdon Press.

Anderson, D. (1983). He's not "cute" anymore. In T. Dougan, L. Isbell, & P. Vyas (Eds.), *We have been there.* (pp. 90–91). Nashville: Abingdon Press.

Bailey, D. B. (1988). Assessing family stress and needs. In D. Bailey and R. Simeonsson, (Eds.). *Family assessment in early intervention.* p. 95–118.

Barnard, K. (1978). *Nursing child assessment feeding scale.* Seattle, WA: Nursing Child Assessment Satellite Training.

Barnard, K. (1978). *Nursing child assessment teaching scale.* Seattle, WA: Nursing Child Assessment Satellite Training.

Beckman, P. J. (1983). Influence of selected child characteristics on stress in families of handicapped infants. *American Journal of Mental Deficiency, 88,* 150–156.

Blacher, J. (1984). A dynamic perspective on the impact of a severely handicapped child on the family. In J. Blacher (Ed.), *Severely handicapped young children and their families.* Orlando, FL: Academic Press.

Bromwich, R. (1981). *Working with parents and infants: An interactional approach.* Baltimore: University Park Press.

Bromwich, R., & Parmelee, A. (1979). An intervention program for pre-term infants. In T. M. Field (Ed.), *Infants born at risk: Behavior and development.* New York: Spectrum.

Brotherson, M. J. (1985). *Parents self report of future planning and its relationship to family functioning and family stress with sons and daughters who are disabled.* Unpublished doctoral dissertation, University of Kansas, Lawrence.

Carey, W. G., & McDevitt, S. C. (1978). Revision of the infants temperament questionnaire. *Pediatrics, 61,* 735–738.

Carney, I. H. (1987). Working with families. In F. Orelove and D. Sobsey (Eds.), *Educating children with multiple disabilities: A transdisciplinary approach.* (pp. 315–338). Baltimore, MD: Paul H. Brookes.

Carney, I. H., Snell, M. E., & Gressard, C. F. (1986). *Parent involvement in I.E.P.'s: The relationship between student age and parent differences.* Unpublished manuscript, University of Virginia, Charlottesville, VA.

Carter, E. A., & McGoldrick, M. (Eds.) (1980). *The family life cycle: A framework for family therapy.* New York: Gardner Press.

Comfort, M. (1988). Assessing parent-child interaction, in D. Bailey and R. Simeonsson (Eds.). *Family assessment in early intervention.* p. 65–94. Columbus, OH: Merrill Publishing Co.

Conner, F., Williamson, G., & Siepp, J. (1978). *Program guide for infants and toddlers with neuromotor and other developmental disabilities* (p. 247–270). New York: Teacher College Press.

Crawley, S. B., & Spiker, D. (1983). Mother-child interaction involving two year olds with Down syndrome: A look at individual differences. *Child Development, 54,* 1312–1323.

David, H. P. (1979). Healthy family functioning: Cross-cultural perspectives: In P. I. Ahmed & G. V. Coelho (Eds.), *Toward a new definition of health.* (pp. 281–319). New York: Plenum Press.

Deal, A. G., Dunst, C. J., & Trivette, C. M. (1989). A flexible and functional approach to developing individualized family support plans. *Infants and Young Children, 1*(4), 32–43.

Diamond, S. (1981). Growing up with parents of a handicapped child: A handicapped person's perspective. In J. L. Paul (Ed.), *Understanding and working with parents of children with special needs.* (pp. 23–50). New York: Holt, Rinehart, & Winston.

Dunst, Trivett, & Deal, (1988). *Enabling and empowering families.* Cambridge, MA: Brookline Books.

Farran, D. C., Kasari, C., Comfort, M., & Jay, S. (1986). *Parent/Caregiver involvement scale.* Honolulu, HI: Center for Development of Early Education, Kamehameha Schools, Kapalama Heights.

Farber, B. (1975). Family adaptations to severely mentally retarded children. In M. J. Begab & S. A. Richardson (Eds.), *The mentally retarded and society: A social science perspective.* Baltimore: University Park Press.

Featherstone, H. (1980). *A difference in the family: Life with a disabled child.* New York: Basic Books.

Fewell, R. (1986). A handicapped child in the family. In R. Fewell & P. Vadasky (Eds.), *Families of handicapped children.* (pp. 3–34). Austin, TX: ProEd.

Fewell, R., Belmonte, J., & Ahlersmeyer, D. (1983). *Questionnaire on family support system.* Unpublished manuscript, Experimental Education Unit, University of Washington, Seattle.

Fraiberg, S. (1970). Intervention in infancy: A program for blind infants. *Journal of the American Academy of Child Psychiatry, 10,* 381–405.

Frederich, W. H. (1979). Predictors of the coping behavior of mothers of handicapped children. *Journal of Consulting and Clinical Psychology, 47,* 1140–1141.

Fullard, W., McDevitt, S. C., & Carey, W. B. (1984). Assessing temperament in one to three-year-old children. *Journal of Pediatric Psychology. 9*(2), 205–217.

Gallagher, J., Cross, A., & Scharfman, W. (1981). The father's role. *Journal of the Division for Early Childhood, 3,* 3–14.

Gath, A. (1977). The impact of an abnormal child upon the parents. *British Journal of Psychiatry, 130,* 405–410.

Gidewall, M. (1987). The other side of the mirror. *Occupational Therapy Forum, 11*(11), 4.

Grossman, F. (1972). *Brothers and sisters of retarded children: An exploratory study.* Syracuse, NY: Syracuse University Press.

Hill, R., & Hansen, D. (1982). The family in disaster. In G. Baker & D. Chapman (Eds.), *Man and society in disaster.* New York: Basic Books.

Huntington, G. S. (1988). Assessing child characteristics that influence family functioning, in D. Bailey and R. Simeonsson (Eds.) *Family assessment in early intervention.* (p. 45–64). Columbus, OH: Merrill Publishing Co.

Johnson, B. H., McGonigel, M. J., Kaufmann, R. K. et al. (1989). *Guidelines and recommended practices for the individualized family service plan.* National Early Childhood Technical Assistance System and Association for the Care of Children's Health.

Kasari, C. (1987). Early intervention and mother-infant interactions in D. Gentry & J. Olson (Eds.) *The parent/family support network series* Warren Center on Human Development, University of Idaho, Moscow, ID.

Kazak, A., & Marvin, R. (1984). Differences, difficulties, and adaptations: Stress and social networks in families with a handicapped child. *Family Relations, 33,* 67–77.

Kogan, K., & Tyler, N. (1973). Mother-child interaction in young physically handicapped children. *American Journal of Mental Deficiency, 77*(5), 492–497.

Kogan, K., Tyler, N., & Turner, P. (1974). The process of interpersonal adaptation between mothers and their cerebral palsied children. *Developmental Medicine and Child Neurology*, 16(9), 518–527.

Lidz, T. (1963). *The family and human adaptation*. New York: International University Press.

Lonsdale, G. (1978). Family life with a handicapped child: The parents speak. *Child Care, Health and Development*, 4, 99–120.

Lynch, E. (1987). Families from different cultures, in D. Gentry & J. Olson (Eds.), *The parent/family support network series*. Warren Center on Human Development, University of Idaho, Moscow, ID.

Lynch, E. W., & Stein, P. (1982). Perspectives on parent participation in special education. *Exceptional Education Quarterly*, 3(2), 56–63.

Lyon, J. (1986). I want to be Zak's mom, not his therapist. *Manassas Parent-Infant Education Program Newsletter*, Manassas, VA.

Lyon, S., & Preis, A. (1983). Working with families of severely handicapped persons. In M. Seligman (Ed.), *The family with a handicapped child*. (pp. 203–232). New York: Grune & Stratton.

Mahoney, G., Powell, A., & Finger, I. (1986). The maternal behavior rating scale. *Topics in Early Childhood Special Education*, 6, 44–56.

Mahoney, G. J., & Powell, A. (1984). *The transactional intervention program: Preliminary teacher's guide*. Woodhaven, Michigan: Woodhaven School District.

McCubbin, H., Joy, C., Cauble, A., Comeau, J., Patterson, J., & Needle, R. (1980). *Family stress, coping and social support*. Springfield, IL: Thomas.

McDevitt, S. C. and Carey, W. B. (1978). The measurement of temperament in 3–7 year old children. *Journal of Child Psychology and Psychiatry*, 19, 245–253.

Michaelis, C. (1980). *Home and school partnerships in exception education*. Rockville, MD: Aspen.

Moeller, C. (1986). The effect of professionals on the family of a handicapped child. In R. Fewell (Ed.), *Families of handicapped children*. Austin, TX: ProEd.

Neugarten, B. (1976). Adaptations and the life cycle. *The Counseling Psychologist*, 6(1), 16–20.

Olson, S., McCubbin, H., Barnes, H., Larsen, A., Muxen, M., & Wilson, M. (1983). *Families: What makes them work*. Beverly Hills: Sage Publications.

Paul, J., & Beckman-Bell, P. (1981). Parent perspectives. In J. L. Paul (Ed.), *Understanding and working with parents of children with special needs*. (pp. 119–153). New York: Holt, Rinehart, & Winston.

Paul, J., & Porter, P. (1981). Parents of handicapped children. In J. L. Paul (Ed.), *Understanding and working with parents of children with special needs*. (p. 1–22). New York: Holt, Rinehart, & Winston.

Peterson, N. L. (1987). *Early intervention for handicapped and at-risk children*. Denver, CO: Love Publishing Co. p. 409–446.

Redman-Bentley, D. (1982). Parent expectations for professionals providing services to their handicapped children. *Physical and Occupational Therapy in Pediatrics*, 2(1), 13–27.

Rosenberg, S., Robinson, C. and Beckman, P. (1984). Teaching skills inventory: A measure of parent performance. *Journal of the Division for Early Childhood*, 8, 107–113.

Shelton, T., Jeppson, E., & Johnson, B. (1987). *Family-centered care for children with special health care needs*. (2nd Ed). Washington, DC: Association for the Care of Children's Health.

Simeonsson, R., Bailey, D., Huntington, G., & Comfort, M. (1986). Testing the concept of goodness of fit in early intervention. *Infant Mental Health Journal*, 7(1), 81–94.

Simeonsson, R., and Huntington, G. S., Short, R. J. and Ware, W. B. (1982). The Carolina record of individual behavior: Characteristics of handicapped infants and children. *Topics in Early Childhood Special Education*, 2(2). 43–55.

Snell, M. E., & Beckman-Brindley, S. (1984). Family involvement in intervention with children having severe handicaps. *Journal of Speech and Hearing*, 3, 213–220.

Stoneman, Z. (1985). Family involvement in early childhood special education programs, in N. H. Fallen, W. Umansky. (Eds.). *Young children with special needs*. Columbus, OH: Merrill Publishing Co.

Suelzle, M., & Keenan, V. (1981). Changes in family support networks over the life cycle of mentally retarded persons. *American Journal of Mental Deficiency*, 86, 267–274.

Thomas, A., Chess, S., & Birch, N. G. (1968). *Temperament and behavior disorders in children*. New York: New York University Press.

Trout, M. D. (1983). Birth of a sick or handicapped infant: Impact on the family. *Child Welfare*, 62, 337–348.

Turnbull, A., Summers, J., & Brotherson, M. (1984). *Working with families with disabled members: A family systems approach*. Lawrence, KS: Kansas University Affiliated Facility.

Turnbull, A. P., & Summers, J. A. (1987). From parent involvement to family support: Evolution to revolution. In S. M. Pueschel, S. Tingey, J. W. Rynders, A. C. Crocker, & D. M. Crutcher (Eds.), *New perspectives on Down's syndrome*. (pp. 289–309). Baltimore: Paul H. Brookes.

Turnbull, A., & Turnbull, R. (1986). *Families, professionals & exceptionalities: A special partnership*. Columbus, OH: Charles E. Merrill Publishers.

Turnbull, H. R. (1985). Jay's story. In H. R. Turnbull & A. P. Turnbull (Eds.), *Parents speak out: Then and now*. (pp. 109–118). Columbus, OH: Charles E. Merrill Publishers.

Vadasy, P., Fewell, R., Meyer, D., & Greenberg, M. (1984). Siblings of handicapped children: A developmental perspective on family interactions. *Family Relations*, 33, 155–167.

Welsh, M., & Odum, C. (1982). Parent involvement in the education of the handicapped child: A review of the literature. *Journal of the Division for Early Childhood*, 3, 15–25.

Zeitlin, S. (1985). *Coping inventory: A measure of adaptive behavior*. Bensenville, IL: Scholastic Testing Service.

Zeitlin, S., Rosenblatt, W., & Williamson, G. (1986). Family stress: A coping model for intervention. *B.C. Journal of Special Education*, 10(3), 231–242.

Zeitlin, S., Williamson, G., & Szczepanski, M. (1989). *Early coping scales: A measure of adaptive behavior*.

Zipper, I., Nash, J., Rounds, K., Weil, M. and Bennett, L. (1990). *Proceeding of the working conference on case management and Public Law 99–457*. Carolina Institute for Research on Infant Personnel Preparation. Frank Porter Graham Child Development Center. Chapel Hill, N.C.

CHAPTER 15

The Medical Perspective

Lillian Gonzalez-Pardo, MD

"The earliest descriptions of the functional deficits to which we now refer as learning disabilities or mental retardation usually included reference to hypothesized organic or physiological mechanisms. This historical precedence in itself does not establish the legitimacy of the physiological approach; after all, the historically preeminent pathophysiology of epilepsy was witchcraft. However, . . . physiological and neurological explanations have, for the most part, stood the test of time. Recent research promises real advances in the application of these principles to real life problems of diagnosis and management of learning disabilities and mental retardation." Rosenberger, 1986

CATEGORIES OF MEDICATIONS COMMONLY USED IN PEDIATRICS THAT MAY AFFECT COGNITION, BEHAVIOR, OR SENSORIMOTOR FUNCTIONS

This section will introduce the medications commonly used in pediatrics, that most occupational therapists may encounter in their practice. The purpose of this section is to discuss certain types of drugs that may affect the occupational therapist's assessment, therapy or management plans. Table 15-1 lists the categories of medication which will be included in this discussion. Certain drugs may affect cognition, behavior, and sensorimotor functions. These drugs may be taken by children for certain medical, or specific clinical indications, and may produce the desired clinical effects; but these same drugs can produce undesirable or intolerable side effects. This section cannot discuss in detail every pharmacologic action, or effect of every medication, and it cannot list all medications in each category.

The use of psychopharmacologic agents in children and adolescents is not without its controversies. The advocates for use of these agents, as well as those who have expressed antimedication viewpoints, are well represented in two excellent references (Solow, 1976; Werry, 1977). It is not the purpose of this section to advocate for or against the use of these medications. The occupational therapist, or practitioners of other disciplines involved in the care of children, must be familiar with their medications, indications for use, and possible effects that may occur with their use. The support staff who cares for individuals who receive these medications can be helpful in monitoring drug effects in children. Cantwell (1978) makes a point about the unreliability of observation made only in the physician's office. Because children may behave differently in different situations, observation in settings other than the office must be done. Objective reporting based on rating scales are much more reliable than anecdotal reports.

Anticonvulsants

Anticonvulsants, sometimes referred to as antiepileptic drugs (AED), are used in a wide variety of clinical types of epilepsy.

An adaptation of the International Classification of Epilepsy is shown in Table 15-2. Table 15-3 contains a categorization of the antiepileptic drugs with the various forms of seizures. Table 15-4 summarizes the side effects of the most commonly used anticonvulsants.

Acute Therapy of Epilepsy

Status epilepticus is defined as a seizure or convulsion lasting longer than 15 to 30 minutes, or recurrent seizures that are so close together that no period of consciousness occurs between seizure periods.

Too often, the acutely convulsing child does not fit the above definition, but is treated aggressively, and consequently develops complications of overmedication—such as respiratory arrest and prolonged sedation. Simple febrile seizures, and seizures occurring as a result of idiopathic epilepsy, will generally last less than 15 minutes, and will stop spontaneously. Since seizure activity in most patients is likely to end spontaneously, therapy should be aimed at stabilizing the patient. (See also the section below on when to call for emergency medical assistance.)

Chronic Therapy of Epilepsy

Most clinical types of epilepsy are treated for a duration of greater than a year to two years, but some types are treated for longer duration, depending on the underlying cause or associated brain abnormality. Maintaining a child on anticonvulsant drug therapy, is a clinical decision that is made after a comprehensive clinical evaluation, that includes a comprehensive medical history, physical examination, and the use of ancillary laboratory procedures. Recognizing the clinical type or classification of seizures is very important in the ultimate choice of antiepileptic drug. A recent trend in antiepileptic drug therapy is monotherapy, that is, to choose a single drug most effective for the particular seizure type. The advantages of monotherapy include: better seizure control, less drug-to-drug interaction, less toxic side effects, lesser dosage of the drug, lower costs, and better compliance.

Anticipatory guidance, and parent and patient education, are as important as the proper choice of anticonvulsant drugs. The use of blood tests to monitor drug levels periodically must

TABLE 15-1. Categories of Medication Included in This Chapter.

Category	Names of Drugs (Generic)	(Trade Name)
A. Anticonvulsants	Carbamazepine	(Tegretol)
	Clonazepam	(Clonopin)
	Ethosuximide	(Zarontin)
	Phenobarbital	
	Phenytoin	(Dilantin)
	Primidone	(Mysoline)
	Valproic Acid	(Depakene, Depakote)
B. Antidepressants	Amitryptyline	(Elavil)
	Imipramine	(Tofranil)
	Lithium	
C. Sedatives Tranquilizers	Barbiturates:	
	Amobarbital	(Amytal)
	Mephobarbital	(Mebaral)
	Phenobarbital	(Nembutal)
	Secobarbital	(Seconal)
	Benzodiazepine:	
	Diazepam	(Valium)
	Chloral Hydrate:	(Noctec)
	Tranquilizers:	
	Chlorpromazine	(Thorazine)
	Thioridazine	(Mallaril)
	Haloperidol	(Haldol)
D. Stimulants	Dextroamphetamine	(Dexedrine)
	Methylphenidate	(Ritalin)
	Pemoline	(Cylert)
E. Miscellaneous	Antihistamines:	
	Chlorpheniramine	(Chlor-Trimeton)
	Cyproheptadine	(Periactin)
	Diphenhydramine	(Benadryl)
	Hydroxyzine	(Atarax, Vistaril)
	Promethazine	(Phenergan)
	Muscle Relaxants:	
	Dantrolene	(Dantrium)
	Lioresal	(Baclofen)

be explained at the beginning. There is some correlation of clinical control of seizures and therapeutic serum levels. However, each patient is different, and therapy must be individualized. The ideal situation is to use the least amount of drug to effectively control the seizures, with the least or no side effects.

Antidepressant/Antimanic Medication

The common antidepressant/antimanic drugs are listed in Table 15-1. The oldest and most popular pediatric use of the tricyclics (e.g., Elavil) is in enuresis (involuntary urination [Thomas, 1985]), but while their symptomatic effect has been established, any curative effect extending beyond one treatment is extremely doubtful.

Tricyclic antidepressants have also been used for children with hyperactivity, but fewer data support the view that they improve cognitive functions and performance. A distinct disadvantage is a negative effect on mood in children, often unpredictable in this age group.

Pharmacologically, these medications are similar to the major tranquilizers, and may produce sedation. In addition, patients may note weakness, tremulousness or agitation. Side effects such as a dry mouth, blurred vision, and constipation

are seen. In large doses, antidepressants may induce severe cardiac arrhythmia resulting in death (Campbell, Green, & Deutsch, 1985).

Lithium is used primarily in manic-depressive disorders, especially in its prophylactic control. Manic-depressive or affective disorders can be described as unipolar or bipolar. Individuals who have episodes in only one of these phases, either manic or depressive, are referred to as having an unipolar type of affective disorder. Individuals who will experience periods of manic, alternating with periods of depression, are called bipolar.

The mild side effects include nausea and fine tremors. More severe side effects include anorexia, vomiting, diarrhea, coarse tremors, weakness, and sometimes hypotonia. Determination of lithium blood levels must be done regularly, because of the narrow margin of the therapeutic and toxic range.

Sedatives/Tranquilizers

Table 15-1 lists the major sedatives and tranquilizers. Barbiturates generally have sedating effects. Phenobarbital, often prescribed for controlling epilepsy, can cause initial sleepiness, but soon becomes tolerated with appropriate anticonvulsant doses. In children, phenobarbital may cause a par-

---

TABLE 15-2. International Classification of Epilepsy (*Epilepsia*, 1981).

I. PARTIAL SEIZURES
  A. Partial Seizures with elementary symptomatology (generally without impairment of consciousness)
    1. With motor symptoms (includes Jacksonian Seizures)
    2. With special sensory or somatosensory symptoms
    3. With autonomic symptoms
    4. Compound forms
  B. Partial seizures with complex symptomatology (generally with impairment of consciousness) (Temporal lobe or psychomotor seizures)
    1. With impairment of consciousness only
    2. With cognitive symptomatology
    3. With affective symptomatology
    4. With "psychosensory" symptomatology
    5. With "psychomotor" symptomatology (automatisms)
    6. Compound forms
  C. Partial seizures secondarily generalized

II. GENERALIZED SEIZURES (bilaterally symmetrical and without local onset)
    1. Absences (petit mal)
    2. Bilateral massive epileptic myoclonus
    3. Infantile spasms
    4. Clonic seizures
    5. Tonic seizures
    6. Tonic-clonic seizures (grand mal)
    7. Atonic seizures
    8. Akinetic seizures

III. UNCLASSIFIED EPILEPTIC SEIZURES (due to incomplete data)

---

brainstem auditory evoked testing (BAER), x-rays, or invasive diagnostic procedures like spinal taps, etc.

Two commonly used major tranquilizers are phenothiazine, chlorpromazine (Thorazine), and thioridazine (Mellaril). They can rapidly control aggressive behavior and are used in acute emergencies and severe emotional disorders. Chronic use of phenothiazines occurs in children with psychosis who are severely disturbed, aggressive, and/or unmanageable. Thioridazine has less serious side effects, and has been used in children with anxiety and hyperactive behavior. Serious side effects of the phenothiazines are dyskinesias, or involuntary movements, and oculogyric crises (eyes are fixed, usually in an upward position, for prolonged periods of time).

Haloperidol (Haldol) chemically is a butyropherone, another major tranquilizer, but different from the phenothiazines. This drug is used for similar indications as the phenothiazines, but is also used in chronic tic disorder, or Tourette's Syndrome. Mild side effects of this drug include sedation, and more serious side effects include orofacial dyskinesia (a type of abnormal involuntary movements of muscles of the face, mouth and tongue).

Stimulants

The three stimulant medications listed in Table 15-1 are the most commonly prescribed for the medical management of hyperactive behavior. They have also been used in children diagnosed as having attention deficit hyperactive disorder (ADHD). The short term efficacy of these agents has been established in diminishing levels of motor activity, and in improving attention span and classroom behavior. However, there is no convincing evidence that stimulant medications are useful in treating learning problems per se (i.e., those who have specific learning disabilities). If attention deficits coexist in children with specific learning disabilities, the stimulant medication may help by enabling the child to be more responsive to the learning situation, when increased motor activity is a distracting factor.

The most common side effects of cerebral stimulants are anorexia and insomnia. Some develop irritability, headaches, and tachycardia. Safer, Allen and Barr (1972) reported growth suppression during prolonged therapy with stimulant medications.

The long term side effects of stimulant medications was reported by Minde, Weiss, and Mendelson (1972). The au-

adoxical hyperactive behavior and sleep disorders. The other forms of barbiturates listed in this chapter Amytal, Nembutal, and Seconal, are used intravenously in anesthesia, or psychiatric interviews; Seconal is a short acting sedative which should not be used on a regular basis for children and adolescents.

The most commonly used benzodiazephine is Diazepam (Valium). It has been used for its anti-anxiety effects, and as adjunct therapy if used orally for some types of epilepsy. Diazepam has a wide margin of safety, and toxic side effects seldom occur unless used in very large doses.

Chloral hydrate is one of the safest and relatively short acting sedatives, often used for procedures that require sedation, such as obtaining electroencephalograms (EEG's),

---

TABLE 15-3. Antiepileptic Drugs Commonly Used for Epilepsy.

Anticonvulsant Drug	Types of Epilepsy			
	Partial	Generalized Tonic	Absence (Petit mal)	Akinetic-Myoclonic
Carbamazepine	*	*		
Clonazepam			*	*
Ethosuximide			*	
Phenobarbitol	*	*		
Phenytoin	*	*		
Primidone	*	*		
Valproic Acid	*	*	*	*
ACTH				*
Diamox (Acetazolamide)				*

TABLE 15-4. Side Effects of Commonly Used Anticonvulsants.*			
Drug	Effects Dependent on Concentration of Drug	Effects Due to Chronic Therapy	Idiosyncratic Effects
Carbamazepine (Tegretol)	• ataxia • nystagmus • sedation • headache	• liver enzymes stimulated to metabolic drug	• decreased white blood cells & platelets • behavior disorders • skin rash • increased atonic seizures
Clonazepam (Clonopin)	• somnolence • confusion • ataxia	• mood disturbance	• anemia—decreased white blood cells • increased salivation • behavioral changes
Ethosuximide (Zarontin)	• ataxia • headache • hiccoughs • nausea & vomiting	• bone marrow depression	• insomnia • increased seizures • nervousness
Phenobarbital	• ataxia • lethargy • apnea • hypotension (low blood pressure)	• decreased intellectual performance	• hyperactivity • behavior & mood disturbance
Phenytoin (Dilantin)	• nausea & vomiting • ataxia • nystagmus • high blood glucose • coma • dysarthria • increased seizures • hallucinations	• excess hair growth • gum enlargement • coarsened facies • acne • peripheral neuropathy	• lymphadenopathy • pseudolymphoma • nephrotic syndrome • Vitamin K deficiency • cerebellar degeneration • hypersensitivity to the drug
Primidone (Mysoline)	• ataxia • lethargy • apnea • hypotension (low blood pressure)	• decreased intellectual performance	• hyperactivity • behavior & mood disturbance
Valproic Acid (Depakene, Depakote)	• nausea & vomiting • ataxia • confusion, apathy • personality changes • tremors	• loss of hair	• liver necrosis with encephalopathy • pancreatitis • high serum ammonia • Reye's-like syndrome • dystonias

Adapted from Ferry, Banner, & Wolf (1986).

thors reported that stimulant medications were helpful in short term therapy, but a five year follow-up study revealed that both treated and untreated children showed a high incidence of emotional disorders, persistent learning problems, and continuing attention deficits, even after the hyperactivity had subsided.

It is important to emphasize that medications must be used only with objective evaluation and adequate follow-up, and used in conjunction with other forms of intervention, such as behavioral management for both the child and parents, including behavioral therapy and appropriate educational intervention.

Kenny and Clemmens (1980) summarized the principal ways in which psychoactive medications (classified in this section as antidepressants, sedatives, tranquilizers and stimulants) may aid in childhood behavior problems as follows:

1. modify behavior such as hyperactivity,
2. decrease impulsivity,
3. prolong attention span,
4. reduce anxiety and psychomotor excitement,
5. reduce depression,
6. make the child more amenable to other therapies,
7. make a child easier to live with, and
8. make the child better able to function.

Miscellaneous

Antihistamines are prescribed for treatment and management of allergic rhinitis, physical allergies, urticaria, nausea and vomiting, motion sickness, and adverse reactions to drugs. Most patients experience sedation, but some children may experience paradoxical stimulation. Antihistamines are often incorporated with other drugs prescribed for treatment of the above mentioned symptoms; they are included in this chapter, to alert those caring for children, who might unknowingly be taking antihistamines, and could develop side effects.

The most common use of Dantrolene and Lioresal, muscle relaxants, is in the control of spasticity. However, there is limited experience of their use in the pediatric age group.

THE CHILD WITH SPECIAL HEALTH CARE NEEDS

As children are removed from large institutions and placed back with families and their communities, more children with developmental disabilities are mainstreamed into public, private, and community-based school systems. Additionally, as hospital-based care of patients is being limited to acute medical care, more and more children with life-sustaining equipment, such as tracheostomy tubes, oxygen tanks, and feeding and/or gastric tubes, are being cared for by their families at home (Burr, Guyer, Todres, Abrahams & Chiodo, 1983). Some of them require home-based programs, but there are those who go to specialized community-based schools.

Because of the presence of these types of children in the schools, there has evolved a category of children being classified in the educational system as "medically fragile," or children with special health care needs. The definition of this group of children is somewhat ambiguous, but could best be defined as children with any or all of the following:

a. Those children with medical diagnoses whose physical conditions are unstable, that may require frequent hospitalizations (greater than two to four times a month), such as those with unstable heart diseases, frequent infections, frequent epilepsy, and childhood cancer requiring chemotherapy and radiation therapy.
b. Those children who have unusual life support equipment to maintain daily function such as those with:
   1. Tracheostomy tubes,
   2. Oxygen tanks,
   3. Gastrostomy or feeding tubes, and
   4. Respirators.
c. Those children whose medical conditions are difficult to manage, and may result in unpredictable mental or physical states such as:
   1. Poorly controlled epilepsy, despite anticonvulsant therapies;
   2. Those who require throat and mouth suction frequently, due to the danger of pulmonary obstruction; and
   3. Those children with metabolic problems, such as difficult to control diabetes mellitus, that may result in either hypoglycemia or hyperglycemia, with resultant coma or loss of consciousness.
d. Those children with chronic medical conditions requiring ongoing medical treatment, such as burn victims, and patients with cystic fibrosis, head trauma, and metabolic disorders such as phenylketonuria (PKU).

Prior to the recent trend of mainstreaming these children with special medical problems, self-contained classrooms served medically stable children who did not require special equipment, other than wheelchairs or braces. Other children were provided with home-based educational services, an expensive form of service provision. These children are now placed in special classrooms or are mainstreamed in regular education.

The Ad Hoc Task Force on Home Care of Chronically Ill Infants and Children of the American Academy of Pediatrics (1984) published guidelines for its program development. The multidisciplinary team approach was emphasized. There are four major categories of services needed to implement home health care for these children:

a. Medical-nursing (including home care equipment);
b. Developmental disciplines (OT, PT [physical therapy], speech, nutrition, social work);
c. Community-based centers—(schools, child care centers, specialized nurseries);
d. Parents and other care-givers, such as foster parents.

Education and training for the family, as well as for professionals and para-professionals, are important in the success of the care plan development. The care plan must include:

1. Case coordinators,
2. A defined back-up system for medical emergency,
3. Family access to a telephone,
4. A plan to monitor the care plan,
5. A primary care physician, and
6. Educational services for school aged children.

The occupational therapist is frequently relied upon by school team members to provide the liaison to the medical services. There are a number of strategies the occupational therapist can use to facilitate positive outcomes when this is the case.

Request for Medical Information

First, and foremost, request a release of the physician's medical records from the parents. Even though parents may have some information about the child's diagnoses, therapy plan, and management, the best way to be properly informed about the child's medical condition, is to get the information from the physician treating the child. Review the information thoroughly and consult a parent, nurse, or physician. Whether you are evaluating the child for an initial assessment, or for ongoing therapy, you need to know the precautions that should be taken to avoid aggravation or precipitation of a medical crisis situation. On the other hand, do not be afraid to approach these children. It is also helpful to have the parents or child's caretaker provide you with the best way to approach these children, without hurting or harming them. Some physicians may have a nurse practitioner, or physician's assistant, who may be familiar with the child as well.

Second, find out the medications that the child is receiving. There are certain effects and side effects of drugs that may affect your assessment and therapy. Please refer to the section on drugs frequently used in children, for further information about effects of these drugs.

Third, you also want to find out whether the physician treating the child is in primary care, such as pediatrics, family practice or general practice, or is in a subspecialty, such as neurology, orthopedics, psychiatry, etc. The primary care physician is more likely to give you information about general health status, such as immunizations, sore throat, upper respiratory infections, ear infections, pneumonia, and urinary tract infections. The subspecialists are more likely to give detailed specific information about their specialty fields. For example, the neurologist may provide diagnosis and management of epilepsy, neuromotor disorders, or developmental problems; it is preferable for children to see a pediatric neurologist whose experience and expertise is with children and young adults. Other specialists, such as orthopedics, can give more specific information about braces, wheelchairs, and other durable medical equipment, or whether surgery could help cure or alleviate a specific orthopedic deformity. Do not hesitate to obtain all of the medical records. Physiatrists (physicians trained in rehabilitation medicine) may be able to give you information on their evaluation and recommended treatment plan. Very few physiatrists specialize in children, as almost always they are general physiatrists whose experience is primarily with adults.

Provide Feedback to the Child's Physician

Part of your role in providing occupational therapy services to children with special health care needs, is to inform the child's physician of your assessment and recommendations. Ask the parents or guardian to release your information to the physician. Most of them will gladly do so, especially when parents or caretakers find it difficult to convey and translate your information to their physicians. Send copies to all physicians involved in the child's care. They may or may not understand your report, but if you make it brief, less technical and succinct, they will appreciate the information, because it provides a broader perspective for the physician.

Participate in Care Plan Development

The complex nature in the care, management, and follow-up of children, with chronic and complicated medical problems, makes it necessary to have consistent follow-up care, with coordination by a care coordinator or a "case manager". It is not unusual for the occupational therapist to participate, and accompany the patient and their parents to the medical specialist for their clinic or office follow-up visits. Direct input and feedback is provided in both directions, and a more effective communication occurs. The participation of the occupational therapist is not only in the direct therapy itself, but also in the overall care plan, as it may occur in the home, the schools, or other community-based programs, such as day care and group homes.

SEEKING MEDICAL ASSISTANCE

When to Call for Emergency Medical Attention

Emergencies are defined as an unforseen combination of circumstances, or the resulting state, that call for immediate action. Medical emergencies may arise at any time. The health and safety of children are the responsibility, not only of the parent, but of the community as well. Emergency services should be available to anyone who needs them. The categories of medical emergencies discussed in this section are divided into immediate and intermediate types of emergencies. A section on special categories is also included.

Who Makes the Call and Who to Call

Depending on the settings in which you evaluate and treat children, the ultimate responsibility of who summons emer-

gency medical care is determined by the hierarchy of medically knowledgeable personnel. The occupational therapist, physical therapist, teacher, or nurse can be called to determine the nature of the emergency, if they have been properly briefed beforehand. If, however, it becomes your responsibility, there are certain guidelines that can be followed as to when to seek emergency medical attention. There are categories of conditions that requires *IMMEDIATE* medical attention, and there are those that require *INTERMEDIATE* medical attention. Table 15-5 lists the primary indicators of the need for *immediate* or *intermediate* medical attention.

Medical Conditions Requiring Immediate Medical Attention

Call 911, if the nature of the condition is immediate or, if in a hospital setting, call the operator for a "Code Blue" team. Cardiorespiratory arrest, shock and status epilepticus and poisonings require immediate attention. Table 15-6 supplies a more detailed description of the situations with clinical signs and appropriate actions.

Medical Conditions Requiring Intermediate Medical Attention

The medical conditions listed in this category are urgent, but not of an emergency nature. A telephone call to the child's parents or caretakers can be initiated, with a recommendation to take the child to their primary care physician, or to an

TABLE 15-5. Categories of Need for Emergency Care.	
Categories	**Indicators**
Immediate Medical Attention: (Dial 911 or call for Code Blue team)	1. Cardiorespiratory arrest 2. Shock 3. *Status epilepticus* or prolonged generalized seizures—greater than 15–20 minutes 4. Poisoning
Intermediate Medical Attention: (Call primary physician or Emergency Room or subspecialists; call for initial telephone consultation).	1. Trauma 2. High fever 3. Persistent cough, vomiting or diarrhea 4. Poorly controlled, frequent seizures 5. Behavior problem

TABLE 15-6. Information Regarding Situations Which Warrant Immediate Medical Attention.

Indicator	Description	Clinical Clues to Diagnosis	What to Do

Cardiorespiratory† Arrest	The child has stopped breathing and/or the heart has also stopped beating.	1. Individual is blue or pale
		2. Individual is unresponsive to tactile or verbal stimuli
		3. No respiratory motion of the chest can be detected
		4. No pulses are palpated
		   Location of pulses:
		   Neck (carotid artery)
		   Wrist (radial artery)
		   Groin (femoral artery)
		5. If basic medical equipment is available:
		   a. no obtainable blood pressure
		   b. no audible heart sounds on the stethoscope
			1. Keep calm
			2. Call for **HELP—911**
			3. Remain with individual
			4. Note time of occurrence
			5. Remember ABC:
			   A. *Airway*—clear mouth and pharynx of vomit, blood, mucous, and saliva
			   —turn patient's head to one side and pull tongue and lower jaw forward and outward with finger
			   —check for foreign bodies in mouth and pharynx
			   B. *Breathing*—while maintaining adequate airway, begin mouth to mouth ventilation at the following frequency:
			   infant—every three seconds 20 times per minute
			   child—every four seconds 15 times per minute
			   adult—every five seconds 12 times per minute The method of doing mouth to mouth ventilation will vary with the circumstances and available equipment as well as resuscitator's experience. Speed is important.
			   C. *Circulation*—After establishing an airway and initiating adequate ventilation, begin external cardiac massage. The patient should be placed on a hard surface. Correct hand position over the sternum should be used on adults.

Shock†	Is a clinical condition when systemic perfusion of tissue becomes inadequate for meeting the body's metabolic needs.
	a. There are three basic *mechanisms* that produce the state of shock:
	   1. Hypovolemic shock, the most common type, is due to loss of circulating blood volume as in trauma, bleeding, severe burns, diarrhea or severe diuresis through urine output. These patients are responsive to volume infusion, usually through intravenous route.
	   2. Cardiogenic shock, is rare in pediatrics but may be caused by congenital heart disease, "cardiac pump" failure from infection of the heart or effusion into the covering of the heart.
	   3. Anaphylaxis from medication such as penicillin; or sepsis or overwhelming infection may also produce a shock state.
		1. Rapid pulse rate or heart rate
		2. Rapid respiration
		3. Temperature instability—high or low temperature
		4. Weak peripheral pulses
		5. Cold and mottled skin
		6. Altered mental status such as confusion, garbled speech and decreasing level of consciousness may occur as decrease in brain perfusion progresses.
			1. Keep calm
			2. Call for **HELP—911** or care unit
			3. Remain with patient
			4. Note time of occurrence
			5. Institute:
			   —Airway
			   —Breathing
			   —Circulation (as in CPR)
			6. Record vital signs (temperature, blood pressure, heart rate and pulse rate) if equipment available

ambulatory or out-patient care type clinic. Ideally, the same physician, or group of physicians, will provide acute, as well as ongoing care for the child.

Several clinical conditions may require intermediate medical attention, including a persistent fever, coughing, vomiting, diarrhea, head trauma, or poorly controlled seizures.

Persistent high fever, especially if unresponsive to antipyretics such as aspirin or acetaminophen (as authorized by the physician), may indicate bacterial or other serious infection that may necessitate comprehensive diagnostic or aggressive therapy. Common infections are: *otitis media*, pharyngitis, gastroenteritis, urinary tract infection, or a lung infection, such as pneumonia.

Persistent cough, vomiting, or diarrhea, which may or may not be accompanied by fever, are indicators of more serious or protracted medical problems that need the physician's care and attention.

Head trauma, with or without loss of consciousness, may need medical assessment and further medical advice, es-

pecially in regards to subsequent clinical observations that may indicate more serious complications.

Frequent poorly controlled seizures, although not as prolonged as *status epilepticus* discussed earlier, may suggest too much, or too little anti-epileptic medications, or other aggravating factors that may be present and need medical attention. Keeping a record of the frequency, duration and description of the seizure is very helpful to the physicians.

The occupational therapist may also encounter behavioral problems in certain settings. Often these problems occur in the schools, the home, hospitals, and other community-based agencies. The levels of intervention that can be instituted depend upon the nature and the severity of the behavior problem. Some behaviors can be handled by the program staff, while others may require additional medical support. Intervention for behavioral problems can include verbal, physical, or chemical actions.

Some of the more common problems encountered in therapy are noncompliance and oppositional behaviors. Behav-

TABLE 15-6. *Continued.*

Indicator	Description	Clinical Clues to Diagnosis	What to Do
Status Epilepticus††	When seizures or convulsions occur for greater than 15 to 30 minutes or occur repetitively so that recovery between seizures is incomplete, the patient is said to be in *status epilepticus*. Usually of the generalized tonic and clonic type, this type of seizure needs immediate medical attention. Common Causes of Status Epilepticus: 1. Patients who are already on antiepileptic drugs who forget to take their medications or are non compliant. 2. Fever infections in patients already prediagnosed with epilepsy. 3. Head trauma. 4. Infections of the brain such as meningitis or encephalitis in patients with no previous history of epilepsy. 5. Metabolic problems such as hypoglycemia, electrolyte imbalance, dehydration, hypoxia, shock.	Depends on the seizure type but generally: 1. Loss of consciousness 2. Alternating increased or tonic extension of extremities with clonic or contraction of muscles. 3. Extension of head and neck often with deviation of eyes upward or sideways rarely downward. 4. There may be loss of bladder or bowel control. 5. The convulsion may terminate by itself, after which the patient is confused, disoriented, unconscious, exhausted or with severe headache.	1. Complex Partial Seizures (Temporal lobe, psychomotor): The person may: have a glassy stare; give no response or inappropriate response when questioned; sit, stand or walk about aimlessly; make lip smacking or chewing motions; fidget with clothes; appear to be drunk, drugged or even psychotic. —Do not try to stop or restrain the person —Try to remove harmful objects from the person's pathway or guide the person away from them —Do not agitate the person After the seizure: The person may be confused or disoriented after regaining consciousness and should not be left alone until fully alert. 2. Generalized tonic-clonic seizure (grand mal). During the seizure: the person may fall, stiffen and make jerking movements. Pale or bluish complexion may result from difficulty breathing. —Help the person into a lying position and put something soft under the head —Remove glasses and loosen any tight clothing —Clear the area of hard or sharp objects —Do not force anything into the person's mouth —Do not try to restrain the person; you cannot stop the seizure —Turn the person on their side After the seizure: The person will awaken confused and disoriented. —Do not offer the person any food or drink until fully awake —Arrange for someone to stay nearby until the person is fully awake. It is rarely necessary to call public authorities unless: —The person does not start breathing after the seizure (begin mouth-to-mouth resuscitation) —The person has one seizure right after another —The person is injured —The person requests an ambulance
Poisonings†	Poisonings in children and adolescents occur frequently and can involve household products, plants, drug ingestions (accidental or intentional), pollutants and others.	It is not possible to discuss these toxic substances individually but some general principles must be discussed. —Raise your level of suspicion for poisoning when a child manifests bizarre clinical and behavioral features, particularly if sudden in onset.	—Identify, whenever possible, the toxic substance and assess the quantity of the substance ingested, assess also the approximate time of ingestion. —Call a Poison Control Center, keep this telephone number handy, because the center can give you some advice over the telephone as to immediate steps that can be taken to prevent further deleterious effects. —Keep syrup of ipecac handy in your home, school or day care center. Certain drugs can be effectively removed by induction of vomiting by syrup of ipecac, but to be certain of the safety for such, call the Poison Control Center for the contraindications to the induction of vomiting. For example, certain substances that are corrosives (liquid drain cleaners) petroleum distillates and pesticides are more dangerous when vomiting is induced. —Always, if in doubt, call the Poison Control Center (keep the telephone number in a prominent accessible location).

† Adapted from: Reece, R. M., (1984). Manual of Emergency Pediatrics.
†† Adapted from: First Aid for Epilepsy. Greater Kansas City Epilepsy League, Kansas City, Missouri. Used with permission. Courtesy of MINCEP, Minnesota Comprehensive Epilepsy Program.

ioral management for these types of behavior can take the form of verbal cueing, or a "time out" procedure. A reward system can be incorporated in this management as part of "catching them being good" (Christopherson, 1988).

Physical isolation may be utilized for those who are physically aggressive to others, or to themselves, and may result in injuries. Occasionally, children are given medications for management. This type of intervention requires a physician's approval and must be monitored *very* closely. The types of medications usually given are those classified as sedatives or tranquilizers. They are often given as a one time dose, or are sometimes prescribed in a p.r.n. (as necessary) dosage. The chronic use of these types of medication must be supervised closely and reevaluated often.

The most serious behavior problems of a psychiatric nature are suicidal behaviors. Suicidal behavior represents a major reason for emergency medical referrals, and must be brought to medical and psychiatric attention. Suicidal attempts, such as drug overdoses and use of lethal weapons, may need initial medical emergency measures, and almost simultaneously, a psychiatric consultation to assist the patient, family, and friends in dealing with the problem.

Other types of behavior problems, such as fire setting, delinquent behavior, and cruelty to animals, can be dealt with on a nonemergency basis. Often, these types of behaviors are of a chronic nature, and are associated with other types of personality disorders, or other types of psychopathology.

DEALING WITH SPECIAL APPARATUS

An increasing number of children who are sent home from hospitals, have continued medical care at home. These children are medically stable, but require continued health supervision because of the specialized nature of their medical problems.

By the time these children are discharged from the acute care hospital, parents and other caretakers have been trained in the use and care of special equipment necessary to maintain nutrition, oxygen, and drainage. Nurses, respiratory therapists, and other personnel participate in the training of the persons responsible for the patient's daily home care. Usually, home health supervision and visits are arranged on a regular basis to monitor any problems or questions that may develop once the patients are home.

Home care for children on respirators was reported by Burr, et al., (1983) in six children with varying medical diagnoses and functional capabilities. At that time, developmental and educational services for these children were limited, and a home bound program was recommended. Home care of the child with a tracheostomy tube has also been reported in children with varied medical conditions, as an alternative to prolonged hospitalization in medically stable children (Foster, 1981). It was emphasized in this report that infant stimulation, and continued occupational and physical therapies, should be continued at home; programs that should have started while in the hospital setting. Home care in these children shortens the hospital stay, allows a return to the home environment sooner, and, hopefully, a more normal lifestyle. Parental support and respite care, may be necessary to lessen the physical and emotional burden on these families who take on the responsibility of the medical care of their children at home.

Coordinated planning, and a multidisciplinary approach to home care of children, is essential to its success. Home-based services must be incorporated into the care plan, and should include not only medical needs, but also developmental, educational, and social support needs. Financial considerations of health care insurers and providers must be discussed with the families. Alternative resources for all medical and support services must be sought and exhausted, to prevent further financial liabilities for families already burdened with physical and emotional stresses (Sporing, Walton, & Cady, 1984).

Children with *spina bifida* can spend considerable time in regular and self-contained classrooms. Some are of normal intelligence, but most have fine motor and visual perception skill deficits, whether they are completely paraplegic or ambulatory with some support. Urinary catherization is sometimes necessary for those who have no bladder control. Often, this procedure is relegated to the parents or the school nurse. There are other medical and surgical ways to divert urine from the bladder, such as an ileal conduit—an operation devised to attach the bladder to a tube that empties into the large intestine, and then into an exterior bag that collects the urine constantly.

Children with hydrocephalus are sometimes managed with a ventriculo-peritoneal (V-P) shunt, surgically placed to divert cerebro-spinal fluid from the ventricles of the brain, to the peritoneal cavity of the abdomen. There are several causes of hydrocephalus, but the V-P shunt is a successful way of arresting or stopping the pressure in the brain. Sometimes a fluid build-up in the brain produces headaches, vomiting, irritability, or behavior changes. It is important to notice these changes, and to report them to the patient's physicians.

MAKING MEDICAL REFERRALS

In the section on emergencies and seeking medical assistance, two categories of immediate and intermediate types of medical condition are described. The types of medical referrals in those instances usually involves the primary care physicians, such as pediatricians and family practice physicians or, as in emergency room settings, the emergency room physicians. This section will cover referrals made to different specialists in medicine, from whom occupational therapists are likely to seek advice or opinion. These specialists are in the fields of neurology, orthopedics, physiatry (rehabilitation medicine), psychiatry, and developmental pediatrics. Other medical specialists, that may also assist in the evaluation of a child with developmental disabilities, are ophthalmologists (eye specialists), and an otolaryngologists (ear, nose and throat specialists).

General Guidelines

There are some general guidelines that would make your referral of benefit to you, the children and their parents. Be specific about your referral questions. The specialist receiving the referral request must know the reason for referral. It is helpful to be specific, if not detailed, in describing your areas of concern. Do not just state "please evaluate." It would be more useful, for example, if motor tone is a concern, to describe your findings. If you are uncertain about a diagnosis, such as cerebral palsy, or feel that a special brace might be helpful for the child's positioning or motor activities, state your observations and questions clearly.

PEDIATRIC NEUROLOGY

For the pediatric neurologist, the most frequent question other professionals ask is regarding the nature of neurological testing.

What is a Neurological Examination?

Neurological examination of infants and children consists of two distinct parts: obtaining an adequate and reliable clinical history, and the actual neurologic examination. The latter part consists of: a) a general physical examination; b) an estimation of development; c) a systematic assessment of motor and sensory functions, cranial nerves, coordination, and reflexes, to determine the intactness of various anatomic parts of the nervous system; d) a mental status examination, and for the school age child, screening tests that would indicate general academic performance.

It is stressed that the clinical history and the actual neurological examination are of equal importance. If a child is sent for neurologic evaluation without a reliable history from parents, caretakers, or a letter or report from the person concerned about the neurological problem, it becomes very difficult for the neurologist to put into perspective the nature of the problem, and how it should relate to the present neurologic assessment of the patient. For example, there are certain types of seizures that fit certain clinical descriptions, but unless this is suspected by the neurologist, or an adequate description is provided, a diagnosis cannot be made on the basis of the examination alone, because in some cases the examination may be entirely normal.

What Does the Neurological Examination Tell You About a Child Medically?

The combined clinical history and actual neurological examination can provide the following information:

1) The medical factors in the child's birth history, and previous illnesses that may be contributing to the present problem. Depending upon the nature and severity of previous medical events, the present problems may be due to an old or static insult to the nervous system.

2) Adequate information concerning the child's family history, and other medical problems, may contribute to finding out the child's present problem. There are certain conditions that are hereditary, or tend to run in families.

3) The diagnosis of seizures, or convulsive disorders or epilepsy, can be made on the basis of an adequate clinical history. Some types of seizures, such as petit mal epilepsy, which is common in the school-age child, may sometimes be described by the teacher or parents as "daydreaming" or "inattention," when in fact the child is having seizures. These are potentially treatable with appropriate medications, and marked improvement in school performance is possible.

4) There are certain types of degenerative neurological disorders, although rare in occurrence, that may initially manifest as deterioration in personality, behavior, and academic performance. These may be associated with specific neurological findings reflecting abnormalities in motor control, sensory systems, cranial nerves, and reflexes. These types of disorders need further diagnostic neurologic work-up.

5) From a neurological standpoint, it is important to establish whether there has been a loss of previously acquired skills, or instead a lack of development of abilities.

6) The general physical examination includes measurements of height, weight, and head circumference. These indicators of physical growth may indicate certain endocrine abnormalities, such as decreased thyroid function. Certain syndromes may suggest chromosomal abnormalities. Some disorders resulting in microcephaly (small head circumference), or macrocephaly (large head), may be secondary to other underlying neurological disorders.

7) Examination for abnormalities of the skin, or other bony abnormalities, may also indicate certain disorders associated with mental retardation syndromes, such as *Tuberous Sclerosis*, Sturge-Weber Syndrome and Neurofibromatosis.

When is it Appropriate to Refer a Child With School-related Problems for a Neurological Examination?

The specific instances in which neurological evaluations are indicated are:

1) Any suspicion of convulsive disorders or seizures as manifested by: a) Frequent short episodes of apparent daydreaming, or loss of contact with the environment, which may suggest petit mal type epilepsy. b) Episodic, unprovoked abnormal behavior, with or without apparent loss of consciousness, which may be followed by headache, sleepiness, or "feeling tired." c) Disorientation in time and space, such as getting lost in the school or classroom, or "forgetting" in the middle of a routine task. d) Frequent attacks of headaches, dizziness, or stomach aches, that are episodic in occurrence, and do not responding to the usual analgesics or medications.

2) Observations of significant changes in personality or behavior, with deterioration or loss of previously acquired skills.

3) A change or deterioration of motor performance associated with incoordination, tremors, or purposeless abnormal movements.

4) For children who have had seizure disorders, whose performance or behavior may suggest overmedication (such as lethargy, incoordination, or changing speech), or inadequate medication (and therefore showing partial or poorly controlled seizures).

5) For children who have a medical history of having been at risk for any insult to the nervous system, such as known birth injury, infections such as meningitis or encephalitis, or history of head injury, who have never been adequately evaluated.

It would be extremely valuable to send any previous educational, or psychological, or other tests on the child to the neurologist prior to the visit. If you have an occupational therapy assessment, send it with your referral or consultation request. Provide your questions, or the focus of your concerns, in a cover letter.

ORTHOPEDICS

Orthopedic evaluations are done by orthopedic surgeons to:

a. Determine if aids to mobility, such as orthopedic devices, braces, special shoes, and other durable medical equipment, such as wheelchairs, prone standers and walkers, may be useful.

b. Determine whether surgery can correct skeletal or muscular deformities resulting from cerebral palsy, particularly the spastic type of cerebral palsy. By tendon or muscle release, lengthening or transfer, joint mobility can be altered so that more functional locomotion and use of extremities can be accomplished. Some patients with cerebral palsy are also at risk for hip dislocation, which is a painful condition for most children. Correction of the dislocated hips can also be achieved with appropriate surgery. Therapists can provide valuable information regarding the timing of these procedures.

REHABILITATION MEDICINE

Rehabilitation medicine or physiatry, is an evolving specialty in pediatrics. Most rehabilitation medicine programs are geared for adults, and have focused on regaining the activities of daily living, therapeutic and motor exercises, and orthotic appliances, such as self-help devices for upper and lower extremities, bracing, splinting, etc. It has been agreed that in children who have not achieved normal development, the word "rehabilitation" is probably not correct. The terminology "infant development" programs is used for "habilitation" of children with developmental delays. To some extent, pediatric physiatry overlaps with orthopedics, in regards to determination of orthotic devices. However, in some tertiary care centers, seating clinics for children are under the management of physiatrists, in conjunction with orthotics specialists, physical therapists, and occupational therapists.

DEVELOPMENTAL PEDIATRICIANS

Developmental pediatricians are physicians trained as pediatricians, who take further training in developmental disabilities. Not all communities will have such specialists, as often they are in teaching facilities, and their practices are in the area of special needs children, and may be part of a multidisciplinary team. After their regular pediatric training, developmental pediatricians receive more comprehensive training and experience with the broad range of developmental disabilities. They become part of the team in specialty clinics, such as the cerebral palsy clinic, cleft lip and palate clinic, and other facial disorders, genetics, neurology and endocrine clinics. As part of their training, they are also made fully aware of the community agencies and facilities that will assist children, and their families, in the long term care and needs of these patients.

HOSPITALIZATION

Occasionally the primary care physician, or the specialty physician will hospitalize a child. Hospitalization of children is a medical decision. This often occurs when diagnostic and treatment procedures cannot be performed on an outpatient basis, such as those of an emergency nature, in which rapid therapy and monitoring is indicated. The emotional and psychological effects of illness on children, and their families, must be adequately addressed. Fear, anxiety, and uncertainty are common reactions experienced by both the children and their families. The physician and the support medical staff must work together to make the hospital stay a beneficial and positive experience for the children and their families.

EXPAND YOUR NEWLY ACQUIRED KNOWLEDGE

1. Identify one drug that is used to increase attention skills. Name two side effects that might occur when using this drug.
2. Design a protocol which identifies when the team would call for emergency support for a child with special health care needs.
3. Create a referral checklist for orthopedic specialty needs; for pediatric neurology needs.

References

Adapted from Commission on Classification and Terminology of the International League Against Epilepsy. (1981). *Epilepsia, 22*: 489–501.

American Academy of Pediatrics (1984). Report of the American Academy of Pediatrics Ad Hoc Task Force on Home Care for Chronically Ill Infants and Children. *Pediatrics, 74*, 434.

Burr, B. H., Guyer, B., Todres, I., Abrahams, B., & Chiodo, T. (1983). Home care for children on respirators. *New England Journal of Medicine, 309*, 1319.

Campbell, M., Green, W. H., & Deutsch, S. I. (1985). *Child and Adolescent Psychopharmacology*, Beverly Hills: Sage Publications.

Cantwell, D. (1978). *Use of psychopharmacologic agents with the emotional disorders of childhood, clinical pharmacology and therapeutics.* Chicago: Yearbook Medical Publishers.

Christopherson, E. (1988). Little People. Kansas City, West Port Publ.

Ferry, P. C., Banner, Jr., W., & Wolf, R. A. (1986). *Seizure Disorder in Children*, Philadelphia: J. B. Lippincott.

Foster, S. & Hoskins, D. (1981). Home Care of the Child with a Tracheostomy Tube, Pediatric Clinics of North America, 28: 855.

Kenny, T. J. & Clemmens, R. L. (1980). Psychotropic drug therapy. In *Behavioral pediatrics and child development: A clinical handbook*. Baltimore: Williams & Wilkins.

Minde, K., Weiss, G., & Mendelson, N. (1972). A five year follow-up of 91 hyperactive school children. *Journal of American Academy of Child Psychiatry, 11*, 595.

Reece, R. M. (Ed.) (1984). *Manual of Emergency Pediatrics*, Chicago: Saunders, 755 pp.

Rosenberger, P. (1986). Neurological assessment. In D. L. Wodrich & J. E. Joy (Ed.) *Multidisciplinary assessment of children with learning disabilities and mental retardation*, (p. 247). Baltimore: Paul H. Brookes Publishing Co.

Safer, D., Allen, R., & Barr, B. (1972). Depression of growth in hyperactive children on stimulant drugs. *New England Journal of Medicine, 287*, 217.

Solow, R. A. (1976). Child and adolescent psychopharmacology in the mid-seventies: Progress or plateau? *Psychiatric Digest, 37*, 15.

Sporing, E. M., Walton, M. K., & Cady, C. E. (1984). *Pediatric Nursing: Policies, Procedures and Personnel*, New Jersey: Medical Economics Publishing, Inc.

Thomas, C. L. (Ed.) (1985). *Taber's cyclopedic medical dictionary*. Philadelphia: F. A. Davis Company, Publishers.

Werry, J. S. (1977). The use of psychotropic drugs in children. *Journal of American Academy of Child Psychiatry, 16*, 446–468.

CHAPTER 16

Tests Used by Other Professionals

Winnie Dunn, PhD, OTR, FAOTA

"Besides talking and thinking differently, each discipline's diagnosticians often act differently . . . Knowledge of the capabilities and limitations of the diagnostic procedures and tools used by each discipline is an important factor in competent multidisciplinary assessment." Wodrich, 1986

Occupational therapists who work in pediatrics will either be a member of an interdisciplinary team, or be in communication with a team that serves the child and family. Therapists who work in clinics, community-based agencies, or schools, will interface with other team members throughout the diagnostic and program planning process. Many times, teams are less effective, because each professional knows about a particular area of expertise, but does not understand information provided by other team members. The purpose of this chapter is to introduce several of the most commonly used psychoeducational tests, and explain important information that an occupational therapist can glean from the test scores, in formulating both an assessment strategy and a program plan.

There are many commercially available tests; some are more carefully designed than others, and some are more frequently used than others. This discussion will be limited to the four most frequently used psychoeducational tests, because these are most likely to be administered at the onset of the diagnostic process to provide direction for further assessment and program planning. They are also well designed test instruments. King-Thomas and Hacker (1987) provide an excellent review of all of the major tests used in pediatrics, and the reader is referred to this text for information on other tests. The following tests will be discussed in this chapter:

- *Kaufman Assessment Battery for Children* (KABC).
- *Wechsler Intelligence Scale for Children*, (Revised) (WISCR) (WPPSI and WAIS-R are similar).
- *Woodcock-Johnson Psycho-Educational Tests Battery* (WJ) (With introduction to the *Woodcock-Johnson*, (Revised), available 1990).
- *Stanford-Binet Intelligence Scale*, (Fourth Edition) (SB).

Most commercially available tests have a mechanism for obtaining a derived score from the raw score performance of the individual. For example, the *Bruininks Oseretsky Test of Motor Proficiency* allows the examiner to obtain a standard score, percentile rank, and stanine score; age equivalent scores are also available (see chapter three for a description). Derived scores allow the examiner to compare the scores on one test to those on another, even though the tests had a different number of items, or a different internal scoring system. It is sometimes very useful for teams to plot the standard scores from all tests onto one chart for comparison; this makes the pattern of strengths and concerns very apparent, and is a concise way of presenting a lot of data. Figure 16-1 summarizes several standard scores that are frequently used in the assessment of children. The bell curve provides a reference point for all of the scales, so it is clear which scores are within or outside normal limits.

KAUFMAN ASSESSMENT BATTERY FOR CHILDREN (KABC)

The KABC was designed by Alan S. Kaufman, Ph.D. and Nadine L. Kaufman, Ph.D., two psychologists who are well experienced in both assessment and test construction. The test is standardized on a large nationwide sample which included both typical children and children with disabilities. It covers the age range of 2½ years to 12½ years. The test battery was designed with the following goals in mind, to:

1. Measure intelligence from a strong theoretical and research base;
2. Separate acquired factual knowledge from the ability to solve unfamiliar problems;
3. Yield scores that translate educational intervention;
4. Include novel tasks;
5. Be easy to administer and objective to score; and
6. Be sensitive to the diverse needs of preschool, minority group, and exceptional children (Kaufman & Kaufman, 1983, p. 5).

The KABC measures intelligence in relation to an individual's style of problem solving and information processing. It was based on the theoretical work of cerebral specialization researchers, and cognitive and neuropsychologists. The Mental Processing component of this test is divided into two primary scales: a sequential and a simultaneous scale. The sequential scale "places a premium on the serial or temporal order of stimuli when solving problems." (p. 2). The simultaneous scale "demands a gestalt-like, frequently spatial, integration of stimuli to solve problems with maximum efficiency." (p. 2). The items are designed to minimize the effects of possible language barriers, cultural diversity, and experience, so that a wide range of children can be accurately assessed on this instrument.

There is also an Achievement Scale on the KABC. The Achievement Scale is made up of items which "assess factual knowledge and skills usually acquired in a school setting or through alertness to the environment." (Kaufman & Kaufman,

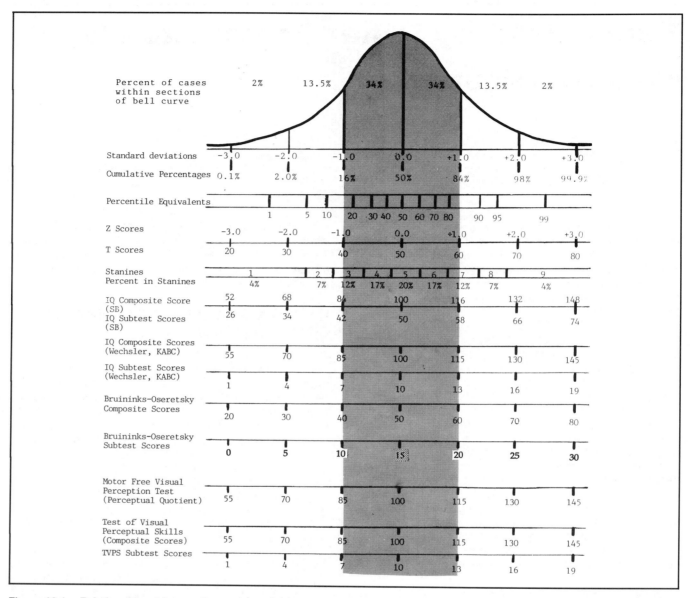

Figure 16-1.   Relationship of frequently used standard scores to the bell curve. Shaded area denotes normal range. *Adapted with permission from Sattler (1988).*

1983, p. 33). By having this scale on the KABC, the diagnostician can make comparisons between ability (mental processing) and achievement, which are necessary for certain educational diagnoses, and has data to suggest directions for intervention planning.

Another nice feature of the KABC is that the authors created a Nonverbal Scale score from the subtests. This is a unique configuration of subtest scores which yields an estimate of intellectual potential in those children who may have communication difficulties. This allows the diagnostician to hypothesize about the effects of language on the child's ability to demonstrate actual ability.

There are sixteen subtests on the KABC. They are designed to yield standard scores to facilitate comparison among the subtests. The subtest demands are summarized briefly in Figure 16-2.

Interpretation of KABC scores requires understanding of the sequential and simultaneous processing concepts. "Each task in the KABC Sequential Processing Scale presents a problem which must be solved by arranging the input in sequential or serial order. Each idea is linearly and temporally related to the preceding one. Although short-term memory is an aspect of each subtest, the unifying process is the sequential handling of the stimuli, regardless of their content, their method of presentation, or the mode of response." (p. 30). Sequential skills are related to many learning tasks. Remembering mathematics facts, or spelling words requires sequential processing. Rules of grammar, systematic hypothesis testing, and multiple step mathematics problems all require sequential skills. The authors also point out the sequential nature of some social skills, such as following the rules of a game, or following adult directions. Children with difficulty on

KABC Assessment

(Not all subtests are given to all age groups)

Sequential Processing Scale

1. *Hand Movements.* Performing a series of hand movements in the same sequence as the examiner performed them.
2. *Number Recall.* Repeating a series of digits in the same sequence as the examiner said them.
3. *Word Order.* Touching a series of silhouettes of common objects in the same sequence as the examiner said the names of the objects. More difficult items include an interference task between the stimulus and response.

Simultaneous Processing Scale

1. *Magic Window.* Identifying a picture that the examiner exposed by slowly moving it behind a narrow window, making the picture only partially visible at any one time.
2. *Face Recognition.* Selecting from a group photograph the one or two faces that were exposed briefly on the preceding page.
3. *Gestalt Closure.* Naming an object or scene pictured in a partially completed "inkblot" drawing.
4. *Triangles.* Assembling several identical triangles into an abstract pattern to match a model.
5. *Matrix Analogies.* Selecting the meaningful picture or abstract design that best completes a visual analogy.
6. *Spatial Memory.* Recalling the placement of pictures on a page that was exposed briefly.
7. *Photo Series.* Placing photographs of an event in chronological order.

Achievement Scale

1. *Expressive Vocabulary.* Naming an object pictured in a photograph.
2. *Faces and Places.* Naming the well-known person, fictional character, or place pictured in a photograph or drawing.
3. *Arithmetic.* Demonstrating knowledge of numbers and mathematical concepts, counting and computational skills, and other school-related arithmetic abilities.
4. *Riddles.* Inferring the name of a concrete or abstract concept when given a list of its characteristics.
5. *Reading/Decoding.* Identifying letters and reading words.
6. *Reading/Understanding.* Demonstrating reading comprehension by following commands that are given in sentences.

Information taken from: *Kaufman Assessment Battery for Children Interpretive Manual.* A. S. Kaufman and N. L. Kaufman. American Guidance Service, Inc.: Circle Pines, Minnesota, 1983. p. 3–5. Used with permission.

Figure 16-2. Description of individual subtests of the Kaufman Assessment Battery for Children.

the Sequential Processing Scale, may have been referred to special education services because of problems in one or more of these skills. The educational environment generally heavily favors the sequential mode of problem solving, and so difficulties in this area are more quickly noticed. The occupational therapist may notice inability to follow a series of directions, poorly organized patterns of movements or clumsiness. When observing closely, the child may have the component parts of a task intact, but has poor ability to sequence that interferes with accurate task performance. Children with attention deficits may have difficulties with sequential processing, because it requires that the individual maintain attention to the stimulus over time, in order to capture which part comes before and after each component. When attention is interrupted frequently, the individual may be able to capture some parts, but may not know how they must be put together.

"The problems presented in the Simultaneous Processing Scale are spatial, analogic, or organizational in nature. The input had to be integrated and synthesized simultaneously to produce the appropriate solution." (p. 30). Simultaneous tasks are more likely to be visual-perceptual in nature, such as in learning the letters and numbers by their shapes, or in gaining important information from the pictures. However, the authors caution that high level intellectual functions are also associated with simultaneous processing; it allows individuals to integrate data from seemingly unrelated sources to create the "big picture." In school, the child with poor simultaneous processing may not be able to capture the main idea in a story, understand mathematical concepts or use charts, graphs and diagrams effectively. The child may be more likely to spell phonetically, and not profit from sight word strategies. Children with difficulty in simultaneous processing may be more rigid and literal in their thinking; they may latch onto small portions of the task, and not understand the overall activity. The occupational therapist may find that this child does not profit from demonstration of the overall task, but rather requires things broken into parts. Table 16-1 presents a summary of the skills & difficulties seen when there is a difference between the sequential & the simultaneous scales on the KABC.

In addition to the processing subscales, the occupational therapist can consider those subtests characteristics that are shared by two or more subtests. Figure 16-3 relates the *primary* task requirements of each subtest with the performance components from AOTA's *Uniform Terminology* (Second Edition) (UT2) (definitions provided in Appendix A) (McGourty, Foto, Marvin, Smith, Smith & Kronsnoble, 1989). There are some task components that are not included on this grid, such as language and auditory perception; these are not the specific area of expertise of the occupational therapist, and so are not part of the UT2 document. Other professionals would be dealing with these factors. The description of the subtests (Figure 16-2) identifies those that are dependent on language and specific areas of auditory perception. Those items marked have been chosen to illustrate the characteristics shared by various subtests, rather than to point out unusual or differentiating features of each subtest. The diagnostic process depends upon finding patterns of performance that can lead to a viable hypothesis about needs and intervention strategies. The therapist can use this figure to analyze the KABC test scores, to determine if a consistent

TABLE 16-1. Examples of skills and difficulties which may be present when a discrepancy exists between the sequential and simultaneous processing scales of the KABC.

Seq > Sim	Sim > Seq
* ability to use stepwise math procedures (e.g., borrowing) * utilizes scientific method * understands chronology of events * good knowledge of grammar rules * rote knowledge of math facts * poor space/time relations * poor sight vocabulary * phonetic speller * difficulty using context	* good math concepts * good overall comprehension * good use of picture cues * uses diagrams, flow charts * uses shapes of letters/words to recognize * poor decoding skills/phonics * doesn't remember details of story * can't recall order of story * failure to understand rules * poor retention of math facts * poor use of steps to solve math problems * poor ability to follow oral directions

KAUFMAN ASSESSMENT BATTERY FOR CHILDREN SUBTESTS

PERFORMANCE COMPONENTS	Hand Movements	Number Recall	Word Order	Magic Window	Face Recognition	Gestalt Closure	Triangles	Metric Analogies	Spatial Memories	Photo Series	Expressive Vocabulary	Faces and Places	Arithmetic	Riddles	Reading/Decoding	Reading Understanding
A. SENSORIMOTOR COMPONENT																
1. Sensory Integration																
a. Sensory Awareness																
b. Sensory Processing																
(1) Tactile																
(2) Proprioceptive																
(3) Vestibular																
(4) Visual	*		*	*	*	*	*	*	*	*	*	*	*		*	*
(5) Auditory		*	*								*	*	*	*	*	*
(6) Gustatory																
(7) Olfactory																
c. Perceptual Skills																
(1) Stereognosis																
(2) Kinesthesia	*															*
(3) Body Scheme	*				*											*
(4) Right-Left Discrimination	*															
(5) Form Constancy			*	*	*	*			*	*	*				*	*
(6) Position in Space	*				*	*	*		*							
(7) Visual-Closure					*		*	*								
(8) Figure Ground						*										
(9) Depth Perception																
(10) Topographical Orientation																
2. Neuromuscular																
a. Reflex																
b. Range of Motion																
c. Muscle Tone																
d. Strength																
e. Endurance																
f. Postural Control																
g. Soft Tissue Integrity																
3. Motor																
a. Activity Tolerance																
b. Gross Motor Coordination																*
c. Crossing the Midline																
d. Laterality																
e. Bilateral Integration																*
f. Praxis																
g. Fine Motor Coordination/ Dexterity		*														*
h. Visual-Motor Integration	*						*									
i. Oral-Motor Control				*	*	*					*		*	*	*	

Figure 16-3. Components of Performance that are represented within the Kaufman Assessment Battery for Children Subtests.

KAUFMAN ASSESSMENT BATTERY FOR CHILDREN SUBTESTS

PERFORMANCE COMPONENTS	Hand Movements	Number Recall	Word Order	Magic Window	Face Recognition	Gestault Closure	Triangles	Metric Analogies	Spatial Memories	Photo Series	Expressive Vocabulary	Faces and Places	Arithmetic	Riddles	Reading/Decoding	Reading Understanding
B. COGNITIVE INTEGRATION AND COGNITIVE COMPONENTS																
1. Level of Arousal																
2. Orientation																
3. Recognition																
4. Attention Span	*	*	*	*	*			*	*	*			*	*	*	*
5. Memory																
a. Short-term	*	*	*	*	*				*							
b. Long-term						*		*		*	*	*	*	*	*	*
c. Remote																
d. Recent																
6. Sequencing	*	*	*							*			*		*	*
7. Categorization								*		*		*		*		
8. Concept Formation								*				*		*		
9. Intellectual Operations in Space							*		*	*			*	*		
10. Problem Solving							*	*					*	*		
11. Generalization of Learning								*		*		*		*		*
12. Integration of Learning																
13. Synthesis of Learning																
C. PSYCHOSOCIAL SKILLS AND PSYCHOLOGICAL COMPONENTS																
1. Psychological																
a. Roles																
b. Values																
c. Interests																
d. Initiation of Activity																
e. Termination of Activity																
f. Self-Concept																
2. Social																
a. Social Conduct																
b. Conversation																
c. Self-Expression																
3. Self-Management																
a. Coping Skills																
b. Time Management							*									
c. Self-Control			*													

Figure 16-3. *Continued.*

pattern of difficulty or strength is present in the child's performance component skills. For example, if a child obtained low scores on Hand Movements and Triangles, both of which require hand manipulations, the occupational therapist might focus on fine motor skills in the evaluation.

The Meaning of Test Scores

The scores on the KABC are normalized standard scores with a mean of 100, and a standard deviation of 15 (this is the same scale that is used on the Wechsler scales). Subtest scores are based on a mean of 10 and a standard deviation of 3. The authors provide specific directions about the interpretation of differences among scores on the KABC. To compare the Sequential and Simultaneous scores, children aged 2 years 6 months, to 4 years 11 months, must have at least a 14 point difference (the .05 significance level); children aged 5 years 0 months to 12 years 5 months must have at least a 12 point difference (the .05 significance level). Differences larger than this are too large to happen by chance, and therefore can be interpreted as a significant finding. If differences are less than this (even by one point), professionals must conclude that the child's problem solving abilities are consistently developed.

To identify significant discrepancies in specific subtest scores, the authors propose that professionals calculate the mean subtest score for all the Mental Processing subtests, and then compare each subtest to that derived mean score. Any score that is 3 or more points different is considered significant;

KABC Kaufman Assessment Battery for Children

by Alan S. Kaufman and Nadeen L. Kaufman

INDIVIDUAL TEST RECORD

Name Pam _____ Sex _____

Parents' names _____

_____

Home address _____

Home phone _____

Grade _____ School _____

Examiner _____

SOCIOCULTURAL INFORMATION (if pertinent)

Race _____

Socioeconomic background _____

_____

_____

	YEAR	MONTH	DAY
Test date	___	___	___
Birth date	___	___	___
Chronological age	8	1	___

Achievement Subtests $\bar{X} = 100; SD = 15$	Standard score ± band of error ___% confidence	Nat'l. %ile rank Table 4	Socio-cultural %ile rank Table 5	S or W Table 11	Other data
11. Expressive Vocabulary	±		/////		
12. Faces & Places	85 ±11	16		W	
13. Arithmetic	88 ±11	21		W	
14. Riddles	117 ±11	87			
15. Reading/ Decoding	120 ±8	91			
16. Reading/ Understanding	100 ±7	50			
Sum of subtest scores	510		Transfer sum to Global Scales. *Sum of subtest scores* column.		

Mental Processing Subtests $\bar{X} = 10; SD = 3$	Scaled Score			Nat'l %ile rank Table 4	S or W Table 11	Other data
	Sequential	Simul-taneous	Non-verbal			
1. Magic Window	/////		/////			
2. Face Recognition	/////					
3. Hand Movements	9	/////	9	37		
4. Gestalt Closure	/////	5		5	W	
5. Number Recall	14	/////		91	S	
6. Triangles	/////	6	6	9	W	
7. Word Order	13	/////		84	S	
8. Matrix Analogies	/////	8	8	25		
9. Spatial Memory	/////	6	6	9	W	
10. Photo Series	/////		10	10	50	
Sum of subtest scores	36	35	39	Transfer sums to Global Scales. *Sum of subtest scores* column.		

Global Scales $\bar{X} = 100; SD = 15$	Sum of subtest scores	Standard score ± band of error % confidence Table 2	Nat'l %ile rank Table 4	Socio-cultural %ile rank Table 5	Other data
Sequential Processing	36	112 ±9			
Simultaneous Processing	35	80 ±8			
Mental Processing Composite	71	91 ±7			
Achievement	510	102 ±5			
Nonverbal		±			

Global Scale Comparisons

Indicate >, <, or ≈   Circle the significance level

Sequential	>	Simultaneous (Table 10)	NS	.05	(.01)
Sequential	≈	Achievement (Table 10)	(NS)	.05	.01
Simultaneous	<	Achievement (Table 10)	NS	.05	(.01)
M P C	<	Achievement (Table 10)	NS	(.05)	.01

AGS ®
© 1983, American Guidance Service, Inc.
Circle Pines, Minnesota 55014
No part of this test record may be photocopied or otherwise reproduced.

Figure 16-4. KABC Assessment Battery for Children. Used with permission from American Guidance Service, Inc. Protocol cover page for the Kaufman Assessment Battery for Children by A. S. Kaufman and N. L. Kaufman. Representative scores for an 8 year, 1 month old girl, Pam.

those that are higher are the child's strengths, while those that are lower are the child's weaknesses. The occupational therapist can review the KABC test scores as part of Type 2 screening, and by using the information summarized in Figure 16-2 can identify appropriate directions for assessment.

Figure 16-4 and Figure 16-5 contain the KABC score sheet and profile respectively. Pam is an eight year, one month old child who is having trouble in school. Her teacher is concerned that she cannot read maps in social studies, and that, although she can do her mathematics facts, she seems to be falling behind in conceptual aspects of mathematics. Her KABC scores are presented in Figures 16-4 and 16-5. The scores reveal that Pam has strengths in Number Recall and

Word Order, and weaknesses in Gestault Closure, Triangles, and Spatial Memory (see the fifth column on the left portion of Figure 16-4). The Global Scale comparisons (bottom right of Figure 16-4) reveal that there are significant discrepancies among the Global scores. These patterns of scores are depicted visually on Figure 16-5 (which is found on the back of the protocol booklet).

When one analyzes the pattern, Pam has significant problems with tests requiring visuospatial processing. It is also interesting to note that the lowest score on her Sequential Scale (an overall *strength*) is Hand Movements. Hand Movements and Triangles both require fine motor competence. This may also be a problem area, and should be investigated further, since these areas seem to be affecting some school performance. The occupational therapist would want to pursue visual perception, visual motor, and fine motor components in follow-up assessments with Pam.

The KABC Interpretive Manual provides a wealth of information about the test, and how to use the scores for designing interventions. The strategies emphasize the balance between remedial and compensatory approaches to problems. For example, a child with strengths in sequential processing, and a weakness in simultaneous processing, needs a balance of activities which take advantage of strong sequential skills to learn new tasks and solve new problems, and activities which

work to remediate the simultaneous problem solving weaknesses that interfere with independent function. It is also appropriate to design compensatory strategies which acknowledge weak areas, and work around them to allow the child to learn in alternate ways. Chapter Six discusses this in more depth.

THE WECHSLER INTELLIGENCE SCALE FOR CHILDREN (REVISED) (WISCR)

The WISCR was designed as an individual intelligence test by David Wechsler, Ph.D. (1974). His work has been a hall-

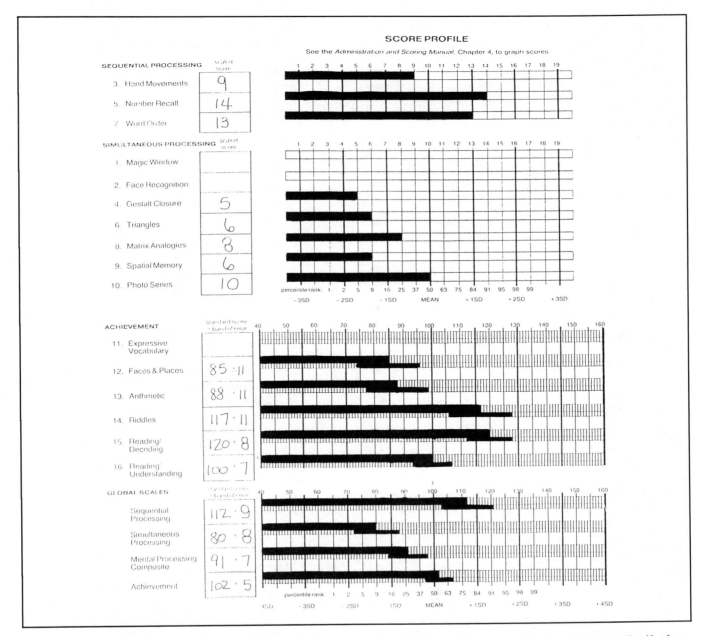

Figure 16-5.   KABC Score Profile. Used with permission from American Guidance Service, Inc. Score profile from the Kaufman Assessment Battery for Children by A. S. Kaufman and N. L. Kaufman. Representative score profile for an 8 year, 1 month old girl, Pam.

mark in the intelligence testing area. He also designed the Wechsler Preschool and Primary Scales of Intelligence (WPPSI), and the Wechsler Adult Intelligence Scales (WAIS) to address younger children and adults. The WISCR spans the 6 year 0 months to 17 years interval. The three tests are very similar, with ten to twelve subtests each, which yield a Full Scale IQ score, a Verbal score and a Performance score. The Wechsler scales are the most widely used intelligence tests (King-Thomas and Hacker, 1987).

The WISCR has been used extensively in the pediatric diagnostic process, and so is probably more familiar to therapists with pediatric experience. The studies that were completed on the WISCR identified three primary factors; the two that are most familiar to professionals are the Verbal Comprehension and Perceptual Organization factors, which are comprised of the subtests on the Verbal and Performance subscales respectively. The third factor, entitled Freedom from Distractibility, is made up of the Arithmetic, Digit Span and Coding subtests. Each of these subtests requires sustained attention to complete the tasks successfully. Figure 16-6 contains a summary of the WISCR subtests.

The Verbal Subscale is comprised of tests with a heavy language component. The individual must listen to the question, and produce an oral response. The auditory channel of communication is heavily tapped on the Verbal Subscale, and so if there is either an auditory processing problem or a language deficit, the individual will score poorly on these subtests. The occupational therapist may notice that the child has a difficult time following oral directions, or may tend to watch others to gain clues about what is expected. Demonstration may be more helpful to a child with Verbal subscale deficits.

The Performance Subscale is comprised of tests which rely heavily on visual perceptual processing. Visual perception and motor manipulation are used on these subtests; since these areas are within the expertise of the occupational therapist, poor scores on this subscale can serve as an indication of the need for the occupational therapist to become involved in the case. Tests of visual perception, visual-motor integration, and fine motor control are appropriate followups.

Meaning of Test Scores

The WISCR IQ scores are based on standard scores with a mean of 100 and a standard deviation of 15 points. This means that a normal score would range from 85 to 115. The subtest scores are based on a mean of 10 and a standard deviation of 3. As with the KABC, the WISCR scores can be analyzed for patterns of performance. The test manual suggests that a 15 point discrepancy between verbal and performance subscale scores, should be considered a significant difference (a pattern that is more unusual than one would expect under normal conditions). Table 16-2 summarizes behaviors associated with higher verbal or higher performance subscale scores. Sattler (1982) suggests a similar procedure for the KABC procedure to analyze subtest differences. Those subtests that are more than 3 points away from the mean of the subtest scores should be considered further. Sattler (1988) provides a detailed discussion of each subtest pattern; therapists who work on teams which use the WISCR a lot, should

---

WISC-R Assessment

Verbal Scale

1. *Information*. 30 questions requiring general knowledge and simple statements of fact (example: Where is Brazil?).
2. *Similarities*. 17 pairs of words that require the child to explain how the 2 items are similar (example: How are a mirror and a window alike?).
3. *Arithmetic*. 18 orally presented (timed) problems to which children must respond verbally without the aid of pencil and paper (example: If apples are priced at 2 for 25 cents, then how many can you buy for $1.00?).
4. *Vocabulary*. 32 words presented orally and requiring practical problem-solving ability (example: What is a garage?).
5. *Comprehension*. 17 problem situations requiring practical problem-solving ability (example: What should you do if someone steals your bicycle?).
6. *Digit Span*. Orally presented sequences of numbers requiring oral repetition (example: Please listen carefully and then say the following numbers: 5-1-6-9.).

Performance Scale

1. *Picture Completion*. 26 drawings of common objects in which children are requested to find an important part that is missing.
2. *Picture Arrangement*. 12 picture series similar to cut-up comic strips that the child is requested to place in correct order so that they make a sensible story.
3. *Block Design*. Picture of an abstract geometric design that the child is asked to replicate by using red and white blocks.
4. *Object Assembly*. Similar to a jigsaw puzzle in that the child is asked to assemble a number of puzzle pieces to make a common object, person, or animal.
5. *Coding*. Requires the child to copy symbols (e.g., vertical lines, circles) that are matched to numbers.
6. *Mazes*. 8 mazes requiring the child to find the most direct route out.

Information taken from: Wodrich, D. L., & Joy, J. E. (1986). *Multidisciplinary assessment of children with learning disabilities and mental retardation.* Baltimore: Paul. H. Brookes Publishing Co., p. 45. Used with permission.

Figure 16-6. Individual subtests for the Weschler Intelligence Scale for Children.

---

familiarize themselves with this reference. Figure 16-7 contains a breakdown of *primary* subtest characteristics when compared to the UT2. Remember, the language and auditory perception detail is not on this figure, since this is not the focus of occupational therapy expertise.

An example of the WISCR profile is depicted in Figure 16-8. Darrel is a six year, five month old boy who is having trouble with his seatwork. It is poorly organized, and he frequently tears his papers up and throws them away. The WISCR

TABLE 16-2. Some hypotheses regarding verbal-performance discrepancies on the Weschler scales.

VS > PS	PS > VS
* language better than perceptual organization	* perceptual organization better than language
* visual motor skills may be deficient	* reading problems
* visual perceptual skills may be deficient	* can't follow oral directions
* auditory processing may be better than visual processing.	* visual processing may be better than auditory processing
* manipulation tasks may be more difficult	* talking, conversation may be more difficult
* may "talk" way out of perceptual tasks	* may prefer drawing, constructing.

WECHSLER INTELLIGENCE SCALE FOR CHILDREN—Revised (WISC-R)

PERFORMANCE COMPONENTS	Information	Similarities	Arithmetic	Vocabulary	Comprehension	Digit Span	Picture Completion	Picture Arrangement	Block Design	Object Assembly	Coding	Mazes
A. SENSORIMOTOR COMPONENT												
1. Sensory Integration												
a. Sensory Awareness												
b. Sensory Processing												
(1) Tactile												
(2) Proprioceptive												
(3) Vestibular												
(4) Visual							*	*	*	*	*	*
(5) Auditory	*	*	*	*	*	*						
(6) Gustatory												
(7) Olfactory												
c. Perceptual Skills												
(1) Stereognosis												
(2) Kinesthesia												
(3) Body Scheme												
(4) Right-Left Discrimination												
(5) Form Constancy							*	*		*	*	
(6) Position in Space								*	*	*		
(7) Visual-Closure							*			*		
(8) Figure Ground												*
(9) Depth Perception												*
(10) Topographical Orientation												
2. Neuromuscular												
a. Reflex												
b. Range of Motion												
c. Muscle tone												
d. Strength												
e. Endurance												
f. Postural Control												
g. Soft Tissue Integrity												
3. Motor												
a. Activity Tolerance												
b. Gross Motor Coordination												
c. Crossing the Midline												
d. Laterality												
e. Bilateral Integration												
f. Praxis												
g. Fine Motor Coordination/ Dexterity									*	*	*	*
h. Visual-Motor Integration										*	*	*
i. Oral-Motor Control	*	*	*	*	*	*						

Figure 16-7. Components of Performance that are represented within the Wechsler Intelligence Scale for Children (Revised).

WECHSLER INTELLIGENCE SCALE FOR CHILDREN—Revised (WISC-R)

PERFORMANCE COMPONENTS	Information	Similarities	Arithmetic	Vocabulary	Comprehension	Digit Span	Picture Completion	Picture Arrangement	Block Design	Object Assembly	Coding	Mazes
B. COGNITIVE INTEGRATION AND COGNITIVE COMPONENTS												
1. Level of Arousal												
2. Orientation												
3. Recognition												
4. Attention Span	*	*	*	*	*	*	*	*	*	*	*	*
5. Memory												
a. Short-term											*	*
b. Long-term	*	*	*	*	*		*	*		*		
c. Remote												
d. Recent												
6. Sequencing			*			*			*		*	*
7. Categorization		*										
8. Concept Formation		*	*	*								
9. Intellectual Operations in Space			*						*	*		*
10. Problem Solving		*	*		*				*			
11. Generalization of Learning					*							
12. Integration of Learning												
13. Synthesis of Learning												
C. PSYCHOSOCIAL SKILLS AND PSYCHOLOGICAL COMPONENTS												
1. Psychological												
a. Roles												
b. Values												
c. Interests												
d. Initiation of Activity												
e. Termination of Activity												
f. Self-Concept												
2. Social												
a. Social Conduct					*							
b. Conversation												
c. Self-Expression												
3. Self Management												
a. Coping Skills												
b. Time Management								*	*	*	*	*
c. Self-Control												

Figure 16-7. *Continued.*

profile reveals a discrepancy between Verbal and Performance IQ's, with Performance significantly lower. He has an average overall IQ score. When examining the subtest score pattern, the significantly lower scores are in Object Assembly, Coding, and Block Design, all of which are timed, and have a motor component. Visual motor integration may be appropriate follow-up evaluation for Darrel.

THE WOODCOCK-JOHNSON PSYCHO-EDUCATIONAL BATTERY (WJ)

The WJ is a comprehensive battery of individually administered tests that cluster into three areas: cognitive ability, achievement and interest. Twelve subtests form the cognitive ability area; the subtests are similar in appearance to other tests of cognitive ability (e.g., WISCR, KABC and Stanford-Binet). Sattler (1988) comments that the Cognitive Abilities full scale score has been shown to rank learning disabled children significantly lower than they would be ranked on the WISC-R (mean 9.1 points over 12 studies). This test is therefore not recommended as a cognitive measure for diagnostic or placement purposes. Ten subtests comprise the achievement area; the titles of the subtests clearly define the various areas of academic performance one sees in a school curriculum. These subtests measure the classic achievement variables well (Sattler, 1988). The last five subtests indicate the individual's preferences for scholastic or nonscholastic activities, and form the interest area. Figures 16-9a and b contain a brief summary of the subtests of the WJ.

The WJ was designed by Richard W. Woodcock, Ph.D.,

WISC-R   RECORD FORM

Wechsler Intelligence Scale
for Children—Revised

NAME ___Darrel_____ AGE _____ SEX _____

ADDRESS_____

PARENT'S NAME _____

SCHOOL _____ GRADE _____

PLACE OF TESTING_____ TESTED BY_____

REFERRED BY_____

WISC-R PROFILE

Clinicians who wish to draw a profile should first transfer the child's *scaled scores* to the row of boxes below. Then mark an X on the dot corresponding to the scaled score for each test, and draw a line connecting the X's.*

VERBAL TESTS   PERFORMANCE TESTS

Information | Similarities | Arithmetic | Vocabulary | Comprehension | Digit Span

Scaled Score: 11 | 12 | 13 | 11 | 12 | 11

Picture Completion | Picture Arrangement | Block Design | Object Assembly | Coding | Mazes

Scaled Score: 12 | 10 | 8 | 6 | 5 | 11

*See Chapter 4 in the manual for a discussion of the significance of differences between scores on the tests.

NOTES

	Year	Month	Day
Date Tested			
Date of Birth			
Age	6	5	

	Raw Score	Scaled Score
VERBAL TESTS		
Information	_____	11
Similarities	_____	12
Arithmetic	_____	13
Vocabulary	_____	11
Comprehension	_____	12
(Digit Span)	(_____)	(11)
Verbal Score	_____	
PERFORMANCE TESTS		
Picture Completion	_____	12
Picture Arrangement	_____	10
Block Design	_____	8
Object Assembly	_____	6
Coding	_____	5
(Mazes)	(_____)	(11)
Performance Score	_____	

	Scaled Score	IQ
Verbal Score	_____	* 111
Performance Score	_____	* 87
Full Scale Score		100

*Prorated from 4 tests, if necessary.

Figure 16-8. WISC-R Record Form. *Reproduced with permission from The Psychological Corporation, Wechsler Intelligence Scale for Children-Revised, 1974.*

and M. Bonner Johnson, Ph.D. in 1977. The WJ contains many forms of scoring, and it is not necessary for the occupational therapist to understand all of them in detail. The WJ also contains summaries of scores which are depicted in profile form on the test protocol; this visual display is very helpful in understanding an individual's performance. Each area contains two profiles of interest: the Percentile Rank Profile and the Subtest Profile.

The Percentile Profile can be found on the cover page of each protocol booklet (the tests of achievement and interest are housed together in the second response booklet). The Percentile Rank Profile from the cognitive ability section is pictured in Figure 16-10. On this profile, the authors have collapsed the individual subtests into groups which seem to tap a similar construct. For example, subtest 2, Spatial Relations and subtest 7, Visual Matching have been combined to form the Perceptual Speed construct on the Cognitive sec-

tion. Some subtests are included on more than one group or cluster, making them non-independent. Some have criticized the authors for creating these groupings; factor analytic studies revealed only two primary factors: verbal and nonverbal/spatial factors (Sattler, 1988). Therefore, one must be cautious about using this type of information since actual validity is unknown.

The examiner plots the individual's score range on the Percentile Profile by coloring in the section of the bar for each construct. The chart has a shaded area for the normal range, and so one can quickly see whether an area is within, above, or below normal limits. As with other tests, discrepancies within the individual's performance provide signals that follow-up may be necessary. The Perceptual Speed construct (See Figure 16-10) contains visual perception items, so a score range that is significantly lower on this composite may trigger the need for occupational therapy involvement. How-

---

Woodcock-Johnson Psycho-Educational Assessment

Part One: Tests of cognitive ability

1. *Subtest 1:* Picture Vocabulary tests the subject's ability to identify pictured objects.

2. *Subtest 2:* Spatial Relations tests the subject's ability to compare shapes visually. The subject's task is to select from a series of shapes the component shapes necessary to make a given whole shape. The shapes become progressively more abstract and complex. The test has a three-minute time limit.

3. *Subtest 3:* Memory for Sentences tests the subject's ability to remember material presented auditorily. In a task such as this, subjects make use of sentence meaning to aid recall.

4. *Subtest 4:* Visual-Auditory Learning tests the subject's ability to associate new visual symbols (rebuses) with familiar words in oral language and to translate series of symbols into verbal sentences. The subtest involves a controlled learning situation, presenting the subject with a miniature learning-to-read task.

5. *Subtest 5:* Blending tests the subject's ability to integrate and then verbalize whole words after hearing components (syllables and/or phonemes) of the words presented sequentially.

6. *Subtest 6:* Quantitative Concepts tests the subject's knowledge of quantitative concepts and vocabulary. No actual calculations or application decisions are involved.

7. *Subtest 7:* Visual Matching tests the subject's ability to identify two numbers that are the same in a row of six numbers. The task proceeds in difficulty from single-digit numbers of five-digit numbers. The test has a two-minute time limit.

8. *Subtest 8:* Antonyms-Synonyms tests the subject's knowledge of word meanings. Part A (Antonyms) requires the subject to state a word whose meaning is the opposite of the presented test word. Part B (Synonyms) requires the subject to state a word whose meaning is the same as the presented word.

9. *Subtest 9:* Analysis-Synthesis tests the subject's ability to analyze the components of an equivalency statement and reintegrate them to determine the components of a novel equivalency statement. Although this is not pointed out to the subject, the task is one of learning a miniature system of mathematics. The subject must be able to identify the colors yellow, black, blue, and red to take the subtest.

10. *Subtest 10:* Numbers Reversed tests the subject's ability to repeat a series of numbers in an order opposite to that in which they are presented. The subtest assesses the subject's ability to hold a sequence of numbers in memory while reorganizing that sequence. Numbers Reversed is more of a perceptual reorganization task than a memory task (in contrast to a numbers forward task).

11. *Subtest 11:* Concept Formation tests the subject's ability to identify rules for concepts when given both instances of the concept and non-instances of the concept. It can be considered a categorical reasoning task.

12. *Subtest 12:* Analogies tests the subject's verbal ability by requiring the subject to complete phrases with words that indicate appropriate analogies. It is largely a relational reasoning task.

Woodcock, R. W., & Johnson, M. B. (1977). Woodcock-Johnson Psycho-Educational Battery. Allen, TX: DLM Teaching Resources. Used with permission.

Figure 16-9a.   Woodcock-Johnson Psycho-Educational Battery—Subtests.

ever, there are other subtests which contain visual perception components as well, so this should not be the only source of information. There are also fine motor components on some of the subtests, and this is not delineated as a construct on this profile. The Percentile Rank Profile provides a quick overview of the individual's performance. The occupational therapist may obtain more helpful clues from the Subtest Profile.

The Subtest Profiles are located on the back page of the protocol booklets (See Figure 16-11). A completed Subtest Profile will also have bands colored in for each subtest. There may be a vertical line drawn on the profile; this line indicates the individual's overall performance, and can be used as a reference point for subtest scores. The authors suggest a rule of thumb for determining whether subtest scores are significantly different. They suggest that a real difference ex-

ists between two scores when "the separation between the two bands is greater than the width of the wider band . . . " (Woodcock & Johnson, 1977, p. 330). Figure 16-11 contains a portion of a Subtest Profile; one can see that the Visual Matching and Spatial Relations subtest bands are significantly lower than the Blending and Memory for Sentences subtests. Neither of these groups is significantly different from the Visual-Auditory Learning subtest. In this pattern, one might hypothesize that visual perception skills are weak, while the auditory mode of processing is stronger; the subtest that falls in between the two groups relies heavily on the stronger and weaker perceptual systems simultaneously.

Figures 16-12 and 16-13 summarize the *primary* performance components for the cognitive and achievement subtests. Remember, the language and auditory processing components will not be well represented here, because UT2

**Woodcock-Johnson
Psycho-Educational Assessment**

Part Two—Tests of Achievement

Subtest 13: Letter-Word Identification
Subtest 14: Word Attack
Subtest 15: Passage Comprehension
Subtest 16: Calculation
Subtest 17: Applied Problems
Subtest 18: Dictation
Subtest 19: Proofing
Subtest 20: Science
Subtest 21: Social Studies
Subtest 22: Humanities

Part Three—Tests of Interest

Subtest 23: Reading Interest
Subtest 24: Mathematics Interest
Subtest 25: Written Language Interest
Subtest 26: Physical Interest
Subtest 27: Social Interest

Woodcock, R. W., & Johnson, M. B. (1977). Woodcock-Johnson Psycho-Educational Battery. Allen, TX: DLM Teaching Resources. Used with permission.

Figure 16-9b. Woodcock-Johnson Psycho-Educational Battery Achievement and Interest subtests.

only covers areas of expertise of the occupational therapist. Figure 16-9a contains subtest descriptions which identify those subtests which rely on language.

The Woodcock-Johnson has recently been revised as the Woodcock-Johnson Psycho-Educational Battery (Revised) (WJ-R). It is available to professionals in 1990, but may not

be fully integrated into school testing programs until the 1990–1991 school year, due to the need for special training. The WJ-R has a more extensive normative group, and is reorganized for more efficient and effective testing. Both the cognitive and achievement sections have been designed to have core subtests (called the standard battery), and supplemental subtests. The standard battery subtests are administered to determine the individual's overall ability; the appropriate supplemental tests are then chosen to provide further data in selected areas of potential concern. Figures 16-14a and b summarize the format of the WJ-R, and provide a brief description of cognitive factors.

An adaptive behavior measure has also been designed to be used with the WJ batteries; it is called *The Scales of Independent Behavior*. The scales are described in Table 16-3. This test is very pertinent to the issues of the occupational therapist and could be used as an adjunct to other evaluation methods.

The occupational therapist gains data pertaining to professional expertise in several cognitive areas. Processing speed and visual processing relate to visual perception and visual-motor skills. Long-term retrieval and fluid reasoning provide insight about specific cognitive processes dealt with by the occupational therapist. The written language sections of the achievement tests can provide insight about fine motor and perceptual motor aspects of writing tasks. Data from these components can narrow the focus of an assessment, or corroborate the occupational therapist's data base. It will be important for occupational therapists to become familiar with the WJ-R, as it becomes the more frequent choice in psychoeducational assessments.

THE STANFORD-BINET INTELLIGENCE SCALE (FOURTH EDITION) (SB4)

The SB4 is the 1986 revision of the 1960 Stanford-Binet Intelligence Scale: Form L-M. This most recent version was

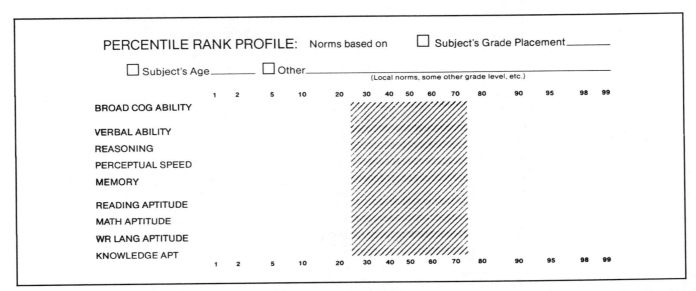

Figure 16-10.   Woodcock-Johnson Psycho-Educational Battery Percentile Rank Profile. *Used with permission by DLM Teaching Resources. Woodcock-Johnson Psycho-Educational Battery (1977) by R. W. Woodcock and M. Bonner Johnson.*

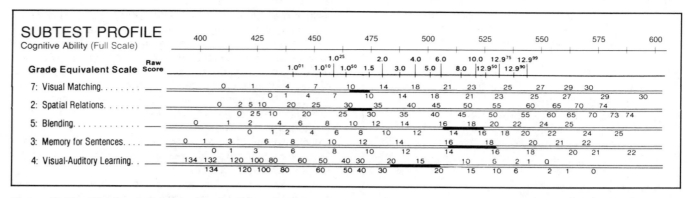

Figure 16-11. Woodcock-Johnson Psycho-Educational Battery Subtest Profile. *Used with permission by DLM Teaching Resources, Allen, TX. Woodcock-Johnson Psycho-Educational Battery Response Booklet (1977) by R. W. Woodcock and M. Bonner Johnson.*

WOODCOCK JOHNSON TESTS OF COGNITIVE ABILITY

PERFORMANCE COMPONENTS	Picture Vocabulary	Spatial Relations	Memory for Sentences	Visual-Auditory Learning	Blending	Quantitative Concepts	Visual Matching	Antonyms/Synonyms	Analysis-Synthesis	Numbers Reversed	Concept Formation	Analogies
A. SENSORIMOTOR COMPONENT												
1. Sensory Integration												
a. Sensory Awareness												
b. Sensory Processing												
(1) Tactile												
(2) Proprioceptive												
(3) Vestibular												
(4) Visual	*			*		*	*		*		*	
(5) Auditory	*	*	*	*	*	*		*	*	*	*	*
(6) Gustatory												
(7) Olfactory												
c. Perceptual Skills												
(1) Stereognosis												
(2) Kinesthesia												
(3) Body Scheme												
(4) Right-Left Discrimination						*						
(5) Form Constancy	*	*		*		*	*		*		*	
(6) Position in Space		*				*			*		*	
(7) Visual-Closure		*										
(8) Figure Ground						*						
(9) Depth Perception												
(10) Topographical Orientation												
2. Neuromuscular												
a. Reflex												
b. Range of Motion												
c. Muscle tone												
d. Strength												
e. Endurance												
f. Postural Control												
g. Soft Tissue Integrity												
3. Motor												
a. Activity Tolerance												
b. Gross Motor Coordination												
c. Crossing the Midline												
d. Laterality												
e. Bilateral Integration												
f. Praxis												
g. Fine Motor Coordination/ Dexterity							*					
h. Visual-Motor Integration							*					
i. Oral-Motor Control	*		*	*	*		*		*	*	*	*

Figure 16-12. Components of Performance that are represented within the Woodcock Johnson Tests of Cognitive Ability.

WOODCOCK JOHNSON TESTS OF COGNITIVE ABILITY

PERFORMANCE COMPONENTS	Picture Vocabulary	Spatial Relations	Memory for Sentences	Visual-Auditory Learning	Blending	Quantitative Concepts	Visual Matching	Antonyms/Synonyms	Analysis-Synthesis	Numbers Reversed	Concept Formation	Analogies
B. COGNITIVE INTEGRATION AND COGNITIVE COMPONENTS												
1. Level of Arousal												
2. Orientation												
3. Recognition												
4. Attention Span		*	*	*	*	*	*		*	*	*	*
5. Memory												
a. Short-term		*	*	*	*		*		*	*	*	
b. Long-term	*					*		*				*
c. Remote												
d. Recent				*					*		*	
6. Sequencing			*		*	*			*	*	*	
7. Categorization						*		*	*		*	*
8. Concept Formation						*		*	*		*	
9. Intellectual Operations in Space		*				*			*		*	
10. Problem Solving						*			*		*	
11. Generalization of Learning				*					—	*	*	
12. Integration of Learning												
13. Synthesis of Learning												
C. PSYCHOSOCIAL SKILLS AND PSYCHOLOGICAL COMPONENTS												
1. Psychological												
a. Roles												
b. Values												
c. Interests												
d. Initiation of Activity												
e. Termination of Activity												
f. Self-Concept												
2. Social												
a. Social Conduct												
b. Conversation												
c. Self-Expression												
3. Self Management												
a. Coping Skills												
b. Time Management												
c. Self-Control				*			*			*	*	*

Figure 16-12. *Continued.*

designed by Robert L. Thorndike, Ph.D., Elizabeth P. Hagen, Ph.D., and Jerome M. Sattler, Ph.D., evaluation specialists. The authors designed a large, national standardization sample to provide stability in the data obtained. The test covers ages two through adult, and scores are based on over 5,000 individuals in 17 age groups (Sattler, 1988). The authors state the purposes of the Fourth Edition, to

1. Help differentiate between students who are mentally retarded and those who have specific learning disabilities;
2. Help educators and psychologists understand why a particular student is having difficulty learning in school;
3. Help identify gifted students; and to
4. Study the development of cognitive skills of individuals from ages 2 to adult. (Thorndike, Hagen, & Sattler, 1986, p. 3).

The Fourth Edition is significantly different from previous editions of the Stanford-Binet tests. The original Stanford-Binet test was published in 1905 by Alfred Binet and Theodore Simon, and marked the beginning of formal and rigorous study of mechanisms for measuring cognitive skills. Earlier versions of the Stanford-Binet tests measured a general ability factor, and did not break performance into its component parts. SB4 breaks the general abilities factor into crystallized abilities, fluid abilities, and short-term memory. The general ability is conceptualized as the processes one uses to design and adapt strategies to solve novel problems. The crystallized abilities represent verbal and quantitative concepts, and assesses how they are used to solve problems. The fluid abilities represent figural, visual, and other nonverbal concepts, and assess how they are used to solve problems. Short-term memory represents the individual's ability to: a) retain new information temporarily before deciding what to do with it, and b) hold information drawn from long-term memory and use it for ongoing tasks. The authors feel that the manner in which an individual uses short-term memory processes can be a significant factor in cognitive efficiency.

WOODCOCK JOHNSON TESTS OF COGNITIVE ABILITY

PERFORMANCE COMPONENTS	Letter/Word Identification	Word Attack	Passage Comprehension	Calculation	Applied Problems	Dictation	Proofing	Science	Social Studies	Humanities	Interest Subtests
A. SENSORIMOTOR COMPONENT											
1. Sensory Integration											
a. Sensory Awareness											
b. Sensory Processing											
(1) Tactile											
(2) Proprioceptive											
(3) Vestibular											
(4) Visual	*	*	*	*	*		*	*	*	*	*
(5) Auditory	*	*	*		*	*	*	*	*	*	*
(6) Gustatory											
(7) Olfactory											
c. Perceptual Skills											
(1) Stereognosis											
(2) Kinesthesia											
(3) Body Scheme											
(4) Right-Left Discrimination				*	*						
(5) Form Constancy	*	*	*	*	*	*	*	*	*	*	
(6) Position in Space				*	*						
(7) Visual-Closure					*						
(8) Figure Ground											
(9) Depth Perception											
(10) Topographical Orientation											
2. Neuromuscular											
a. Reflex											
b. Range of Motion											
c. Muscle Tone											
d. Strength											
e. Endurance											
f. Postural Control											
g. Soft Tissue Integrity											
3. Motor											
a. Activity Tolerance											
b. Gross Motor Coordination											
c. Crossing the Midline											
d. Laterality											
e. Bilateral Integration											
f. Praxis											
g. Fine Motor Coordination/ Dexterity				*	*						
h. Visual-Motor Integration				*	*						
i. Oral-Motor Control	*	*	*		*		*	*	*	*	*

Figure 16-13. Components of Performance that are represented within the Woodcock Johnson Tests of Cognitive Ability.

There are fifteen subtests on the SB4. They fall into four categories: Verbal Reasoning, Abstract/Visual Reasoning, Quantitative Reasoning and Short-term Memory. The authors conducted factor analyses to confirm the organization of the subtests within these categories. There is preliminary evidence to suggest that there is a relationship between the subtests and these categories, although some of the subtests did not demonstrate an association with any of the categories, and were only associated with the general abilities factor. Sattler (1988) reports additional principal components factor

WOODCOCK JOHNSON TESTS OF COGNITIVE ABILITY

PERFORMANCE COMPONENTS	Letter/Word Identification	Word Attack	Passage Comprehension	Calculation	Applied Problems	Dictation	Proofing	Science	Social Studies	Humanities	Interest Subtests
B. COGNITIVE INTEGRATION AND COGNITIVE COMPONENTS											
1. Level of Arousal											
2. Orientation											
3. Recognition	*										
4. Attention Span		*	*	*	*	*	*				
5. Memory											
a. Short-term						*					
b. Long-term	*	*	*	*	*		*	*	*	*	
c. Remote											
d. Recent											
6. Sequencing				*	*						
7. Categorization			*	*	*			*	*	*	
8. Concept Formation		*		*	*			*	*	*	
9. Intellectual Operations in Space				*	*						
10. Problem Solving				*	*		*				
11. Generalization of Learning											
12. Integration of Learning											
13. Synthesis of Learning											
C. PSYCHOSOCIAL SKILLS AND PSYCHOLOGICAL COMPONENTS											
1. Psychological											
a. Roles											*
b. Values											*
c. Interests											*
d. Initiation of Activity											
e. Termination of Activity											
f. Self-Concept											
2. Social											
a. Social Conduct											
b. Conversation											
c. Self-Expression											
3. Self-Management											
a. Coping Skills											
b. Time Management											
c. Self-Control				*	*						

Figure 16-13. *Continued.*

analyses which support these categories. Figure 16-15 summarizes the *primary* occupational therapy performance components necessary for each subtest on the SB4.

Meaning of Test Scores

The SB4 is designed to have a standard score mean of 100 with a standard deviation of 16. This means that a score of 85 on the WISCR is equivalent to an SB4 score of 84. The SB4 calls the composite ability scores Standard Age Scores (SAS). These scores can be found on the cover page of the Record Booklet (see Figure 16-16), and are called: Verbal Reasoning SAS, Abstract/Visual Reasoning SAS, Quantitative Reasoning SAS and Short-term Memory SAS. The total test Composite SAS is marked with an asterisk. Another helpful feature of this cover page is the behavioral checklist provided on the lower left corner. The occupational therapist can glean useful information about the child from these impressions which are recorded by the psychological examiner. Subtest scores can be compared on the inside front cover, using the Profile Analysis (Figure 16-17). The Standard Age Scores are plotted on this profile, and so can be compared to one another quickly. The subtests are designed to have a mean of 50 and a standard deviation of 8. Although the man-

Woodcock-Johnson Psycho-Educational Assessment

The WJ-R Tests of Cognitive Ability is divided into a Standard Battery and a Supplemental Battery. Depending on the purpose and extent of the assessment, the Standard can be used alone, or in conjunction with the Supplemental Battery. This design gives you great flexibility in making WJ-R meet your assessment needs. If your time is limited, simply use the Standard Battery, which allows you to look at all seven cognitive abilities in less than 40 minutes! If you desire to measure any factor in-depth, just choose the appropriate tests from the Supplemental Battery. The chart below shows which tests from the Standard and Supplemental Batteries measure each of the seven cognitive factors.

Cognitive Factors	Explanation	Subtests in Standard Battery	Subtests in Supplemental Battery
Long-term Retrieval	Retrieving information stored much earlier	1. Memory for Names	8. Visual-Auditory Learning 15. Delayed Recall-Memory for Names 16. Delayed Recall-Visual Auditory Learning
Short-term Memory	Storing information and retrieving immediately or within a few seconds	2. Memory for Sentences	9. Memory for Words 17. Numbers Reversed
Processing Speed	Working quickly, particularly under pressure to maintain focused attention	3. Visual Matching	10. Cross Out
Auditory Processing	Fluently perceiving patterns among auditory stimuli	4. Incomplete Words	11. Sound Blending 18. Sound Patterns
Visual Processing	Fluently manipulating stimuli that is usually visual in the mind's eye	5. Visual Closure	12. Picture Recognition 19. Spatial Relations
Comprehension-Knowledge	Known as crystallized intelligence, it represents a person's breadth and depth of knowledge of a culture	6. Picture Vocabulary	13. Oral Vocabulary 20. Listening Comprehension 21. Verbal Analogies
Fluid Reasoning	Reasoning in a novel situation	7. Analysis-Synthesis	14. Concept Formation 19. Spatial Relations 21. Verbal Analogies

Adapted from promotional materials for the Woodcock-Johnson Psycho-educational Battery-Revised, DLM Teaching Resources, 1989.

Figure 16-14a.   Cognitive subtests of the Woodcock-Johnson Psycho-Educational Battery (Revised).

WJ Assessment

Content/Curricular Areas	Subtests in Standard Battery	Subtests in Supplemental Battery
Reading	22. Letter-Word Identification 23. Passage Comprehension	31. Word Attack 32. Reading Vocabulary
Mathematics	24. Calculation 25. Applied Problems	33. Quantitative Concepts
Written Language	26. Dictation 27. Writing Samples	34. Proofing 35. Writing Fluency P. Punctuation and Capitalization S. Spelling U. Usage H. Handwriting
Knowledge	28. Science 29. Social Studies 30. Humanities	

Adapted from promotional materials for the Woodcock-Johnson Psycho-educational Battery-Revised. DLM Teaching Resources, 1989.

Figure 16-14b.   Achievement subtests of the Woodcock-Johnson Psycho-Educational Battery (Revised).

TABLE 16-3.   Subscales of the Scales of Independent Behavior.

Subscale A: **Gross-Motor Skills.** The 17 tasks in this subscale sample skills from below one year, such as sitting without support, to mature adult fitness, such as regular strenuous physical activities for strength and endurance. The items in this subscale access skills using large muscles of the arms, legs, or the entire body in tasks involving balance, coordination, strength, and endurance.

Subscale B: **Fine-Motor Skills.** This subscale evaluates performance on 17 tasks that require eye-hand coordination using small muscles of the fingers, hands, and arms. The skills sampled range from those typically developed in infancy, such as picking up small objects, to those acquired after age 12, such as assembling objects with small parts.

Subscale C: **Social Interaction.** This subscale evaluates performance on 16 tasks that require social interaction with other people. Tasks range in difficulty from socialization appropriate in infancy, such as handing toys to another person, to more complex interactions involving entertaining and making plans to attend social activities outside the home.

Subscale D: **Language Comprehension.** This subscale evaluates performance on 16 tasks involving understanding of signals, signs, or speech and in deriving information from spoken and written language. The tasks included in this subscale range in difficulty from basic skills observed in infants, such as recognizing one's name, to more complex levels that include searching for and securing information through reading or listening.

Subscale E: **Language Expression.** This subscale evaluates performance on 17 tasks that involve talking and other forms of expression. Provision is made for assessing the skills of subjects who use nonoral methods of communication (sign language or language boards). The tasks range in difficulty from those typically mastered in infancy or early childhood, such as indicating "yes" or "no" and repeating common words, to the more complex skills involved in preparing and delivering formal reports to other people.

Subscale F: **Eating and Meal Preparation.** This subscale includes 16 tasks that evaluate performance in eating and preparation of meals. Initial tasks are appropriate for infants and assess simple eating and drinking skills; more advanced items test mastery of tasks involved in meal preparation.

Subscale G: **Toileting.** This subscale includes 14 tasks that evaluate performance in using the toilet and bathroom. The range of skills in this subscale is relatively more restricted than other subscales. The tasks range in difficulty from infancy and early childhood, such as staying dry or using the toilet regularly without accidents, to later childhood activities such as selecting and using appropriate bathroom facilities outside the home.

Subscale H: **Dressing.** This subscale includes 18 tasks that evaluate performance in dressing. These tasks range from simple levels for very young children, such as removing clothing, to complex skills requiring appropriate selection and maintenance of clothes.

Subscale I: **Personal Self-Care.** The 15 tasks in this subscale evaluate performance in basic grooming and health maintenance skills. The tasks range in difficulty from skills normally mastered by young children, such as using a toothbrush or wiping one's face with a washcloth, to adult skills to seeking professional assistance to treat illness or maintain health.

Subscale J: **Domestic Skills.** This subscale evaluates performance on 16 tasks needed in maintaining a home environment. The tasks range in difficulty from the early childhood level, such as putting a dish in or near the sink, to complex maintenance tasks, such as routine painting or repairs.

Subscale K: **Time and Punctuality.** This subscale includes 15 tasks that evaluate time concepts and use of time. The tasks range in difficulty from assessing the concept of time of day to keeping appointments.

Subscale L: **Money and Value.** This subscale evaluates skills on 17 tasks related to determining the value of items and using money. The tasks range in difficulty from skills generally mastered in early childhood, such as saving small amounts of money or selecting particular coins, to complex consumer decisions involving investments and use of credit.

Subscale M: **Work Skills.** The 16 tasks in this subscale evaluate work habits and selected prevocational skills. These skills are generally more developmentally advanced than most of the other subscales. They range from simple work tasks, such as indicating when a chore is finished, to prevocational skills, such as completing employment applications and job resumes.

Subscale N: **Home/Community Orientation.** This subscale evaluates performance on 16 tasks involving getting around the home and neighborhood and traveling in the community. Starting with very simple tasks that assess the subject's concept and use of space within the home environment, the subscale progresses to advanced tasks that assess more complex travel skills involving the location of important sites within the subject's home community.

Scale PB: **Problem Behaviors.** In addition to evaluating functional independence and adaptive behaviors, the SIB includes a scale for identifying problem behaviors that often limit personal adaptation and community adjustment.

Taken from: Bruininks, R. H., Woodcock, R. W., Weatherman, R. F., & Hill, B. K. (1984). *Interviewer's Manual, Scales of independent behavior.* Allen, TX: DLM Teaching Resources, p. 5 & 6. Used with permission.

---

ual does not specify the criteria for significant differences, scores which are more than 8 points apart, are more than one standard deviation away from each other. The child's scores presented in Figure 16-17 would indicate the need for further investigation of visual perceptual skills.

Sattler (1988) advocates a similar interpretation strategy for the SB4, as is used in the WISC-R. The factor scores can be compared first (verbal comprehension, non-verbal reasoning, and memory). Sattler (1988) reports exact differences that are necessary for significance, but minimum differences range between 8 and 15 points. For example, the Verbal Comprehension and Non-Verbal Reasoning factors are sig-

nificantly different (at the .05 level), if they are 12 or more points apart on an eight-year-old child. Subtest scores can also be compared to their corresponding factor score (Sattler, 1988). In this comparison, one is trying to determine whether one subtest is significantly different from its group. For example, the Pattern Analysis subtest would have to be 5.30 points lower than the mean of the Non-Verbal Reasoning subtest scores, to be considered significantly discrepant. Smaller differences are not generally considered significant. Sattler (1988) provides exact comparison data. Finally, subtest scores can be compared to each other. Scores that are at least 6–10 points apart are considered significant (at the

STANFORD-BINET INTELLIGENCE SCALE 4th Ed.

PERFORMANCE COMPONENTS	1	2	3	4	5	6	7	8	9	10	11	12	13	14	15
A. SENSORIMOTOR COMPONENT															
1. Sensory Integration															
a. Sensory Awareness															
b. Sensory Processing															
(1) Tactile															
(2) Proprioceptive															
(3) Vestibular															
(4) Visual	*		*		*	*	*	*	*		*	*			*
(5) Auditory	*	*	*	*				*	*	*		*	*		
(6) Gustatory															
(7) Olfactory															
c. Perceptual Skills															
(1) Stereognosis															
(2) Kinesthesia					*										
(3) Body Scheme										*					
(4) Right-Left Discrimination					*	*	*	*			*				
(5) Form Constancy	*		*	*	*	*	*	*	*		*				
(6) Position in Space			*		*	*	*	*			*	*		*	*
(7) Visual-Closure			*					*							
(8) Figure Ground			*					*							
(9) Depth Perception			*				*								
(10) Topographical Orientation															*
2. Neuromuscular															
a. Reflex															
b. Range of Motion															
c. Muscle tone															
d. Strength															
e. Endurance															
f. Postural Control															
g. Soft Tissue Integrity															
3. Motor															
a. Activity Tolerance															
b. Gross Motor Coordination															
c. Crossing the Midline															
d. Laterality															
e. Bilateral Integration															
f. Praxis															
g. Fine Motor Coordination/ Dexterity					*	*						*			
h. Visual-Motor Integration					*	*						*			*
i. Oral-Motor Control	*	*	*	*				*	*	*			*	*	

Figure 16-15. Components of Performance that are represented within the Stanford-Binet Fourth Edition Subtests.

.05 level). As with other comparisons, Sattler (1988) provides exact amounts for each subtest pair.

SUMMARY

Occupational therapists have a great deal of expertise in comprehensive assessment, and can enhance those skills by becoming familiar with the tests used frequently by others on their interdisciplinary team. This chapter merely provides an introduction; test manuals, the team members themselves, and a number of assessment textbooks can provide additional information on tests of interest. Jerome Sattler's book, *Assessment of Children* (1988), is an excellent desk reference, both for the major psycho-educational tests, and for the principles and ethics of assessment.

STANFORD-BINET INTELLIGENCE SCALE 4th Ed.

	1	2	3	4	5	6	7	8	9	10	11	12	13	14	15
PERFORMANCE COMPONENTS															
B. COGNITIVE INTEGRATION AND COGNITIVE COMPONENTS															
1. Level of Arousal															
2. Orientation															
3. Recognition	*														
4. Attention Span	*	*		*	*	*	*	*	*	*	*	*	*	*	*
5. Memory															
a. Short-term							*	*	*	*	*	*	*	*	*
b. Long-term	*	*	*	*					*		..				
c. Remote		*		*											
d. Recent															
6. Sequencing						*			*	*	*	*	*	*	*
7. Categorization		*	*	*					*	*	*				
8. Concept Formation	*	*	*	*	*				*		*				
9. Intellectual Operations in Space		*	*	*		*	*				*				
10. Problem Solving		*	*	*		*	*	*	*		*				
11. Generalization of Learning		*	*	*							*				
12. Integration of Learning				*	*										
13. Synthesis of Learning															
C. PSYCHOSOCIAL SKILLS AND PSYCHOLOGICAL COMPONENTS															
1. Psychological															
a. Roles		*													
b. Values		*													
c. Interests		*													
d. Initiation of Activity															
e. Termination of Activity															
f. Self-Concept															
2. Social															
a. Social Conduct		*	*												
b. Conversation															
c. Self-Expression															
3. Self Management															
a. Coping Skills															
b. Time Management						*				*	*			*	
c. Self-Control		*													

Figure 16-15. *Continued.*

EXPAND YOUR NEWLY ACQUIRED KNOWLEDGE

1. Name four subtest scores on the WISC-R that might serve as clues that the student is having problems which can be addressed by the occupational therapist. Describe what each subtest score means, and name one assessment strategy you might use to follow up on that concern.

2. Consider the sequential and simultaneous subtest scores on the KABC. Describe two strategies you could use during therapeutic intervention which would accommodate the following patterns:
   a. high sequential, low simultaneous scores
   b. low sequential, high simultaneous scores

3. Name the cognitive subtests on the Woodcock-Johnson Psychoeducational Test Battery that might indicate problems with visual perceptual processing. Describe the perceptual components that are tapped in each. How would you follow up on these findings.

9-74539

STANFORD-BINET INTELLIGENCE SCALE

RECORD BOOKLET

Stanford-Binet Intelligence Scale: Fourth Edition

Name ____________________

____________________ Sex ______

Ethnicity NA H B W/NH O/AA PI Other ______

	YEAR	MONTH	DAY
Date of Testing			
Birth Date			
Age			

School ____________________

Grade ____________________

Examiner ____________________

Father's Occupation: ____________________

Mother's Occupation: ____________________

FACTORS AFFECTING TEST PERFORMANCE

Overall Rating of Conditions

Optimal — Good — Average — Detrimental — Seriously detrimental

	RAW SCORE	STANDARD AGE SCORE *
Verbal Reasoning		
1 Vocabulary		
6 Comprehension		
7 Absurdities		
14 Verbal Relations		
Sum of Subtest SAS's		
Verbal Reasoning SAS		
Abstract/Visual Reasoning		
5 Pattern Analysis		
9 Copying		
11 Matrices		
13 Paper Folding & Cutting		
Sum of Subtest SAS's		
Abstract/Visual Reasoning SAS		
Quantitative Reasoning		
3 Quantitative		
12 Number Series		
15 Equation Building		
Sum of Subtest SAS's		
Quantitative Reasoning SAS		
Short-Term Memory		
2 Bead Memory		
4 Memory For Sentences		
8 Memory For Digits		
10 Memory For Objects		
Sum of Subtest SAS's		
Short-Term Memory SAS		
Sum of Area SAS's		

COMPOSITE SCORE *

Test Composite .... ______

Partial Composite .... ______

Partial Composite based on ____________________

	1 2 3 4 5	
Attention		
a) Absorbed by task		Easily distracted
Reactions During Test Performance		
a) Normal activity level		Abnormal activity level
b) Initiates activity		Waits to be told
c) Quick to respond		Urging needed
Emotional Independence		
a) Socially confident		Insecure
b) Realistically self-confident		Distrusts own ability
c) Comfortable in adult company		Ill-at-ease
d) Assured		Anxious
Problem-Solving Behavior		
a) Persistent		Gives up easily
b) Reacts to failure realistically		Reacts to failure unrealistically
c) Eager to continue		Seeks to terminate
d) Challenged by hard tasks		Prefers only easy tasks
Independence of Examiner Support		
a) Needs minimum of commendation		Needs constant praise and encouragement
Expressive Language		
a) Excellent articulation		Very poor articulation
Receptive Language		
a) Excellent sound discrimination		Very poor sound discrimination
Was it difficult to establish rapport with this person? Easy		Difficult

*** Be sure that all Standard Age Scores (SAS's) are based on the tables in the *Guide* with the number 9-74502 on the cover.**

The Riverside Publishing Company

Robert L. Thorndike
Elizabeth P. Hagen
Jerome M. Sattler

Figure 16-16. Stanford-Binet Intelligence Scale Record Booklet . *Reprinted with permission of The Riverside Publishing Company from the Stanford-Binet Intelligence Scale Technical Manual: Fourth Edition by R. L. Thorndike, E. P. Hagen, and J. M. Sattler. The Riverside Publishing Company, 8420 W. Bryn Mawr Avenue, Chicago, IL 60631, 1986.*

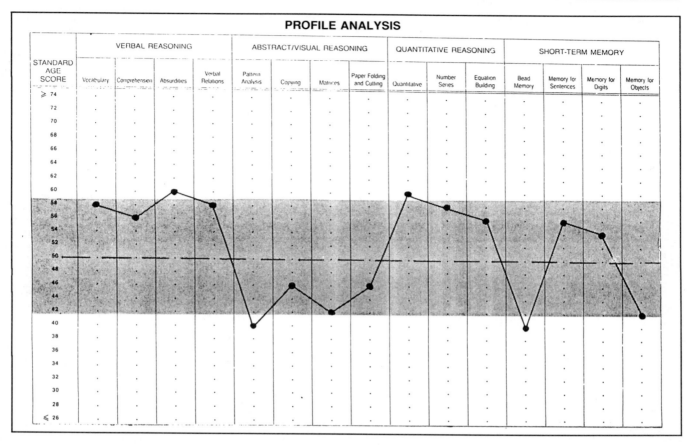

Figure 16-17. Stanford-Binet Profile Analysis. *Reprinted with permission of The Riverside Publishing Company from the Stanford-Binet Intelligence Scale Technical Manual: Fourth Edition by R. L. Thorndike, E. P. Hagen, and J. M. Sattler, The Riverside Publishing Company, 8420 W. Bryn Mawr Avenue, Chicago, IL 60631, 1986.*

References

Kaufman, A. S., & Kaufman, N. L. (1983). *Kaufman assessment battery for children—Interpretive manual*. Circle Pines, MN: American Guidance Service.

King-Thomas, L., & Hacker, B. J. (1987). *A therapist's guide to pediatric assessment*. Boston: Little, Brown and Company.

McGourty, L., Foto, M., Marvin, J., Smith, N., Smith, R., & Kronsnoble, S. (1989). *Uniform terminology for occupational therapy*, (2nd Edition). Rockville, MD: American Occupational Therapy Association.

Sattler, J. (1982). *Assessment of children's intelligence and special abilities*, (2nd Edition). Boston, (2nd Edition). Allyn and Bacon, Inc.

Sattler, J. (1988). *Assessment of children*, (3rd Edition). San Diego: Jerome M. Sattler Publisher.

Thorndike, R. L., Hagen, E. P., & Sattler, J. M. (1986). *Technical Manual, Stanford-Binet Intelligence Scale*, (4th Edition). Chicago: The Riverside Publishing Company.

Wechsler, D. (1974). Manual for the Wechsler intelligence scale for children, (Revised). San Antonio, TX: The Psychological Corporation.

Wodrich, D. L. (1986). The terminology and purposes of assessment. In D. L. Wodrich & J. E. Joy (Ed.), *Multidisciplinary assessment of children with learning disabilities and mental retardation*, (p. 2, 24). Baltimore: Paul H. Brookes Publishing Co.

Wodrich, D. L., & Joy, J. E. (1986). *Multidisciplinary assessment of children with learning disabilities and mental retardation*. Baltimore: Paul H. Brookes Publishing Co.

Woodcock, R. W., & Johnson, M. B. (1977). *Woodcock-Johnson psycho-educational battery*. Allen, TX: DLM Teaching Resources.

Appendices

Uniform Terminology for Occupational Therapy—Second Edition

Uniform Terminology for Occupational Therapy—Second Edition delineates and defines OCCUPATIONAL PERFORMANCE AREAS and OCCUPATIONAL PERFORMANCE COMPONENTS that are addressed in occupational therapy direct service. These definitions are provided to facilitate the uniform use of terminology and definitions throughout the profession. The original document, *Occupational Therapy Product Output Reporting System and Uniform Terminology for Reporting Occupational Therapy Services*, which was published in 1979, helped create a base of consistent terminology that was used in many of the official documents of The American Occupational Therapy Association, Inc. (AOTA), in occupational therapy education curricula, and in a variety of occupational therapy practice settings. In order to remain current with practice, the first document was revised over a period of several years with extensive feedback from the profession. The revisions were completed in 1988. It is recognized and recommended that a document of this nature be updated periodically so that occupational therapy is defined in accordance with current theory and practice.

GUIDELINES FOR USE

Uniform Terminology—Second Edition may be used in a variety of ways. It defines occupational therapy practice, which includes OCCUPATIONAL PERFORMANCE AREAS and OCCUPATIONAL PERFORMANCE COMPONENTS. In addition, it will be useful to occupational therapists for (a) documentation, (b) charge systems, (c) education, (d) program development, (e) marketing, and (f) research. Examples of how OCCUPATIONAL PERFORMANCE AREAS and OCCUPATIONAL PERFORMANCE COMPONENTS translate into practice are provided below. It is not the intent of this document to define specific occupational therapy programs nor specific occupational therapy interventions. Some examples of the differences between OCCUPATIONAL PERFORMANCE AREAS and OCCUPATIONAL PERFORMANCE COMPONENTS and programs and interventions are

1. An individual who is injured on the job may be able to return to work, which is an OCCUPATIONAL PERFORMANCE AREA. In order to achieve the outcome of returning to work, the individual may need to address specific PERFORMANCE COMPONENTS such as strength, endurance, and time management. The oc-cupational therapist, in cooperation with the vocational team, utilizes planned interventions to achieve the desired outcome. These interventions may include activities such as an exercise program, body mechanics instruction, and job modification, and may be provided in a work-hardening program.

2. An individual with severe physical limitations may need and desire the opportunity to live within a community-integrated setting, which represents the OCCUPATIONAL PERFORMANCE AREAS of activities of daily living and work. In order to achieve the outcome of community living, the individual may need to address specific PERFORMANCE COMPONENTS, such as normalizing muscle tone, gross motor coordination, postural control, and self-management. The occupational therapist, in cooperation with the team, utilizes planned interventions to achieve the desired outcome. Interventions may include neuromuscular facilitation, object manipulation, instruction in use of adaptive equipment, use of environmental control systems, and functional positioning for eating. These interventions may be provided in a community-based independent living program.

3. A child with learning disabilities may need to perform educational activities within a public school setting. Since learning is a student's work, this educational activity would be considered the OCCUPATIONAL PERFORMANCE AREA for this individual. In order to achieve the educational outcome of efficient and effective completion of written classroom work, the child may need to address specific OCCUPATIONAL PERFORMANCE COMPONENTS, including sensory processing, perceptual skills, postural control, and motor skills. The occupational therapist, in cooperation with the team, utilizes planned interventions to achieve the desired outcome. Interventions may include activities such as adapting the student's seating to improve postural control and stability and practicing motor control and coordination. This program could be provided by school district personnel or through contracted services.

4. An infant with cerebral palsy may need to participate in developmental activities to engage in the OCCUPATIONAL PERFORMANCE AREAS of activities of daily living and play. The developmental outcomes may be achieved by addressing specific PERFORMANCE COMPONENTS such as sensory awareness and neu-

romuscular control. The occupational therapist, in cooperation with the team, utilizes planned interventions to achieve the desired outcomes. Interventions may include activities such as seating and positioning for play, neuromuscular facilitation techniques to enable eating, and parent training. These interventions may be provided in a home-based occupational therapy program.

5. An adult with schizophrenia may need and desire to live independently in the community, which represents the OCCUPATIONAL PERFORMANCE AREAS of activities of daily living, work activities, and play or leisure activities. The specific OCCUPATIONAL PERFORMANCE AREAS may be medication routine, functional mobility, home management, vocational exploration, play or leisure performance, and social skills. In order to achieve the outcome of living alone, the individual may need to address specific PERFORMANCE COMPONENTS such as topographical orientation, memory, categorization, problem solving, interests, social conduct, and time management. The occupational therapist, in cooperation with the team, utilizes planned interventions to achieve the desired outcome. Interventions may include activities such as training in the use of public transportation, instruction in budgeting skills, selection of and participation in social activities, and instruction in social conduct. These interventions may be provided in a community-based mental health program.

6. An individual who abuses substances may need to reestablish family roles and responsibilities, which represents the OCCUPATIONAL PERFORMANCE AREAS of activities of daily living and work. In order to achieve the outcome of family participation, the individual may need to address the PERFORMANCE COMPONENTS of roles, values, social conduct, self-expression, coping skills, and self-control. The occupational therapist, in cooperation with the team, utilizes planned intervention to achieve the desired outcomes. Interventions may include role and value clarification exercises, role-playing, instruction in stress management techniques, and parenting skills. These interventions may be provided in an inpatient acute care unit.

Because of the extensive use of the original document (*Uniform Terminology for Reporting Occupational Therapy Services*, 1979) in official documents, this revision is a second edition and does not completely replace the 1979 version. This follows the practice that other professions, such as medicine, pursue with their documents. Examples are the *Physician's Current Procedural Terminology First–Fourth Editions (CPT 1–4)* and the *Diagnostic and Statistical Manual First–Third Editions (DSM-I–III-R)*. Therefore, this document is presented as *Uniform Terminology for Occupational Therapy—Second Edition*.

BACKGROUND

Task Force Charge

In 1983, the Representative Assembly of the American Occupational Therapy Association charged the Commission on Practice to form a task force to revise the *Occupational Therapy Product Output Reporting System and Uniform Terminology for Reporting Occupational Therapy Services*. The document had been approved by the Representative Assembly in 1979 and needed to be updated to reflect current practice.

Background Information

The *Occupational Therapy Product Output Reporting System and Uniform Terminology for Reporting Occupational Therapy Services* (hereafter to be referred to as *Product Output Reporting System* or *Uniform Terminology*) document was originally developed in response to the Medicare-Medicaid Anti-Fraud and Abuse Amendments of 1977 (Public Law 95–142), which required the Secretary of the Department of Health and Human Services to establish regulations for uniform reporting systems for all departments in hospitals. The AOTA developed the documents in hospitals. The AOTA developed the documents to create a uniform reporting system for occupational therapy departments. Although the Department of Health and Human Services never adopted the system because of antitrust concerns relating to price fixing, occupational therapists have used the documents extensively in the profession.

Three states, Maryland, California, and Washington, have used the *Product Output Reporting System* as a basis for statewide reporting systems. AOTA's official documents have relied on the definitions to create uniformity. Many occupational therapy schools and departments have used the definitions to guide education and documentation. Although the initial need was for reimbursement reporting systems, the profession has used the documents primarily to facilitate uniformity in definitions.

Task Force Formation

In 1983, Linda Kohlman McGourty, a member of the AOTA Commission on Practice, was appointed by the commission's chair, John Farace, to chair the Uniform Terminology Task Force. Initially, a notice was placed in the *Occupational Therapy Newspaper* for people to submit feedback for the revisions. Many responses were received. Before the task force was appointed in 1984, Maryland, California, and Washington adopted reimbursement systems based on the *Product Output Reporting System*. Therefore, to increase the quantity and quality of input for the revisions, it was decided to postpone the formation of the task force until these states had had an opportunity to use the systems.

In 1985, a second notice was placed in the *Occupational Therapy News* requesting feedback, and a task force was appointed. The following people were selected to serve on the task force:

Linda Kohlman McGourty, MOT, OTR, Washington (Chair)
Roger Smith, MOT, OTR, Wisconsin
Jane Marvin, OTR, California
Nancy Mahon Smith, MBA, OTR, Maryland and Arkansas
Mary Foto, OTR, California

These people were selected based on the following criteria:

1. Geographical representation
2. Professional expertise
3. Participation in other current AOTA projects

4. Knowledge of reimbursement systems
5. Interest in serving on the task force

Development of the Uniform Terminology—Second Edition

The task force met in 1986 and 1987 to develop drafts of the revisions. A draft from the task force was submitted to the Commission on Practice in May of 1987. Listed below are several decisions that were made in the revision process by the task force and the Commission on Practice.

1. To not replace the original document (*Uniform Terminology for Reporting Occupational Therapy Services*, 1979) because of the number of official documents based on it and the need to retain a *Product Output Reporting System* as an official document of the AOTA.
2. To limit the revised document to defining OCCUPATIONAL PERFORMANCE AREAS and OCCUPATIONAL PERFORMANCE COMPONENTS for occupational therapy intervention (i.e., indirect services were deleted and the *Product Output Reporting System* was not revised) to make the project manageable.
3. To coordinate the revision process with other current AOTA projects such as the Professional and Technical Role Analysis (PATRA) and the Occupational Therapy Comprehensive Functional Assessment of the American Occupational Therapy Foundation (AOTF).
4. To develop a document that reflects current areas of practice and facilitates uniformity of definitions in the profession.
5. To recommend that the AOTA develop a companion document to define techniques, modalities, and activities used in occupational therapy intervention and a document to define specific programs that are offered by occupational therapy departments. The Commission on Practice subsequently developed educational materials to assist in the application of uniform terminology to practice.

Several drafts of the revised *Uniform Terminology—Second Edition* document were reviewed by appropriate AOTA commissions and committees and by a selected review network based on geographical representation, professional expertise, and demonstrated leadership in the field. Excellent responses were received, and the feedback was incorporated into the final document by the Commission on Practice.

OUTLINE

OCCUPATIONAL THERAPY ASSESSMENT

OCCUPATIONAL THERAPY INTERVENTION

I. OCCUPATIONAL THERAPY PERFORMANCE AREAS
  A. Activities of Daily Living
    1. Grooming
    2. Oral Hygiene
    3. Bathing
    4. Toilet Hygiene
    5. Dressing
    6. Feeding and Eating
    7. Medication Routine
    8. Socialization
    9. Functional Communication
    10. Functional Mobility
    11. Sexual Expression
  B. Work Activities
    1. Home Management
      a. Clothing Care
      b. Cleaning
      c. Meal Preparation and Cleanup
      d. Shopping
      e. Money Management
      f. Household Maintenance
      g. Safety Procedures
    2. Care of Others
    3. Educational Activities
    4. Vocational Activities
      a. Vocational Exploration
      b. Job Acquisition
      c. Work or Job Performance
      d. Retirement Planning
  C. Play or Leisure Activities
    1. Play or Leisure Exploration
    2. Play or Leisure Performance

II. PERFORMANCE COMPONENTS
  A. Sensory Motor Component
    1. Sensory Integration
      a. Sensory Awareness
      b. Sensory Processing
        (1) Tactile
        (2) Proprioceptive
        (3) Vesticular
        (4) Visual
        (5) Auditory
        (6) Gustatory
        (7) Olfactory
      c. Perceptual Skills
        (1) Stereognosis
        (2) Kinesthesia
        (3) Body Scheme
        (4) Right–Left Discrimination
        (5) Form Constancy
        (6) Position in Space
        (7) Visual Closure
        (8) Figure–Ground
        (9) Depth Perception
        (10) Topographical Orientation
    2. Neuromuscular
      a. Reflex
      b. Range of Motion
      c. Muscle Tone
      d. Strength
      e. Endurance
      f. Postural Control
      g. Soft Tissue Integrity
    3. Motor
      a. Activity Tolerance
      b. Gross Motor Coordination
      c. Crossing the Midline
      d. Laterality

    e. Bilateral Integration
    f. Praxis
    g. Fine Motor Coordination/Dexterity
    h. Visual-Motor Integration
    i. Oral-Motor Control
  B. Cognitive Integration and Cognitive Components
    1. Level of Arousal
    2. Orientation
    3. Recognition
    4. Attention Span
    5. Memory
      a. Short-Term
      b. Long-Term
      c. Remote
      d. Recent
    6. Sequencing
    7. Categorization
    8. Concept Formation
    9. Intellectual Operations in Space
   10. Problem Solving
   11. Generalization of Learning
   12. Integration of Learning
   13. Synthesis of Learning
  C. Psychosocial Skills and Psychological Components
    1. Psychological
      a. Roles
      b. Values
      c. Interests
      d. Initiation of Activity
      e. Termination of Activity
      f. Self-Concept
    2. Social
      a. Social Conduct
      b. Conversation
      c. Self-Expression
    3. Self-Management
      a. Coping Skills
      b. Time Management
      c. Self-Control

OCCUPATIONAL THERAPY ASSESSMENT

Assessment is the planned process of obtaining, interpreting, and documenting the functional status of the individual. The purpose of the assessment is to identify the individual's abilities and limitations, including deficits, delays, or maladaptive behavior that can be addressed in occupational therapy intervention. Data can be gathered through a review of records, observation, interview, and the administration of test procedures. Such procedures include, but are not limited to, the use of standardized tests, questionnaires, performance checklists, activities, and tasks designed to evaluate specific performance abilities.

OCCUPATIONAL THERAPY INTERVENTION

Occupational therapy addresses function and uses specific procedures and activities to (a) develop, maintain, improve, and/or restore the performance of necessary functions; (b) compensate for dysfunction; (c) minimize or prevent debilitation; and/or (d) promote health and wellness. Categories

of function are defined as OCCUPATIONAL PERFORMANCE AREAS and PERFORMANCE COMPONENTS. OCCUPATIONAL PERFORMANCE AREAS include activities of daily living, work activities, and play/leisure activities. Performance components refer to the functional abilities required for occupational performance, including sensory motor, cognitive, and psychological components. Deficits or delays in these OCCUPATIONAL PERFORMANCE AREAS may be addressed by occupational therapy intervention.

I. OCCUPATIONAL PERFORMANCE AREAS
  A. Activities of Daily Living
    1. *Grooming*—Obtain and use supplies to shave; apply and remove cosmetics; wash, comb, style, and brush hair; care for nails; care for skin; and apply deodorant.
    2. *Oral Hygiene*—Obtain and use supplies; clean mouth and teeth; remove, clean, and reinsert dentures.
    3. *Bathing*—Obtain and use supplies; soap, rinse, and dry all body parts; maintain bathing position; transfer to and from bathing position.
    4. *Toilet Hygiene*—Obtain and use supplies; clean self; transfer to and from, and maintain toileting position on, bedpan, toilet, or commode.
    5. *Dressing*—Select appropriate clothing; obtain clothing from storage area; dress and undress in a sequential fashion; and fasten and adjust clothing and shoes. Don and doff assistive or adaptive equipment, prostheses, or orthoses.
    6. *Feeding and Eating*—Set up food; use appropriate utensils and tableware; bring food or drink to mouth; suck, masticate, cough, and swallow.
    7. *Medication Routine*—Obtain medication; open and close containers; and take prescribed quantities as scheduled.
    8. *Socialization*—Interact in appropriate contextual and cultured ways.
    9. *Functional Communication*—Use equipment or systems to enhance or provide communication, such as writing equipment, telephones, typewriters, communication boards, call lights, emergency systems, braille writers, augmentative communication systems, and computers.
   10. *Functional Mobility*—Move from one position or place to another, such as in bed mobility, wheelchair mobility, transfers (bed, car, tub, toilet, chair), and functional ambulation, with or without adaptive aids, driving, and use of public transportation.
   11. *Sexual Expression*—Recognize, communicate, and perform desired sexual activities.
  B. Work Activities
    1. *Home Management*
      a. *Clothing Care*—Obtain and use supplies, launder, iron, store, and mend.
      b. *Cleaning*—Obtain and use supplies, pick up, vacuum, sweep, dust, scrub, mop, make bed, and remove trash.
      c. *Meal Preparation and Cleanup*—Plan nutritious meals and prepare food; open and close containers, cabinets, and drawers; use kitchen

utensils and appliances; and clean up and store food.

   d. *Shopping*—Select and purchase items and perform money transactions.

   e. *Money Management*—Budget, pay bills, and use bank systems.

   f. *Household Maintenance*—Maintain home, yard, garden appliances, and household items, and/or obtain appropriate assistance.

   g. *Safety Procedures*—Know and perform prevention and emergency procedures to maintain a safe environment and prevent injuries.

2. *Care of Others*—Provide for children, spouse, parents, or others, such as the physical care, nurturance, communication, and use of age-appropriate activities.

3. *Educational Activities*—Participate in a school environment and school-sponsored activities (such as field trips, work-study, and extracurricular activities).

4. *Vocational Activities*

   a. *Vocational Exploration*—Determine aptitudes, interests, skills, and appropriate vocational pursuits.

   b. *Job Acquisition*—Identify and select work opportunities and complete application and interview processes.

   c. *Work or Job Performance*—Perform job tasks in a timely and effective manner, incorporating necessary work behaviors such as grooming, interpersonal skills, punctuality, and adherence to safety procedures.

   d. *Retirement Planning*—Determine aptitudes, interests, skills, and identify appropriate avocational pursuits.

C. Play or Leisure Activities

1. *Play or Leisure Exploration*—Identify interests, skills, opportunities, and appropriate play or leisure activities.

2. *Play or Leisure Performance*—Participate in play or leisure activities, using physical and psychosocial skills.

   a. Maintain a balance of play or leisure activities with work and activities of daily living.

   b. Obtain, utilize, and maintain equipment and supplies.

II. PERFORMANCE COMPONENTS

A. Sensory Motor Component

1. *Sensory Integration*

   a. *Sensory Awareness*—Receive and differentiate sensory stimuli.

   b. *Sensory Processing*—Interpret sensory stimuli.

     (1) *Tactile*—Interpret light touch, pressure, temperature, pain, vibration, and two-point stimuli through skin contact/receptors.

     (2) *Proprioceptive*—Interpret stimuli originating in muscles, joints, and other internal tissues to give information about the position of one body part in relationship to another.

     (3) *Vestibular*—Interpret stimuli from the inner ear receptors regarding head position and movement.

     (4) *Visual*—Interpret stimuli through the eyes, including peripheral vision and acuity, awareness of color, depth, and figure-ground.

     (5) *Auditory*—Interpret sounds, localize sounds, and discriminate background sounds.

     (6) *Gustatory*—Interpret tastes.

     (7) *Olfactory*—Interpret odors.

   c. *Perceptual Skills*

     (1) *Stereognosis*—Identify objects through the sense of touch.

     (2) *Kinesthesia*—Identify the excursion and direction of joint movement.

     (3) *Body Scheme*—Acquire an internal awareness of the body and the relationship of body parts to each other.

     (4) *Right–Left Discrimination*—Differentiate one side of the body from the other.

     (5) *Form Constancy*—Recognize forms and objects as the same in various environments, positions, and sizes.

     (6) *Position in Space*—Determine the spatial relationship of figures and objects to self or other forms and objects.

     (7) *Visual Closure*—Identify forms or objects from incomplete presentations.

     (8) *Figure–Ground*—Differentiate between foreground and background forms and objects.

     (9) *Depth Perception*—Determine the relative distance between objects, figures, or landmarks and the observer.

     (10) *Topographical Orientation*—Determine the location of objects and settings and the route to the location.

2. *Neuromuscular*

   a. *Reflex*—Present an involuntary muscle response elicited by sensory input.

   b. *Range of Motion*—Move body parts through an arc.

   c. *Muscle tone*—Demonstrate a degree of tension or resistance in a muscle.

   d. *Strength*—Demonstrate a degree of muscle power when movement is resisted as with weight or gravity.

   e. *Endurance*—Sustain cardiac, pulmonary, and musculoskeletal exertion over time.

   f. *Postural Control*—Position and maintain head, neck, trunk, and limb alignment with appropriate weight shifting, midline orientation, and righting reactions for function.

   g. *Soft Tissue Integrity*—Maintain anatomical and physiological condition of interstitial tissue and skin.

3. *Motor*
   a. *Activity Tolerance*—Sustain a purposeful activity over time.
   b. *Gross Motor Coordination*—Use large muscle groups for controlled movements.
   c. *Crossing the Midline*—Move limbs and eyes across the sagittal plane of the body.
   d. *Laterality*—Use a preferred unilateral body part for activities requiring a high level of skill.
   e. *Bilateral Integration*—Interact with both body sides in a coordinated manner during activity.
   f. *Praxis*—Conceive and plan a new motor act in response to an environmental demand.
   g. *Fine Motor Coordination/Dexterity*—Use small muscle groups for controlled movements, particularly in object manipulation.
   h. *Visual-Motor Integration*—Coordinate the interaction of visual information with body movement during activity.
   i. *Oral-Motor Control*—Coordinate oropharyngeal musculature for controlled movements.

B. Cognitive Integration and Cognitive Components
   1. *Level of Arousal*—Demonstrate alertness and responsiveness to environmental stimuli.
   2. *Orientation*—Identify person, place, time, and situation.
   3. *Recognition*—Identify familiar faces, objects, and other previously presented materials.
   4. *Attention Span*—Focus on a task over time.
   5. *Memory*
      a. *Short-Term*—Recall information for brief periods of time.
      b. *Long-Term*—Recall information for long periods of time.
      c. *Remote*—Recall events from distant past.
      d. *Recent*—Recall events from immediate past.
   6. *Sequencing*—Place information, concepts, and actions in order.
   7. *Categorization*—Identify similarities of and differences between environmental information.
   8. *Concept Formation*—Organize a variety of information to form thoughts and ideas.
   9. *Intellectual Operations in Space*—Mentally manipulate spatial relationships.
   10. *Problem Solving*—Recognize a problem, define a problem, identify alternative plans, select a plan, organize steps in a plan, implement a plan, and evaluate the outcome.
   11. *Generalization of Learning*—Apply previously learned concepts and behaviors to similar situations.
   12. *Integration of Learning*—Incorporate previously acquired concepts and behavior into a variety of new situations.
   13. *Synthesis of Learning*—Restructure previously learned concepts and behaviors into new patterns.

C. Psychosocial Skills and Psychological Components
   1. *Psychological*
      a. *Roles*—Identify functions one assumes or acquires in society (e.g., worker, student, parent, church member).
      b. *Values*—Identify ideas or beliefs that are intrinsically important.
      c. *Interests*—Identify mental or physical activities that create pleasure and maintain attention.
      d. *Initiation of Activity*—Engage in a physical or mental activity.
      e. *Termination of Activity*—Stop an activity at an appropriate time.
      f. *Self-Concept*—Develop value of physical and emotional self.
   2. *Social*
      a. *Social Conduct*—Interact using manners, personal space, eye contact, gestures, active listening, and self-expression appropriate to one's environment.
      b. *Conversation*—Use verbal and nonverbal communication to interact in a variety of settings.
      c. *Self-Expression*—Use a variety of styles and skills to express thoughts, feelings, and needs.
   3. *Self-Management*
      a. *Coping Skills*—Identify and manage stress and related reactors.
      b. *Time Management*—Plan and participate in a balance of self-care, work, leisure, and rest activities to promote satisfaction and health.
      c. *Self-Control*—Modulate and modify one's own behavior in response to environmental needs, demands, and constraints.

References

American Medical Association. (1966–1988). *Physicians' current procedural terminology first–fourth editions (CPT 1–4)*. Chicago: Author.

American Occupational Therapy Association. (1979). *Occupational therapy output reporting system and uniform terminology for reporting occupational therapy services*. Rockville, MD: Author.

American Psychiatric Association. (1952–1987). *Diagnostic and statistical manual of mental disorders first–third editions (DSM-I-III-R)*. Washington, DC: Author.

Medicare–Medicaid Anti-Fraud and Abuse Amendments (Public Law 95–142). (1977), 42 U.S.C. §1305.

Prepared by the Uniform Terminology Task Force (Linda Kohlman McGourty, MOT, OTR, Chair, and Mary Foto, OTR, Jane K. Marvin, MA, OTR, CIRS, Nancy Mahan Smith, MBA, OTR, and Roger O. Smith, MOT, OTR, task force members) and members of the Commission on Practice, with contributions from Susan Kronsnoble, OTR, for the Commission on Practice (L. Randy Strickland, EdD, OTR, FAOTA, Chair).

Approved by the Representative Assembly April 1989).

Guidelines for Occupational Therapy Documentation

Guidelines for Occupational Therapy Documentation

These guidelines are provided to assist members of the American Occupational Therapy Association (AOTA) in documenting occupational therapy services. Occupational therapy personnel shall document the type and frequency of services provided within the time frames established by facilities, government agencies, and accreditation organizations.

The purpose of documentation is to do the following:

1. Provide a serial and legal record of the patient's condition and the course of therapeutic intervention from admission to discharge.
2. Serve as an information source for patient care.
3. Facilitate communication among health care professionals who contribute to the patient's care.
4. Furnish data for use in treatment, education, research, and reimbursement.

Types of Documentation

The various types of documentation are

1. initial note
2. assessment notes and reports
3. treatment plans and goals
4. progress notes
5. treatment records
6. discharge summaries
7. consultation reports
8. special reports (e.g., referrals to other programs and agencies, summary reports for legal reasons, home programs, and correspondence)
9. critical incidence reports or notes

Table 1
Components of Total Occupational Therapy or Facility Record for Each Patient

CONTENT	CLARIFICATION
A. Identification and Background Information	
1. Name, age, sex, date of admission, treatment diagnosis, and date of onset of current diagnosis.	Name may be omitted depending on the facility and department policies and procedures.
2. Referral source, services requested, and date of referral to occupational therapy.	Include who requested occupational therapy services, what specific services were requested, and the date.
3. Pertinent history that indicates prior levels of function and support systems.	Include applicable developmental, educational, vocational, socioeconomic, and medical history (may be brief).
4. Secondary problems or preexisting conditions.	Include any additional problems or conditions that may affect patient function or treatment outcomes.
5. Precautions and contraindications.	May be identified by referral source or occupational therapy staff.
B. Assessment and Reassessment	
Refer to the Uniform Occupational Therapy Checklist (AOTA, 1979) for specific skills and performance.	Independent living/daily living skills and performance components
	Sensorimotor skills and performance components
	Cognitive skills and performance components
	Psychosocial skills and performance components
	Therapeutic adaptations and prevention
1. Tests and evaluations administered and the results.	State name and type of evaluation, date administered, and results, and whether assessment or reassessment.
2. Summary and analysis of assessment findings.	State facts in an objective manner. Analysis of objective findings should include measurable data to define the patient's assets and deficits.
3. References to other pertinent reports and information.	Include any additional sources of data or evaluation results that help formulate the total assessment of the patient.
4. Occupational therapy problem list.	This list should be compatible with a master problem list developed by the health care team or other health care professionals (when available).
5. Recommendations for occupational therapy services.	State whether occupational therapy services are recommended or not.
C. Treatment Planning	
1. Short- and long-term goals.	Define clearly the goals established by the patient, family, and therapist. These goals should be measurable and related to the occupational therapy problem list.
2. Activities and/or treatment procedures.	State clearly the specific methods to be used in the intervention and relate the methods to the problems identified on the occupational therapy problem list.
3. Type, amount, and frequency of treatment.	State skill and performance areas to be addressed and estimate the number, duration, and frequency of treatment sessions to accomplish goals.
4. Anticipated time to achieve goals.	State the anticipated number of therapy sessions or days of therapy to reach the desired outcome. This information may be an overall statement not necessarily written for each goal.
5. Statement of potential functional outcome.	State the anticipated outcome and clearly relate it to the long-term goals.

D. Treatment Implementation

1. Activities, procedures, and modalities used.	State the specific media and methods used.
2. Patient's response to treatment and the progress toward goal attainment as related to problem list.	State the patient's physical and behavioral response to therapy and whether the goals are being achieved.
3. Goal modification when indicated by the response to treatment.	If the goals have been modified in the treatment process, state the new goals and rationale for changes.
4. Change in anticipated time to achieve goals.	If for any reason the treatment time frame is altered, include the reason for the change and the new anticipated time frame.
5. Attendance and participation with treatment plan (attendance could be a check format).	State if the patient is following through with treatment plan.
6. Statement of reason for patient missing treatment.	Write the reasons for treatment not occurring as scheduled.
7. Assistive/adaptive equipment, orthotics, and prosthetics if issued or fabricated, and specific instructions for the application and/or use of the item.	State the device, note whether it was fabricated, sold, rented, or loaned, and state the effectiveness of the device.
8. Patient-related conferences and communication.	If occupational therapy personnel participated in a conference or made a pertinent contact with a family member, agency, or health care professional, state this information with a brief summary of the conference or communication.
9. Home programs.	Include a copy of the home program as established with the patient in the patient record.

E. Discontinuation of Services

1. Summary of assessment and treatment implementation.	State clearly and concisely a summary of the total occupational therapy intervention process, the number of sessions, the goals achieved, and the functional outcome. Compare the initial and discharge status.
2. Home programs.	Include the actual written home program that is to be followed after discharge.
3. Follow-up plans.	State the schedule and specific plans.
4. Recommendations.	State any recommendations pertaining to the patient's future needs.
5. Referral(s) to other health care providers and community agencies.	Make referral(s) or recommendations for referral(s) when additional or new services are needed.

Protocol for Documentation

Each patient referred to occupational therapy must have a case record maintained as a permanent file. The record should be

1. organized
2. legible
3. concise
4. clear
5. accurate
6. complete
7. current
8. objective (clear distinction made between facts and opinions)
9. correct in grammar and spelling

Fundamental Elements of Documentation

The following ten elements should be present:

1. patient's full name and case number on each page of documentation;
2. date stated as month, day, and year for each entry;
3. identification of type of documentation and department name;
4. signature with a minimum of first name, last name, and professional designation;
5. signature of the recorder directly at the end of the note without space left between the body of the note and the signature;
6. countersignature by a registered occupational therapist (OTR) on documentation written by students and certified occupational therapy assistants (COTA) if required by law or the facility;
7. compliance with confidentiality standards;
8. acceptable terminology as defined by the facility;
9. facility approved abbreviations;
10. errors corrected by drawing a single line through an error, and the correction initialed (liquid correction fluid and erasures are not acceptable), or facility requirements followed.

Content of Documentation

The following components should be included in the total occupational therapy or facility record for each patient (see Table 1). Each occupational therapy department must determine the type and frequency of documentation and must abide by the written policies and procedures of the individual facility.

Reference

American Occupational Therapy Association. (1979). *Uniform terminology for reporting occupational services*. Rockville, MD: Author.

Related Readings

Discharge planning policy and procedure manual. (Available from Spain Rehabilitation Center, University of Alabama Hospitals, 619 South 19th Street, Birmingham, AL 35233.)

Forms and procedures for documentation of occupational therapy services. (Available from Northwest Hospital, Occupational Therapy Department, 1551 North 120th, Seattle, WA 98133.)

Hopkins, H. L., & Smith, H. D. (1983). *Willard and Spackman's occupational therapy* (6th ed.). Philadelphia: Lippincott. (pp. 312–313, 774–775, 823–824, 864)

I'm glad you asked. (1983, October). *Occupational Therapy Newspaper*, p. 13.

Inaba, M., & Jones, S. (1977). Medical documentation for third-party payers. *Physical Therapy, 57*(7), 791–794.

Joint Commission on Accreditation of Hospitals. (1983). *Consolidated standards manual/83: for child, adolescent, and adult psychiatric, alcoholism, and drug abuse facilities*. (Available from author, 875 North Michigan Avenue, Chicago, IL 60611.)

Joint Commission on Accreditation of Hospitals. (1984a). *Accreditation manual for hospitals—1984*. (Available from author, 875 North Michigan Avenue, Chicago, IL 60611.)

Joint Commission on Accreditation of Hospitals. (1984b). *Accreditation manual for long-term care facilities*. (Available from author, 875 North Michigan Avenue, Chicago, IL 60611.)

Kuntavanish, A. (1980). *Occupational therapy documentation guidelines handout*. (Available from Greater Southeast Community Hospital, 1310 Southern Avenue, SE, Washington, DC 20032.)

Llorens, L. A., & Shuster, J. J. (1977). Occupational therapy sequential client care recording system: A comparative study. *American Journal of Occupational Therapy, 31*(6), 367–371.

Occupational therapy department progress note requirements. (1984). (Available from Haverford State Hospital, 3500 Darby Road, Haverford, PA 19041.)

Occupational therapy—Documentation procedures. (Available from Saint Bernadine Hospital, 2101 North Waterman Avenue, San Bernardino, CA 92404.)

Occupational therapy. Guidelines for utilization of specialized rehabilitation services in home health agencies. (1976). (Available from Task Force of the Home Health Agency Assembly of New Jersey, Inc., and New Jersey Occupational Therapy Association, PO Box 773, Union, NJ 07083.)

Occupational therapy—Policies and procedures for documentation. (Available from Michael Reese Hospital and Medical Center, 2929 South Ellis Avenue, Chicago, IL 60616.)

Occupational therapy treatment documentation for inpatients and outpatients 1983. (1983). (Available from Providence Hospital, PO Box 1067, Everett, WA 98206.)

Standards for services for developmentally disabled individuals. (1984). (Available from Accreditation Council for Services for Mentally Retarded and Other Developmentally Disabled Persons, 5101 Wisconsin Avenue, NW, Washington, DC 20016.)

Standards manual for facilities serving people with disabilities, 1982. (1982). (Available from Commission on Accreditation of Rehabilitation Facilities, 2500 North Pantano Road, Tucson, AZ 85715.)

Standards of practice for occupational therapy services. In *Division policy and procedures manual.* (Available from John F. Marr Division, Saint Elizabeth's Hospital, 2700 Martin Luther King, Jr. Avenue, SE, Washington, DC 20032.)

Steffli, B. M., & Eide, I. (1978). *Discharge planning handbook.* Thorofare, NJ: Charles B. Slack.

Prepared by the Documentation Task Force (Linda Kohlman McGourty, MOT, OTR, chair, Mary Foto, OTR, Susan Kronsnoble, OTR, Carole Lossing, OTR, Sharon Rask, OTR, and Christine de Renne Stephan, OTR) for the Commission on Practice (Esther Bell, MA, OTR, FAOTA, chair).

Approved by the Representative Assembly April 1986.

NOTE: From "Guidelines for Occupational Therapy Documentation" by the AOTA Documentation Task Force (Linda Kohlman McGourty, Chair), 1986, <u>American Journal of Occupational Therapy</u>, <u>40</u>: 830–832. Copyright 1986 by AOTA. Reprinted by permission.

Individualized Educational Plans

The first one is computer generated.
The second one is a traditional format.
The key features of the IEP are marked as follows:

1. current levels of performance.
2. annual goals and short term objectives.
3. special education and related services involvement, and the extent of participation in the regular classroom.
4. amount of regular classroom placement.
5. projected dates for initiation and anticipated duration of services.
6. evaluation procedures, criteria and schedules for measuring objectives on at least an annual basis.

```
            INDIVIDUAL EDUCATION PROGRAM (IEP)


      Name:  Laura Riggs
      Chronological age:  6 yrs, 2 mos, 26 da
      Parents:  John & Sally Riggs
                8500 Clay
                Maryville, OK 00000
                (609) 422-7196 (Home)
                (609) 422-7626 (Mom's work)
                (609) 422-6291 (Dad's work)


      Exceptionality:  DD
      School(s):  Trailwood Elementary
      Grade:  1st


      AREA                1     Assessment LEVEL        INDICATOR

      PHYSICAL

      Physical health           normal                  observation
                                                        parent report
      Vision                    passed/no glasses       school nurse
      Hearing                   passed @ 20 decibels    school nurse


      COMMUNICATION
      Speech/language           10%ile (receptive &     TELD
                                expressive

      PSYCH
      Verbal intelligence       40%ile                  WISC-R
      Performance intelligence  35%ile                  WISC-R
      Full scale                35%ile                  WISC-R


      EDUCATIONAL /DEV.
      Total reading             10%ile                  CAT
      Total math                40%ile                  CAT
      Total language            10%ile                  CAT
      Total battery             20%ile                  CAT


      OTHER
      Gross, fine, and visual   10% for CA              Bruininks
      motor skills                                       Oseretsky
      Visual percept            2y 6m DELAY             Beery Test of
                                                        Visual Percep
                                                        (Non-Motor)
```

2   ANNUAL GOALS

1.   Increase reading level
2.   Increase expressive and receptive language
3.   Increase neuromuscular function in the areas of fine, gross and
      visual motor skills to enhance classroom performance and percep-
      tual skills.

      Vocational goals and P.E. have been considered.

3   SERVICES TO BE PROVIDED

Excep Del. Type	Service Provider (First Mid Last)	Min/Days Day	No. /wk	Initiation wks	End Date	Date
S/L	L. Durham	40	2	36	10/26/90	10/26/91
OT	R. Rogis	30	2	36	10/26/90	10/26/91
Reading Spec.	M. Shipley	30	2	36	10/26/90	10/26/91

4 L. Riggs is in the Regular Classroom 80% of the time.

SPECIAL RECOMMENDATIONS:
LAURA SHOULD BE SEATED AT THE FRONT OF THE ROOM TO REDUCE THE AFFECTS
OF HER FUNCTIONAL VISUAL DEFICITS WHEN COPYING FROM THE BOARD. A PEN-
CIL GRIP SHOULD ALSO BE IMPLEMENTED TO IMPROVE PREHENSION PATTERNS.

GOAL 1:   PROGRAMMED BY READING SPECIALIST
GOAL 2:   PROGRAMMED BY SPEECH/LANGUAGE
GOAL 3:   INCREASE NEUROMUSCULAR FUNCTION IN THE AREAS OF FINE, GROSS
AND VISUAL MOTOR SKILLS TO ENHANCE CLASSROOM PERFORMANCE AND PERCEPTUAL
ABILITY.

2 GIVEN DEMONSTRATION STUDENT WILL TANDEM WALK ACROSS AN 3 FT BALANCE BEAM
WITH NOT MORE THAN 2 MISSTEPS, 8 OF 10 TRIALS, 5 INTERMITTENT SESSIONS.

     Baseline: 0/10 Date 9/20/90   Provider_____
6 Target: 8/10 Date 1/26/91
     GIVEN VERBAL INSTRUCTIONS, STUDENT WILL WALK UP/DOWN STAIRS ALTERNATING
     FEET IN REGULAR RHYTHM 10 OF 10 TRIALS, 5 INTERMITTENT SESSIONS

     Baseline: 5/10 Date 9/20/90   Provider_____
     Target: 10/10 Date 5/20/91

     Strategies: GROSS MOTOR

     Materials: Balance beam
                 Stairs
                 Tape

GIVEN VERBAL INSTRUCTION STUDENT WILL BE ABLE TO CUT OUT A 4 INCH
square WITH NOT MORE THAN 3, 1/2 INCH ERRORS, 4 OF 5 TRAILS, 5
INTERMITTENT SESSIONS.

     Baseline: 0/5   Date 9/20/90   Provider: _____
     Target: 4/5   Date 1/26/91

GIVEN VERBAL INSTRUCTIONS AND DEMONSTRATION STUDENT WILL BE ABLE
TO SEPARATE 20 REGULAR SIZED PLAYING CARDS, BY COLOR, INTO TWO
SEPARATE STACKS IN 15 SECS. OR LESS 5 INTERMITTENT SESSIONS.

     Baseline: 8/20   Date 9/27/90   Provider: _____
     Target: 20/20 Date 5/20/91

INDIVIDUAL EDUCATION PROGRAM

STUDENT: _Riggs, Laura_   DATE OF BIRTH: _3/6/84_   PARENT: _John & Sally Riggs_

AGE: _6 yr 2 m_ GRADE: _1st_   ATTENDANCE CENTER: _Trailwood Elementary_   NEW ☒   UP DATE ☐

PRIMARY EXCEPTIONALITY: _developm. delayed_

Summary of Educational Performance/Learner characteristics (strength & weakness):

1

Physical health normal - observation, parent report
Vision - passed, school nurse
Hearing - passed, school nurse
Communication - receptive & expressive 10%ile (TELD)
Psych: full scale 35%ile, Verbal subtest 40%ile, Performance subtest 35% (WISC-R)
Reading 10%ile (CAT); math 40%ile (CAT); Language - 10%ile (CAT)
Gross, fine, & visual motor - 10%ile (Bruininks Oseretsky)
Visual Perception - 2 yr 6 m delay (Test of Visual Perc - non-motor)

Special Educational & Related Services Needed:

3

Speech/Language	40 min/day, 36 weeks (10/26/90 - 10/26/91)
Occupational Therapy	30 min/day, 36 weeks (10/26/90 - 10/26/91)
Reading Specialist	30 min/day, 36 weeks (10/26/90 - 10/26/91)

5 Services to be provided (date & duration):

Annual Goals:

2

1. Increase reading level
2. Increase expressive and receptive language

3. Increase neuromuscular function in the areas of fine, gross and visual motor skills to enhance classroom motor performance and perceptual abilities.

Recommended Daily Schedule:

4

8:30-9:00 Reading Specialist
9:00-11:00 Classroom - math, social studies, gym
11:30-11:40 Speech/Language

12:30-1:00 Occupational Therapy
1:00-3:30 Classroom - writing, reading, recess

Regular classroom 80%

Sally Riggs
John Riggs
(PARENT SIGNATURE)   (DATE)

Parents present at conference   yes (X)   no ( )
When not present, follow up dates _____
_____

Method of follow up _____

	SIGNATURE	POSITION		SIGNATURE	POSITION
1.	Sara Trippe, PhD	Psych	5.	_____ Scott	teacher
2.	Ann Jones, OTR	OT	6.	Will Wright	reading spec
3.	Laura Smith	Speech	7.		
4.	Carl Johnson	Princip.	8.		

NAME: Riggs, Laura

DATE: 10/1/90

I.E.P. FOR YEAR 90-91

ANNUAL GOAL: Increase neuromuscular function in the areas of fine, gross and visual motor skills to enhance classroom motor performance and perceptual abilities

INITIATION DATE	TARGET DATE	SHORT-TERM OBJECTIVES INCLUDING EVALUATION PROCEDURE AND COMPLETION CRITERIA	SPECIAL METHODS AND MATERIALS	REVIEW DATE	COMPLETION DATE	COMMENTS
10/26/90	1/26/91	Given demonstration, student will tandem walk on 8 ft. balance beam with not more than 2 missteps, 8 of 10 trials, 5 intermittent sessions.	balance beam tape	1/26/91		
1/26/91	5/20/91	Given verbal instructions, student will walk up/down stairs alternating feet in regular rhythm 10 of 10 trials, 5 intermittent sessions.	stairs to stage stairs to balcony	5/20/91		
10/26/90	1/26/91	Given demonstration, student will cut out a 4 inch square with not more than 3 errors of 1/2 inch, 4 of 5 trials, 5 intermittent sessions	scissors patterns	1/26/91		
1/26/91	5/20/91	Given demonstration, student will be able to separate 20 regular size playing cards by color into two separate stacks in 30 seconds or less, 5 intermittent sessions.	deck of cards	5/20/91		
1/26/91	5/20/91	Given verbal instructions and demonstration, student will be able to copy ten capital letters from the chalkboard (seated 10 feet from chalkboard, letters each 6" tall) in 30 seconds or less, 5 intermittent sessions	large-rule tablet paper large pencil	5/20/91		
1/26/91	5/20/91	Given clothing with buttons (1/2" or smaller), the student will fasten 4 buttons on own clothing independently in 9 of 10 attempts in 30 seconds.		5/20/91		

D—Sources Relative to Efficacy
E—Resources for Writers

SOURCES RELATIVE TO EFFICACY

American Occupational Therapy Association (1985). Study suggests occupational therapy benefits schizophrenics. *Efficacy Data Brief*, 1(1). Rockville, MD: author.

American Occupational Therapy Association (1986). Occupational therapy found to be among significant predictors of long-term outcomes in spinal cord injury. *Efficacy Data Brief*, 2(1). Rockville, MD: author.

American Occupational Therapy Association (1986). Rehabilitation including occupational therapy improves function, may reduce costs in multiple sclerosis care. *Efficacy Data Brief*, 2(2). Rockville, MD: author.

American Occupational Therapy Association (1986). Elderly treated in special unit including occupational therapy, have more community placements, fewer readmissions. *Efficacy Data Brief*, 2(3). Rockville, MD: author.

American Occupational Therapy Association (1988). Intensive multidisciplinary rehabilitation of stroke patients increases independence, decreases living costs, study shows. *Efficacy Data Brief*, 3(1). Rockville, MD: author.

American Occupational Therapy Association (1988). Stroke patients achieve greater return to independent living in special unit: Role of occupational therapy is noteworthy. *Efficacy Data Brief*, 3(2). Rockville, MD: author.

American Occupational Therapy Association (1988). Outpatient stroke therapy improves functional ability, reduces deterioration, investigation suggests. *Efficacy Data Brief*, 3(3). Rockville, MD: author.

American Occupational Therapy Association (1988). Use of splints and pressure garments is related to decreased incidence of contractures and surgery in burn patients. *Efficacy Data Brief*, 3(4). Rockville, MD: author.

American Occupational Therapy Association (1988). Research supports efficacy of sensory integration procedures. *Efficacy Data Brief*, 3(5). Rockville, MD: author.

Bair, J., & Gwin, C. H. (1985). *A productivity systems guide for occupational therapy*. Rockville, MD: American Occupational Therapy Association.

Joe, B. E., & Ostrow, P. (1987). *Quality assurance monitoring in occupational therapy*. Rockville, MD: American Occupational Therapy Association.

Ostrow, P. C., Williamson, J. W., & Joe, B. E. (1983). *Quality assurance primer*. Rockville, MD: American Occupational Therapy Association.

RESOURCES FOR WRITERS

Baker, S. (1981). *The practical stylist* (5th ed.). New York: Harper & Row.

Bernstein, T. M. (1982). *The careful writer: A modern guide to English usage* (7th ed.). New York: Atheneum.

Manhard, S. J. (1987). *The goof-proofer*. New York: Macmillan Publishing Company.

Strunk, Jr., W. & White, E. B. (1979). *The elements of style*. New York: Macmillian Publishing Company.

SOAP Notes and Problem Oriented Medical Record (non-SOAP)

SOAP Plan of Care

Identifying information:

Date of order:

Date of first contact:

Evaluations administered:

SUBJECTIVE: Pertinent data from the patient. Paraphrase or quote key ideas if possible. The record should be representative of the key communication themes and issues. It is from the perspective of the patient (or family if the patient is unable to communicate). If the patient is unresponsible, state this briefly. It can include, but is not limited to: current complains or symptoms, view of self, patient goals, orientation to the past and present, and self-assessment of abilities and disabilities.

OBJECTIVE: Factual observations and evaluation findings are reported. The information includes evaluation results and functional levels of performance.

ASSESSMENT: This section provides a brief summary or interpretation of the findings from S and O. Do not restate the specific findings from the O section. Professional judgment, based on collected data, leads to the development of a numbered problem list.

PLAN: The plan follows the numbered problem list (every problem listed has a plan). The plan includes the long term goals, the short term goals, and the plan for intervention.

SOAP Plan of Care

Identifying information: *Megan Roberts, a six year old female was thrown from a moving vehicle upon impact, on 6-21-90 sustaining a right subdural hematoma and a fractured right tibia and fibula. The hematoma was surgically evacuated on 6-21-90 and the fractures were set 6-23-89. Patient was non-responsive until 6-26-89.*

Date of order: *6-28-89 A. F. Joe : OT for rehab evaluation and tt.*

Date of first contact: *6-28-89*

Evaluations administered: *chart review, observation, parents interview, cognitive function evaluation, U.E. ROM, sensory awareness screening.*

S: *Patient "no, no, no"*

   Mother: "She's more easily upset today. Had a restless night."

O: *RUE: Active and passive ROM within normal limits (observation).*
   LUE: Marked spasticity/rigidity. Passive ROM within normal limits with inhibition techniques with the exception of elbow extension (-40°).
   Cognitive level IV (Ranchos). Unable to determine tactile, proprioception, or visual processing due to agitation.

A: 1. *Soft tissue integrity deficits © elbow.*
   2. *Muscle tone and reflexes increased © UE*
   3. *Attention span deficits*
   4. *Feeding deficits*

P: 1. *Increase © elbow extension to 0° and maintain © UE PROM*
   2. *Decrease muscle tone and reflex response so that M.R. can purposely reach mouth bilaterally 8 of 10 trials.*
   3. *With a low stimulus environment, increase attention to task to 5 minutes in 4 of 5 tt. sessions.*
   4. *Presented one small serving dish at a time with one food at a time, M.R. will successfully manage finger foods with 100% accuracy during three of four meals.*

                                   Marla Jones, OTR
                                   6-29-90

SOAP Progress Note:

Identifying information:

SUBJECTIVE: (see Plan of Care)

OBJECTIVE: Each numbered problem appears individually, with an update of data from reassessment and observation.

ASSESSMENT: Provide a brief summary of the patient's overall status and limitations. Do not reiterate the findings reported in the O section. List any new problems which are identified, adding them sequentially to the existing problem list.

PLAN: If the patient's condition warrants a continuation of
the current plan, state "Plan continued".   If the patient's
condition warrants a change, state the change clearly.
Changes may be a change in intervention techniques, or simply
a change in treatment frequency, duration, or length.

SOAP Progress Note:

Identifying information: *Megan Roberts*

S: "*nope , go , nope*"
   Mother "*We're exhausted, but she's sleeping a little better. Sometimes I think she knows us.*"

O: 1. *Soft tissue integrity deficit @ elbow improved. PROM = -10° extension.*
   2. *Muscle tone & reflexes increased @ LE - no change. Inhibition required to maintain PROM. Flexor tone predominates.*
   3. *Attention span deficits: During AM tx patient has elicited 3 min attention span for four consecutive days during slow sensory-motor activities (eg. rocking on reach ball).*

A: 4. *Feeding deficits. On 7-6-90 patient reached her mouth with two french fries. (2 of 10 attempts).*
   M. R. continues to function cognitively on Ranchos level IV with some level V behaviors as she begins to interact inconsistently with the environment. A gradual decrease in the intensity of agitation is accompanied by a preference for slow, rhythmic gross motor activities.

P: *Plan continued.*
                              Marla Jones, OTR
                              7-6-90

SOAP Discharge Note:

| Initial   visit:_____ | Final |

visit:_____

| Diagnosis:_____ | Referred |

by:_____

| Referral   date:_____ | Referred |

for:_____

SUBJECTIVE: same as plan of care

OBJECTIVE: Address every problem dealt with during the course
of treatment as described in the progress note section.   Additionally state specifically if the problem was "resolved"
or "not resolved".

ASSESSMENT: List the primary deficits and special circumstances. Briefly state the rehabilitation prognosis.

PLAN: The plan has three parts.   1) Patient discharged to

_____. OR Treatment discontinued due

to _____. 2) Recommendations: i.e.

referrals to other agencies and/or any suggestions to the pa-

tient or family. It may be appropriate to state "none". 3)

Follow-up: State what will be done after

discharge/discontinuation. It can be phone contact, outpa-

tient therapy, or "none".

SOAP Discharge Note: Megan Roberts

Initial visit: _6-28-90_____ Final visit: __9-16-90_____

Diagnosis: _closed head injury_ Referred by: _Dr. F. Joe_____

Referral date: _6-28-90_____ Referred for: _O.T. for rehab eval. and tx._

S: "I'm hungry." "I hurt."

O: 1. Resolved; soft tissue integrity. PROM ® UE within normal limits.
Directed self ranging, and bilateral activities demonstrate no ® elbow limitation.

2. Resolved; directed bilateral activities show M.R. able to reach her mouth 10/10 trials (passive).

3. Attention span deficit - client meets original goal (5 min.) but new goal 30 min. is not resolved.

4. Feeding deficits; Criteria reached (finger foods) and new goal is use of utensils with 50% accuracy. Not resolved.

A: Megan continues to make steady progress and the following problems are priority for tx. in out patient program.
1. Poor activity tolerance (30 min.)
2. Poor visual motor integration (evaluation enclosed)
3. Poor attention span (30 min.)
4. Poor feeding behavior
5. Poor selfcare (dressing, bathing)

P: Patient is discharged to home with parents and siblings to begin day program at City Center Rehabilitation Unit on 9-20-90. Out patient program in O.T. to begin 9-20-90. Case manager at CCRU attended team meeting 9-15-90 for full report. To follow up, as M.R.'s O.T. program will be managed at CCRU.

Marla Jones, OTR
9-18-90

Problem Oriented Medical Record
Program Plan

Patient's Name_____ Hospital Number_____ Age____

Diagnosis_____ Referral Source_____

Referral Date_____ Initial O.T. Contact_____

Patient Information

<u>Evaluation Techniques</u>   Results
_____Initial Interview
_____Observation   _____
_____Chart Review   _____
_____Others: _____
                                      _____
                                      _____
Problems Found   _____
                                      _____
                                      _____
_____   _____
_____   _____
_____   _____
_____   _____
_____   _____
_____   _____
_____   _____

Short term goals
_____
_____
_____
_____

Long term goals
_____
_____
_____

Treatment Plan
_____
_____
_____
_____

_____Unable to determine at this time

Occupational therapist signature_____
                            Date _____
Physician signature_____
                            Date _____

Problem Oriented Medical Record
Program Plan

Patient's Name _Megan Roberts_   Hospital Number _52-693_ Age _6_

Diagnosis _subdural hematoma_   Referral Source _Dr. F. Joe_

Referral Date _6-28-89_   Initial O.T. Contact _6-28-89_

Patient Information _The patient was thrown from a moving vehicle (6-21-89) upon impact, sustaining a right subdural hematoma (which was evacuated surgically 6-21-90). She also sustained ft tibia & fibula. She was non responsive until 6-23-89. Lives with both parents and two younger sisters._

Evaluation Techniques   Results

_6-28_ Initial Interview   _Dependent in all functional_
_6-28_ Observation   _activities of self care._
_6-28_ Chart Review   _Cognitive Level II (Ranchos). Unable_
_____ Others: _to determine tactile, proprioceptive,_
                            or visual processing due to agitation.
                            RUE: Active and passive ROM
Problems Found   _within normal limits._
                            LUE: Severe spasticity/rigidity.
                            Passive ROM within normal
1. soft tissue integrity _limits with inhibition techniques_
   deficits ⓇL elbow   _with the exception of elbow_
2. Muscle tone and reflexes _flexion (-40°)._
   increased Ⓛ UE
3. Attention span deficits
4. Feeding deficits

Short term goals
1. Increase Ⓛ elbow extension to 0° and maintain Ⓛ UE PROM
2. Decrease muscle tone & reflex responses so that M.R. can purposely
   reach mouth bilaterally 8 of 10 trials
3. With a low stimulus environment, MR will attend to task for 5 minutes
   in 4 of 5 tx. sessions.

Long term goals
Return to home environment with independence in feeding, bathing,
dressing, & toiletting. Out-patient tx. for cognitive deficits
& Ⓛ UE function.

Treatment Plan
Self-care: to begin ē feeding and progress to bathing
Inhib/facil techniques incorporated into games to
normalize muscle tone and increase Ⓛ UE use.
Monitor attention span and begin orientation activities.

_____ Unable to determine at this time

Occupational therapist signature _Marla Jones, OTR_
                          Date _6-29-90_
Physician signature _S. Joe, MD_
                          Date _June 30, 1989_

Problem Oriented Medical Record
Progress/Discharge Note

Patient's Name_____Hospital Number_____Age____
Diagnosis_____Referral Source_____
Subjective information:

<u>Problem</u>   <u>Progress</u>   <u>Plan</u>

_____

___progress   Occupational Therapy Signature_____
___discharge   Date_____

Problem Oriented Medical Record
Progress/Discharge Note

Patient's Name _Megan Roberts_ Hospital Number _52-693_ Age _6_
Diagnosis _subdural hematoma_ Referral Source _Dr. F. Goe_
Subjective information:
 Patient: "No, no, no".
 Mother: "She's more easily upset today. Had a restless night."

Problem	Progress	Plan
1. Soft tissue integrity deficit Ⓛ elbow	Ⓛ elbow PROM improved from -40° (6-28-90) to -10°(7-6-90) in extension.	Continue inhibition techniques with PROM.
2. Muscle tone and reflexes increased Ⓛ UE	No change. Inhibition techniques are required to maintain PROM. Flexor tone predominates.	"
3. Attention span deficits	During AM TX, M.R. has elicited 3 min. attention span for 4 consecutive days during slow sensory-motor activities (e.g. rocking or beach ball). Agitation is decreasing.	Continue slow-rhythmic activities to increase attention span.
4. Feeding deficits	The first successful participation by M.R. in feeding occurred 7-6-90. She reached the mouth with 2 french fries (2 of 10 attempts for 20% accuracy).	Continue to work toward successful finger feeding before introducing utensils.

✔ progress
___ discharge

Occupational Therapy Signature _Marla Jones_
Date _7-6-90_

Problem Oriented Medical Record
Progress/Discharge Note

Patient's Name _Megan Roberts_ Hospital Number _52-693_ Age _6_
Diagnosis _Subdural hematoma_ Referral Source _O. F. Joe_
Subjective information: "I'm hungry".
                       "I hurt."

Problem	Progress	Plan
1. Soft tissue integrity deficit, © elbow.	Resolved. PROM within normal limits	none
2. Muscle tone and reflexes increased © UE	Resolved. Directed bilateral activities show good functional use of BUE's	none
3. Attention span deficit	M.R. met original goal of 5 min. attention span, but upgraded goal of 30 minutes has not been met. Not resolved.	
4. Feeding deficits	Finger feeding criterion goal reached. Currently uses utensils with 50% accuracy. Not resolved.	
5. Bathing/dressing deficits	M.R. continues to need verbal sequencing prompts throughout. Needs reminders for safety. Not resolved.	

M.R. is discharged to home with parents and siblings to begin day program at City Center Rehabilitation Unit 9-20-90. Outpatient program in O.T. to begin 9-20-90. Case manager at CCRU attended 9-15-90 team meeting for full report. No follow-up, as M.R.'s O.T. program will be managed at CCRU.

___progress   Occupational Therapy Signature _Marla Jones, OTR_
✓discharge   Date _9-18-90_

Index

Page numbers in *italics* denote figures; those followed by "t" denote tables.